Pathology of the
Urinary Bladder

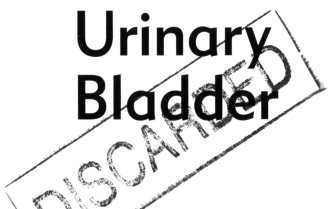

*To my wife, Joan, for your enduring loyalty;
and to Katharine and Alexander for continuing to allow
me those rare but necessary moments of peace and quiet
in the turmoil of daily life that have enabled me to
concentrate on producing this book.*

Christopher S. Foster

*To my wife, Karen, for your love and encouragement
that has enabled me to reach high while helping me
keep my feet on the ground.
To my children Marty, Merrill, Mickey, Alex and David
who make my life so full of wonderful days.*

Jeffrey S. Ross

MPP

42

Christopher S. Foster MD PhD FRCPath

Professor of Cellular Pathology and Molecular Genetics
School of Clinical Laboratory Sciences
The University of Liverpool
Royal Liverpool University Hospital
Liverpool
UK

Jeffrey S. Ross MD

Cyrus Strong Merrill Professor and Chairman
Department of Pathology and Laboratory Medicine
Albany Medical College;
Senior Scientitic Fellow Millennium Pharmaceuticals Inc.
Albany, New York
USA

Pathology of the Urinary Bladder

MAJOR PROBLEMS IN PATHOLOGY

SAUNDERS

Philadelphia Edinburgh London New York Oxford
St Louis Sydney Toronto 2004

SAUNDERS
An imprint of Elsevier Inc
The Curtis Centre
Independence Square west
Philadelphia, PA 19106

First published 2004

ISBN 0721692125

British Library Cataloguing in Publication Data
A catalogue record for this book is available from the British Library

Library of Congress Cataloging in Publication Data
A catalog record for this book is available from the Library of
Congress

Notice
Medical knowledge is constantly changing. Standard safety
precautions must be followed, but as new research and clinical
experience broaden our knowledge, changes in treatment and drug
therapy may become necessary or appropriate. Readers are advised
to check the most current product information provided by the
manufacturer of each drug to be administered to verify the
recommended dose, the method and duration of administration,
and contraindications. It is the responsibility of the practitioner,
relying on experience and knowledge of the patient, to determine
dosages and the best treatment for each individual patient. Neither
the Publisher nor the editors assumes any liability for any injury
and/or damage to persons or property arising from this publication.
The Publisher

Printed in China

Last digit is the print number : 9 8 7 6 5 4 3 2 1

Commissioning Editor: Michael Houston
Project Development Manager: Joanne Scott
Project Manager: Jess Thompson
Illustration Manager: Mick Ruddy
Design Manager: Sarah Russell
Illustrator: Tim Loughhead

The
publisher's
policy is to use
**paper manufactured
from sustainable forests**

Contents

Preface

Diseases of the human urinary bladder, whether benign or malignant, are collectively responsible for significant morbidity and mortality in men and women of all ages in all countries throughout the world. Accurate diagnosis of bladder disease is usually not facile, frequently requiring acquisition and analysis of simultaneous data from clinical chemistry, radiology, urology, microbiology and, ultimately, the surgical pathology laboratory. Even following detailed histopathologic examination of biopsy tissues taken from precisely defined microanatomic sites within the bladder, informed opinions as to the diagnostic or prognostic significance of particular morphologic features frequently remain controversial, to the extent that distinction of benign reactive or inflammatory disease from malignant neoplastic disease may not be possible. This is the current clinicopathologic context within which this book has been conceived and written. The subject of bladder disease, particularly bladder cancer, is complex and is fraught with doubts, uncertainties, and apparent contradictions. The natural biology of bladder neoplasia, which has been poorly understood, is gradually becoming clearer, as those proteins and their associated gene sequences that determine clinically important phenotypes and genotypes are identified, become assessed as prognostic indicators, and are evaluated for their clinical relevance.

We have taken this opportunity to assemble a wide spectrum of expert, and occasionally divergent, opinions on those topics we consider to be of the greatest importance in understanding and resolving fundamental diagnostic problems in bladder pathology. The roots of this understanding are buried deep within the normal embryology, developmental biology, anatomy and physiology of the urinary bladder, and without which there cannot be a firm or reliable foundation upon which to base modern concepts of bladder disease diagnosis, pathogenesis, or treatment. Modern immunohistochemical amd molecular biological analytical techniques offer promise in accurately identifying intrinsic regions of benign and malignant disease and provide pathologists with tissues that, in the near future, will allow molecular-genetic mapping of different phenotypic and genotypic subtypes of bladder cancer. While, as yet, rudimentary and preliminary in the depth of knowledge and under-standing provided, we have included sections detailing the current status of molecular genetics in bladder cancer as well as in the embryology and developmental biology of the urinary bladder. We anticipate rapid advances in this field with identification of gene sequences which, when employed as diagnostic probes, will reveal the emergence of behavioral (e.g., metastatic) or therapeutically responsive subtypes during progression of bladder cancer not only refining diagnosis, but also influencing differential or selective approaches to the clinical management of individual patients.

Despite the intrigue and lure of modern molecular genetics, we emphasize that high-quality informed microscopic morphological analysis remains fundamental and the 'gold standard' of urinary bladder histomorphological diagnosis. To evaluate the tissue diagnosis of bladder disease, we have assembled a comprehensive collection of highly informed opinions on bladder pathology. Within the chapters dealing with strictly morphologic aspects of diagnostic bladder histopathology, particularly bladder neoplasia, there is intrinsic repetition and redundancy between certain parts of several of the contributions. This we not only accept as inevitable, particularly in the circumstance that there are no absolute or incontrovertible relationships between morphologic appearances and behavioural or prognostic phenotypes, but also we welcome as reinforcing some of the most important aspects of bladder histopathology. Repetition among authors should signify enlightened agreement, rather than unquestioning acceptance of current dogma. In contrast, apparent conflict between opinions emphasizes real differences of interpretation among experienced diagnostic pathologists, and hence highlights the most important problems yet to be answered in the diagnostic surgical pathology of the human bladder. We anticipate that the current rate at which the fields of human urinary bladder biology, physiology and surgical pathology are evolving will ensure rapid resolution of many of these important and fundamental issues within the foreseeable future.

Christopher S. Foster
Jeffrey S. Ross
2004

List of Contributors

Manal Ismail Abd-Elghany MBBCh MSc PhD
Lecturer of Pathology
Faculty of Medicine
Department of Pathology
El-Minia University
El-Minia
Egypt

Mahul B. Amin MD
Director of Surgical Pathology and Professor
Department of Pathology, Urology, Hematology
and Oncology;
Associate Director
Cancer Pathogenomics
Winship Cancer Institute
Emory University Hospital
School of Medicine
Atlanta, GA
USA

Karl-Erik Andersson MD PhD
Professor of Clinical Pharmacology
Department of Clinical Pharmacology
Lund University Hospital
Lund
Sweden

Georg Bartsch MD
Professor and Chairman
Department of Urology
University of Innsbruck
Innsbruck
Austria

Gail Bentley MD
Assistant Professor
Department of Pathology
Wayne State University
Karmanos Cancer Institute and Harper
University Hospital
Detroit, MI
USA

Christer Busch MD PhD
Professor of Urologic Pathology
Department of Pathology
University Hospital
Uppsala
Sweden

Stephen J. Cina MD
Staff Pathologist
Wilford Hall Medical Center
Lackland Air Force Base, TX
USA

Michael B. Cohen MD
Professor and Chairman
Department of Pathology
University of Iowa Healthcare
Iowa City, IA
USA

Carlos Cordon-Cardo MD PhD
Director
Division of Molecular Pathology
Memorial Sloan-Kettering Cancer Center
New York, NY
USA

Philip Cornford BSc MBBS FRCS(Urol) MD FEBU
Consultant Urologist and Honorary Senior Lecturer
Department of Urology
Royal Liverpool University Hospital NHS Trust
Liverpool
UK

Frans M. J. Debruyne MD PhD
Professor
Head of Urology
Department of Urology
University Hospital Nijmegen
Nijmegen
The Netherlands

Anthony D. Desmond MBBS FRCS
Consultant Urological Surgeon
Urology Directorate
Royal Liverpool and Broadgreen University Hospital
NHS Trust
Liverpool
UK

Andrew Dodson FIBMS
Diagnostic Developments Manager
Department of Cellular Pathology and Molecular Genetics
School of Clinical Laboratory Sciences
The University of Liverpool
Royal Liverpool University Hospital
Liverpool
UK

John N. Eble MD MBA FRCPA
Nordschow Professor and Chairman
Department of Pathology and Laboratory Medicine
Roudebush VAMC
Indianapolis, IN
USA

Jonathan I. Epstein MD
Professor of Pathology Urology Oncology
Department of Pathology
The Johns Hopkins Medical Institutions
Baltimore, MD
USA

Magnus Fall MD PhD
Professor
Department of Urology
Sahlgrenska University Hospital
Goteborg
Sweden

Mark Fordham FRCS
Consultant Urological Surgeon
Department of Urology
Royal Liverpool and Broadgreen University Hospital
NHS Trust
Broadgreen Hospital
Liverpool
UK

Christopher S. Foster MD PhD FRCPath
Professor of Cellular Pathology and Molecular Genetics
School of Clinical Laboratory Sciences
The University of Liverpool
Royal Liverpool University Hospital
Liverpool
UK

Christine Gosden PhD FRCPath
Professor of Medical Genetics
Department of Cellular and Molecular Pathology
Royal Liverpool and Broadgreen University Hospital
NHS Trust
Liverpool
UK

David Grignon MD
Professor and Chair
Department of Pathology
Wayne State University
Gordon H Scott Hall of Basic Medical Sciences
Detroit, MI
USA

Jonathan H. Hughes MD PhD
Pathologist
Laboratory Medicine Consultants Ltd
Las Vegas, NV
USA

Pradip Javle FRCS
Consultant Urologist
Micheal Heal Department of Urology
Leighton Hospital
Crewe
UK

Sonny L. Johansson MD PhD
Professor Director of Anatomic Pathology
Department of Pathology and Microbiology
Nebraska Medical Center
Omaha, NE
USA

Youqiang Ke PhD DVM
Reader in Cancer Biology
The Molecular Pathology Laboratories
School of Clinical Laboratory Sciences
Faculty of Medicine
University of Liverpool
Liverpool
UK

George Kokai MD DS MRCPath
Consultant Paediatric Pathologist
Department of Paediatric Histopathology
Alder Hey Children's Hospital
Liverpool
UK

Robert M. Levin PhD
Director of Research
Albany College of Pharmacy
Albany, NY
USA

Sanjay Logani MD
Assistant Professor of Pathology
Emory University School of Medicine
1364 Clifton Road
Atlanta, GA
USA

Penelope A. Longhurst PhD
Research Associate Professor of Pharmacology
Department of Basic and Pharmaceutical Sciences
Albany College of Pharmacy
Albany, NY
USA

Paul Mansour MB ChB FRCPath
Consultant Cellular Pathologist
Southport and Ormskirk Hospital NHS Trust
Department of Cellular Pathology
Southport and Formby District General Hospital
Southport
UK

Rolando A. Milord MD
Fellow in Urologic Pathology
The Johns Hopkins Medical Institutions
Baltimore, MD
USA

Rodolfo Montironi MD FRCPath
Institute of Pathological Anatomy and Histopathology
School of Medicine
Polytechnic University of the March Region (Ancona)
Umberto 1° Regional Hospital
Torrette di Ancona
Italy

Hind Nassar MD
Surgical Pathology Fellow
Harper Hospital
Pathology Department
Detroit, MI
USA

Keith Parsons FRCS
Consultant Urological Surgeon
Department of Urology
Royal Liverpool and Broadgreen University Hospital
NHS Trust
Liverpool
UK

Ralph Peeker MD PhD
Associate Professor
Department of Urology
Sahlgrenska University Hospital
Göteborg
Sweden

Joe Philip AFRCSI
Research Fellow in Virology
Michael Heal Department of Urology
Leighton Hospital
Crewe
UK

Jae Y. Ro MD
Chairman/Director of Pathology
Asian Medical Center
Ulsan University School of Medicine
Songpa-gu
Seoul
Korea

Hermann Rogatsch MD
Associate Professor of Pathology
Institute of Pathology
University of Innsbruck
Innsbruck
Austria

Jeffrey S. Ross MD
Cyrus Strong Merrill Professor and Chairman
Department of Pathology and Laboratory Medicine
Albany Medical College;
Senior Scientific Fellow Millennium
Pharmaceuticals Inc.
Albany, NY
USA

Wael Sakr MD
Professor of Pathology
Vice Chair, Anatomic Pathology
Department of Pathology
Wayne State University School of Medicine
Harper University Hospital
Detroit, MI
USA

Marta Sánchez-Carbayo MSc PhD
Research Associate
Division of Molecular Pathology
Memorial Sloan-Kettering Cancer Center
New York, NY
USA

Jack A. Schalken PhD
Professor
Head of Urological Research
Department of Urology
University Hospital Nijmegen
Nijmegen
The Netherlands

Gurpreet Singh FRCS (Urology)
Consultant Neurourologist
Southport and Ormskirk Hospital
Southport
UK

Bakulesh M. Soni MBBS MS
Consultant in Spinal Injuries
District General Hospital
Southport
Honorary Lecturer Neurological Sciences
University of Liverpool
Liverpool
UK

Arnulf Stenzl MD
Professor of Urology
Chairman of Urology
Department of Urology
University of Tuebingen
Tubingen
Germany

Hannes Strasser MD
Associate Professor
Department of Urology
University of Innsbruck
Innsbruck
Austria

Pheroze Tamboli MD
Assistant Professor of Pathology
Department of Pathology
The University of Texas M. D. Anderson Cancer Center
Houston, TX
USA

Jennifer Temple BSc (Hons)
Department of Cellular Pathology and Molecular Genetics
School of Clinical Laboratory Sciences
The University of Liverpool
Royal Liverpool University Hospital
Liverpool
UK

Subramanian Vaidyanathan MBBS MS MCh PhD
Staff Physician
Regional Spinal Injuries Centre
District General Hospital
Southport
UK

Jessica L. J. Vriesema MD PhD
Resident Urology
Department of Urology
University Hospital Nijmegen
Nijmegen
The Netherlands

Bengt Uvelius MD PhD
Consultant in Urology
Department of Urology
Lund University Hospital
Lund
Sweden

Johannus A. Witjes PhD
Professor of Oncological Urology
Department of Urology
University Hospital Nijmegen
Nijmegen
The Netherlands

Acknowledgements

Setting the format in the first volume of the new series of *Major Problems in Pathology* is a very exciting and challenging event. This book on *Pathology of the Urinary Bladder* provides that detailed format.

In addition to the authors, who have provided a wealth of detailed information relating to their individual fields of interest and expertise, we acknowledge and are indebted, to Mrs. Jill Gosney who painstakingly proof read, corrected and edited all of the manuscripts at both the pre- and post-formatting stages during the genesis of this book. She was the focus of communication between authors, editors and publishers. Without her support and attention to detail, we would not have attained the high level of quality that is now apparent. With respect to the illustrations, Mr. A. J. C. Williams devoted much time and energy to ensuring that the detail of every illustration was as precise as possible. There is no doubt that his expertise and professionalism has significantly contributed to the very high quality of illustrations present throughout the book. These two persons have set extremely high standards with respect to care and attention to detail, which will result in a first-class series of *Major Problems in Pathology*.

As Editors, we are grateful to the constant support and assistance of the Publishers, Elsevier in London and in Edinburgh during the evolution of this innovative and challenging project.

Christopher S. Foster
Jeffrey S. Ross
2004

In Memoriam

Fathollah K. Mostofi
(1911–2003)

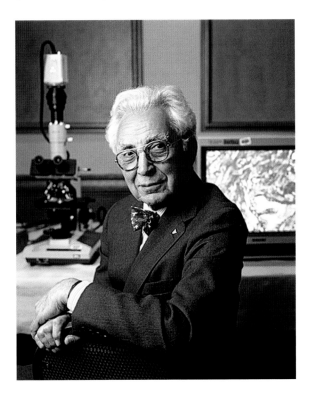

Fathollah K. Mostofi MD, one of the world's leading experts and founder member of the field of genitourinary pathology died of congestive cardiac failure on April 6, 2003 at the age of 91. His first publications[1,2] in 1954, began to outline his concepts with respect to bladder epithelium. Over the next half-century, his constant and tireless work to better understand the origins and development of bladder neoplasia were accompanied by his co-authorship of more than 200 articles and 15 books on genitourinary pathology, principally on the bladder.

It was our privilege to know "Kash" Mostofi for almost 20 years, initially as a revered mentor and later as a friend and colleague. In the world of bladder pathology, Kash was an authority of significant stature having contributed to much of the early understanding of bladder neoplasia, yet continuing to modulate some of his initial concepts as he embraced the emerging new technologies of monoclonal antibodies, image analysis, molecular genetics and oligonucleotide arrays. In this respect, Kash Mostofi was almost unique in having initiated much of the preliminary work that formed the foundation of current concepts of bladder cancer pathology and yet continuing to work actively and providing original insights to the field, some half a century later. It was to provide such a "long view" that Kash Mostofi had agreed to write a section for this book. It was intended that his contribution would provide the perspective against which the expertise of others could be arranged. Unfortunately, as we are all aware, events overtook Kash such that his contribution was never completed and therefore, is not contained within this book. Instead, we acknowledge the very significant role played by Kash to developing the field of bladder pathology. We particularly wish to remember that many of the ideas and concepts that have formed the basis of various different sections of this book originated from the work Dr. Mostofi performed many years ago.

1) Dean AL, Mostofi FK, Thomson RV, and Clark ML: A restudy of the first 1400 tumors in the bladder tumor registry, Armed Forces Institute of Pathology. American Journal of Urology 71:571-590, 1954.
2) Mostofi FK: Potentialities of bladder epithelium. Journal of Urology 71:705-714, 1954.

1

EMBRYOLOGY AND ANATOMY OF THE URINARY BLADDER

Christopher S. Foster, Andrew Dodson, Anthony D. Desmond and Mark Fordham

INTRODUCTION

In the adult human of both genders, the fully developed urinary bladder is a hollow muscular organ located entirely within the pelvis immediately behind the pubic symphysis until distended, its main function being that of a reservoir to retain urine prior to voiding. When full of urine, the bladder rises above the symphysis to impinge upon the abdominal space.[1] The shape of the empty bladder comprises an upward-pointing apex, a superior surface, two infralateral (anterolateral) surfaces, a posterior surface and a neck. The apex reaches a short distance above the pubic bone and ends as the urachus which, in the embryo, arises as the allantoic diverticulum and forms the cranial portion of the developing bladder.[2,3] In extra-embryonic life, this becomes a fibrous cord which extends from the apex of the bladder to the umbilicus, between the peritoneum and the fascia transversalis. Only the superior surface of the bladder is covered by peritoneum, although in the male a small part of the base also has a peritoneal covering. The neck of the bladder, its most inferior part, leads to the urethra.

The human urinary bladder is, both embryologically and physiologically, an extremely complex organ, being composed of many different tissue types from diverse embryologic origins.[4,5] To comprehend fully the micro-anatomic tissue structure of the mature adult urinary bladder, a detailed understanding of the embryonic origins of the different tissue components is essential.[6] Some of these embryonic components (e.g. Wolffian ducts) originate in mesoderm whereas analogous tubular structures (e.g. Müllerian ducts) originate in endoderm, each utilizing different modes of morphogenesis. Other structures, including the embryonic bladder itself, are initially lined by epithelium of mesenchymal origin, but later undergo replacement by cells of epithelial endodermal origin.[7,8]

EMBRYOLOGY

From the fourth to the beginning of the seventh week of intrauterine life, in both genders, the terminal hindgut becomes subdivided by descent of the urorectal septum (Fig. 1.1) into the cloaca[9] to form the anorectal canal posteriorly, and the primitive urogenital sinus anteriorly.[10] The cloacal membrane is then divided by the urorectal septum into the urogenital membrane anteriorly, and the anal membrane posteriorly.[10,11]

Mesonephric ducts (Wolffian ducts)

The mesonephric (Wolffian) duct originates in the mesodermal cells of the intermediate cell mass in each lateral compartment of the thoracic and lumbar regions of the developing embryo of both genders (Fig. 1.2a). At the same time, migration of primordial germ cells influences differentiation within the evolving mesonephric ridge forming the gonad.[12] The Wolffian duct arises simultaneously, but independently, from the tubules comprising the mesonephros. The lateral ends of these ducts then fuse with the mesonephric duct to form a continuum.[13] The mesonephric duct initially develops

as a solid rod of cells within the intermediate cell mass but becomes canalized through the combined effects of cell migration and apoptosis – ultimately, in the male, to form the vas deferens and the canal of the epididymis, and in the female to form Gartner's duct. While undergoing morphogenesis, the developing mesonephric duct, on each side, extends to fuse with, and to penetrate, the cloaca in its anterior aspect. Thereafter, the ureteric bud arises as an outgrowth of the mesonephric duct near its opening into the cloaca. In both genders, the mesonephric duct undergoes modification after giving rise to the embryonic ureteric diverticula. The metanephros develops, in part, from the mesonephric ureteric bud (Figure 1) and in part, from the adjacent lumbosacral mesoderm of the intermediate cell mass. The latter, initiating differentiation of the metanephros, ultimately become the ureter, pelvis and major and minor calyces of the kidney. The ureteric diverticulum is drawn cranially to produce the ureter, the pelvis of the ureter and the major and minor calyces as well as the collecting ducts of the developing kidney. Inferiorly, the developing ureteric bud becomes integrated into the developing bladder where, as the lower end of the ureter, it forms part of the trigone and is thus anchored into the bladder wall.[14–16]

During the seventh week of intrauterine life in the male, synthesis and release of testosterone by cells of the genital ridge induce differentiation of testicular tissue as well as development of other internal and

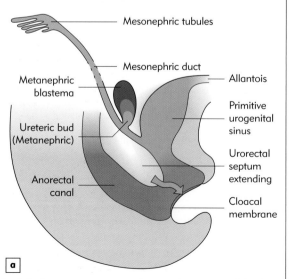

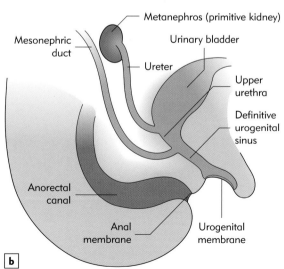

Fig. 1.1 Successive stages in the morphogenesis of the lower urinary/genital system in both genders, occurring from the fourth to the beginning of the seventh week post implantation. **(a)** Descent of the urorectal septum to fuse with the cloacal membrane divides the primitive hindgut into **(b)** the anterior urogenital sinus and the posterior anorectal canal.

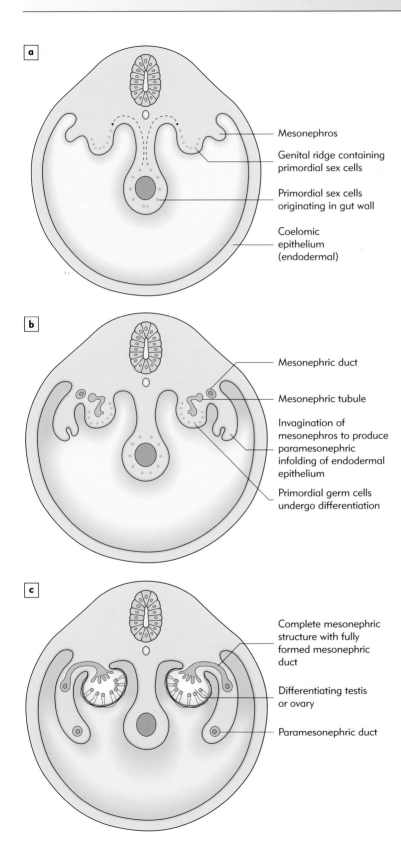

a
- Mesonephros
- Genital ridge containing primordial sex cells
- Primordial sex cells originating in gut wall
- Coelomic epithelium (endodermal)

b
- Mesonephric duct
- Mesonephric tubule
- Invagination of mesonephros to produce paramesonephric infolding of endodermal epithelium
- Primordial germ cells undergo differentiation

c
- Complete mesonephric structure with fully formed mesonephric duct
- Differentiating testis or ovary
- Paramesonephric duct

Fig. 1.2 Transverse section of human embryo during the fifth week post implantation. The primordial sex cells migrate to the genital ridge along the medial region of the mesonephros. **(a)** During the fifth to sixth weeks, mesodermal cells of the intermediate cell mass in the thoracic and lumbar regions undergo differentiation to form two epithelial structures. A longitudinal mesonephric duct (Wolffian duct) develops dorsolaterally while a series of discrete tubules develop transversely within the region of the genital ridge. These tubules fuse, at their lateral ends, with the Wolffian duct to form the integrated mesonephros. **(b, c)** By the seventh week, in male embryos, testosterone is secreted by cells of the genital ridge. This hormone simultaneously suppresses the development of female genital organs, and the definitive genders now diverge. However, the presence of differentiating testicular or ovarian epithelium promotes further development of the mesonephros (Wolffian duct) into the vas deferens and epididymis of male. In the female, the Wolffian duct degenerates leaving vestigial structures such as Gartner's duct cysts.

external tissues of the male reproductive system.[17] At the same time, the hormone suppresses development of female genital tissues.[18] Thereafter, in the male, the upper (cranial) end of the mesonephric duct associates with the developing testis and joins to the efferent ductules of the testis to become the duct of the epididymis, the vas deferens and the ejaculatory duct, the latter opening into the developing prostatic urethra at the site which will become the verumontanum. From the ejaculatory duct, a further outgrowth develops as the seminal vesicle. In the female, the mesonephric duct involutes with its cells becoming absorbed into surrounding structures or eradicated by apoptosis. Small remnants persist as the duct of the paroophoron. The caudal end may persist and extend from the epoophoron to the hymen as Gartner's duct.

Paramesonephric ducts (Müllerian ducts)

The paramesonephric (Müllerian) ducts form simultaneously on both sides of the human embryo during the sixth week of intrauterine life, identically in both genders (Fig. 1.2b). The ducts develop from coelomic endodermal epithelium that invaginates longitudinally into adjacent mesenchymal cells of the intermediate cell mass, lateral to the metanephros that is already present. Morphogenesis of the tubular paramesonephric ducts employs a mechanism distinct from that responsible for development of the mesonephric duct (Fig. 1.2c). Rather than originating as a solid core that becomes hollow by cell migration and apoptosis, the paramesonephric duct is tubular from the outset, being formed by folding and invagination of the planar structure at the

wall of the coelomic cavity on each side of the developing embryo. The cranial aspect of each developing paramesonephric tube remains patent as an abdominal ostium to become the fimbriae of the uterine (Fallopian) tube. The two laterally placed caudal ends develop a solid bud of cells that extend into the pelvis and converge towards the midline to lie adjacent to each other. Around the eighth week, these fuse to form a solid bud. During the ninth week, the single fused solid tip of this bud anneals with the posterior wall of the urogenital sinus in the midline.

Until the end of ninth week of intrauterine life, development and deployment of the paramesonephric ducts are identical, but thereafter the fate of these structures is different in the two genders. In the male embryo, the paramesonephric ducts begin to degenerate from the twelfth week onwards, leaving small residual components at the cranial and caudal ends. The cranial end persists as the appendix testis whereas the caudal end forms the prostatic utricle. In the female embryo, the paramesonephric ducts form the uterine (Fallopian) tube, uterus and part of the upper vagina.

Vestiges of Wolffian and Müllerian ducts

Typically, failure of complete degeneration of the early embryonic structures results in formation of cysts during later life (Fig. 1.3). In the male, cysts of Wolffian origin may arise in the superior and inferior aberrant ductules of the testis and the appendix of the epididymis. Cysts of the appendix testis are probably of Müllerian origin. In the female, sites of cysts of Wolffian origin include the tubules and ductus of the epo-

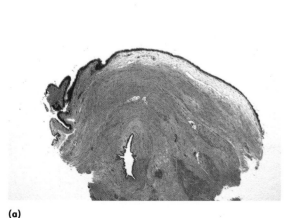

(a)

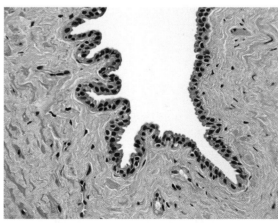

(b)

Fig. 1.3 (a, b) Vestigial suburothelial cyst occurring in the region of the membranous urethra in a male. The structure is histologically similar to that of the vas deferens and is of likely Wolffian origin.

ophoron and paroophoron. Gartner's duct cysts adjacent to the vagina are probably of Wolffian origin. Since the Müllerian ducts form the uterine tube and the uterus of the female, vestigial remnants that become cystic are extremely uncommon. However, there is some evidence that, in the female, multicentric clear cell adenocarcinoma of the lower urinary tract may be of Müllerian origin.[19]

The allantois is a diverticulum that grows ventrally, initially from the yolk sac but later following differential growth with folding of the embryo, from the primitive urogenital sinus. The allantois extends into the body stalk (later to become the umbilical cord) as a continuation of the developing urinary bladder. In the embryo, the developing bladder is connected to the allantois by the urachus, an intra-embryonic canal that initially connects the cloaca with the allantois. In the adult, the bladder is connected to the umbilicus by the median umbilical ligament formed by obliteration of the lumen of the urachus. Pathologic aspects of the urachus and its vestiges are considered in Chapter 5. Persistent remnants of the urachus are recognized to predispose to carcinoma of both adeno- and papillary type.[20]

Bladder, ureters and urethra

When it first opens to the outside, anteriorly and inferiorly, the urogenital sinus (the ventral division of the cloaca) is tubular and continuous with the allantois. At this stage, the urogenital sinus is divided into a ventral or pelvic portion, to become the bladder proper, and a

urethral portion (which receives the mesonephric and the fused Müllerian ducts) and later becomes the prostatic and membranous urethras in the male and the whole of the urethra in the female. Above the openings of the mesonephric ducts is the vesicourethral canal. Below this level is the definitive urogenital sinus. With further development, the location of the mesonephric duct orifices changes following gradual absorption of the terminal segments of the ducts into the wall of the sinus. Consequently, the ureters (initially outbuddings of the mesonephric ducts) enter the bladder separately.[21] Later, the ureteric orifices migrate cranially and laterally, while the mesonephric ducts enter the upper part of the urethra that develops from morphogenesis of the definitive urogenital sinus. Since both the mesonephric ducts and the ureters are mesodermal in origin, the whole of the mucosa of the embryonic bladder, including its lining, is of mesodermal origin at its inception.[8] However, this mesodermal lining is later replaced by ingrowth of epithelium of endodermal origin to cover the entire inner surface of the urinary bladder.[22,23] Hence, the vesicourethral canal gives rise to the urinary bladder and to the upper segment of the urethra.[22]

Development of the definitive urogenital sinus is different in the two genders.[24] In the male (Fig. 1.4), two distinct regions arise:[25] a short pelvic portion forms the lower part of the prostatic and the membranous urethras while the distal portion later forms the penile urethra. In the female (Fig. 1.5), the definitive urogenital sinus forms a small portion of the urethra, the lower one-fifth of the vagina[26] and the vestibule. After

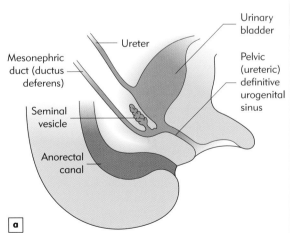
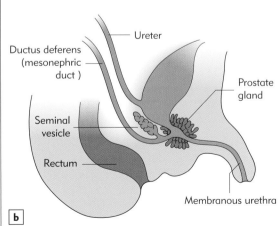

Fig. 1.4 (a, b) Differentiation of the urogenital sinus and adjacent structures in the male (weeks 7–10). Outgrowth of epithelium from the pelvic portion of the definitive urogenital sinus gives rise to the prostate gland. Simultaneously, the seminal vesicle develops as a cranial bud from the mesonephric (Wolffian) duct as this differentiates into the ductus deferens.

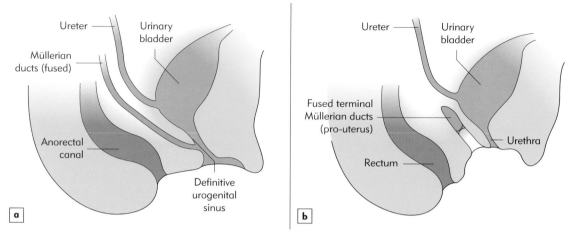

Fig. 1.5 (a, b) Differentiation of the urogenital sinus and adjacent structures in the female (weeks 7–10). The Müllerian ducts, fused in the midline, anneal with the posterior wall of the urogenital sinus in the midline to form the uterus and possibly the upper part of the vagina. Vestiges of the involuted Wolffian (mesonephric) duct system may persist as epoophoron and paroophoron cysts.

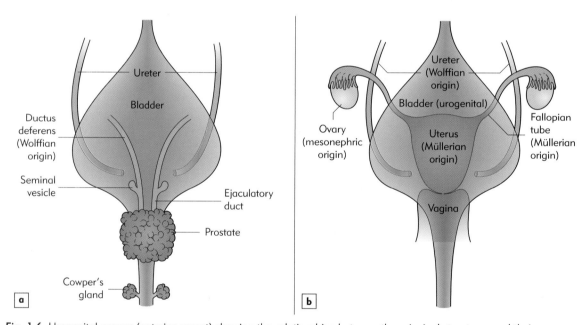

Fig. 1.6 Urogenital organs (anterior aspect) showing the relationships between the principal structures and their embryonic origins: **(a)** male, **(b)** female. The developing metanephric components are not included to assist clarity of these illustrations.

the eighth week, the ventral part of the urogenital sinus expands to form an epithelial sac, the apex of which tapers into an elongated narrowed urachus. The splanchnic mesoderm surrounding both segments then begins to differentiate into interlacing bands of smooth muscle fibers and an outer fibroconnective tissue coat so that, by the beginning of the twelfth week, the layers characteristic of the adult urethra and bladder are established.

At the end of the twelfth week of intrauterine life, the epithelium of the cranial portion of the urethra begins to proliferate and forms a number of outbuddings which penetrate into adjacent mesenchyme.[27,28] In the male, these buds form the primitive prostate gland, whereas in the female they give rise to the urethral and paraurethral glands (Fig. 1.6). The muscular connective tissue that forms the tunica muscularis (detrusor muscle) and the urethral musculature has the same embryonic origin, constituting one uninterrupted structure. In the male, this structure is complicated by the simultaneous development of the prostate gland.[29] This arrangement is particularly apparent in the female, where the urinary bladder and urethra comprise a single continuous tubular unit. Expansion of the upper part will form the bladder.

MOLECULAR BIOLOGY

During the first 5 weeks of gestation, development of embryos that are *potentially* male or female is identical and hence indistinguishable.[30] Synthesis and secretion of testosterone together with Müllerian inhibiting substance are regulating factors in the determination of male phenotypic differentiation and require an endocrinologically active testis. Thus, some preceding factor(s) are required before release of testosterone to initiate virilization of the Wolffian duct system with subsequent formation of structures recognized as epididymis, vas deferens and seminal vesicle. Dihydrotestosterone, synthesized from testosterone, induces development of the prostate and male external genitalia. The molecular mechanisms by which testosterone and dihydrotestosterone influence fetal development appear to involve the same high-affinity androgen receptor protein that transports both molecules to the nucleus of target cells.[31] Conversely, the differential effect of the two variants of the same distinct hormones strongly suggests the possibility of subtle variation in the structure of the receptor protein, with the possibility of more than one receptor. The androgen receptor is encoded by a gene located at Xq11.2–q12. Current analysis of the human genome suggests the possibility of two splice variants of this receptor protein. The human genome database is presently known to include at least 142 different genes, excluding the classical androgen receptor, that contain androgen-binding or response elements. Some, such as the anti-Müllerian hormone located on chromosome 19p13.2–13.3, have functions relating to the control of embryologic differentiation. Many of the others have important regulatory functions not hitherto associated with embryologic differentiation or the regulation of urogenital morphogenesis.

In response to a signal from a dominant-acting gene on the Y chromosome, primordial cells in the embryonic genital ridge differentiate into Sertoli cells. This influences newly migrated germ cells to differentiate into spermatogonia, thereby creating pro-testicular tissue. Several genes (including SRY, WT1, SOX9, SF1, XH2 and DAX1[32] and DMRT1[33]) have been identified, which – acting together or independently – control testicular differentiation. Cells of the pro-testicular tissue thereafter secrete a second spectrum of hormones in this differentiation cascade that lead to development of the majority of male sexual characteristics.[34] Sertoli cells secrete Müllerian inhibitor factor (MIF) causing regression of the Müllerian ducts together with any residual oogonia. Differentiated Leydig cells secrete testosterone that promotes secondary differentiation and growth of Wolffian duct structures. Dihydrotestosterone, elaborated by metabolism of testosterone, possibly by a variety of different cells outwith Leydig cells, initiates and promotes growth of the prostate and phallus as well as fusion of labioscrotal folds.

Wnt-4 is initially required in developing embryos of both genders to initiate and modulate formation of Müllerian ducts. Thereafter, in the developing ovary, Wnt-4 suppresses development of Leydig cells. Female sexual development is crucially dependent upon Wnt-4 signaling. Female embryos containing mutated Wnt-4 are masculinized with absence of Müllerian ducts, although Wolffian ducts continue to develop. Consequently, Wnt-4-mutant females are able to activate testosterone biosynthesis ectopically.[35]

In both genders, development of the urogenital system is the vectorial consequence of many interacting factors, both humoral and physical (structural). Several of the known factors, especially the appearance of stromal cells expressing unique phenotypic properties, can only participate in coordinated urological differentiation if their own earlier evolution has occurred correctly.[36] Such differentiation processes include transdifferentiation from a mesenchymal to a epithelial phenotype. The identity of a few individual factors critical to such processes is now becoming recognized, although their mechanisms of interaction are presently uncertain. For example, PATCHED – the human ortholog of the Drosophila gene known as Sonic hedgehog (Shh) and located on chromosome 9q22.3 – is expressed in urogenital sinus epithelium.[37] Initial upregulation of Shh expression in male embryos depends upon testosterone – and hence all of the preceding biological requirements for synthesis of that hormone and its appropriate receptor(s). However, several splice variants of PATCHED are recognized to have distinct roles[38] and to be involved in the genesis of superficial bladder cancer.[39] At the same time, transcription factor Pax-2 is critically required for differentiation of the epithelia comprising the ureter, Müllerian duct and Wolffian duct as well as the nephrogenic mesenchyme.[40]

With respect to development of the Müllerian ducts, although their location and the time course of their appearance have been known for many years, the molecular and cell-biological factors regulating their genesis remain unknown. Development of the Wolffian duct, and subsequently differentiation of the ureteric bud and ureter from the Wolffian duct,[13] require appropriate control of growth factor FGF-3 expression.[41] All of these structures do not appear in isolation but are intimate and integral components of the complex interaction that results in accurate development of the functional urogenital system. In one of the most recently reported studies of human embryos, the caudal ends of developing Müllerian ducts have been shown to be intimately connected to the Wolffian ducts (i.e. these two systems should no longer be considered as *indepen*dent but as *inter*dependent), opening of the Müllerian ducts into the coelomic cavity being formed as a result of invagination of coelomic epithelium.[42] These invaginations grow rapidly and involve coordinated epithelial cell proliferation together with simultaneous epithelial–mesenchymal interaction to produce functional ducts. Following caudal fusion, the two Müllerian ducts then bifurcate, each to unite separately with its corresponding ipsilateral Wolffian duct. At these sites there is, at least initially, an epithelial composite comprising endodermally derived epithelium (Müllerian) with epithelium derived by transdifferentiation of mesenchyme from the inner cell mass (Wolffian). It is likely that the point of fusion between these two duct systems is defined by the synchronous interaction of chemotactic, hormonal and physical factors. From current knowledge of heterogeneous composites, it is likely that this site of interaction will be the location of tissue malformation and/or predisposition to certain diseases presently undefined.

MICROANATOMY

General composition

The wall of the fully developed urinary bladder comprises six identifiable layers of tissue. The first three layers – an inner lining of transitional epithelium (urothelium), a thin underlying layer of loose connective tissue and a discontinuous layer of smooth muscle (muscularis mucosae) – together form a modified mucosa (Fig. 1.7a, b). Beneath the muscularis mucosae is a variably thick region of fibrovascular connective tissue. The fibrous composition of this region is more substantive than that of the mucosa, providing support

and resilience to the mucosa as well as to the contained vascular and neural connective tissue elements. The tunica muscularis (detrusor) is composed of bands and cords of smooth muscle arranged in intersecting planes that allow a smooth and uniform circumferential pressure to be applied throughout the bladder wall when contracting and expelling the luminal contents. In the majority of the bladder, there is no distinctive anatomic distribution of inner radial and outer longitudinal fibers, such as occurs in the gastrointestinal tract (Fig. 1.7c). However, at the bladder neck and in the region of the urethra, true inner radial and outer longitudinal coats can be defined. External to the muscle is a variable amount of fibro-adipose connective tissue.

Although these layers can be considered generally as structures of distinct composition, the reality is that the micro-anatomic structure of the urinary bladder is not as clearly defined as that of other hollow viscera, such as the gastrointestinal tract. While this has given cause to much controversy, particularly with respect to nomenclature of the mucosa, there is a certain pragmatic value in employing a terminology which, although imprecise, is generally understood by urologists and pathologists alike, and which forms the basis of intelligible communication.

Lining of the bladder

The interior of the bladder is completely covered by urothelium (transitional epithelium), several layers in depth.[43] There is a loose underlying connective tissue that allows considerable distortion of the entire mucosa which contributes to its folded contours when the bladder is empty, but becomes smooth, flat and variably distended when the bladder distends with urine. This arrangement pertains to all regions except the trigone, where the loose subepithelial connective tissue is attenuated and mucosa is firmly adherent to the underlying superficial musculature of the trigone.

Bladder musculature

The bladder wall has been described as containing three muscular coats. However, this is true only around the upper urethra and bladder outlet. In the region of the neck of the bladder, anterior to the developing prostate, embryonic muscle undergoes transdifferentiation from a smooth phenotype to a skeletal phenotype, being one of the two sites in the developing embryo (the other being the esophagus) in which this phenomenon is

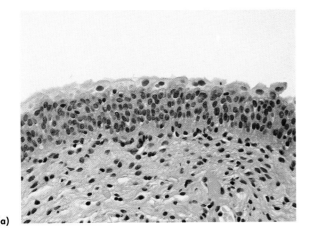

(a)

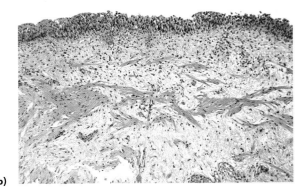

(b)

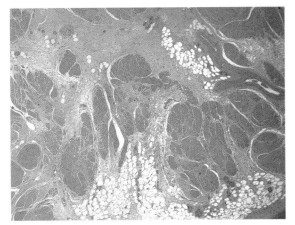

(c)

Fig. 1.7 (a) Vertical section through normal urothelium revealing the strata of epithelial cells from the basal layer through 5–7 layers of maturation to the overlying flattened 'umbrella' cells. In the normal (non-neoplastic) urothelium, the basal layer of epithelial cells expresses Bcl-2 while all the epithelial cells express RB1 and PTEN at varying intensities. HER2/*neu* and p53 are not expressed by normal urothelial cells. Ki67, indicating proliferation, may not be expressed in a single field of this size. **(b)** Transverse section through urinary bladder mucosa clearly showing the layers of the urothelium (dysplastic) underlying connective tissue, incomplete strands of muscularis mucosae and additional fibrovascular connective tissue before reaching the detrusor muscle below. The subepithelial connective tissue immediately beneath the urothelium contains a rich plexus of neurons that is invisible without special immunohistochemical staining (see Chapter 20). The muscularis mucosae is a tenuous and incomplete layer in which muscle fibers and bundles ramify at oblique angles to each other. These appearances are in stark contrast to the muscularis mucosae of the gastrointestinal tract. **(c)** Section through the outer half of the detrusor muscle showing the intersecting bundles and fascicles of smooth muscle cells surrounded by fibrous connective tissue that is more resilient than that found within the mucosa; between the muscle weave convoluted nerve bundles and blood vessels. Adipose connective tissue is variable in quantity and distribution, frequently being present throughout all layers of the detrusor to reach the lower zone of the mucosa.

presently recognized to occur (Fig. 1.8). Throughout the remainder of the bladder, there is no distinct layering with respect to radial and longitudinal deployment and muscle bundles, which interweave freely from one level to another. The bladder musculature is arranged in relatively coarse bundles separated by resilient but distensible fibrovascular/neural connective tissue, with no planar sheet formation. The longitudinal axes of the bundles transect each other with no specific orientation. However, around the bladder neck, where distinct layers can be separated, definitive longitudinal and circular arrangements can be identified.

In the region of the bladder neck, the muscle bundles on the inner region of the bladder are arranged radially,

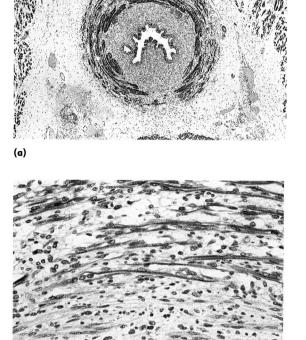

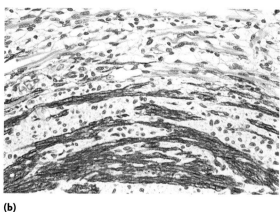

(a)

(b)

(c)

Fig. 1.8 (a) Bladder neck at 16 weeks post implantation indicating the distribution of the developing muscle. **(b)** Following transdifferentiation, the inner muscle bands retain a smooth muscle phenotype, as defined by expression of the PCKδ isoenzyme. **(c)** The outer muscle basal transdifferentiation to a skeletal muscle phenotype as defined by expression of the PCKμ isoenzyme and the appearance of eon-striations.

all converging toward the internal meatus.[44] These form a definite inner coat, which continues beyond the internal meatus into the urethra where the bundles become aligned along its inner aspect as the urethral inner longitudinal muscle layer.[45] In the middle portion of the bladder, other muscle bundles condense in a circular orientation. These bundles separate from each other as they extend outwards, merging with intervening muscle bundles extending laterally and dorsally to fuse with the lateral border and the dorsal aspect of the deep trigone. Some bundles continue to extend behind the deep trigone before fusing with it.

The muscle fibers of the outer wall of the bladder contribute to the outer longitudinal coat in the region of the bladder neck above the level of the internal meatus; these bundles form a complete sheet of radially arranged muscles. In the male, a few dorsal and longitudinal fibers fuse with the deep surface of the apex of the trigone while others penetrate the base of the prostate gland to mix with its musculature. Other bundles descend to loop around the proximal urethra before reverting to its outer surface, thus forming a contractile

'sling'. In the female, the arrangement is essentially the same, except that instead of penetrating the substance of the prostate, the fibers end in the vesicovaginal septum. This arrangement is very close to the original description of the ventral outer loop.[46] However, it is not the only loop around the urethra.[47] Definitive muscle bundles from the ventral outer longitudinal coats extend downward and dorsally around the sides of the proximal urethra to loop around its dorsal surface. Thus, there are many loops around the urethra, all of them in direct continuation with the outer longitudinal coat of the bladder, although none is continuous with the middle circular layer. From this muscular arrangement, the only fibers that could exert any action as a sphincter are the semicircular fibers surrounding the proximal part of the male urethra and the entire female urethra. No separate anatomic entity located at the level of the internal meatus or at any other level can be delineated as the internal sphincter. The sphincteric mechanism is not localized in one place or at one level but involves the entire prostatomembranous urethra in the male[48] and the entire urethral length in the female.

The trigone

Two layers – superficial and deep – can be identified.

- The *superficial trigone* comprises muscle fibers that originate as the longitudinal fibers of the intravesical ureter and diverge at the ureteral orifice to continue into the base of the bladder to become the superficial trigone.[49] Some fibers extend across the base of the trigone between the two ureters; the remainder extend medially to converge at the internal meatus before extending downward into the urethra in the midline posteriorly. In the male, these fibers terminate at the level of the verumontanum to join the musculature of the ejaculatory ducts. In the female, homologous fibers terminate at the level of the external meatus.

- The *deep trigone* comprises all the fibers comprising Waldeyer's sheath and extends downwards into the base of the bladder. Waldeyer's sheath comprises a specialized complex of fibromuscular connective tissue containing smooth muscle cells. The sheath occurs in continuity with the ureteric tunica adventitia and surrounds the pelvic ureter, particularly its intravesical compartment. The precise origin of Waldeyer's sheath is embryologically uncertain. Potentially, it could be of detrusor or ureteral origin, or it could arise from previously undifferentiated cells of mesenchymal origin lying between the two differentiated tissues of detrusor smooth muscle and periureteral fibrous connective tissue. In the adult of either gender, the upper muscle cells of Waldeyer's sheath fuse with, and are in continuity with, the periureteric muscle cells. Within the pelvic segment, the lower cells of Waldeyer's sheath lie close to the ureter in its intramural portion. However, as the ureter becomes submucosal, the muscle fibers diverge and loop around the ureter to join together, immediately beneath the opening of the ureter.[50] This identifiable collection of fibromuscular connective tissue extends downwards, deep to the superficial trigone in a flattened arrangement rather than as a tubular structure. These cells of the former sheath terminate at the level of the internal meatus. This component of Waldeyer's sheath provides additional anchorage of the ureter to the detrusor.

With respect to the deep trigone, the salient difference from the superficial trigone is that the tubular sheath becomes flattened so that its muscle bundles become compacted and more firmly bound together. This change in distribution begins just in front of the ureteral orifice. The upper fibers extend medially to meet those originating from the other side, thus forming the base of the trigonal structure. The lower fibers proceed obliquely medially and downwards to join and fuse with the fibers from the other side. The deep trigone ends at the internal meatus as a dense fibromuscular structure. There is no muscular communication between the planes occupied by the superficial and deep layers of the trigone. Behind the upper segment, the deep trigone is loosely adherent to detrusor circular muscle. However, in its lower segment, it is increasingly more adherent and firmly attached to the underlying detrusor and middle circular layer of the bladder. The superficial trigone adheres firmly to the overlying mucosal layer because the connective tissue is attenuated. The two layers of the trigone are in direct continuation with the lower ureter, with no interruption or loss of any of the musculature. The musculature of the ureter has not been interrupted, but has progressed from a tubular to a planar structure.

INNERVATION

The bladder and urethra receive a rich nerve supply from both sympathetic and parasympathetic divisions of the autonomic nervous system. The sympathetic nerve supply originates from the lower thoracic and upper lumbar segments (T11–T12 and L1–L2). These fibers descend in the sympathetic trunk into the lumbar splanchnic nerves to reach the superior hypogastric plexus, an inferior extension of the aortic plexus. The aortic plexus separates into a right and a left plexus (hypogastric nerves) which extend inferiorly to join the pelvic plexus arising from the pelvic parasympathetic innervation. Together, these nerves extend toward the bladder and urethra.

The parasympathetic nerve supply arises from sacral segments S2–S4 and forms the rich pelvic parasympathetic plexus, joined by the hypogastric plexus. Vesical branches emerge from this plexus towards the bladder base. The vesical plexus, the principal extension of the pelvic plexus, joins the lateral aspect of the bladder, simultaneously innervating both the bladder and the urethra. In the male, a separate segment extends to the prostate, forming the prostatic plexus. The cavernous nerves emerge from the prostatic plexus to supply the penile erectile tissue in the male or the clitoris in the female. These nerves carry both efferent and afferent pathways, and are combined motor and sensory.

Branches of the vesical plexus ramify in the extra-vesical connective tissue and penetrate the muscular coat as they extend throughout the bladder wall. Ganglia are present along the nerve trunks of the vesical plexus and also in its deeper branches. In a manner not dissimilar to the gastrointestinal tract, repetitive branching produces progressively smaller nerves that are distributed throughout the muscular coat. Sympathetic nerve fibers are more frequent in the bladder base and proximal urethra than in the bladder dome and lateral walls. Within the bladder wall, the nerves appear to be erratically distinguished (folded), thus enabling them to straighten without stretching during bladder extension. The motor nerve supply to the detrusor muscle is primarily the pelvic parasympathetic plexus whereas the motor nerve supply to the trigone and the lower end of the ureters is of sympathetic origin.

It is believed that the sensations of stretch and fullness in the bladder are carried along the pelvic parasympathetic innervation and that sensations of pain, touch and temperature are carried along the sympathetic innervation. The sympathetic adrenergic nerve endings are both alpha- and beta-adrenergic, with alpha-adrenergic predominance in the bladder base and proximal urethra, and beta-adrenergic preponderance in the bladder dome and lateral wall. The functional value of this arrangement is discussed in the section on neurogenic bladder in Chapter 4; physiologic aspects of the microneuroanatomy are discussed in Chapter 3.

The adjacent bladder wall

The ureter, wrapped with its sheath, pierces the bladder wall to gain access to the inner aspect of the bladder and is completely surrounded by detrusor muscle.[14] The latter contributes a few fibers to the ureteral sheath. Thus, the initial connection between ureter and bladder is established and some fixation is imparted to the sheath while the ureter is otherwise free to slide in and out within it. If it were not for its fixation to Waldeyer's sheath cranially and the internal meatus and proximal urethra distally, the ureter could easily pull out from within the bladder. The site of penetration of the detrusor by the ureter (the ureteral hiatus) is probably the weakest part of the bladder wall.[51] As the ureter penetrates the bladder, it lies submucosally, with the detrusor musculature behind. It maintains its tubular shape for a distance (the submucosal ureter) before it loses its lumen and becomes part of the trigone, both superficial and deep. The detrusor lies behind the submucosal ureter as well as behind the trigone. The trigone is superimposed over the detrusor which, at that level, is composed of two layers. Immediately behind the deep trigone, some detrusor circular fibers fuse with it; the remainder are unattached to the trigone but form a definite layer of circular orientation deeper to the deep trigone. Still deeper, the detrusor outer longitudinal muscular coat is very well developed posteriorly and forms a complete sheet behind the deep trigone. Through the connection between the deep trigone and the detrusor circular fibers, the trigone gains its firm fixation. In the midline posteriorly, at the level of the trigone and from the inside outwards, four layers can be distinguished:

- the superficial trigone
- the deep trigone
- the detrusor circular coat
- the detrusor outer longitudinal coat.

CONCLUSION

This brief overview of the embryology and micro-anatomy of the human urinary bladder highlights the complex interrelationships between different tissues that occur during morphogenesis of this structure. While the events responsible for evolution of the various structures are now known, the molecular genetic and biochemical factors responsible for initiating and modulating these interactive events are only just being identified. Although (as yet) unclear, many of the pathologic processes (whether infective, inflammatory or neoplastic) that affect the urogenital system may derive in part from the embryologic origin of its various components.[52] Further consideration of such relationships is presently beyond the scope of this work. Nevertheless, abnormal embryologic development is already recognized as an important cause of some category of known urinary bladder pathology,[53] as considered in Chapter 5 and Chapter 6. It is predicted that, within the near future, substantive progress will be made in identifying the aberrant molecular genetic factors that are (singly or together) responsible for other urinary bladder pathologies. The predisposition of certain individuals to particular diseases will become apparent such that biologically appropriate close monitoring of such individuals will retard or abolish evolution of those diseases that can be predicted with accuracy.

REFERENCES

1. Worthen N, Bustillo M. Effect of urinary bladder fullness on fundal height measurements. Am J Obstet Gynecol 1980;138:759–762.

2. Thambi Dorai CR. Umbilical evagination of the bladder with omphacele minor. Paediatr Surg Int 2000;16:128–129.

3. Favre R, Kohler M, Gasser B, et al. Early fetal megacystis between 11 and 15 weeks of gestation. Ultrasound Obstet Gynecol 1999;14:402–406.

4. Shapiro E. New concepts on the normal and abnormal developing bladder. Adv Exp Med Biol 1999;462:193–199.

5. Nguyen HT, Kogan BA. Fetal bladder physiology. Adv Exp Med Biol 1999;462:121–128.

6. O'Rahilly R, Muecke EC. The timing and sequence of events in the development of the human urinary system during the embryonic period proper. Z Anat Entwicklungsgesch 1972;138:99–109.

7. Gyllensten L. Contributions to embryology of the urinary bladder: development of definitive relations between openings of the Wolffian ducts and ureters. Acta Anat 1949;7:305.

8. Cunha GR. Overview of epithelial–mesenchymal interactions in the bladder. Adv Exp Med Biol 1999;462:3–5.

9. Okonkwo JE, Crocker KM. Cloacal dysgenesis. Obstet Gynecol 1977;50:97–101.

10. Jo Mauch T, Albertine KH. Urorectal septum malformation sequence: insights into pathogenesis. Anat Rec 2002;268:405–410.

11. Warne S, Chitty LS, Wilcox DT. Prenatal diagnosis of cloacal anomalies. BJU Int 2002;89:78–81.

12. Witschi E. Migration of the germ cells of human embryos from the yolk sac to the primitive gonadal folds. Contrib Embryol 1948;32:67.

13. Baker LA, Gomez RA. Embryonic development of the ureter. Semin Nephrol 1998;18:569–584.

14. Batourina E, Choi C, Paragas N, et al. Distal ureter morphogenesis depends on epithelial cell remodeling mediated by vitamin A and Ret. Nat Genet 2002;32:109–115.

15. Itatani H, Koide T, Okuyama A, et al. Development of the ureterovesical junction in human fetus: in consideration of the vesicoureteral reflux. Invest Urol 1977;15:232–238.

16. Oswald J, Brenner E, Deibl M, et al. Longitudinal and thickness measurement of the normal distal and intravesical ureter in human fetuses. J Urol 2003;169:1501–1504.

17. Jost A. The role of fetal hormones in prenatal development. Harvey Lect 1961;55:201.

18. Jost A. Development of sexual characteristics. Science 1970;6:67.

19. Mai KT, Yazdi HM, Perkins DG, et al. Multicentric clear cell adenocarcinoma in the urinary bladder and the urethral diverticulum: evidence of origin of clear cell adenocarcinoma in the female lower urinary tract from Mullerian duct remnants. Histopathology 2000;36:380–382.

20. Isotalo PA, Robertson SJ, Futter NG. Urinary bladder urachal remnants underlying papillary urothelial carcinoma. Arch Pathol Lab Med 2002;126:1252–1253.

21. Eccles MR, Jacobs GH. The genetics of primary vesico-ureteric reflux. Ann Acad Med Singapore 2000;29:337–345.

22. De La Rosette J, Smedts F, Schoots C, et al. Changing patterns of keratin expression could be associated with functional maturation of the developing human bladder. J Urol 2002;168:709–717.

23. Aboseif S, El-Sakka A, Young P, et al. Mesenchymal reprogramming of adult human epithelial differentiation. Differentiation 1999;65:113–118.

24. Cunha GR, Chung LW, Shannon JM, et al. Stromal–epithelial interactions in sex differentiation. Biol Reprod 1980;22:19–42.

25. Kurzrock EA, Baskin LS, Cunha GR. Ontogeny of the male urethra: theory of endodermal differentiation. Differentiation 1999;64:115–122.

26. Bulmer D. The development of the human vagina. J Anat 1957;91:490.

27. Yi ES, Shabaik AS, Lacey DL, et al. Keratinocyte growth factor causes proliferation of urothelium in vivo. J Urol 1995;154:1566–1570.

28. Southgate J, Hutton KA, Thomas DF, et al. Normal human urothelial cells in vitro: proliferation and induction of stratification. Lab Invest 1994;71:583–594.

29. Volmar KE, Fritsch MK, Perlman EJ, et al. Patterns of congenital lower urinary tract obstructive uropathy: relation to abnormal prostate and bladder development and the prune belly syndrome. Pediatr Dev Pathol 2001;4:467–472.

30. Puerta-Fonolla AJ. Morphogenesis of the human genital tract. Ital J Anat Embryol 1998;103:3–15.

31. Wilson JD, Griffin JE, Leshin M, George FW. Role of gonadal hormones in development of the sexual phenotypes. Hum Genet 1981;58:78–84.

32. Merchant-Larios H, Moreno-Mendoza N. Onset of sex differentiation: dialog between genes and cells. Arch Med Res 2001;32:553–558.

33. Raymond CS, Kettlewell JR, Hirsch B, et al. Expression of Dmrt1 in the genital ridge of mouse and chicken embryos suggests a role in vertebrate sexual development. Dev Biol 1999;215:208–220.

34. Ostrer H. Sexual differentiation. Semin Reprod Med 2000;18:41–49.

35. Vainio S, Heikkila M, Kispert A, et al. Female development in mammals is regulated by Wnt-4 signalling. Nature 1999;397:405–409.

36. Zhau HE, Hong SJ, Chung LW. A fetal rat urogenital sinus mesenchymal cell line (rUGM): accelerated growth and conferral of androgen-induced growth responsiveness upon a human bladder cancer epithelial cell line in vivo. Int J Cancer 1994;56:706–714.

37. Podlasek CA, Barnett DH, Clemens JQ, et al. Prostate development requires Sonic hedgehog expressed by the urogenital sinus epithelium. Dev Biol 1999;209:28–39.

38. Rahnama F, Toftgard R, Zaphiropoulos PG. Distinct roles of PTCH2 splice variants in hedgehog signaling. Biochem J 2004; 378(Pt 2):325–34.

39. LaRue H, Simoneau M, Aboulkassim TO, et al. The PATCHED/Sonic hedgehog signalling pathway in superficial bladder cancer. Med Sci (Paris) 2003;19:920–925.

40. Kuschert S, Rowitch DH, Haenig B, et al. Characterization of Pax-2 regulatory sequences that direct transgene expression in the Wolfffian duct and its derivatives. Dev Biol 2001;229:128–140.

41. Chua SS, Ma ZQ, Gong L, et al. Ectopic expression of FGF-3 results in abnormal prostate and Wolffian duct development. Oncogene 2002;21:1899–1908.

42. Hashimoto R. Development of the human Mullerian duct in the sexually undifferentiated stage. Anat Rec 2003;272A:514–519.

43. Hoyes AD, Ramus NI, Martin BG. Fine structure of the epithelium of the human fetal bladder. J Anat 1972;111:415–425.

44. Droes JT. Observations on the musculature of the urinary bladder and the urethra of the human foetus. Br J Urol 1974;46:179–185.

45. Koide T, Okuyama A, Itatani H, et al. Muscular development of the bladder neck in the human fetus. Invest Urol 1979;17:50–54.

46. Wesson MB. Anatomical, embryological and physiological studies of the trigone and neck of the bladder. J Urol 1920;4:279.

47. Bourdelat D, Barbet JP, Butler-Browne GS. Fetal development of the urethral sphincter. Eur J Pediatr Surg 1992;2:35–38.

48. Oelrich TM. The urethral sphincter muscle in the male. Am J Anat 1980;158:229–246.

49. Tacciuoli M, Lotti T, de Matteis A, et al. Development of the smooth muscle of the ureter and vesical trigone: histological investigation in human fetus. Eur Urol 1975;1:282–286.

50. Tanagho EA, Pugh RCB. The anatomy and function of the ureterovesical junction. Br J Urol 1963;35:151.

51. Berrocal T, Lopez-Pereira P, Arjonilla A, et al. Anomalies of the distal ureter, bladder and urethra in children: embryologic, radiologic and pathologic features. Radiographics 2002;22:1139–1164.

52. Ariel I, de Groot N, Hochberg A. Imprinted H19 gene expression in embryogenesis and human cancer: the oncofetal connection. Am J Med Genet 2000;91:46–50.

53. Cooper MJ, Fischer M, Komitowski D, et al. Developmentally imprinted genes as markers for bladder tumor progression. J Urol 1996;155:2120–2127.

2

SURGICAL ANATOMY OF THE LOWER URINARY TRACT

Hannes Strasser, Georg Bartsch and Arnulf Stenzl

INTRODUCTION

In the past few years clinical, sonographic, urodynamic and anatomic studies have allowed a better understanding of the pathophysiology of urinary incontinence. In spite of these investigations, the exact role of the smooth muscle wall of the urethra and the urethral rhabdosphincter remains a controversial issue in urologic literature.

For understanding of normal micturition and continence, precise knowledge of the neuroanatomy of the lower urinary tract is an essential prerequisite. In order to reassess the topography of the muscular structures and the nerves supplying the different portions of the sphincter complex, two extensive combined anatomic–histologic studies of the urethra and the rhabdosphincter in both men and women were therefore performed.

The urethra, the rhabdosphincter and their innervation were examined by means of anatomic dissections and serial anatomic as well as histologic sections of 28 anonymous specimens (14 male, 14 female, including 11 fetuses) that were available for scientific investigation. Fetal studies were included because, owing to the larger proportions, the pelvic autonomic nervous system in the fetus is much easier to identify than in adult specimens. Magnifying lenses and a dissecting microscope were employed for the preparation of the nerves supplying the urethra and the rhabdosphincter. The pelvic plexus and the pudendal nerves were dissected along their complete course. In addition to the normal hematoxylin–eosin staining, azan staining and a variation of the Masson–Goldner staining were used in the histologic sections.

ANATOMY OF THE MALE URETHRA AND RHABDOSPHINCTER

Membranous urethra

The membranous urethra is the thickest segment of the urethra. It is approximately 1.5 cm long and descends with a ventral concavity between the apex of the prostate and the bulb of the penis. It is a muscular organ that contains smooth muscle fibers.

The autonomic innervation of the membranous urethra arises from the pelvic plexus which is located on either side of the rectovesical pouch lateral and cranial to the rectum and the seminal vesicles. The right and the left pelvic plexus give off nerve fibers to both prostatic plexuses which are directly adjacent to the seminal vesicles. The cavernous nerves then course caudally as part of the 'neurovascular bundle' which lies in the triangle of connective tissue between the levator ani muscle, the prostate and the rectum. Lateral to the membranous urethra, these nerve fibers pass the urogenital hiatus, finally reaching the corpora cavernosa. The membranous urethra is innervated by branches derived from the prostatic plexus as well as the cavernous nerves. All nerve fibers supplying the membranous urethra run dorsolateral to the urethra to reach the periurethral connective tissue (Figs 2.1, 2.2).

Rhabdosphincter

The rhabdosphincter forms a muscular coat ventral and lateral to the membranous urethra and prostate, the core of which is an omega-shaped loop around the membranous urethra. The muscle fibers in this region are arranged on the ventral and lateral aspects of the membranous urethra. Both ends of the omega-shaped sphincter insert at the perineal body. The sphincter loop is continuous with muscle bundles which run along the anterior and lateral aspects of the prostate and extend cranially to the bladder neck (Fig. 2.3).

Pudendal nerve

The pudendal nerve accompanies the internal pudendal vessels in the pudendal canal on the lateral wall of the ischiorectal fossa. Its branches supplying the rhabdosphincter can be prepared with the help of magnifying lenses. These branches are given off lateral to the rhabdosphincter and reach the muscle at its dorsolateral aspects. The mean distance from the membran-

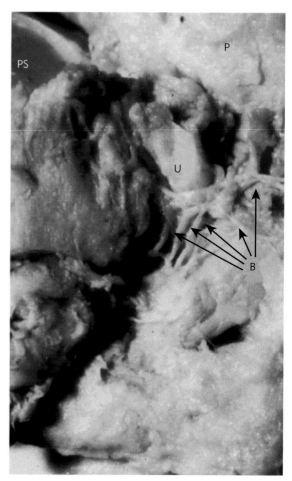

Fig. 2.1 Fetal male specimen, lateral view. B, branches of the pelvic plexus innervating the urethra (marked by arrows); P, prostate; PS, pubic symphysis; U, urethra.

ous urethra to the point of entry of these fine fibers into the rhabdosphincter is 0.5–1.1 cm (Fig. 2.4).

ANATOMY OF THE FEMALE URETHRA AND RHABDOSPHINCTER

Membranous urethra

In the cranial and most of the middle third of the urethra, three smooth muscle layers forming an outer and an inner longitudinal as well as a middle transverse layer can be found. The inner longitudinal layer is delicate, thinning out towards the external meatus.

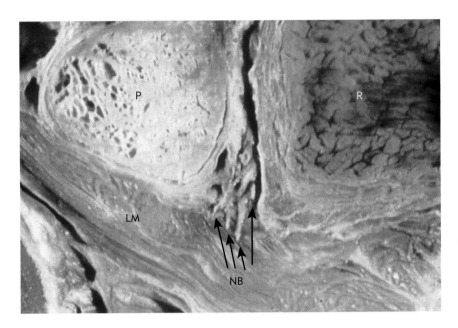

Fig. 2.2 Anatomic specimen, male, lateral view. LM, levator ani muscle; NB, neurovascular bundle (marked by arrows); P, prostate; R, rectum.

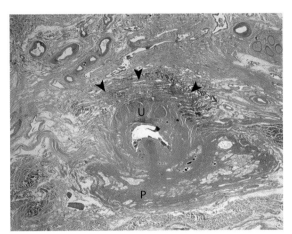

Fig. 2.3 Histologic section of male rhabdosphincter (marked by arrowheads). P, apex of the prostate; U, urethra.

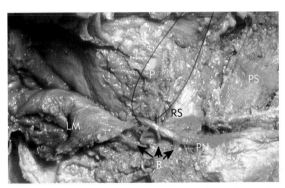

Fig. 2.4 Pudendal nerve, male specimen, lateral view. B, branches of the pudendal nerve innervating the rhabdosphincter (marked by arrows); LM, levator ani muscle; P, prostate; PN, pudendal nerve; PS, pubic symphysis; RS, rhabdosphincter.

Rhabdosphincter

The rhabdosphincter can be identified in the middle and caudal third of the urethra, its major portion being located at the ventral and lateral aspects of the urethra. Dorsally, collagenous connective tissue can be found. As in the male, the rhabdosphincter in the female has an omega-like shape in transverse section (Fig. 2.5), which is in contrast to other studies that describe the striated sphincter as having a nearly ring-shaped configuration.

There is no clearly defined boundary between the smooth muscle layers cranially and the striated musculature caudally. A gradual transition in the middle third of the urethra with intermingling of fibers of smooth and striated musculature can be observed, a finding that has been described previously.

Autonomic innervation

The autonomic fibers that supply the pelvic visceral organs emerge from the pelvic plexus and course in a

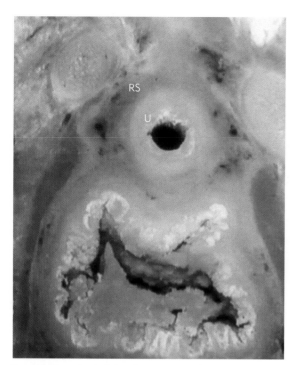

Fig. 2.5 Female rhabdosphincter, cranial view.
RS, rhabdosphincter; U, urethra.

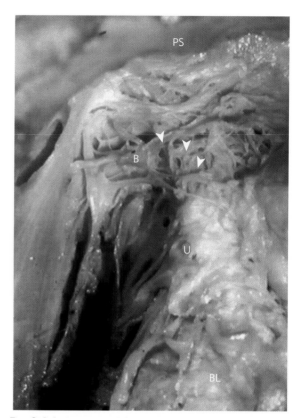

Fig. 2.6 Innervation of the proximal female urethra.
B, branches of the pelvic plexus innervating the proximal
urethra (marked by arrowheads); BL, bladder; PS, pubic
symphysis; U, urethra.

sagittal layer of connective tissue containing vessels and
nerves lateral to the rectum. The cranial portion of the
pelvic plexus is located close to the lateral margin of
the rectouterine pouch, while its ventral and caudal
portions extend to the lateral aspects of the cervix. The
nerve fibers supplying the urethra can be traced from
the pelvic plexus along the lateral aspects of the uterus
and the vagina all the way to the bladder neck and the
cranial urethra (Fig. 2.6). Some of these thin fibers,
branching off from a relatively thick fiber at the lower
margin of the lateral vaginal wall, enter the bladder
neck and the cranial portion of the urethra at the dorsolateral aspects.

Pudendal nerve

The pudendal nerve gives off the inferior rectal nerves,
perineal nerves and the dorsal nerve of the clitoris.
Arising from the terminal branch of the pudendal
nerve, several thin branches can be found that run to
the rhabdosphincter which they enter at its dorsolateral
aspects.

CONCLUSION

The urethral sphincter system consists of the smooth
muscle wall of the urethra which is innervated by the
autonomic nervous system as well as the striated
rhabdosphincter which is supplied by somatic nerves.[1–6]
There is general agreement that the autonomic nerve
fibers serving the smooth muscle sphincter originate
from the pelvic plexus. The innervation of the rhabdosphincter has been a matter of controversy but most
authors now agree that the latter is supplied by
branches of the pudendal nerve.[4–6]

The circular orientation of the striated muscle fibers
of the omega-shaped rhabdosphincter, the largest
muscular component of the urethra, indicates that it
really acts as a sphincter. Gosling et al. found type I
fibers exclusively in the human rhabdosphincter,[7]
whereas other authors recorded up to 42% type II

fibers.[8] Although ATPase was used in each case, there were slight variations in the technique used and the interpretation of the fiber type depends on the method used. Muscle fibers identified histochemically as type I fibers are functionally slow-twitch fibers which use oxidative phosphorylation to obtain energy and are able to maintain tone over prolonged time periods without fatigue.

Although there is much controversy about whether the smooth muscle wall of the urethra or the rhabdosphincter is more important for urinary control, better understanding of the anatomy of urinary control now suggests that an intact rhabdosphincter is essential for urinary continence following radical prostatectomy and cystectomy. Clinical and sonographic data have also supported this notion as weakness of the rhabdosphincter appears to be the most common reason for postprostatectomy urinary incontinence.[9–13] Furthermore, recent investigations suggest that the rhabdosphincter plays a crucial role in urinary stress incontinence in females as well as in urinary incontinence with advancing age.[14,15]

Clinical experience has shown that in women undergoing caudal urethrectomy for complicated diverticula or tumors, continence may be maintained unless a major portion of the middle third of the urethra is removed.[16,17] It has long been assumed that in women the bladder neck and an adequate length of cranial urethra are necessary for maintaining urinary continence. However, more recent studies have shown that female patients with an orthotopic neobladder following radical cystectomy with removal of the bladder neck and a segment of cranial urethra remained continent and were able to empty their urinary reservoirs.[18,19] No prominent sphincteric structure is present in the bladder neck and the cranial urethra of women.

The autonomic nerves predominantly innervate and regulate the cranial part of the urethra. These findings and the results of animal experiments support earlier publications that any complete autonomic denervation of the urethra in patients undergoing cystectomy and subsequent orthotopic urinary diversion may result in long-term smooth muscle dysfunction.[20,21] This may lead to spasticity or rigidity of the urethra and may impair postoperative continence and voiding due to the absence of the tonus-regulating function of the autonomic nerves.

Functional studies performed in sheep confirm the anatomic findings. The smooth muscle of the bladder neck and the urethra is innervated by autonomic nerves, while the rhabdosphincter is innervated by the pudendal nerve. Unilateral dissection of nerves leads to a reduced ipsilateral electromyographic (EMG) reaction. After bilateral dissection, however, the EMG signals disappear completely in the proximal urethra. Any stimulation of the pudendal nerve does not lead to a response in the proximal urethral segment.[21]

These findings may be another hint that – especially in the female patient – preservation of autonomic nerves is beneficial in orthotopic neobladder reconstruction.[19,20] Urinary continence after any bladder substitution can be maintained despite removal of the bladder neck and the adjacent proximal urethra. The bulk of the rhabdosphincter lies in the mid to caudal third of the urethra and is not removed in proximal urethrectomy as described above. Its innervation via the pudendal nerve is not disturbed during this type of surgery. There is an appreciable risk, however, of dissecting the autonomic nerves to the urethra originating in both pelvic plexuses when performing a subtotal vaginectomy and resection of the bladder neck including a wide margin of the surrounding tissue. Therefore, the nerve supply to the remaining smooth musculature of the bladder neck and the urethra may well be compromised during cystectomy. Attempted nerve preservation in male patients will not only lead to preservation of potency but has also been shown clinically to be advantageous for continence. The role of the vasculature has also been discussed.[22]

It is not yet clear how many of these autonomic nerves are needed for satisfactory function of urethral smooth musculature, and the extent to which these nerves can be spared during cystectomy cannot be defined intra-operatively. However, the latest scientific data suggest that most of the autonomic innervation of the remnant urethra should stay intact to ensure that both muscular resistance and relaxation are preserved postoperatively despite the removal of a safe segment of the proximal urethra for oncologic reasons.

REFERENCES

1. Colleselli K, Strasser H, Moriggl B, et al. Anatomical approach in surgery on the membranous urethra. World J Urol 1990;7:189.
2. Walsh PC, Lepor H, Eggleston JC. Radical prostatectomy with preservation of sexual function: anatomical and pathological considerations. Prostate 1983;4:473–485.
3. Myers RP. Male urethral sphincteric anatomy and radical prostatectomy. Urol Clin North Am 1991;18:211–217.

4. Strasser H, Klima G, Poisel S, et al. Anatomy and innervation of the rhabdosphincter of the male urethra. Prostate 1996;28:24–31.

5. Tanagho EA. Anatomy of the lower urinary tract. In: Walsh PC, Retik AB, Stamey TA, Vaughan ED Jr (eds) Campbell´s Urology, 6th edn. Philadelphia: W.B. Saunders, 1992, p 40.

6. Colleselli K, Stenzl A, Eder R, et al. The female urethral sphincter: a morphological and topographical study. J Urol 1998;160:49–54.

7. Gosling JA, Dixon JS, Critchley HOD, Thompson SA. A comparative study of the human external sphincter and periurethral levator ani muscles. Br J Urol 1981;53:35–41.

8. Schroder HD, Reske-Nielsen E. Fiber type in the striated urethral and anal sphincters. Acta Neuropathol 1983;60:278–282.

9. Presti JC Jr, Schmidt RA, Narayan PA, et al. Pathophysiology of urinary incontinence after radical prostatectomy. J Urol 1990;143:975–978.

10. Steiner MS, Morton RA, Walsh PC. Impact of anatomical radical prostatectomy on urinary incontinence. J Urol 1991;145:512–514, discussion 514–515.

11. Helweg G, Strasser H, Knapp R, et al. Transurethral sonomorphologic evaluation of the male external sphincter of the urethra. Eur Radiol 1994;4:525.

12. Strasser H, Frauscher F, Helweg G, et al. Transurethral ultrasound: evaluation of anatomy and function of the rhabdosphincter of the male urethra. J Urol 1998;159:100–104, discussion 104–105.

13. Ficazzola MA, Nitti VW. The etiology of post-radical prostatectomy incontinence and correlation of symptoms with urodynamic findings. J Urol 1998;160:1317–1320.

14. Frauscher F, Helweg G, Strasser H, et al. Intraurethral ultrasound: diagnostic evaluation of the striated urethral sphincter in incontinent females. Eur Radiol 1998;8:50–53.

15. Strasser H, Tiefenthaler M, Steinlechner M, et al. Urinary incontinence in the elderly and age-dependent apoptosis of rhabdosphincter cells. Lancet 1999;354:918–919.

16. Spence HM, Duckett JW Jr. Diverticulum of the female urethra: clinical aspects and presentation of a simple operative technique for cure. J Urol 1970;194:432–437.

17. Neuwirth H, Stenzl A, deKernion JB. Urethral cancer. In: Haskell C (ed) Cancer Treatment. Philadelphia: W.B. Saunders, 1990, p. 762.

18. Stein JP, Stenzl A, Esrig D, et al. Lower urinary tract reconstruction following cystectomy in women using the Kock ileal reservoir with bilateral ureteroileal urethrostomy: initial clinical experience. J Urol 1994;152:1404–1408.

19. Stenzl A, Colleselli K, Bartsch G. Update of urethra-sparing approaches in cystectomy in women. World J Urol 1997;15:134–138.

20. Stenzl A, Colleselli K, Poisel S, et al. Rationale and technique of nerve sparing radical cystectomy before an orthotopic neobladder procedure in women. J Urol 1995;154:2044–2049.

21. Strasser H, Ninkovic M, Hess M, et al. Anatomic and functional studies of the male and female urethral sphincter. World J Urol 2000;18:324-329.

22. Colleselli K, Stenzl A, Toerek R, et al. Blood supply of the male rhabdosphincter. Eur Urol 1998;33 (Suppl. 1):69.

3

NEUROTRANSMISSION AND ACTIVATION OF THE BLADDER

Karl-Erik Andersson

INTRODUCTION

The normal bladder functions – storage and elimination of urine – are dependent on neural circuits in the brain and spinal cord that coordinate the activity of the detrusor and that of the smooth and striated muscles of the outflow region. This chapter will briefly review the principles of nervous control of micturition, and then focus on the peripheral mechanisms involved in the activation of the bladder, and on how these mechanisms can be changed in different disease states.

CENTRAL NERVOUS CONTROL

The central nervous mechanisms for regulation of micturition are still incompletely known. Normally, the micturition reflex is mediated by a spinobulbospinal pathway, passing through relay centers in the brain (Fig. 3.1). In principle, the central pathways are organized as on–off switching circuits.[1] The reflex circuits involved consist of five basic components (Table 3.1). Studies in humans and animals have identified three areas in the brainstem and diencephalon that are specifically implicated in micturition control:

- Barrington's nucleus or the pontine micturition center (PMC) in the dorsomedial pontine tegmentum, which directly excites bladder motoneurons and indirectly inhibits urethral sphincter motoneurons via inhibitory interneurons in the medial sacral cord
- the periaqueductal gray (PAG) receiving bladder filling information
- the pre-optic area of the hypothalamus possibly involved in determining the beginning of micturition.

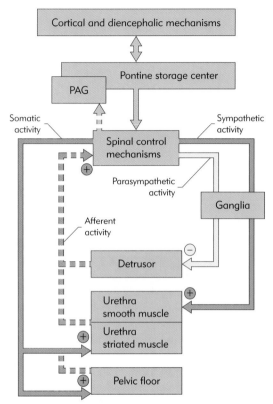

Table 3.1 Basic components of reflexes that control micturition

- Primary afferent neurons
- Spinal interneurons
- Neurons in the brain that modulate spinal reflexes
- Spinal efferent neurons
- Peripheral efferent neurons

Fig. 3.1 Urine storage reflexes. During filling, there is continuous and increasing afferent activity (interrupted line, +) from the bladder. There is no spinal parasympathetic outflow (light blue line, –) that can contract the bladder. The sympathetic outflow to urethral smooth muscle, and the somatic outflow to urethral and pelvic floor striated muscles (continuous dark blue lines, +), keep the outflow region closed. Whether or not the sympathetic innervation to the bladder (not indicated) contributes to bladder relaxation during filling in humans has not been established. PAG, periaqueductal gray.

According to positron emission tomography (PET) scan studies in humans, these supraspinal regions are active during micturition.[2,3]

PERIPHERAL NERVOUS CONTROL

The peripheral nervous mechanisms for bladder emptying and urine storage involve a complex pattern of efferent and afferent signaling in *parasympathetic*, *sympathetic* and *somatic* nerves (Figs 3.1, 3.2). These nerves are parts of reflex pathways which either maintain the bladder in a relaxed state (enabling urine storage at low intravesical pressure) or initiate

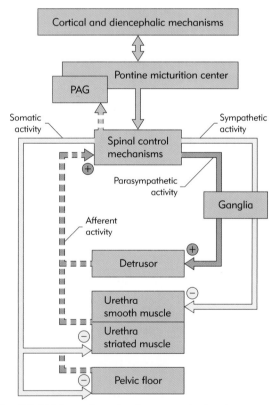

Fig. 3.2 Voiding reflexes involve supraspinal pathways, and are under voluntary control. During bladder emptying, the spinal parasympathetic outflow (continuous dark blue line, +) is activated, leading to bladder contraction. Simultaneously, the sympathetic outflow to urethral smooth muscle, and the somatic outflow to urethral and pelvic floor striated muscles (light blue lines, –) are turned off, and the outflow region relaxes. There is activity in afferent nerves (interrupted line, +). PAG, periaqueductal gray.

micturition by relaxing the outflow region and contracting the bladder smooth muscle.

Parasympathetic innervation

Contraction of the detrusor smooth muscle and relaxation of the outflow region result from activation of parasympathetic neurons located in the sacral parasympathetic nucleus in the spinal cord at the level of S2–S4.[4] The axons pass through the pelvic nerve and synapse with the postganglionic nerves in the pelvic plexus, in ganglia on the surface of the bladder (vesical ganglia) or within the walls of the bladder and urethra (intramural ganglia).[5] The preganglionic neurotransmission is predominantly mediated by acetylcholine (ACh) acting on nicotinic receptors, although the transmission can be modulated by adrenergic, muscarinic, purinergic and peptidergic presynaptic receptors.[4] The postganglionic neurons in the pelvic nerve mediate the excitatory input to the human detrusor smooth muscle by releasing ACh acting on muscarinic receptors. However, an atropine-resistant component has been demonstrated, particularly in functionally and morphologically altered human bladder tissue (see below).

The pelvic nerve also conveys parasympathetic fibers to the outflow region and the urethra. These fibers exert an inhibitory effect and thereby relax the outflow region. This is mediated partly by nitric oxide,[6] although other transmitters might be involved.[7–9]

Sympathetic innervation

Most of the sympathetic innervation of the bladder and urethra originates from the intermediolateral nuclei in the thoracolumbar region (T10–L2) of the spinal cord. The axons travel either through the inferior mesenteric ganglia and the hypogastric nerve, or pass through the paravertebral chain and enter the pelvic nerve. Thus, sympathetic signals are conveyed in both the hypogastric and pelvic nerves.

The predominant effects of the sympathetic innervation of the lower urinary tract in humans are inhibition of the parasympathetic pathways at spinal and ganglion levels, and mediation of contraction of the bladder base and the urethra. However, in several animals, the adrenergic innervation of the detrusor is believed to inactivate the contractile mechanisms in the detrusor directly.[10] Norepinephrine (noradrenaline) is released in response to electrical stimulation of detrusor tissues in vitro, and the normal response of detrusor tissues to released norepinephrine is relaxation.[10]

Sensory (somatic) innervation

Most of the sensory innervation of the bladder and urethra reaches the spinal cord via the pelvic nerve and dorsal root ganglia. In addition, some afferents travel in the hypogastric nerve. The sensory nerves of the striated muscle in the rhabdosphincter travel in the pudendal nerve to the sacral region of the spinal cord.[5] The most important afferents for the micturition process are myelinated Aδ-fibers and unmyelinated C-fibers traveling in the pelvic nerve to the sacral spinal cord, conveying information from receptors in the bladder wall to the spinal cord. The Aδ-fibers respond to passive distension and active contraction, thus conveying information about bladder filling.[11]

The activation threshold for Aδ-fibers is 5–15 mm H_2O, which is the intravesical pressure at which humans report the first sensation of bladder filling.[4] C-fibers have a high mechanical threshold and respond primarily to chemical irritation of the bladder mucosa[12] or cold.[13] Following chemical irritation, the C-fiber afferents exhibit spontaneous firing when the bladder is empty and increased firing during bladder distension.[12] These fibers are normally inactive and are therefore termed 'silent fibers'.

NEUROTRANSMISSION: CHOLINERGIC MECHANISMS

Cholinergic nerves

Although histochemical methods that stain for ACh-esterase (AChE) are not specific for ACh-containing nerves,[5] they have been used as an indirect indicator of cholinergic nerves. The vesicular ACh transporter (VAChT) is a marker specific for cholinergic nerve terminals.[14] In rats, for example, bladder smooth muscle bundles were supplied with a very high number of VAChT-positive terminals also containing neuropeptide Y (NPY), nitric oxide synthase (NOS) and vasoactive intestinal polypeptide (VIP).[15] Similar findings have been made in the bladders of neonates and children.[16] The muscle coat of the bladder showed a rich cholinergic innervation and small VAChT-immunoreactive neurons were found scattered throughout the detrusor muscle. VAChT-immunoreactive nerves were also observed in a suburothelial location in the bladder. The function of these nerves is unclear, but a sensory function or a neurotrophic role with respect to the urothelium cannot be excluded.[16]

Muscarinic receptors

Molecular cloning studies have revealed five distinct genes for muscarinic acetylcholine receptors (mAChRs) in rats and humans, and it is now generally accepted that five receptor subtypes correspond to these gene products.[17,18] Muscarinic receptors are coupled to G-proteins. The signal transduction systems involved varies, but M_1, M_3 and M_5 preferentially couple to phosphoinositide hydrolysis leading to mobilization of intracellular calcium, whereas activation of muscarinic M_2 and M_4 receptors inhibits adenylyl cyclase activity. It has been suggested that muscarinic receptor stimulation may also inhibit K_{ATP} channels in smooth muscle cells from urinary bladder through activation of protein kinase C.[19]

Bladder

Detrusor smooth muscle from various species contains muscarinic receptors of the M_2 and M_3 subtypes.[20] In the human bladder, the occurrence of mRNAs encoding M_2 and M_3 subtypes has been demonstrated, whereas no mRNA encoding M_1 receptors was found.[21]

The M_3 receptors in the human bladder are believed to cause a direct smooth muscle contraction through phosphoinositide hydrolysis,[22] whereas the role for the M_2 receptors is not clarified. However, it has been suggested that M_2 receptors may oppose sympathetically induced smooth muscle relaxation, mediated by β-adrenoceptors, since activation of M_2 receptors results in inhibition of adenylyl cyclase.[23] Contractile mechanisms involving M_2 muscarinic receptors, such as activation of a non-specific cationic channel and inactivation of potassium channels, may be operative in the bladder.[20] However, there is general agreement that M_3 receptors are mainly responsible for the normal micturition contraction.[20] Even in the obstructed rat bladder, M_3 receptors were found to play a predominant role in mediating detrusor contraction.[24] On the other hand, in certain disease states, M_2 receptors may contribute to contraction of the bladder. Thus, in the denervated rat bladder, a combination of M_2 and M_3 – mediated contractile responses.[25,26]

Muscarinic receptors may also be located on the presynaptic nerve terminals and participate in the regulation of transmitter release. The inhibitory prejunctional muscarinic receptors have been classified as muscarinic M_2 in the rabbit[27] and rat,[28] and M_4 in the guinea-pig urinary bladder.[29] Prejunctional facilitatory muscarinic receptors appear to be of the M_1 subtype in the rat and rabbit urinary bladder.[27,28] Prejunctional muscarinic facilitation has also been detected in human bladders.[30] The muscarinic facilitatory mechanism seems to be upregulated in hyperactive bladders from chronic spinal cord transected rats. The facilitation in these preparations is primarily mediated by M_3 muscarinic receptors.[30]

Muscarinic receptor functions may be changed in different urologic disorders, such as outflow obstruction, bladder overactivity without overt neurogenic cause, neurogenic bladder and diabetes. However, it is not always clear what the changes mean in terms of changes in detrusor function.

Outflow obstruction

There is good evidence that outflow obstruction may change the cholinergic functions of the bladder. Thus, detrusor denervation as a consequence of outflow obstruction has been demonstrated in several species including humans.[31–34] In pigs with experimental outflow obstruction, Sibley[35] found that the detrusor response to intramural nerve stimulation was decreased, and that there was a supersensitivity to ACh. Similar changes were found in the bladders of patients with bladder instability and outflow obstruction.[36] Sibley[32] suggested the supersensitivity to be due to partial denervation of the bladder, one consequence of which may be detrusor overactivity. On the other hand, Yokoyama et al.[37] found that the responses to ACh of detrusor strips from patients with bladder overactivity were not significantly different from those without. The reasons for these conflicting results are unclear, but may be partly explained by the occurrence of 'patchy denervation' (see below).

Immunohistologic investigations of the obstructed mouse bladder (also exhibiting bladder overactivity) revealed that the nerve distribution patterns were markedly changed. In large parts of the detrusor, the smooth muscle bundles were completely devoid of accompanying VAChT-immunoreactive varicose terminals. In other parts, the densities of nerve structures were nearly normal.[34]

The obstructed human bladder often shows an increased (up to ≈50%) atropine-resistant contractile component.[35,38,39] This may be taken as indirect evidence of changes in the cholinergic functions of the bladder, since normally the atropine-resistant component is almost negligible.[10,39,40] Alternatively, there may be an upregulation of the non-adrenergic, non-cholinergic (NANC) component of contraction (see below).

Detrusor overactivity

Turner and Brading[41] suggested that, in the unstable (overactive) bladder, alterations of the smooth muscle are seen, which may be a consequence of 'patchy denervation' of the detrusor. This was supported by recent studies on human overactive bladders.[42,43] Kinder and Mundy[44] compared detrusor muscle from human normal, idiopathic unstable and hyperreflexic (neurologic damage) bladders. They found no significant differences in the degree of inhibition of electrically induced contractions produced by tetrodotoxin or atropine in detrusor strips from any of these bladders, and no significant differences in the concentration–response curves for ACh. Bayliss et al.[39] found no atropine resistance in bladders with neuropathic overactivity, but could demonstrate atropine-resistant contractions in those with idiopathic overactivity. In overactive bladders without associated neurologic disorders, a decreased number of muscarinic receptors was demonstrated,[45] but the relation to overactivity remains unclear.

Neurogenic bladder

Conflicting results concerning changes in the cholinergic functions in neurogenic bladders have been reported. In patients with myelomeningocele and detrusor dysfunction, Gup et al.[46] found no supersensitivity to carbachol and no changes in the binding properties of the muscarinic receptors. However, German et al.[47] found that isolated detrusor strips from patients with neurogenic detrusor overactivity were supersensitive to both carbachol and KCl, but responded in a way similar to normal controls to intramural nerve stimulation. The results were interpreted to suggest a state of post-junctional supersensitivity of the detrusor secondary to a partial parasympathetic denervation.[47] An atropine-resistant component of the contraction of the human neurogenic bladder has been reported by some investigators,[48] but not by others.[39]

Diabetes

Patients with diabetes mellitus and voiding dysfunction show a variety of urodynamic abnormalities, including neurogenic detrusor overactivity and impaired detrusor contractility.[49] In bladders from diabetic animals, an increased density of muscarinic receptors accompanied by an enhanced muscarinic receptor-mediated phosphoinositide hydrolysis was found.[50,51] An upregulation of M_2 receptor mRNA has been demonstrated in rats with streptozotocin-induced diabetes,[52] and also that a supersensitivity of postjunctional muscarinic receptors may develop.[53] However, it is unclear what these receptor changes mean for the functional bladder disorders seen in diabetic animals. If found also in humans, they could contribute to voiding dysfunction and lower urinary tract symptoms. Interestingly, an aldose reductase inhibitor reduced the increase in muscarinic receptors and normalized the increased contractile response to ACh seen in rats with streptozotocin-induced diabetes.[54]

NEUROTRANSMISSION: ADRENERGIC MECHANISMS

Adrenergic nerves

Fluorescence histochemical studies have shown that the body of the detrusor receives a relatively sparse innervation by noradrenergic nerves. The density of noradrenergic nerves increases markedly towards the bladder neck where the smooth muscle receives a dense noradrenergic nerve supply, particularly in the male. The importance of the noradrenergic innervation of the bladder body has been questioned since patients with a deficiency in dopamine β-hydroxylase, the enzyme that converts dopamine to norepinephrine, void normally.[55] Noradrenergic nerves also occur in the submucosa of the bladder, only some of which are related to the vascular supply.[56] Their functional significance remains to be clarified.

α-Adrenoceptors

In the human detrusor, β-adrenoceptors (ARs) dominate over α-ARs and the normal response to norepinephrine is relaxation.[10,57] Goepel et al. found that the number of α-ARs in the human detrusor was low, the order of abundance being $\beta > \alpha_2 >> \alpha_1$. They found the amount of α_1-ARs too small for a reliable quantification.[58] Levin et al.,[59] on the other hand, found that in the human bladder neck region the predominating postjunctional α-AR subtype appeared to be α_1. Walden et al.[60] reported a predominance of α_{1A}-AR mRNA in the human bladder dome, trigone and bladder base. This contrasts with the findings of Malloy et al.[61] who established that among the high-affinity receptors for prazosin, only α_{1A} and α_{1D} mRNAs were expressed in the human bladder. The total α_1-AR expression was low – 6.3 ± 1.0 mol/mg. The relation between the different subtypes was α_{1D}: 66% and α_{1A}: 34%, with no expression of $\alpha 1B$.

Even if the α-ARs have no significant role in normal bladder contraction, there is evidence that this may change after, for example, bladder outlet obstruction, parasympathetic decentralization, and in hyperactive bladders.

Outflow obstruction

Whether or not outflow obstruction changes the function of bladder α-ARs seems controversial. Perlberg and Caine[62] showed that norepinephrine caused contraction instead of the normal relaxant response in bladder strips from patients with benign prostatic obstruction. On the other hand, a change in α-AR function was not confirmed by Smith and Chapple[63] who found that only 5 of 72 human bladder strips responded to phenylephrine, results that are not in agreement with the view of a change in α-AR function. Dog detrusor muscle, which is normally relaxed by norepinephrine, responded with contraction in 7 out of 12 dogs with bladder outlet obstruction.[64] However, this was suggested to be dependent on a decrease in β-AR function rather than to an increase in α-AR function. In rat outflow obstruction, Mattiasson et al.[65] found that the number of α-ARs in the detrusor, as determined by [^{3}H]dihydroergocryptine binding, was decreased, and that α-AR-mediated contraction was impaired. In contrast, Saito et al.[66] found that in mildly obstructed rats, there was an increased detrusor response to phenylephrine, suggesting an enhanced α-AR function. A significant subtype (selective α_{1D}-AR mRNA) up-regulation was found in rats with outflow obstruction,[67] but functional correlates were not reported. Factors such as the degree and duration of obstruction may have an important influence on the α-ARs in the detrusor, but the functional consequences have not yet been established.

Neurogenic bladder

In parasympathetically decentralized cat bladder, a change in AR-mediated function was reported, with a shift from a β-AR-dominated relaxant influence in the normal bladder to an α-AR-dominated response after decentralization.[68] However, other investigators were unable to confirm this finding.[69,70] The discrepancy in results is difficult to explain, but is probably attributable to differences in experimental approaches.

Detrusor overactivity

Detrusor tissue from patients with detrusor overactivity (without neurologic disorders) had an almost four-fold increase in the density of α-ARs compared to the density in controls.[45] The importance of this finding for detrusor overactivity is, however, unclear.

β-Adrenoceptors

The β-ARs of the human bladder were shown to have functional characteristics typical of neither β_1- nor β_2-ARs.[71,72] Both normal and neurogenic human detrusors are able to express β_1-, β_2- and β_3-AR mRNAs, and selective β_3-AR agonists effectively relax both types of detrusor muscle.[73,74] Thus, it seems that atypical β-AR-mediated responses reported in early studies of β-AR antagonists are mediated by β_3-ARs. It may be speculated that in detrusor overactivity, there is a lack of an inhibitory β-AR-mediated norepinephrine response.

NON-ADRENERGIC, NON-CHOLINERGIC MECHANISMS

Atropine resistance and NANC activation

In most mammalian species, part of the neuronally induced bladder contraction is resistant to atropine.[10] Several explanations for this phenomenon have been proposed,[75] one being the occurrence of an NANC transmitter. The proportion of NANC-mediated response to the total contraction seems to vary with species and the frequency of stimulation. Thus, in rats and guinea-pigs, atropine has little effect on the response to single nerve stimuli, but at 20 Hz, it inhibits about 25% of the response. Corresponding figures for rabbit and pig were 40% and 75%, respectively.[76] In strips of normal human bladders, the reported degrees of atropine resistance have varied from a few per cent to up to 50%.[35,38–40,77–80]

Luheshi and Zar[81] investigated whether the full atropine sensitivity of the human detrusor, reported by some investigators, was due to a genuine absence of a non-cholinergic element in its motor transmission, or was dependent on the experimental protocols. Using a specially designed stimulation protocol, they found that part of the electrically induced response (about 30%) was resistant to atropine. Most probably, normal human detrusor muscle exhibits little atropine resistance. This does not exclude that atropine resistance can increase in morphologically and/or functionally changed bladders, and that it plays a role in the activation of the bladder.

Outflow obstruction

As mentioned previously, the atropine-resistant component of bladder contraction may change with outflow obstruction. Thus, Sjögren et al.[38] found that in detrusor strips from male patients with a diagnosis of unstable bladder, and in particular from patients with bladder hypertrophy, an atropine-resistant component of up to 50% of the electrically induced contraction could be demonstrated. Atropine resistance associated with outflow obstruction has been demonstrated by other investigators.[35,39,63]

Other disorders

A significant degree of atropine resistance (about 40%) has also been reported to occur in interstitial cystitis[82] and in neurogenic bladders.[83] To what extent the NANC component contributes to the voiding contraction in these conditions remains to be established.

NANC NEUROTRANSMISSION: ATP

Evidence has been presented[79,80,82] that the atropine-resistant contractile component evoked in human detrusor by electrical stimulation can be abolished by α,β-methylene ATP, suggesting that the NANC mediator is ATP. However, this has been questioned.[40]

Husted et al.[84] showed that ATP not only produced a concentration-dependent contraction in isolated human detrusor muscle, but also that ATP influenced the responses to transmural nerve stimulation, probably by both pre- and postjunctional effects. The contractile effects of ATP are mediated through stimulation of P2X receptors. Hardy et al.[85] demonstrated the presence of the P2X1 receptor subtype in the human bladder, using reverse transcriptase polymerase chain reaction (RT-PCR), and confirmed that activation of purinergic P2X receptors (putatively P2X1) may be important in the initiation of contraction in human detrusor. Purinergic transmission seemed to be more important in muscle taken from patients with bladder instability. Their results also indicated the possibility that human bladder expresses multiple isoforms of the P2X1 receptor which may be potential sites for modifying or regulating putative purinergic activation of the human bladder. Supporting such a concept, mice deficient in P2X3

receptors exhibited a marked urinary bladder hyporeflexia, characterized by decreased voiding frequency and increased bladder capacity, but normal bladder pressures.[86]

Immunohistochemical studies localized P2X3 receptors to nerve fibers innervating the urinary bladder of wild-type mice, and showed that loss of this receptor subtype did not alter sensory neuron innervation density. P2X3 receptors thus seem to be critical for peripheral afferent pathways controlling urinary bladder volume reflexes.

Available results suggest that ATP may contribute to excitatory neurotransmission in the bladder by stimulation of both detrusor and afferent nerves. The importance of this for the emptying contraction of the human bladder under normal and pathophysiologic conditions remains to be established.

NANC NEUROTRANSMISSION: NO

Nitrergic nerves

Evidence has accumulated that L-arginine-derived nitric oxide (NO) is responsible for the main part of the inhibitory NANC responses in the lower urinary tract.[10] In biopsies taken from the lateral wall and trigone regions of the human bladder, a plexus of NADPH-diaphorase containing nerve fibers was found.[87] Samples from the lateral bladder wall contained many NADPH-reactive nerve terminals, particularly in the subepithelial region immediately beneath the urothelium; occasionally they penetrated into the epithelial layer.

Immunohistochemical investigations of pig bladder revealed that the density of NOS immunoreactivity was higher in trigonal and urethral tissue than in the detrusor.[88]

Functional effects of NO

Klarskov[89] reported an NANC-mediated relaxation of human detrusor muscle preparations in response to electrical stimulation. The relaxation was seen only occasionally, and was short lasting and fading. Its tetrodotoxin sensitivity was apparently not tested. In small biopsy preparations of the human detrusor, James et al.[90] found that electrical stimulation evoked relaxations sensitive to N^G-nitro-L-arginine, but insensitive to tetrodotoxin. They suggested that NO might be generated from the detrusor muscle and be an important factor for bladder relaxation during the filling phase. However, Elliott and Castleden[91] were unable to demonstrate a nerve-mediated relaxation in human detrusor muscle.

If NO has an important role in bladder relaxation, it may be expected that the detrusor muscle has a high sensitivity to agents acting by increasing the intracellular concentrations of cyclic guanosine monophosphate (cGMP). In the pig detrusor, the NO donor (SIN-1) and NO relaxed carbachol and endothelin-1 contracted preparations by approximately 60%. However, isoprenaline was about 1000 times more potent than SIN-1 and NO and caused complete relaxation. Nitroprusside, SIN-1 and NO were only moderately effective in relaxing isolated rat, pig and rabbit detrusor muscle, compared to their effects on the urethral muscle.[89,92,93] These results agree favorably with those of Morita et al.[94] who found that, in rabbits, cGMP is mainly related to urethral relaxation and cyclic adenosine monophosphate (cAMP) to urinary bladder relaxation.

Theoretically, NO-release from inhibitory nerves to the detrusor could be one factor keeping the bladder relaxed during filling. In fact, NO has been suggested to have such a function in the stomach, i.e. as a mediator of adaptive relaxation to accommodate food or fluid.[95] However, available results suggest that it is unlikely that NO has a role as a neurotransmitter causing direct relaxation of the detrusor smooth muscle, since the detrusor sensitivity to NO and agents acting via the cGMP system is low. This does not exclude the fact that NO may modulate the effects of other transmitters, or that it has a role in afferent neurotransmission.

Outflow obstruction

In male neuronal NOS (nNOS)-deficient mice, Burnett et al.[96] found markedly dilated bladders with muscular hypertrophy, findings compatible with deficient urethral relaxation and increased outflow resistance. Supporting the premise that the bladder changes were caused by disturbances in outflow relaxation, the decrease in tension produced by low frequency stimulation of nerves of isolated urethral preparations from wild-type controls was absent in preparations from nNOS-deficient mice. In contrast to these findings, Sutherland et al.,[97] investigating female nNOS-deficient mice with voiding, urodynamic and muscle strip testing, as well as histologic examination, found no marked differences between these animals and normal controls. NO-mediated smooth muscle relaxation is mediated by cGMP through activation of cGMP-dependent protein

kinase I (cGKI). cGKI-deficient mice, male or female, showed no sign of bladder hypertrophy.[98] The role of NO (or lack of it) in the development of bladder hypertrophy associated with outflow obstruction in humans has not yet been established.

Detrusor overactivity

Evidence that baseline NOS activity prevents uninhibited bladder contractions also exists from urodynamic studies performed in a fetal lamb model.[99] If the nitrergic nerves observed in the detrusor, and particularly within and beneath the urothelium, are afferent terminals, NO may be involved in the regulation of the threshold for bladder afferent firing. Supporting such a view, intravesical oxyhemoglobin (a nitric oxide scavenger) induced bladder overactivity in normal rats.[100] It was suggested that intravesical oxyhemoglobin induced detrusor overactivity by interfering with NO generated in the urothelium or suburothelially, and that NO may be involved in the regulation of the threshold for afferent firing in the bladder. Inhibition of the L-arginine/NO pathway by NOS inhibitors also leads to detrusor overactivity and decreased bladder capacity.[101] Furthermore, cGKI-deficient mice showed detrusor overactivity characterized by decreased inter-contraction intervals and non-voiding bladder contractions.[98] This further supports the view that the L-arginine/NO pathway is involved in the control of detrusor activity.

NANC NEUROTRANSMISSION: NEUROPEPTIDES

Tachykinins

The functional roles of the many neuropeptides that have been demonstrated to be synthesized, stored and released in the human lower urinary tract[102,103] have not been established. As discussed by Maggi,[102,103] neuropeptide-containing, capsaicin-sensitive primary afferents in the bladder and urethra may have not only a sensory function, but also a local effector or efferent function. In addition, they may play a role as neurotransmitters and/or neuromodulators in the bladder ganglia and at the neuromuscular junctions. As a result, the peptides may be involved in the mediation of various effects, including micturition reflex activation, smooth muscle contraction, potentiation of efferent neurotransmission, and changes in vascular tone and permeability. Evidence for this is based mainly on experiments in animals. Studies on isolated human bladder muscle strips have failed to reveal any specific local motor response attributable to a capsaicin-sensitive innervation.[102] However, cystometric evidence that capsaicin-sensitive nerves may modulate the afferent branch of the micturition reflex in humans has been presented.[104] In a small number of patients suffering from bladder hypersensitivity disorders, intra-vesical capsaicin produced a long-lasting, symptomatic improvement.

Substance P (SP) and various related peptides have been shown to have contractile effects in isolated bladder smooth muscle from various species, and the potential role of SP in the atropine-resistant component of the contractile response induced by electrical stimulation has been studied by several investigators.[10] With few exceptions, these studies did not favor the view that SP, released from postganglionic nerve terminals, has an excitatory transmitter role. On the other hand, evidence has been presented that SP may play a role in the afferent, sensory branch of the micturition reflex.[10]

Several tachykinins are present in sensory nerves of the urinary bladder in rat and other mammalian species, including humans. Receptor subtypes were identified in urinary bladders of several mammals, both in vitro and in vivo. In the rat urinary bladder three receptor types, classified as NK_1, NK_2 and NK_3, have been demonstrated, as evidenced by radioligand binding, and autoradiographic and functional experiments.[102,103]

The existence of two different receptors for tachy-kinins in the rat bladder, whose activation was responsible for initiation of the micturition reflex and direct smooth muscle contraction, respectively, has been suggested.[105] However, evidence has been presented that, at the peripheral level, neither NK_1 nor NK_2 receptors have any importance for normal initiation of the micturition reflex in the rat.[106] This does not exclude that they have such a role in, for example, detrusor overactivity induced by irritants.

Tachykinins have contractile effects in the human bladder.[102,107] The potency of neurokinins was shown to be NKA > NKB >> SP. This, and results with subtype selective agonists,[107] suggested that the tachykinin receptor-mediating contraction in the human bladder is of the NK_2 type.

Detrusor overactivity

Bladder outflow obstruction, which is often associated with overactivity, causes a reduction in the density of neuropeptide-containing nerves.[108] On the other hand, in bladder tissue from women with idiopathic detrusor overactivity, a significant increase in the density of subepithelial, presumptive sensory nerves compared to stable controls was reported.[109] Capsaicin-sensitive afferents may be a part of a spinal, vesicovesical exci-tatory (short-loop) reflex providing a neurogenic mechanism for idiopathic and/or neurogenic detrusor overactivity.[102]

Evidence in support of a role of capsaicin-sensitive nerves in the pathogenesis of neurogenic detrusor overactivity in humans has been presented,[110,111] and intravesical capsaicin and resiniferatoxin (which by stimulation of vanilloid receptors desensitize a sub-population of afferent nerves) have been shown to improve bladder control of patients with neurogenic bladders.[111–113]

Vasoactive intestinal polypeptide

Vasoactive intestinal polypeptide (VIP) was shown to inhibit spontaneous contractile activity in isolated detrusor muscle from several animal species and from humans, but to have little effect on contractions induced by muscarinic receptor stimulation or by electrical stimulation of nerves.[10] In isolated rat bladder, VIP had no effect; however, in isolated guinea-pig bladder, VIP produced contraction. Stimulation of the pelvic nerves in cats increased the VIP output from the bladder, and increased bladder blood flow, although only moderately.[114] Intravenous VIP induced bladder relaxation in dogs.[115] On the other hand, VIP given intravenously to patients in a dose causing increases in heart rate had no effect on cystometric parameters.[116] Plasma concentrations of VIP were obtained which, in other clinical investigations, had been sufficient to cause relaxation of smooth muscle.[116]

Outflow obstruction

In rats with infravesical outflow obstruction, bladder hypertrophy and detrusor overactivity, the concentra-tions of VIP in the middle and lower parts of obstructed bladders were higher than in controls.[117] Neither in the hypertrophic, nor in the normal isolated rat bladder, did VIP have relaxant or contractant effects, and the peptide did not influence contractions induced by electrical stimulation.[117,118] This does not support the view that lack of VIP is associated with detrusor overactivity, at least not in the rat.

Detrusor overactivity

VIP levels were markedly reduced in patients suffering from idiopathic[108,119] or neurogenic detrusor overactivity.[120] These results were interpreted to suggest that VIP (or rather lack of it) may be involved in some forms of detrusor overactivity.

Neuropeptide Y

The human bladder is richly endowed with neuropeptide Y (NPY)-containing nerves.[121-124] It seems that NPY can be found in adrenergic as well as cholinergic nerves. In neonates and children, Dixon et al.[16] found small ganglia were scattered throughout the detrusor muscle of the urinary bladder. Approximately 75% of the intramural neurons were VAChT immunoreactive, whereas approximately 95% contained NPY and approximately 40% contained NOS. VAChT-immunoreactive nerves were also observed in a subepithelial location in all the organs examined, the majority containing NPY, whereas a small proportion contained NOS. The number of NPY-containing nerves did not change in the obstructed human bladder, where a general loss of sensory peptides was demonstated.[108]

The presence of functional NPY receptors in human bladder was investigated by Davis et al.[125] using peptide YY (PYY) as the agonist and [^{125}I]PYY as the radioligand. No quantifiable specific [^{125}I]PYY binding was detected in human bladder, and PYY caused no contraction of bladder preparations; furthermore, field stimulation-induced contraction was not affected by PYY. The authors concluded that the human bladder expresses only very few (if any) functional NPY receptors. This is in contrast to findings in animal bladders. NPY-containing nerves were shown to be present in abundance in the rat detrusor.[10] Iravani and Zar[126] found that exogenously added NPY contracted strips of rat detrusor and potentiated non-cholinergic motor transmission, the effects of which were blocked by nifedipine. It was concluded that the abundant presence of NPY-like immunoreactive nerve fibers in the detrusor muscle was consistent with a motor transmitter function of the peptide in the rat bladder. These results are not in agreement with those of Zoubek et al.[127] who found that porcine NPY did not induce any direct contractile effect in isolated strips of rat detrusor. On the other hand, porcine NPY had a marked inhibitory effect on the cholinergic component of electrically induced contractions in rat bladder strips, particularly at low (< 10 Hz) frequencies of stimulation. In the isolated guinea-pig detrusor, NPY had no effects per se, but decreased the electrically induced NANC response.[128]

Thus, available information on the effects of NPY on detrusors from different species is conflicting. Even if it has been suggested that NPY may have an important role in the neural control of the lower urinary tract in the rat,[129] there is no convincing information that this is the case in humans.

CONCLUSION

There is abundant evidence that cholinergic neurotransmission is predominant in the activation of the human detrusor, both normally and in dysfunctional states. This may not be the case in animals, which should be considered when animal models are used for study of bladder function. Release of ACh, which stimulates M_2 and M_3 receptors on the detrusor smooth muscle cells, will lead to bladder contraction. Other neurotransmitters/modulators (e.g. ATP) have been demonstrated in the bladder of both animals and humans, but their roles in the human bladder, normally and in different bladder disorders, remain to be established.

REFERENCES

1. de Groat WC, Downie JW, Levin RM, et al. Basic neurophysiology and neuropharmacology. In: Abrams P, Khoury S, Wein A (eds) Incontinence, 1st International Consultation on Incontinence. Plymouth: Plymbridge Distributors, 1999, pp. 105–154
2. Blok BF, Sturms LM, Holstege G. Brain activation during micturition in women. Brain 1998;121:2033–2042.
3. Nour S, Svarer C, Kristensen JK, et al. Cerebral activation during micturition in normal men. Brain 2000;123:781–789.
4. de Groat WC, Booth AM, Yoshimura N. Neurophysiology of micturition and its modification in animal models of human disease. In: Maggi CA (ed.) Nervous Control of the Urogenital System. The Autonomic Nervous System series, Vol. 6. Reading: Harwood Academic, 1993, pp 227–289.
5. Lincoln J, Burnstock G. Autonomic innervation of the urinary bladder and urethra. In: Maggi CA (ed.) Nervous Control of the Urogenital System. The Autonomic Nervous System series, Vol. 6. Reading: Harwood Academic, 1993, pp 33–68.
6. Andersson KE, Persson K. Nitric oxide synthase and the lower urinary tract: possible implications for physiology and pathophysiology. Scand J Urol Nephrol 1995;175 (Suppl.):43–53.
7. Bridgewater M, Brading AF. Evidence for a non-nitrergic inhibitory innervation in the pig urethra. Neurourol Urodyn 1993;12:357–358.
8. Hashimoto S, Kigoshi S, Muramatsu I. Nitric oxide-dependent and -independent neurogenic relaxation of isolated dog urethra. Eur J Pharmacol 1993;231:209–214.

9. Werkström V, Persson K, Ny L, et al. Factors involved in the relaxation of female pig urethra evoked by electrical field stimulation. Br J Pharmacol 1995;116:1599–1604.

10. Andersson K-E. Pharmacology of lower urinary tract smooth muscles and penile erectile tissues. Pharmacol Rev 1993;45:253–308.

11. Janig W, Morrison JF. Functional properties of spinal visceral afferents supplying abdominal and pelvic organs, with special emphasis on visceral nociception. Prog Brain Res 1986;67:87–114.

12. Habler HJ, Janig W, Koltzenburg M. Activation of unmyelinated afferent fibres by mechanical stimuli and inflammation of the urinary bladder in the cat. J Physiol 1990;425:545–562.

13. Fall M, Lindstrom S, Mazieres L. A bladder-to-bladder cooling reflex in the cat. J Physiol 1990;427:281–300.

14. Arvidsson U, Reidl M, Elde R, et al. Vesicular acetylcholine transporter (VAChT) protein: a novel and unique marker for cholinergic neurons in the central and peripheral nervous systems. J Comp Neurol 1997;378:454–467.

15. Persson K, Andersson K-E, Alm P. Choline acetyltransferase and vesicular acetylcholine transporter protein in neurons innervating the rat lower urinary tract. Proc Soc Neurosci 1997;596:9 (abstract).

16. Dixon JS, Jen PYP, Gosling JA. The distribution of vesicular acetylcholine transporter in the human male genitourinary organs and its co-localization with neuropeptide Y and nitric oxide synthase. Neurourol Urodyn 2000;19:185–194.

17. Eglen RM, Hegde S, Watson N. Muscarinic receptor subtypes and smooth muscle function. Pharmacol Rev 1996;48:531–565.

18. Caulfield MP, Birdsall NJM. International Union of Pharmacology. XVII. Classification of muscarinic acetyl-choline receptors. Pharmacol Rev 1998;50:279–290.

19. Bonev AD, Nelson MT. Muscarinic inhibition of ATP-sensitive K^+ channels by protein kinase C in urinary bladder smooth muscle. Am J Physiol 1993;265:C1723–1728.

20. Hegde SS, Eglen RM. Muscarinic receptor subtypes modulating smooth muscle contractility in the urinary bladder. Life Sci 1999;64:419–428.

21. Yamaguchi O, Shisda K, Tamura K, et al. Evaluation of mRNAs encoding muscarinic receptor subtypes in human detrusor muscle. J Urol 1996;156:1208–1213.

22. Harriss DR, Marsh KA, Birmingham AT, Hill SJ. Expression of muscarinic M3-receptors coupled to inositol phospholipid hydrolysis in human detrusor cultured smooth muscle cells. J Urol 1995;154:1241–1245.

23. Hegde SS, Choppin A, Bonhaus D, et al. Functional role of M_2 and M_3 muscarinic receptors in the urinary bladder of rats in vitro and in vivo. Br J Pharmacol 1997;120:1409–1418.

24. Krichevsky VP, Pagala MK, Vaydovsky I, et al. Function of M3 muscarinic receptors in the rat urinary bladder following partial outlet obstruction. J Urol 1999;161:644–650.

25. Braverman AS, Luthin GR, Ruggieri MR. M2 muscarinic receptor contributes to contraction of the denervated rat urinary bladder. Am J Physiol 1998;275:R1654–R1660.

26. Braverman A, Legos J, Young W, et al. M2 receptors in genito-urinary smooth muscle pathology. Life Sci 1999;64:429–436.

27. Tobin G, Sjögren C. In vivo and in vitro effects of muscarinic receptor antagonists on contractions and release of [^{3}H]acetylcholine in the rabbit urinary bladder. Eur J Pharmacol 1995;28:1–8.

28. Somogyi GT, de Groat WC. Evidence for inhibitory nicotinic and facilitatory muscarinic receptors in cholinergic nerve terminals of the rat urinary bladder. J Auton Nerv Syst 1992;37:89–98.

29. Alberts P. Classification of the presynaptic muscarinic receptor that regulates ^{3}H-acetylcholine secretion in the guinea pig urinary bladder in vitro. J Pharmacol Exp Ther 1995;4:458–468.

30. Somogyi GT, de Groat WC. Function, signal transduction mechanisms and plasticity of presynaptic muscarinic receptors in the urinary bladder. Life Sci 1999;64:411–418.

31. Gosling JA, Gilpin SA, Dixon JS, et al. Decrease in the autonomic innervation of human detrusor muscle in outflow obstruction. J Urol 1986;136:501–504.

32. Sibley GN. The physiological response of the detrusor muscle to experimental bladder outflow obstruction in the pig. Br J Urol 1987;60:332–336.

33. Speakman MJ, Brading AF, Gilpin CJ, et al. Bladder outflow obstruction – a cause of denervation supersensitivity. J Urol 1987;138:1461–1466.

34. Pandita RK, Fujiwara M, Alm P, et al. Cystometric evaluation of bladder function in non-anesthetized mice with and without bladder outlet obstruction. J Urol 2000;164(4):1385–1389.

35. Sibley GN. A comparison of spontaneous and nerve-mediated activity in bladder muscle from man, pig and rabbit. J Physiol (Lond) 1984;354:431–443.

36. Harrison SCV, Hunnam GR, Farman P, et al. Bladder instability and denervation in patients with bladder outflow obstruction. Br J Urol 1987;60:519–522.

37. Yokoyama O, Nagano K, Kawaguchi K, et al. The response of the detrusor muscle to acetylcholine in patients with infravesical obstruction. Urol Res 1991;19:117–121.

38. Sjögren C, Andersson KE, Husted S, et al. Atropine resistance of transmurally stimulated isolated human bladder muscle. J Urol 1982;128:1368–1371.

39. Bayliss M, Wu C, Newgreen D, et al. A quantitative study of atropine-resistant contractile responses in human detrusor smooth muscle, from stable, unstable and obstructed bladders. J Urol 1999;162:1833–1839.

40. Tagliani M, Candura SM, Di Nucci A, et al. A re-appraisal of the nature of the atropine-resistant contraction to electrical field stimulation in the human isolated detrusor muscle. Naunyn Schmiedebergs Arch Pharmacol 1997;356:750–755.

41. Turner WH, Brading AF. Smooth muscle of the bladder in the normal and the diseased state: pathophysiology,

diagnosis and treatment. Pharmacol Ther 1997;75:77–110.

42. Charlton RG, Morley AR, Chambers P, et al. Focal changes in nerve, muscle and connective tissue in normal and unstable human bladder. BJU Int 1999;84:953–960.

43. Mills IW, Greenland JE, McMurray G, et al. Studies of the pathophysiology of idiopathic detrusor instability: the physiological properties of the detrusor smooth muscle and its pattern of innervation. J Urol 2000;163:646–651.

44. Kinder RB, Mundy AR. Pathophysiology of idiopathic detrusor instability and detrusor hyperreflexia. An in vitro study of human detrusor muscle. Br J Urol 1987;60:509–515.

45. Restorick JM, Mundy AR. The density of cholinergic and alpha and beta adrenergic receptors in the normal and hyper-reflexic human detrusor. Br J Urol 1987;63:32–35.

46. Gup DI, Baumann M, Lepor H, et al. Muscarinic cholinergic receptors in normal pediatric and myelodysplastic bladders. J Urol 1989;142:595–599.

47. German K, Bedwani J, Davies J, et al. Physiological and morphometric studies into the pathophysiology of detrusor hyperrflexia in neuropathic patients. J Urol 1995;153:1678–1683.

48. Saito M, Kondo A, Kato T, et al. Response of the human neurogenic bladder induced by intramural nerve stimulation. Nippon Hinyokika Gakkai Zasshi 1993;84:507–513.

49. Kaplan SA, Te AE, Blaivas JG. Urodynamic findings in patients with diabetic cystopathy. J Urol 1995;153:342–344.

50. Latifpour J, Gousse A, Kondo S, et al. Effects of experimental diabetes on biochemical and functional characteristics of bladder muscarinic receptors. J Pharmacol Exp Ther 1989;248:81–88.

51. Mimata H, Wheeler MA, Fukumoto Y, et al. Enhancement of muscarinic receptor-coupled phosphatidyl inositol hydrolysis in diabetic bladder. Mol Cell Biochem 1995;152:71–76.

52. Tong YC, Chin WT, Cheng JT. Alterations in urinary bladder M2-muscarinic receptor protein and mRNA in 2-week streptozotocin-induced diabetic rats. Neurosci Lett 1999;277:173–176.

53. Hashitani H, Suzuki H. Altered electrical properties of bladder smooth muscle in streptozotocin-induced diabetic rats. Br J Urol 1996;77:798–804.

54. Kanda M, Eto K, Tanabe N, et al. Effects of ONO-2235, an aldose reductase inhibitor, on muscarinic receptors and contractile response of the urinary bladder in rats with streptozotocin-induced diabetes. Jpn J Pharmacol 1997;73:221–228.

55. Gary T, Robertson D. Lessons learned from dopamine β-hydroxylase deficiency in humans. News Physiol Sci 1994;9:35–39.

56. Gosling JA, Dixon JS, Jen PYP. The distribution of noradrenergic nerves in the human lower urinary tract. Eur Urol 1999;38 (Suppl. 1):23–30.

57. Åmark P. The effect of noradrenaline on the contractile response of the urinary bladder. Scand J Urol Nephrol 1986;20:203–207.

58. Goepel M, Wittmann A, Rubben H, et al. Comparison of adrenoceptor subtype expression in porcine and human bladder and prostate. Urol Res 1997;25(3):199–206.

59. Levin RM, Ruggieri MR, Wein AJ. Identification of receptor subtypes in the rabbit and human urinary bladder by selective radio-ligand binding. J Urol 1988;139(4):844–848.

60. Walden PD, Durkin MM, Lepor H, et al. Localization of mRNA and receptor binding sites for the alpha 1a-adrenoceptor subtype in the rat, monkey and human urinary bladder and prostate. J Urol 1997;157(3):1032–1038.

61. Malloy BJ, Price DT, Price RR, et al. Alpha1-adrenergic receptor subtypes in human detrusor. J Urol 1998;160(3 Pt 1):937–943.

62. Perlberg S, Caine M. Adrenergic response of bladder muscle in prostatic obstruction. Its relation to detrusor instability. Urology 1982;20(5):524–527.

63. Smith DJ, Chapple CR. In vitro response of human bladder smooth muscle in unstable obstructed male bladders: a study of pathophysiological causes? Neurourol Urodyn 1994;34:14–15.

64. Rohner TJ, Hannigan JD, Sanford EJ. Altered in vitro adrenergic responses of dog detrusor muscle after chronic bladder outlet obstruction. Urology 1978;11(4):357–361.

65. Mattiasson A, Ekström J, Larsson B, et al. Changes in the nervous control of the rat urinary bladder induced by outflow obstruction. Neurourol Urodyn 1987;6:37–45.

66. Saito M, Wein AJ, Levin RM. Effect of partial outlet obstruction on contractility: comparison between severe and mild obstruction. Neurourol Urodyn 1993;12(6):573–583.

67. Hampel C, Dolber PC, Savic SL, et al. Changes in α1 adrenergic (AR) subtype gene expression during bladder outlet obstruction of rats. J Urol 2000;163:228 (abstract 1015).

68. Norlen L, Dahlstrom A, Sundin T, et al. The adrenergic innervation and adrenergic receptor activity of the feline urinary bladder and urethra in the normal state and after hypogastric and/or parasympathetic denervation. Scand J Urol Nephrol 1976;10(3):177–184.

69. Malkowicz SB, Atta MA, Elbadawi A, et al. The effect of parasympathetic decentralization on the feline urinary bladder. J Urol 1985;133(3):521–523.

70. Andersson KE, Atta MA, Elbadawi A, et al. Effects of parasympathetic decentralization on some nerve-mediated functions in the feline urinary bladder. Acta Physiol Scand 1991;141(1):11–18.

71. Nergardh A, Boreus LO, Naglo AS. Characterization of the adrenergic beta-receptor in the urinary bladder of man and cat. Acta Pharmacol Toxicol 1977;40(1):14–21.

72. Larsen JJ. Alpha and beta-adrenoceptors in the detrusor muscle and bladder base of the pig and beta-adrenoceptors in the detrusor muscle of man. Br J Pharmacol 1979;65(2):215–222.

73. Igawa Y, Yamazaki Y, Takeda H, et al. Functional and molecular biological evidence for a possible beta 3-adrenoceptor in the human detrusor muscle. Br J Pharmacol 1999;126(3):819–825.

74. Takeda M, Obara K, Mizusawa T, et al. Evidence for beta 3-adrenoceptor subtypes in relaxation of the human urinary bladder detrusor: analysis by molecular biological and pharmacological methods. J Pharmacol Exp Ther 1999;288(3):1367–1373.

75. Taira N. The autonomic pharmacology of the bladder. Annu Rev Pharmacol 1972;12:197–208.

76. Brading AF, Inoue R. Ion channels and excitatory transmission in the smooth muscle of the urinary bladder. Z Kardiol 1991;80 (Suppl. 7):47–53.

77. Cowan WD, Daniel EE. Human female bladder and its noncholinergic contractile function. Can J Physiol Pharmacol 1983;61(11):1236–1346.

78. Kinder RB, Mundy AR. Atropine blockade of nerve-mediated stimulation of the human detrusor. Br J Urol 1985;57(4):418–421.

79. Hoyle CH, Chapple C, Burnstock G. Isolated human bladder: evidence for an adenine dinucleotide acting on P2X-purinoceptors and for purinergic transmission. Eur J Pharmacol 1989;174(1):115–118.

80. Ruggieri MR, Whitmore KE, Levin RM. Bladder purinergic receptors. J Urol 1990;144(1):176–181.

81. Luheshi GN, Zar MA. Presence of non-cholinergic motor transmission in human isolated bladder. J Pharm Pharmacol 1990;42(3):223–224.

82. Palea S, Artibani W, Ostardo E, et al. Evidence for purinergic neurotransmission in human urinary bladder affected by interstitial cystitis. J Urol 1993;150(6):2007–2012.

83. Wammack R, Weihe E, Dienes H-P, Hohenfellner R. Die Neurogene Blase in vitro. Akt Urol 1995;26:16–18.

84. Husted S, Sjögren C, Andersson KE. Direct effects of adenosine and adenine nucleotides on isolated human urinary bladder and their influence on electrically induced contractions. J Urol 1983;130(2):392–398.

85. Hardy LA, Harvey IJ, Chambers P, et al. A putative alternatively spliced variant of the P2X(1) purinoreceptor in human bladder. Exp Physiol 2000;85:461–463.

86. Cockayne DA, Hamilton SG, Zhu QM, et al. Urinary bladder hyporeflexia and reduced pain-related behaviour in P2X3-deficient mice. Nature 2000;407:1011–1015.

87. Smet PJ, Edyvane KA, Jonavicius J, et al. Colocalization of nitric oxide synthase with vasoactive intestinal peptide, neuropeptide Y, and tyrosine hydroxylase in nerves supplying the human ureter. J Urol 1994;152(4):1292–1296.

88. Persson K, Alm P, Johansson K, et al. Nitric oxide synthase in pig lower urinary tract: immunohistochemistry, NADPH diaphorase histochemistry and functional effects. Br J Pharmacol 1993;110(2):521–530.

89. Klarskov P. Influence of prostaglandins and ketoprofen on contractile responses of human and pig detrusor and trigone muscles in vitro. Pharmacol Toxicol 1987;61(1):37–41.

90. James MJ, Birmingham AT, Hill SJ. Partial mediation by nitric oxide of the relaxation of human isolated detrusor strips in response to electrical field stimulation. Br J Clin Pharmacol 1993;35(4):366–372.

91. Elliott RA, Castleden CM. Nerve mediated relaxation in human detrusor muscle. Br J Clin Pharmacol 1993;36:479.

92. Persson K, Andersson KE. Nitric oxide and relaxation of pig lower urinary tract. Br J Pharmacol 1992;106(2):416–422.

93. Persson K, Andersson KE. Non-adrenergic, non-cholinergic relaxation and levels of cyclic nucleotides in rabbit lower urinary tract. Eur J Pharmacol 1994;268(2):159–167.

94. Morita T, Tsujii T, Dokita S. Regional difference in functional roles of cAMP and cGMP in lower urinary tract smooth muscle contractility. Urol Int 1992;49(4):191–195.

95. Desai KM, Sessa WC, Vane JR. Involvement of nitric oxide in the reflex relaxation of the stomach to accommodate food or fluid. Nature 1991;351:477–479.

96. Burnett AL, Calvin DC, Chamness SL, et al. Urinary bladder–urethral sphincter dysfunction in mice with targeted disruption of neuronal nitric oxide synthase models idiopathic voiding disorders in humans. Nat Med 1997;3(5):571–574.

97. Sutherland RS, Kogan BA, Piechota HJ, et al. Vesicourethral function in mice with genetic disruption of neuronal nitric oxide synthase. J Urol 1997;157(3):1109–1116.

98. Persson K, Pandita RK, Aszodi A, et al. Functional characteristics of urinary tract smooth muscles in mice lacking cGMP protein kinase type I. Am J Physiol Regul Integr Comp Physiol 2000;279(3):R1112–1120.

99. Mevorach RA, Bogaert GA, Kogan BA. Role of nitric oxide in fetal lower urinary tract function. J Urol 1994;152(2 Pt 1):510–514.

100. Pandita RK, Mizusawa H, Andersson KE. Intravesical oxyhemoglobin initiates bladder overactivity in conscious, normal rats. J Urol 2000;164:545–550.

101. Persson K, Igawa Y, Mattiasson A, et al. Effects of inhibition of the L-arginine/nitric oxide pathway in the rat lower urinary tract in vivo and in vitro. Br J Pharmacol 1992;107(1):178–184.

102. Maggi CA. The dual, sensory and 'efferent' function of the capsaicin-sensitive primary sensory neurons in the urinary bladder and urethra. In: Maggi CA (ed.) Nervous Control of the Urogenital System. The Autonomic Nervous System series, Vol. 6. Reading: Harwood Academic, 1993, pp 383–422.

103. Maggi CA. The mammalian tachykinin receptors. Gen Pharmacol 1995;26(5):911–944.

104. Maggi CA, Barbanti G, Santicioli P, et al. Cystometric evidence that capsaicin-sensitive nerves modulate the afferent branch of micturition reflex in humans. J Urol 1989;142:150–154.

105. Maggi CA, Santicioli P, Giuliani S, et al. Activation of micturition reflex by substance P and substance K: indirect evidence for the existence of multiple tachykinin

receptors in the rat urinary bladder. J Pharmacol Exp Ther 1986;238(1):259–266.

106. Lecci A, Giuliani S, Patacchini R, et al. Evidence against a peripheral role of tachykinins in the initiation of micturition reflex in rats. J Pharmacol Exp Ther 1993;264(3):1327–1332.

107. Giuliani S, Patacchini R, Barbanti G, et al. Characterization of the tachykinin neurokinin-2 receptor in the human urinary bladder by means of selective receptor antagonists and peptidase inhibitors. J Pharmacol Exp Ther 1993;267(2):590–595.

108. Chapple CR, Milner P, Moss HE, et al. Loss of sensory neuropeptides in the obstructed human bladder. Br J Urol 1992;70(4):373–381.

109. Moore KH, Gilpin SA, Dixon JS, et al. Increase in presumptive sensory nerves of the urinary bladder in idiopathic detrusor instability. Br J Urol 1992;70(4):370–372.

110. Fowler CJ, Jewkes D, McDonald WI, et al. Intravesical capsaicin for neurogenic bladder dysfunction. Lancet. 1992;339(8803):1239.

111. De Ridder D, Baert L. Vanilloids and the overactive bladder. BJU Int 2000;86(2):172–180.

112. Cruz F. Desensitization of bladder sensory fibers by intravesical capsaicin or capsaicin analogs. A new strategy for treatment of urge incontinence in patients with spinal detrusor hyperreflexia or bladder hypersensitivity disorders. Int Urogynecol J Pelvic Floor Dysfunct 1998;9(4):214–220.

113. Fowler CJ. Intravesical treatment of overactive bladder. Urology 2000;55 (Suppl. 5A):60–64.

114. Andersson PO, Bloom SR, Mattiasson A, et al. Bladder vasodilatation and release of vasoactive intestinal polypeptide from the urinary bladder of the cat in response to pelvic nerve stimulation. J Urol 1987;138(3):671–673.

115. Andersson PO, Sjögren C, Uvnas B, et al. Urinary bladder and urethral responses to pelvic and hypogastric nerve stimulation and their relation to vasoactive intestinal polypeptide in the anaesthetized dog. Acta Physiol Scand 1990;138(3):409–416.

116. Klarskov P, Holm-Bentzen M, Norgaard T, et al. Vasoactive intestinal polypeptide concentration in human bladder neck smooth muscle and its influence on urodynamic parameters. Br J Urol 1987;60(2):113–118.

117. Andersson PO, Andersson KE, Fahrenkrug J, et al. Contents and effects of substance P and vasoactive intestinal polypeptide in the bladder of rats with and without infravesical outflow obstruction. J Urol 1988;140(1):168–172.

118. Igawa Y, Persson K, Andersson KE, et al. Facilitatory effect of vasoactive intestinal polypeptide on spinal and peripheral micturition reflex pathways in conscious rats with and without detrusor instability. J Urol 1993;149(4):884–889.

119. Gu J, Restorick JM, Blank MA, et al. Vasoactive intestinal polypeptide in the normal and unstable bladder. Br J Urol 1983;55(6):645–647.

120. Kinder RB, Restorick JM, Mundy AR. Vasoactive intestinal polypeptide in the hyper-reflexic neuropathic bladder. Br J Urol 1985;57(3):289–291.

121. Gu J, Blank MA, Huang WM, et al. Peptide-containing nerves in human urinary bladder. Urology 1984;24(4):353–357.

122. Iwasa A. Distribution of neuropeptide Y (NPY) and its binding sites in human lower urinary tract. Histological analysis. Nippon Hinyokika Gakkai Zasshi 1993;84(6):1000–1006 (in Japanese).

123. Crowe R, Noble J, Robson T, et al. An increase of neuropeptide Y but not nitric oxide synthase-immunoreactive nerves in the bladder neck from male patients with bladder neck dyssynergia. J Urol 1995;154(3):1231–1236.

124. Dixon JS, Jen PY, Gosling JA. A double-label immunohistochemical study of intramural ganglia from the human male urinary bladder neck. J Anat 1997;190 (Pt 1):125–134.

125. Davis B, Goepel M, Bein S, et al. Lack of neuropeptide Y receptor detection in human bladder and prostate. BJU Int 2000;85(7):918–924.

126. Iravani MM, Zar MA. Neuropeptide Y in rat detrusor and its effect on nerve-mediated and acetylcholine-evoked contractions. Br J Pharmacol 1994;113(1):95–102.

127. Zoubek J, Somogyi GT, de Groat WC. A comparison of inhibitory effects of neuropeptide Y on rat urinary bladder, urethra, and vas deferens. Am J Physiol 1993;265(3 Pt 2):R537–543.

128. Lundberg JM, Hua XY, Franco-Cereceda A. Effects of neuropeptide Y (NPY) on mechanical activity and neurotransmission in the heart, vas deferens and urinary bladder of the guinea-pig. Acta Physiol Scand 1984;121(4):325–332.

129. Tran LV, Somogyi GT, de Groat WC. Inhibitory effect of neuropeptide Y on adrenergic and cholinergic transmission in rat urinary bladder and urethra. Am J Physiol 1994;266(4 Pt 2):R1411–1417.

4

REGULATION OF BLADDER FUNCTION

Bengt Uvelius, Robert M. Levin and Penelope A. Longhurst

Efficient bladder function depends on the coordination of a variety of different cellular and biochemical processes. In this chapter we will describe the mechanisms responsible for normal bladder function and indicate how they may be altered by some disease states. Because of space restrictions, only a limited number of studies can be cited and wherever possible we have relied on the use of review articles.

MORPHOLOGY OF THE DETRUSOR MUSCLE

The smooth muscle cells in the detrusor are long and spindle shaped, with a central nucleus. Depending on the degree of stretch, their length varies from 100 to 700 microns.[1] The diameter also varies with the degree of stretch but is less than 5–6 microns in the nuclear region (Fig. 4.1).

The cytoplasm contains many myofilaments. The membranes contain regularly spaced dense bands, with membrane vesicles (caveolae) between them. Dense bodies are scattered in the cytoplasm. Mitochondria (responsible for oxidative phosphorylation) and sarcoplasmic reticulum (involved in protein synthesis and storage of intracellular Ca^{2+}) are also present, but constitute only a few per cent of the cell volume

The smooth muscles cells are arranged in bundles. In human detrusor the muscle bundles are large, often up to a few millimeters in diameter.[2] In smaller mammals the bundles are smaller and often only 100 microns in diameter when relaxed.[1] The muscle is generally not arranged in distinct layers. Intermediate junctions are seen between the cells[3] and constitute areas of mechanical coupling. There are no classical gap junctions between the detrusor muscle cells[3] but recently interstitial cells have been demonstrated histochemically in

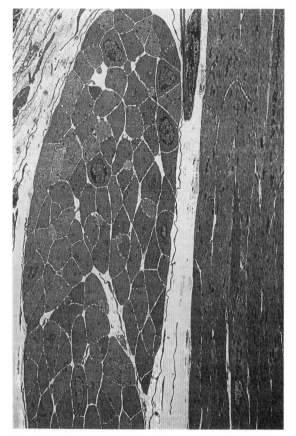

Fig. 4.1 Electron micrograph of the musculature of a moderately distended guinea pig bladder. A bundle of muscle cells in transverse section (to the left) and one in almost longitudinal section (to the right) can be observed. (Reproduced with permission from Uvelius & Gabella.[1])

the bladder wall.[4] Typical gap junctions have been demonstrated by electron microscopy between the interstitial cells[5] and it is thus possible that the interstitial cellular network may operate as a functional syncytium integrating signals and responses in the bladder wall.

CONTRACTILE PROTEINS AND DETRUSOR MECHANICS

The contractile machinery of the detrusor smooth muscle cells is similar to that of other smooth muscles.[6] There are two contractile filaments:

* *Thin filaments*, whose major component is actin, are anchored to the dense bodies (which contain alpha-actinin). The dense bands are related to the dense bodies, but are attached to the inner surface of the cell membrane.
* *Thick filaments*, whose major component is myosin.

The cells also contain intermediate filaments (diameter intermediate to thin and thick filaments). In mature smooth muscle the intermediate filaments mainly contain desmin, but in developing smooth muscle vimentin seems to be dominant. The intermediate filaments do not participate in contraction but seem to constitute a cytoskeleton.[7]

Each myosin molecule contains two polypeptide chains that for most of their length are wound around each other. The free N-terminal regions are arranged as globular myosin heads.[8] These heads (or cross-bridges) can, when the system is activated, attach to sites on the thin filament. Next, a translatory movement is performed, upon which the attachment is broken. The myosin head is then tilted back to its original position by energy released from hydrolysis of one molecule of ATP. Repeated cross-bridge cyclings produce a sustained contraction, the force output depending on the number of cross-bridges that are active at the same time. When the load is lower than the isometric, the thick and thin filaments slide past each other and result in tissue shortening: the lower the load, the higher the shortening velocity becomes. Maximum shortening velocity against zero load is proportional to the maximum turnover rate of the cross-bridges.

The relation between force and shortening velocity (v) is hyperbolic (Fig. 4.2), and can be approximated by the Hill[9] equation:

$$v = b(1 - P/P_0)/(P/P_0 + a/P_0)$$

where P_0 is the isometric force and a and b are constants.

In clinical urodynamics, this equation is transformed to a similar equation describing the hyperbolic relationship between detrusor pressure and flow rate (the so-called urethral resistance relation, URR).

The contractile machinery is activated by Ca^{2+} ions through two different mechanisms:[8]

* The myosin molecule contains a 20 kDa regulatory light chain situated in the head region. In the presence of Ca^{2+}, a Ca^{2+}–calmodulin-dependent myosin light chain (MLC) kinase will phosphorylate the MLC and activate the myosin head.
* The inhibitory action of caldesmon (a thin filament-associated protein) on actin–myosin interaction is reversed in the presence of Ca^{2+}. The Ca^{2+} comes

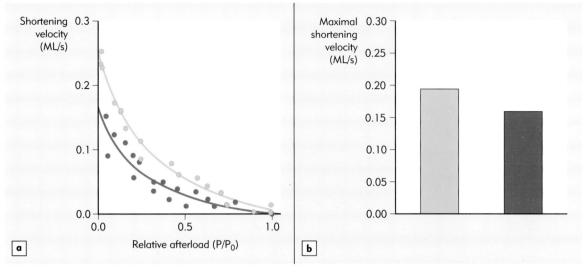

Fig. 4.2 Force–velocity relationships of detrusor muscle from control and obstructed rat bladders. **(a)** The shortening velocity, in muscle lengths (ML) per second, is plotted against the relative afterload (P/P_0). Filled pink and filled purple circles show data from a control and a hypertrophic preparation, respectively. Fits to the Hill[9] equation are shown. **(b)** The summarized V_{max} data of control (filled pink) and hypertrophic (filled purple) muscles. The obstructed detrusor specimens had a significantly lower V_{max}. (From Sjuve R, Haase H, Morano I, et al. Contraction kinetics and myosin isoform composition in smooth muscle from hypertrophied rat urinary bladder. J Cell Biochem 1996;63:86–93.[10] Copyright © 1996. Reprinted by permission of Wiley-Liss, Inc., a subsidiary of John Wiley & Sons, Inc.)

from the intercellular space and enters the cell during the action potential, or is released from the sarcoplasmic reticulum.

There is a characteristic relationship between cell length and force production. The active force at a certain cell length is influenced by, for example, the overlap between thin and thick filaments. The length–active tension relation (Fig. 4.3) in detrusor muscle (as in smooth muscle in general) shows that it can produce active force over a large length range.[11] One reason for this might be that the thin filaments can successively interact with a number of thick filaments during the shortening of the cell.

Maximum shortening velocity (V_{max}) varies from one smooth muscle organ to another. Detrusor muscle is a fast smooth muscle with a V_{max} of 0.2–0.3 muscle lengths per second.[10] In addition to the 20 kDa light chains described above, the myosin heads also contain a 17 kDa light chain (LC17). This exists as one acidic (LC17a) and one basic (LC17b) isoform. Muscles with a high relative amount of LC17a have a high V_{max}.[12] Another factor that influences V_{max} is the relative number of myosin heads that have a 7-amino acid insert.[8,10] The higher the relative number of myosin heads with insert, the higher the V_{max}. Compared to

other smooth muscles, detrusor muscle has a relatively high amount of LC17a and number of myosin heads with the insert.

The length–passive tension relationship describes the mechanical properties of the passive muscle. Passive tension increases exponentially with stretch but is normally low over the ascending part of the length–active tension curve, where the bladder muscle cells usually work. The muscle also exhibits viscoelastic properties (e.g. displays stress–relaxation), whereby a rapid stretch of detrusor is followed by a partial viscoelastic relaxation of stress.

DETRUSOR FUNCTION

As described in Chapter 3, the neurogenic response of urinary bladder body strips is complex, consisting of a rapid phasic component and a sustained tonic component. There is now general agreement that the rapid phasic component, which is lost after desensitization of P2X receptors, results primarily from ATP release, and that the tonic component, which is reduced after blockade of muscarinic receptors, results from acetylcholine (ACh) release.[13] Norepinephrine (noradrenaline) is also released from bladder strips during electrical field

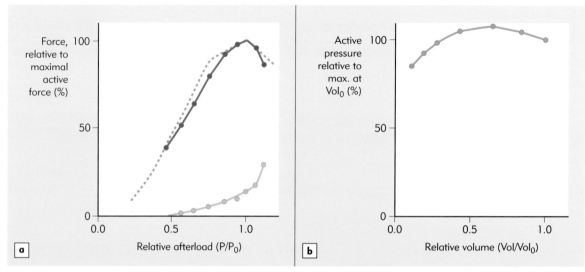

Fig. 4.3 **(a)** Length dependence of active (purple circles) and passive (pink circles) force of intact human detrusor muscle strips in vitro. Length expressed relative to optimum length (l_0) for active force. The dotted line shows length–active force data from rabbit detrusor muscle. **(b)** Volume–pressure relation of the urinary bladder calculated from the data in **(a)**, and using the law of Laplace (V_0 is the volume corresponding to l_0). (Reproduced with permission from Malmqvist et al.[11])

stimulation. Although it is difficult to demonstrate any functional effect of neuronally released norepinephrine, bladder body strips normally respond to norepinephrine with a relaxation as a result of stimulation of β-adrenergic receptors.

Muscarinic receptors

Stimulation of muscarinic receptors by ACh released from parasympathetic nerves is probably the primary stimulus for bladder emptying, particularly in the human bladder. Like many other smooth muscles, the bladder contains a heterogeneous population of muscarinic receptors. Using receptor binding and molecular techniques, M_2 receptors have been shown to be present at a three- to ten-fold greater density than M_3 receptors. However, the muscarinic receptor responsible for the functional response to acetylcholine is the M_3 receptor.[14–16] Bladders from knockout mice lacking the M_3 receptor contract poorly (or not at all) to the nonselective muscarinic agonist, carbachol.[17] As a result, male M_3 knockout mice develop urinary retention and bladder hypertrophy due to an inability of the bladder smooth muscle to contract sufficiently in vivo to overcome the urethral resistance. In contrast, bladder strips from M_2-receptor knockout mice contract in response to carbachol in a manner similar to that of

wild-type controls.[18] However, the strips from the M_2 knockouts are slightly but significantly less sensitive to carbachol.

The direct contractile response of bladder strips to muscarinic stimulation results from stimulation of phospholipase C causing release of Ca^{2+} from intracellular stores and hydrolysis of phosphatidylinositol (PI) to inositol 1,4,5-triphosphate (IP_3) and diacylglycerol (DAG). Carbachol-stimulated PI hydrolysis in bladders is antagonized by M_3, but not by M_2, antagonists. In contrast, M_2 receptor stimulation is coupled through an inhibitory G protein (Gi) to inhibition of adenylate cyclase (AC).[19] Recent studies suggest that rather than having a direct contractile effect, stimulation of bladder M_2 receptors decreases cyclic adenosine 5′-monophosphate (cAMP) formation by inhibiting AC.[16] β-Adrenergic receptors predominate over α-adrenergic receptors in the bladder body, where their tonic stimulation by norepinephrine released from sympathetic nerve endings is thought to promote bladder filling by activating AC, increasing cAMP, and relaxing detrusor smooth muscle. Thus, during voiding, ACh released from parasympathetic nerves stimulates M_3 receptors to contract the bladder and, as a result of concurrent M_2-receptor stimulation, inhibits β-adrenergic-induced cAMP formation and relaxation (Fig. 4.4).[20] This physiologic antagonism of M_2 muscari-

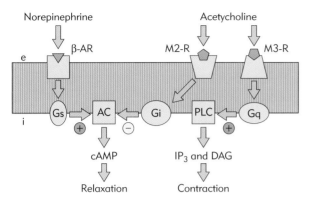

Fig. 4.4 Schematic representation of the proposed interactions between beta-adrenergic and muscarinic cholinergic stimulation of detrusor smooth muscle (see text for explanation of abbreviations). (Adapted from Eglen et al.[20] with permission from Elsevier.) AR: adrenergic receptor; e: extracellular; Gq: pertussis toxin-insensitive G protein; GS: stimulatory G protein; i: intra-cellular; R: receptor. (+) Indicates the pathway is stimulated, (−) that the pathway is inhibited.

nic and β-adrenergic activation is thought to result in more efficient voiding.

Stimulation of the bladder by ACh also results in activation of ion channels and release of Ca^{2+} from intracellular stores. The depolarizing phase of the action potential of bladder smooth muscle results from activation of an inward Ca^{2+} current; repolarization is dependent on an outward K^+ current. Tetrodotoxin has no effects on the bladder action potential, suggesting that the fast Na^+ channel has no role in bladder smooth muscle activation.[13]

Inhibitory prejunctional M_2 receptors in bladder smooth muscle may modulate ACh release under normal conditions.[21] However, the physiologic relevance of activation of these prejunctional receptors relative to the probably much greater contribution of postjunctional M_2 receptors is still unclear. Higher concentrations of ACh, such as those found after inhibition of acetyl cholinesterase by physostigmine, activate facilitatory presynaptic M_1 receptors. Somogyi and de Groat speculate that activation of these M_1 receptors may be of importance in pathologic conditions such as the neurogenic hyperreflexic bladder where neural firing and transmitter release are increased.[21] However, this has not been investigated.

ATP receptors

The bladder contains a heterogeneous population of ATP receptors. Contractile responses to ATP result from stimulation of P2X ATP receptors which are transmitter-gated ion channels; relaxation results from stimulation of G protein-coupled P2Y receptors.[22,23] mRNA for the P2X1 receptor subtype is expressed in bladder and P2X1 immunoreactivity is associated with

bladder smooth muscle membranes.[24–26] Other subtypes of P2X and P2Y receptors may play a role in the functional responses to ATP, but it has been difficult to characterize the receptors pharmacologically.

α- and β-Adrenergic receptors

Adrenergic receptor subtypes are differentially distributed within the bladder. As described above, β-adrenergic receptors coupled to AC predominate in the bladder body where their stimulation causes detrusor relaxation. mRNA for β_1-, β_2- and β_3-receptor subtypes is expressed in detrusor smooth muscle but β_3-receptors mediate relaxation of human bladder strips in response to adrenergic stimulation.[27,28] However β_1- and β_2-receptors may also mediate relaxation in bladders from other species. In contrast, α-adrenergic receptors coupled to PI hydrolysis predominate in the bladder base, trigone and urethra, where their stimulation causes smooth muscle contraction. The α_{1d}-receptor subtype predominates in human detrusor (60–70% of total); α_{1a}-receptors (30–40%) are also present.[29] In contrast, α_{1a}-receptors predominate in human prostate and are responsible for contraction in response to adrenergic stimulation.[30,31] Because irritative bladder symptoms caused by outlet obstruction are relieved by non-selective α-adrenergic antagonists, Malloy et al. suggest that detrusor α_{1D}-receptors are responsible for irritative symptoms.[29] Prejunctional α_1- and α_2-adrenergic receptors are also found in bladder dome where they modulate release of acetylcholine and norepinephrine.[32,33] Interestingly, the functional α_1-receptor subtypes on the detrusor smooth muscle and cholinergic nerve terminals in the rat bladder have been shown to be different; prejunctional α_{1A}-receptors on cholinergic nerve terminals facilitate ACh release, while postjunctional α_{1B}- and/or α_{1D}-receptors mediate smooth muscle contraction.[34]

DETRUSOR METABOLISM

Smooth muscle has low phosphagen reserves. This is mainly due to its low levels of creatine phosphate. The rabbit bladder contains 1.2 μmol/g ATP and 1.5 μmol/g creatine phosphate.[35] A basal ATP turnover rate of 0.9 μmol/min at 27°C (which corresponds to 2 μmol/min at 37°C) for the rabbit bladder[36] and 3 μmol/min for the rat detrusor[37] has been reported.

The small phosphagen reserves indicate that the activity of the detrusor muscle is dependent on an instantaneous production of ATP. If the oxygen tension is lowered during a contraction, the contractile amplitude immediately decreases.[38] If oxygen is readministered, force immediately begins to increase and reaches the original value.

Although detrusor muscle can oxidize fatty acids, glucose metabolism provides most of the energy for ATP synthesis.[39] The metabolism of glucose can be considered to take place in two consecutive steps:

1. via glycolysis to pyruvate, a chain of reactions not dependent on oxygen and with a low net production of ATP
2. via the citric acid cycle producing CO_2 and H_2O as end products, and with a high oxygen-dependent production of ATP.

The glycolysis is dependent on access to NAD. This is normally generated in the citric acid cycle, and also by the conversion of pyruvate to lactate, a reaction catalyzed by lactate dehydrogenase. The basal metabolic rate is high in the detrusor, and there is considerable lactate production, even when oxygen is available.[37] (This so-called aerobic glycolysis is also common in other smooth muscles.) Both oxygen consumption and lactate production increase when the bladder strips are contracting. In the relaxed muscle about 5% of the ATP is produced by glycolysis and 95% by oxidative metabolism. In the contracting muscle the relative amount of ATP produced by glycolysis doubles.

Lactate dehydrogenase (LDH) consists of four subunits composed of two different polypeptide chains (M and H). Five different forms of LDH exist: M4, M3H, M2H2, MH3 and H4. Compared to the H subunit, the M form has a lower degree of substrate inhibition by pyruvate and product inhibition by lactate and would therefore be less affected by hypoxia or inhibition of mitochondrial function. In normal detrusor muscle, the M form accounts for almost 70% of total LDH.[40] This may be one explanation for the limited inhibition of detrusor contractile force by lowering oxygen tension (in anoxic conditions contractile force still amounts to 40% of maximum[37]).

DETRUSOR BLOOD FLOW

Normal function of the detrusor is dependent on an adequate supply of oxygen and nutrients. Evaluation of blood flow to the detrusor during bladder filling has provided conflicting results. In part, this may be because of problems encountered in correlating absolute bladder blood flow at a single time point with what occurs during the normal, dynamic natural filling situation, to differences in the techniques of blood flow measurement, and to differences in the rates of bladder filling. Laser Doppler flowmetry studies in anesthetized humans during cystometry have shown that bladder perfusion increases[41] or decreases[42] after filling to capacity. However, in conscious pigs, blood flow is found to be unaltered during compliant filling and decreases only transiently during voiding.[43] Thus, the blood supply to the bladder is able to adapt to distension during a normal micturition cycle.

EFFECTS OF AGING

Detrusor morphology

Aging in otherwise healthy bladders seems to have little influence on the ultrastructure of the detrusor[44,45] except for a widening of the dense bands and a decreased number of caveolae between the dense bands. The caveolae are believed to be involved in Ca^{2+} regulation.

Contractile proteins and detrusor mechanics

Aging has no effects on detrusor concentrations of actin-, myosin- or intermediate-filament proteins.[46]

Little is known about changes in the mechanical properties of the aged detrusor smooth muscle. Intact smooth muscle strips from aged rats have decreases in maximum velocity of shortening (V_{max}) and isometric force.[47] In detrusor muscle where the cell membranes were permeabilized by a detergent, and where the contractile machinery could be activated maximally, there was no difference in either V_{max} or isometric force.[46] This suggests that the effects of aging on V_{max} and isometric force do not result from a direct effect on the contractile proteins, but are due to alterations in the activation systems (function of nerve terminals, receptor function, and/or Ca^{2+} handling of the detrusor muscle cells).

Detrusor function

Urodynamic studies in humans are difficult to evaluate to assess possible effects of aging on detrusor muscle function. In experimental animals, several functional changes have been reported to occur, for example, decreased response to cholinergic[47] and β-adrenergic agonists.[48] The decreased responsiveness to β-adrenergic stimulation may result from a decreased β-receptor density and a reduced formation of cAMP, perhaps related to changes in the stimulatory G protein (Gs) or the catalytic subunit of AC.[48] The detrusor sensitivity to muscarinic stimulation either does not change with increasing age[49,50] or decreases.[47] Sneddon and McLees found that bladders from neonatal rabbits were significantly more responsive to P2X agonists than those from adults and suggest that the relative contributions of cholinergic and purinergic mechanisms to neurogenic contraction are influenced during development.[51]

Detrusor metabolism

Little is known about the metabolic properties of aged detrusor muscle. Detrusor muscle from aged rats exhibits a lower basal metabolic rate and a reduced contribution of aerobic glycolysis to total metabolic energy production during both relaxation and contraction under normoxic conditions than does muscle from young adult animals.[47] When stimulated under anoxic conditions they were, however, able to increase their rate of lactate production to the same levels as young adult detrusor muscles. More recently, Lin and co-workers demonstrated that bladders from young rats were more resistant to fatigue resulting from repetitive stimulation than bladders from elderly rats.[52] This decreased contractility in the older bladders was associated with a decrease in ATP and creatine phosphate concentrations.

Detrusor blood flow

In the rat, blood flow to the detrusor was significantly lower in 24-month-old rats when compared to 6-month-old rats.[53] The decreased blood flow in the older rats correlated with decreased voiding pressures and decreased in vitro responses to bethanechol and low-frequency field stimulation.

EFFECTS OF OBSTRUCTION

Detrusor morphology

The most striking effect of outlet obstruction on the detrusor muscle is the pronounced hypertrophy of the muscle cells.[3,54] In the obstructed rat bladder the contour of the muscle cells was variable; cells were found to be polygonal, crescent-like, flattened out, indented by other cells or wedge shaped, in contrast to the ovoid shape of normal detrusor muscle cells. The dense bands occupied a higher proportion of the cell membrane than in control cells. Similar changes are found in obstructed rabbit[55] and human[54] bladder, although hypertrophic muscle cells are not always found in the obstructed human bladder.[56]

There is an increase in total amount of detrusor collagen in obstructed bladder.[57] In rabbit bladder[55] and in some specimens from obstructed human bladder[54] there are signs of intercellular fibrosis, with an increased distance between contiguous smooth muscle cells. Such changes might be secondary to degenerative phenomena related to, for example, disturbed cell metabolism. They are not found in the obstructed rat bladder.

Contractile proteins and detrusor mechanics

Obstruction induces a considerable net synthesis of contractile and cytoskeletal proteins.[58] Myosin synthesis does not keep pace with actin, so the myosin/actin ratio decreases. There are changes in actin and myosin isoforms in obstructed detrusor from rat,[58] rabbit[59] and man,[60] but the functional significance is not clear.

The hypertrophic detrusor muscle has an increased desmin concentration.[58] This corresponds well with an increased number of intermediate filaments observed in other hypertrophic smooth muscles. It may be that an enforced cytoskeleton is necessary when the cell volume increases.

The obstructed rat detrusor has a doubled relative amount of LC17b and a 50% decrease in myosin heads with the 7-amino acid insert.[10] This corresponds well with the lower V_{max} observed in obstructed detrusor (see Fig. 4.2). The rate of contraction of the hypertrophic detrusor muscle cell is slower than that of the control, perhaps as an adaptation to the prolonged, high-pressure micturitions (slow muscles are more 'economical' with ATP consumption than fast muscles).

In the obstructed bladder there is considerable remodeling of the contractile machinery. The length–active tension relationship (expressed relative to bladder circumference) is shifted to the right, i.e. maximum active force is produced at a length corresponding to a larger circumference.[61] This remodeling, which decreases active force at small circumferences, may be one causative factor for the development of residual urine (for metabolic factors, see below). Maximum active force is lower than in normal muscle.[37] This could be due to the changed myosin/actin ratio mentioned above.[58] The low active force in smooth muscle in general compared to skeletal muscle has been suggested as being due to its low myosin/actin ratio.

Detrusor function

Functional changes have been reported for bladders subjected to outlet obstruction but in only a few studies have the mechanisms responsible been studied. An increase in contractility is usually seen in animal bladders which respond to obstruction with small increases in mass (i.e. are compensated), while bladders which are greatly hypertrophic become dysfunctional (or decompensated). An increase in atropine resistance has been reported in bladders from patients with benign prostatic hyperplasia (BPH) resulting from an increased sensitivity to ATP.[62] Atropine resistance is also found in bladder strips from patients with detrusor instability or instability secondary to BPH.[63]

Alterations in adrenergic responsiveness of detrusor muscle are also associated with obstruction. Both in dogs[64] and in humans[65] the normal β-receptor mediated relaxant response of detrusor strips to norepinephrine was converted to an α-receptor mediated contractile response. Similarly, Moore et al. found that the ability of rat bladder strips to relax in response to norepinephrine was inversely related to the bladder mass; severely obstructed bladders tended to contract in response to norepinephrine while less severely obstructed bladders relaxed.[66]

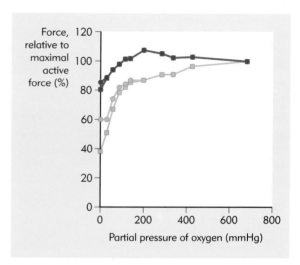

Fig. 4.5 Phasic (circles) and sustained (squares) contractions of detrusor muscle from control (filled pink) and from obstructed rat bladders (filled purple) in vitro. Contractile force of the muscle from obstructed bladders is less affected than the control muscle by lowering oxygen tension. (Adapted from Arner et al.[37])

Detrusor metabolism

During outlet obstruction, metabolism of both rat and rabbit bladders is shifted to more glycolysis with lactate formation and less glucose oxidation. Uvelius and Arner[67] favor the idea that this shift is an adaptation to glycolysis as a major process for ATP production during the prolonged micturition when detrusor pressures often exceed arterial pressures. The LDH isoform pattern is shifted towards more M4, making the active force more resistant to a hypoxic environment (Fig. 4.5). On the other hand, Levin et al.[68] suggest that the shift of glucose metabolism to lactate production is secondary to mitochondrial dysfunction, and is responsible for the decreased contractility observed in obstructed rabbit bladders which others explained by a decreased myosin/actin ratio (see above). The decreased mitochondrial function could also contribute to the development of residual urine (cf. the rightward shift of the length–active tension curve mentioned above). Obstructed rat bladders have a considerable residual urine but do not seem to have much mitochondrial dysfunction.[69]

Detrusor blood flow

As described above for normal blood flow, few studies are available that monitor dynamic blood flow during the micturition cycle. In animals, absolute bladder blood flow increases during the first 24 hours after outlet obstruction[70,71] but returns to normal values within 7 days.[71,72] However, in hypertrophic (i.e. decompensated) bladders, absolute blood flow decreases after chronic outlet obstruction.[73] In contrast to the transient decrease in bladder wall blood flow and oxygen tension observed during a normal micturition cycle in conscious pigs, after outlet obstruction the prolonged increase in intravesical pressure during micturition is associated with a significantly greater and prolonged decrease in blood flow and oxygen tension.[74] Thus the reduced blood flow and decreased oxygen supply to the bladder wall during outlet obstruction may contribute to the biochemical and cellular changes associated with outlet obstruction.

EFFECTS OF DIABETES

Detrusor morphology

The morphologic characteristics of the hypertrophic detrusor smooth muscle cells in diabetic rats are similar to those reported after outlet obstruction (see above). It should be noted that the degree of hypertrophy induced by diabetes is generally considerably less (two- to three-fold increase in bladder mass) than that caused by obstruction (two- to ten-fold increase). The bladder wall thickness, bladder diameter and muscle wall area are significantly greater in diabetic rats compared to controls.[75] The contour of the detrusor muscle cells in diabetic rats is irregular, with a cross-sectional area approximately twice that of controls, but the muscle cell length is shorter.[75,76] The relative amount of smooth muscle in bladders from diabetic rats is unchanged compared to controls.[77] Fibrosis or other degenerative phenomena have not been noted, but histologic observations have not been made at time points longer than 8 weeks' duration of diabetes.

Similar to the findings in obstructed bladders, diabetes causes an increase in the total amount of detrusor collagen but a decrease in the concentration; this is prevented by insulin treatment.[76,78] Collagen fibrils were noted predominantly in the loose connective tissue between the smooth muscle bundles.[76]

Contractile proteins and detrusor mechanics

Little work has been done to examine the effects of diabetes on detrusor contractile or cytoskeletal proteins.

Koo et al. showed that expression of rat bladder β-actin mRNA was increased during the first 2 weeks after induction of diabetes but returned to control levels by 6 weeks.[79] This differs from the effects of outlet obstruction, which stimulates a decrease in rabbit bladder β-actin mRNA expression.[59]

Similar to the changes reported for obstructed bladders (see above), remodeling of the bladder wall occurs in diabetic rats.[80,81] Chronic diabetes causes a rightward shift of both the passive and active length–tension relations.[78,80,81] Both are normalized by insulin.[78] Maximum active force has been reported to be lower[80,81] or higher[78] in bladders from diabetic rats; these discrepancies may be related to the method of data expression used.

Detrusor function

Functional changes are associated with the bladder hypertrophy caused by diabetes mellitus in animal models, but there is no good agreement as to whether responses are increased or decreased. Binding studies show there is an upregulation of muscarinic receptors in bladders from diabetic rats associated with an increased responsiveness to carbachol[82] but no change in subtype selectivity.[83] However, Tong et al. report increases in both protein and mRNA for the m_2 receptor in bladders from diabetic rats.[84] Functional studies have not yet been performed to establish whether there are changes in responsiveness to M_2 or M_3 receptor stimulation in diabetes. Bladders from diabetic rats are also more responsive to the relaxant effects of isoproterenol;[82,85] this is associated with an overall increase in β-receptor density.[82]

Detrusor metabolism

The decline in circulating insulin levels associated with diabetes mellitus causes decreases in skeletal muscle and adipose tissue glucose uptake, decreases in glycogen synthesis, and increases in glycogenolysis and gluconeogenesis. Despite the limited influence of insulin on glucose uptake and metabolism by smooth muscle cells, diabetes-induced alterations in bladder glucose metabolism and energy utilization have been reported. There are no differences in ATP or creatine phosphate content in bladders from control and diabetic rats, and removing glucose from the bathing medium causes similar declines in contractility of bladder strips from both groups.[86]

Arner et al. showed that reducing the oxygen tension causes similar reductions in force generation of bladder strips from diabetic and control rats.[77] There were no differences in lactate production by controls or diabetics under normoxia or anoxia. In contrast, Waring and Wendt reported that bladders from diabetic rats had a reduced ability to contract under anoxic conditions compared to controls.[87] This was associated with decreases in lactate formation by the diabetic bladders, suggesting that bladders from diabetics have a greater energy limitation because of diminished anaerobic ATP production.

LDH activity is two-fold higher in bladders from diabetic rats, accompanied by decreases in the relative proportion of the M3H and M2H2 isozymes.[77] However, the relative amount of the M form is unchanged, in contrast to the findings in obstructed bladders (see above[67]). Thus, the increased enzymatic activity reported by Arner et al. could not be related to the observed metabolic changes in bladders from diabetic rats.

NEUROGENIC BLADDER

Detrusor morphology and function

Neuropathic bladders from patients with spina bifida have increased collagen infiltration of the detrusor muscle.[88] This infiltration is mainly by type III collagen.[89,90] The density of cholinergic nerves in such bladders is decreased, leading to a decreased contractile response to nerve stimulation and a possible development of postjunctional supersensitivity to muscarinic agonists.[90] The smooth muscle cells are hypertrophied in denervated rat bladder.[91]

A detailed description is, however, lacking regarding ultrastructural changes in neuropathic bladders. After denervation, the response of rat bladders to adrenergic stimulation changes from the usual inhibitory β-response to an excitatory α-response, but returns to normal after reinnervation.[92] The postjunctional supersensitivity to cholinergic muscarinic stimulation which occurs after removal of the pelvic ganglion[93] has also been attributed to an increase in the density of M_2 receptors.[94]

Contractile proteins

The detrusor muscle from denervated rat bladder has the same content and concentration of contractile and cytoskeletal proteins as bladders with intact innervation subjected to outlet obstruction.[95] This shows that the stimulus for the smooth muscle cells to hypertrophy and the synthesis of these proteins is not dependent on the presence of functioning nerves.

REFERENCES

1. Uvelius B, Gabella G. Relation between cell length and force production in urinary bladder smooth muscle. Acta Physiol Scand 1980;110:357–365.
2. Brading A. Physiology of bladder smooth muscle. In: Torrens M, Morrison JFB (eds) The Physiology of the Lower Urinary Tract. New York: Springer-Verlag, 1987, p 161.
3. Gabella G, Uvelius B. Urinary bladder of rat: fine structure of normal and hypertrophic musculature. Cell Tissue Res 1990;262:67–79.
4. McCloskey KD, Gurney AM. Kit positive cells in the guinea pig bladder. J Urol 2002;168:832–836.
5. Sui GP, Rothery S, Dupont E, et al. Gap junctions and connexin expression in human suburothelial interstitial cells. BJU Int 2002;90:118–129.
6. Brading A, Fry CH, Maggi CA, et al. Cellular biology. In: First WHO Consultation on Incontinence. Geneva: WHO, 1998, p 57.
7. Small JV, Sobieszek A. The contractile apparatus of smooth muscle. Int Rev Cytol 1980;64:241.
8. Chacko S, DiSanto M, Menon C, et al. Contractile protein changes in urinary bladder smooth muscle following outlet obstruction. Adv Exp Med Biol 1999;462:137–153.
9. Hill AV. The heat of shortening and the dynamic constants of muscle. Proc R Soc Lond [Biol] 1938;126:136.
10. Sjuve R, Haase H, Morano I, et al. Contraction kinetics and myosin isoform composition in smooth muscle from hypertrophied rat urinary bladder. J Cell Biochem 1996;63:86–93.
11. Malmqvist U, Arner A, Uvelius B. Mechanics and Ca^{2+}-sensitivity of human detrusor muscle bundles studied in vitro. Acta Physiol Scand 1991;143:373–380.
12. Malmqvist U, Arner A. Correlation between isoform composition of the 17 kDa myosin light chain and maximal shortening velocity in smooth muscle. Pflugers Arch 1991;418:523–530.
13. Andersson K-E. Pharmacology of lower urinary tract smooth muscles and penile erectile tissues. Pharmacol Rev 1993;45:253–308.
14. Longhurst PA, Leggett RE, Briscoe JAK. Characterization of the functional muscarinic receptors in the rat bladder. Br J Pharmacol 1995;116:2279–2285.
15. Wang P, Luthin GR, Ruggieri MR. Muscarinic acetylcholine receptor subtypes mediating urinary bladder contractility and coupling to GTP binding proteins. J Pharmacol Exp Ther 1995;273:959–966.
16. Hegde SS, Choppin A, Bonhaus D, et al. Functional role of M_2 and M_3 muscarinic receptors in the urinary bladder of

rats in vitro and in vivo. Br J Pharmacol 1997;120:1409–1418.

17. Matsui M, Motomura D, Karasawa H, et al. Multiple functional defects in peripheral autonomic organs in mice lacking muscarinic acetylcholine receptor gene for the M3 subtype. Proc Natl Acad Sci USA 2000;97:9579–9584.

18. Stengel PW, Gomeza J, Wess J, Cohen ML. M_2 and M_4 receptor knockout mice: muscarinic receptor function in cardiac and smooth muscle in vitro. J Pharmacol Exp Ther 2000;292:877–885.

19. Noronha-Blob L, Lowe V, Patton A, et al. Muscarinic receptors: relationships among phosphoinositide breakdown, adenylate cyclase inhibition, in vitro detrusor muscle contractions and in vivo cystometrogram studies in guinea pig bladder. J Pharmacol Exp Ther 1989;249:843–851.

20. Eglen RM, Reddy H, Watson N, et al. Muscarinic acetylcholine receptor subtypes in smooth muscle. Trends Pharmacol Sci 1994;15:114–119.

21. Somogyi GT, de Groat WC. Evidence for inhibitory nicotinic and facilatory muscarinic receptors in cholinergic nerve terminals of the rat urinary bladder. J Auton Nerv Syst 1992;37:89–97.

22. Bolego C, Pinna C, Abbracchio MP, et al. The biphasic response of rat vesical smooth muscle to ATP. Br J Pharmacol 1995;114:1557–1562.

23. McMurray G, Dass N, Brading AF. Purinoceptor subtypes mediating contraction and relaxation of marmoset urinary bladder smooth muscle. Br J Pharmacol 1998;123:1579–1586.

24. Longhurst PA, Schwegel T, Folander K, et al. The human P_{2X1} receptor: molecular cloning, tissue distribution, and localization to chromosome 17. Biochem Biophys Acta 1996;1308:185–188.

25. Michel AD, Lundstrom K, Buell GN, et al. A comparison of the binding characteristics of recombinant P_{2X1} and P_{2X2} purinoceptors. Br J Pharmacol 1996;118:1806–1812.

26. Lee HY, Bardini M, Burnstock G. Distribution of P2X receptors in the urinary bladder and the ureter of the rat. J Urol 2000;163:2002–2007.

27. Igawa Y, Yamazaki Z, Takeda H, et al. Functional and molecular biological evidence for a possible β3-adrenoceptor in the human detrusor muscle. Br J Pharmacol 1999;126:819–825.

28. Takeda M, Obara K, Mizusawa T, et al. Evidence for β3-adrenoceptor subtypes in relaxation of the human urinary bladder detrusor: analysis by molecular biological and pharmacological methods. J Pharmacol Exp Ther 1999;288:1367–1373.

29. Malloy BJ, Price DT, Price RR, et al. α_1-Adrenergic receptor subtypes in human detrusor. J Urol 1998;160:937–943.

30. Price D, Schwinn DA, Lomasney J, et al. Identification, quantification, and localization of mRNA for three distinct alpha₁ adrenergic receptor subtypes in human prostate. J Urol 1993;150:546–551.

31. Forray C, Bard JA, Wetzel JM, et al. The α_1-adrenergic receptor that mediates smooth muscle contraction in

human prostate has the pharmacological properties of the cloned human alpha₁c subtype. Mol Pharmacol 1994;45:703–708.

32. Maggi CA, Santicioli P, Furio M, et al. Dual effects of clonidine on micturition reflex in urethane anesthetized rats. J Pharmacol Exp Ther 1985;235:528–536.

33. de Groat WC, Yoshiyama M, Ramage AG, et al. Modulation of voiding and storage reflexes by activation of α_1-adrenoceptors. Eur Urol 1999;36:68–73.

34. Szell EA, Yamamoto T, de Groat WC, Somogyi GT. Smooth muscle and parasympathetic nerve terminals in the rat urinary bladder have different subtypes of α_1-adrenoceptors. Br J Pharmacol 2000;130:1685–1691.

35. Kato K, Lin AT-L, Haugaard N, et al. Effects of outlet obstruction on glucose metabolism of the rabbit urinary bladder. J Urol 1990;143:844–847.

36. Wendt IR, Gibbs CL. Energy expenditure of longitudinal smooth muscle of rabbit urinary bladder. Am J Physiol 1987;252:C88–96.

37. Arner A, Malmqvist U, Uvelius B. Metabolism and force in hypertrophic smooth muscle from rat urinary bladder. Am J Physiol 1990;258:C923–932.

38. Uvelius B, Arner A. Changed metabolism of detrusor muscle cells from obstructed rat urinary bladder. Scand J Urol Nephrol Suppl 1997;184:59–65.

39. Hypolite JA, Haugaard N, Wein AJ, et al. Comparison of palmitic acid and glucose metabolism in the rabbit urinary bladder. Neurourol Urodyn 1989;8:599.

40. Polyanska M, Arner A, Malmquist U, Uvelius B. Lactate dehydrogenase activity and isoform distribution in the rat urinary bladder: effects of outlet obstruction and its removal. J Urol 1993;150:543–545.

41. Irwin P, Galloway NTM. Impaired bladder perfusion in interstitial cystitis: a study of blood supply using laser Doppler flowmetry. J Urol 1993;149:890–892.

42. Batista JE, Wagner JR, Azadzoi IM, et al. Direct measurement of blood flow in the human bladder. J Urol 1996;155:630–633.

43. Greenland JE, Brading AF. Urinary bladder blood flow changes during the micturition cycle in a conscious pig model. J Urol 1996;156:1858–1861.

44. Elbadawi A, Yalla SV, Resnick NM. Structural basis of geriatric voiding dysfunction. II. Aging detrusor: normal versus impaired contractility. J Urol 1993;150:1657–1667.

45. Hald T, Brading AF, Elbadawi A, et al. Pathology and pathophysiology. In: Cockett ATK, Khoury S, Aso Y, et al. (eds) The 3rd International Consultation on Benign Prostatic Hyperplasia (BPH). Jersey: Scientific Communication International, 1995, p 125.

46. Sjuve R, Uvelius B, Arner A. Old age does not affect shortening velocity or content of contractile and cytoskeletal proteins in the rat detrusor smooth muscle. Urol Res 1997;25:67–70.

47. Munro DD, Wendt IR. Contractile and metabolic properties of longitudinal smooth muscle from rat urinary bladder and the effects of aging. J Urol 1993;150:529–536.

48. Nishimoto T, Latifpour J, Wheeler MA, et al. Age-dependent alterations in β-adrenergic responsiveness of rat detrusor smooth muscle. J Urol 1995;153:1701–1705.

49. Ordway GA, Esbenshade TA, Kolta MG, et al. Effect of age on cholinergic muscarinic responsiveness and receptors in the rat urinary bladder. J Urol 1986;136:492–496.

50. Saito M, Kondo A, Gotoh M, et al. Age-related changes in the response of the rat urinary bladder to neurotransmitters. Neurourol Urodyn 1993;12:191.

51. Sneddon P, McLees A. Purinergic and cholinergic contractions in adult and neonatal rabbit bladder. Eur J Pharmacol 1992;214:7–12.

52. Lin ATL, Yang CH, Chang LS. Impact of aging on rat urinary bladder fatigue. J Urol 1997;157:1990–1994.

53. Saito M, Ohmura M, Kondo A. Effect of ageing on blood flow to the bladder and bladder function. Urol Int 1999;62:93–98.

54. Elbadawi A, Yalla SV, Resnick NM. Structural basis of geriatric voiding dysfunction. IV. Bladder outlet obstruction. J Urol 1993;150:1681–1695.

55. Gosling JA, Kung LS, Dixon JS, et al. Correlation between the structure and function of the rabbit urinary bladder following partial outlet obstruction. J Urol 2000;163:1349–1356.

56. Gosling JA, Dixon JS. Structure of trabeculated detrusor smooth muscle in cases of prostatic hypertrophy. Urol Int 1980;35:351–355.

57. Uvelius B, Mattiasson A. Collagen content in the rat urinary bladder subjected to infravesical outflow obstruction. J Urol 1984;132:587–590.

58. Malmqvist U, Arner A, Uvelius B. Contractile and cytoskeletal proteins in smooth muscle during hypertrophy and its reversal. Am J Physiol 1991;260:C1085–1093.

59. Kim YS, Wang Z, Levin RM, Chacko S. Alterations in the expression of the β-cytoplasmic and the γ-smooth muscle actins in hypertrophied urinary bladder smooth muscle. Mol Cell Biochem 1994;131:115–124.

60. Malmqvist U, Arner A, Uvelius B. Cytoskeletal and contractile proteins in detrusor smooth muscle from bladders with outlet obstruction – a comparative study in rat and man. Scand J Urol Nephrol 1991;25:261–267.

61. Mattiasson A, Uvelius B. Changes in contractile properties in hypertrophic rat urinary bladder. J Urol 1982;128:1340–1342.

62. Husted S, Sjögren C, Andersson K-E. Direct effects of adenosine and adenine nucleotides on isolated human urinary bladder and their influence on electrically induced contractions. J Urol 1983;130:392–398.

63. Bayliss M, Wu C, Newgreen D, et al. A quantitative study of atropine-resistant contractile responses in human detrusor smooth muscle, from stable, unstable and obstructed bladders. J Urol 1999;162:1833–1839.

64. Rohner TJ Jr, Hannigan JD, Sanford EJ. Altered in vitro adrenergic responses of dog detrusor muscle after chronic bladder outlet obstruction. Urology 1978;11:357–361.

65. Perlberg S, Caine M. Adrenergic response of bladder muscle in prostatic obstruction. Its relation to detrusor instability. Urology 1982;20:524–527.

66. Moore CK, Levendusky M, Longhurst PA. Relationship between mass of obstructed rat bladders and responsiveness to adrenergic stimulation. J Urol 2002;168:1621–1625.

67. Uvelius B, Arner A. Metabolism of detrusor smooth muscle in normal and obstructed urinary bladder. Adv Exp Med Biol 1995;385:29–39, discussion 75–79.

68. Levin RM, Monson FC, Haugaard N, et al. Genetic and cellular characteristics of bladder outlet obstruction. Urol Clin North Am 1995;22:263–283.

69. Damaser MS, Haugaard N, Uvelius B. Partial obstruction of the rat urinary bladder: effects on mitochondria and mitochondrial glucose metabolism in detrusor smooth muscle cells. Neurourol Urodyn 1997;16:601–607.

70. Shabsigh A, Hayek OR, Weiner D, et al. Acute increase in blood flow to the rat bladder subsequent to partial bladder outlet obstruction. Neurourol Urodyn 2000;19:195–206, discussion 206–208.

71. Lieb J, Chichester P, Kogan B, et al. Rabbit urinary bladder blood flow changes during the initial stage of partial outlet obstruction. J Urol 2000;164:1390–1397.

72. Lin AT, Chen MT, Yang CH, Chang LS. Blood flow of the urinary bladder: effects of outlet obstruction and correlation with bioenergetic metabolism. Neurourol Urodyn 1995;14:285–292.

73. Schröder A, Chichester P, Kogan BA, et al. Effect of chronic bladder outlet obstruction on the blood flow of the rabbit urinary bladder. J Urol 2001;165:640–646.

74. Brading AF. Alterations in the physiological properties of urinary bladder smooth muscle caused by bladder emptying against an obstruction. Scand J Urol Nephrol Suppl 1997;184:51–58.

75. Lincoln J, Haven AJ, Sawyer M, Burnstock G. The smooth muscle of rat bladder in the early stages of streptozotocin-induced diabetes. Br J Urol 1984;56:24–30.

76. Uvelius B. Detrusor smooth muscle in rats with alloxan-induced diabetes. J Urol 1986;136:949–952.

77. Arner A, Malmqvist U, Österman A, Uvelius B. Energy turnover and lactate dehydrogenase activity in detrusor smooth muscle from rats with streptozotocin-induced diabetes. Acta Physiol Scand 1993;147:375–383.

78. Eika B, Levin RM, Longhurst PA. Collagen and bladder function in streptozotocin-diabetic rats: effects of insulin and aminoguanidine. J Urol 1992;148:167–172.

79. Koo HP, Santarosa RP, Buttyan R, et al. Early molecular changes associated with streptozotocin-induced diabetic bladder hypertrophy in the rat. Urol Res 1993;21:375–381.

80. Andersson P-O, Malmgren A, Uvelius B. Cystometrical and in vitro evaluation of urinary bladder function in rats with streptozotocin-induced diabetes. J Urol 1988;139:1359–1362.

81. Malmgren A, Andersson PO, Uvelius B. Bladder function in rats with short- and long-term diabetes; effects of age and muscarinic blockade. J Urol 1989;142:1608–1614.

82. Latifpour J, Nishimoto T, Marian MJ, et al. Differential regulation of bladder beta-adrenergic and muscarinic cholinergic receptors in experimental diabetes. Diabetes 1991;40:1150–1156.

83. Fukomoto Y, Yoshida M, Weiss RM, et al. Reversibility of diabetes- and diuresis-induced alterations in rat bladder dome muscarinic receptors. Diabetes 1994;43:819–826.

84. Tong YC, Chin WT, Cheng JT. Alterations in urinary bladder M_2-muscarinic receptor protein and mRNA in 2-week streptozotocin-induced diabetic rats. Neurosci Lett 1999;277:173–176.

85. Kudlacz EM, Gerald MC, Wallace LJ. Effects of diabetes and diuresis on contraction and relaxation mechanisms in rat urinary bladder. Diabetes 1989;38:278–284

86. Longhurst PA, Briscoe JAK, Leggett RE, et al. The influence of diabetes mellitus on glucose utilization by the rat urinary bladder. Metabolism 1993;42:749–755.

87. Waring JV, Wendt IR. Effects of anoxia on force, intracellular calcium and lactate production of urinary bladder smooth muscle from control and diabetic rats. J Urol 2000;163:1357–1363.

88. Shapiro E, Becich MJ, Perlman E, Lepor H. Bladder wall abnormalities in myelodysplastic bladders: a computer assisted morphometric analysis. J Urol 1991;145:1024–1029.

89. Ewalt DH, Howard PS, Blyth B, et al. Is lamina propria matrix responsible for normal bladder compliance? J Urol 1992;148:544–549.

90. German K, Bedwani J, Davies J, et al. Physiological and morphometric studies into the pathophysiology of detrusor hyperreflexia in neuropathic patients. J Urol 1995;153:1678–1683.

91. Ekström J, Uvelius B. Changes in length and volume of smooth muscle cells of the hypertrophied rat urinary bladder. Acta Physiol Scand 1983;118:305–308.

92. Elmér M. Responses of the denervated rat urinary bladder to alfa adrenoceptor stimulation. Acta Physiol Scand 1976;98:440–444.

93. Elmér M. Action of drugs on the innervated and denervated urinary bladder of the rat. Acta Physiol Scand 1974;91:289–297.

94. Braverman AS, Luthin GR, Ruggieri MR. M-2 muscarinic receptor contributes to contraction of the denervated rat urinary bladder. Am J Physiol 1998;275:R1654–1660.

95. Berggren T, Uvelius B, Arner A. Denervation and outlet obstruction induce a net synthesis of contractile and cytoskeletal proteins in the urinary bladder of the male rat. Urol Res 1996;24:135–140.

5

PATHOLOGY OF THE URACHUS
John N. Eble

INTRODUCTION

The first observation of urachal disease is generally attributed to Bartolomeo Cabriolus, whose 1550 *Alphabet Anatomique* contained a description of a patient with a patent urachus. Over the next four and one half centuries, case reports and small collections of cases have been reported by pathologists and surgeons from around the world. While the reader is referred to the appropriate specialized reports in the sections of this chapter, three more comprehensive reviews deserve mention here.[1-3] The first is *Embryology, Anatomy, and Diseases of the Umbilicus Together with Diseases of the Urachus*.[2] This book, written by Thomas S. Cullen and illustrated by Max Brödel, was published in 1916. Cullen's review of the early literature, together with Brödel's incomparable illustrations of original dissections, gives a foundation for understanding urachal anatomy and pathology which is not available elsewhere. The monograph *Patologia dell'Uraco*, published by Vio, Battisti and Torchi in 1967,[3] and the 1978 thesis of Bucchiere,[1] are not readily available to most readers but do constitute the two most comprehensive and detailed treatises on urachal diseases of the last 50 years.

THE NORMAL URACHUS

Embryology and gross anatomy

Early in embryonic life, the allantois projects outwards from the yolk sac into the body stalk, the structure which later forms the umbilical cord. The origin of the allantois is in the portion of the yolk sac which subsequently gives rise to the cloacal portion of the hindgut. As the urinary bladder differentiates from the cloaca, the allantois remains connected to the apex of the bladder (Fig. 5.1).[2] The urachus is the intra-abdominal structure containing the allantois and

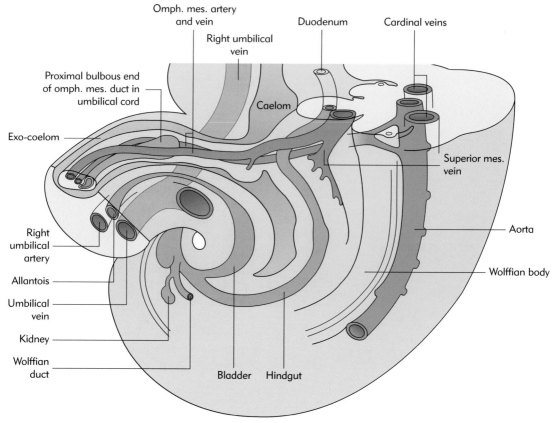

Omph. mes. artery and vein

Right umbilical vein

Duodenum

Cardinal veins

Proximal bulbous end of omph. mes. duct in umbilical cord

Caelom

Exo-coelom

Superior mes. vein

Right umbilical artery

Aorta

Allantois

Wolffian body

Umbilical vein

Kidney

Wolffian duct

Bladder   Hindgut

Fig. 5.1 Diagram of the relationships of the allantois, urinary bladder, and hindgut to the embryo and body stalk in a 7 mm embryo. (Adapted from Cullen.[2])

connecting the apex of the urinary bladder to the body wall at the umbilicus (Fig. 5.2). The relative contributions of the allantois and the cloaca to the urachus have been debated and are still unclear.[4–6] As the embryo grows longer, the urachus grows to maintain its connection with the bladder dome and body stalk (Fig. 5.3). By the beginning of the sixth month, the urachus has become an elongated structure, little more than a millimeter in diameter, connecting the urinary bladder to the body wall at the location of the umbilicus. At birth, the dome of the bladder and the umbilicus are close together (Fig. 5.4) and the urachus is only 2.5–3 mm long with a diameter of 1 mm throughout most of its course and a diameter of 3 mm as it joins the bladder.[4] To put this in perspective, the urachus must be viewed in comparison with the neighboring umbilical arteries which are 5–7 mm in diameter, and the umbilical vein which is 10 mm in diameter. At its superior end, the urachus usually divides into three fibrous strands. Two

of these attach to the adventitia of the umbilical arteries and the middle one passes through the body wall into the umbilical cord where it breaks up into a number of fine strands about 10 mm from the surface of the body.[4] Those fibrous strands are the last remnants of the allantois.

The urachus lies in a space between the anterior abdominal wall and the peritoneum, bounded anteriorly and posteriorly by the umbilicovesical fascia. Laterally, it is between the two umbilical arteries which are surrounded by umbilicovesical fascia. Inferiorly, the umbilicovesical fascial layers spread out over the surface of the dome of the bladder. The space thus defined – the space of Retzius – is roughly pyramidal and the fascial planes separate it from the peritoneum and other structures (Fig. 5.5). After birth, the apex of the urinary bladder descends into the pelvis, drawing the urachus with it. Since the urachus is attached to the adventitia of the obliterated umbilical arteries, its descent brings

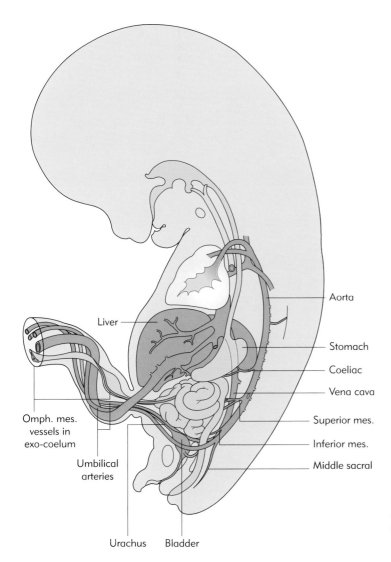

Liver

Omph. mes.
vessels in
exo-coelum

Umbilical
arteries

Urachus   Bladder

Aorta

Stomach

Coeliac

Vena cava

Superior mes.

Inferior mes.

Middle sacral

Fig. 5.2 Diagram of the relationship of the urachus to the urinary bladder and umbilical cord in a 45 mm embryo. (Adapted from Cullen.[2])

them along as well. Attached superiorly to the fibrous tissue which closes the umbilical fascial tunnel, the adventitia of the arteries is teased out into a complex of fibrous strands – the plexus of Luschka. The urachus is involved in this teasing process and Begg noted that this may account for the irregular distribution of epithelial elements or rests seen in many specimens.[4]

Based on the relationship of the urachus to the umbilical arteries, four anatomic variants were recognized by Hammond et al. in adults and children.[7] In type I, the urachus is well defined and extends from the bladder to the umbilicus, separate from the umbilical arteries. The type II variant consists of union of the urachus with one of the umbilical arteries and their joint continuation to

the umbilicus. When the urachus and both umbilical arteries join and continue to the umbilicus as a cord (the ligamentum commune) the variant is type III. Type IV consists of a short tubular urachus which ends before fusing with either umbilical artery. Hammond et al. found type I in 7 of 20 adult specimens, type II in 4 of 20, type III in 4 of 20, and type IV in 5 of 20 adult specimens.[7] In a study of 81 specimens, Blichert-Toft et al. found 7 of type I (2 adults, 1 child and 4 stillborn infants), 10 of type II, 20 of type III, and 44 of type IV.[8] Inasmuch as the bladder had yet to descend into the pelvis in the 4 stillborns, it was to be expected that all would be of type I, the fetal type. Both studies demonstrate that the fetal type of anatomy may persist into

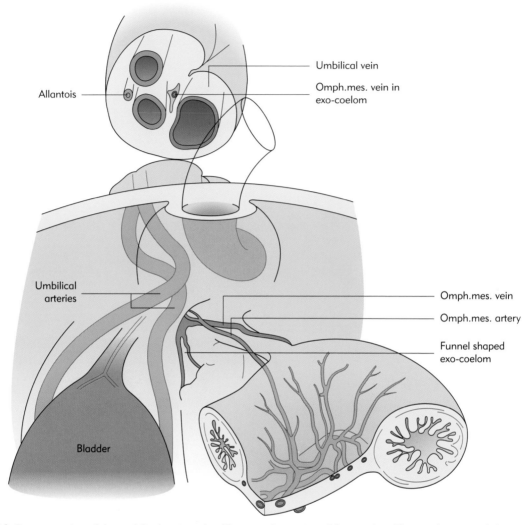

Fig. 5.3 Reconstruction of the umbilical region of a 45 mm embryo, viewed from within. The urachus extends between the umbilical arteries to the umbilicus. (Adapted from Cullen.[2])

adulthood but they disagree on the prevalence of that variant.

In the adult, the urachus outside the urinary bladder wall ranges in length from 2 to 15 cm but most often is from 5 to 5.5 cm long.[4,8] At its junction with the urinary bladder, the urachus is most often from 4 to 8 mm broad and tapers from that to about 2 mm at its superior end.[8] For clinical and pathologic purposes, it is convenient to divide the urachus into three parts: supravesical, intramural and intramucosal. When there is no communication with the bladder lumen, only the

intramural and supravesical portions are present. Tubular urachal remnants lined by epithelium are found within the wall of the urinary bladder in approximately one-third of the adult population, and are evenly distributed between men and women.[9]

Schubert et al. classified the architecture of the intramural urachal canals into three types, ranging from simple tubular canals to more complex passages.[9] The mucosal portion may consist of a wide diverticular opening (a papilla) or a small opening flush with the mucosal surface. An example of a urachus terminating

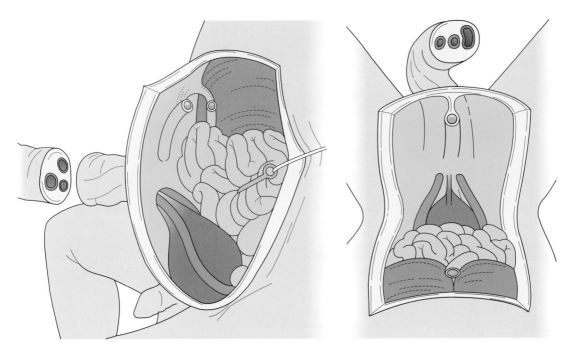

Fig. 5.4 Side and posterior views of the umbilical region in a fetus near term. Note that the urinary bladder has yet to descend and that its apex is close to the umbilicus. (Adapted from Cullen.[2])

in a papilla in the mucosa of the urinary bladder is illustrated in Figure 5.6. Wutz considered that an opening into the bladder lumen existed in most cases and that there was a small fold of mucosa which covered the opening and prevented the efflux of urine into the urachus.[10] This 'valve of Wutz' has been the subject of much controversy, with Begg finding only one example of this structure in his series of dissections and Hammond et al. finding none.[4,7] Bucchiere concluded that the valve exists but is particularly difficult to demonstrate in fixed specimens.[1] Begg did find that a delicate orifice existed in one-third of his specimens but that in the remaining two-thirds, microscopic sections confirmed that no orifice was present.[4] Hammond et al. found such communications in only 10% of their specimens.[7]

Histology of the urachus

The microscopic structure of the urachus consists of a central lumen surrounded by an epithelial lining. This is surrounded by a coat of dense fibrous tissue which in turn is surrounded by loose connective tissue. These structures are surrounded by an array of bundles of smooth muscle which lastly are enveloped in an adventitia of connective tissue.[4] The whole is found in a zone of areolar tissue between the transversalis fascia and the peritoneum. The persistence of the epithelial lining was early called into question but the studies of Begg and later investigators amply demonstrated that an epithelial lining frequently persists into adulthood.[4,8,9] Blichert-Toft et al. found that epithelium was present in six of seven examples of the type I anatomic variant and that it extended at least half the distance to the umbilicus and in three instances to the level of the umbilicus.[8] However, in 44 examples of the type IV variant, they found that only 16 had epithelium and in most of those the epithelium was limited to the region of the apex of the urinary bladder.

In their study of intramural urachal remnants, Schubert et al. found that 68% were lined by urothelium (Fig. 5.7), while in the remainder columnar epithelium was found either adjacent to urothelium or as a simple layer of columnar cells which sometimes formed papillary projections.[9] Columnar epithelium with mucous goblet cells was reported by Tyler as lining part of the urachus of a newborn boy.[11] From these studies, it is apparent that mucus-secreting columnar epithelium

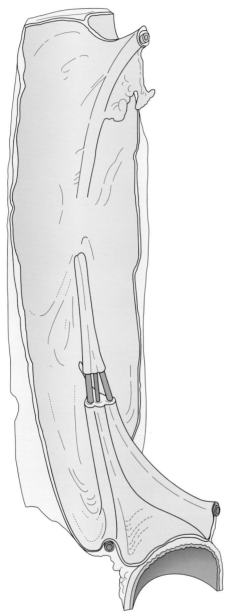

Fig. 5.5 Umbilicovesical fascia investing the umbilical arteries and urachus and reflecting on the dome of the urinary bladder and abdominal wall to define the space of Retzius. (Adapted from Cullen.[2])

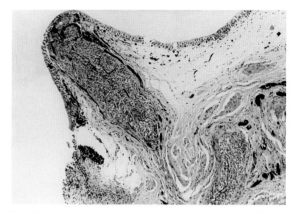

Fig. 5.6 Intramucosal urachus terminating in a papilla. H&E ×0.5.

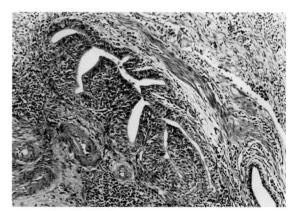

Fig. 5.7 Urothelium lining the urachal canal. Muscle fibers of the urachus are visible to the right and above the canal. H&E ×63.

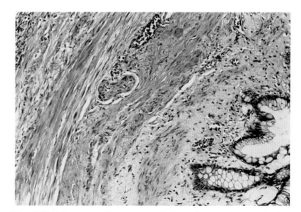

Fig. 5.8 Mucous columnar epithelium lining the urachal canal. The subepithelial connective tissue, muscle and adventitial layers are visible. H&E ×63.

(Fig. 5.8), while not the most common epithelial lining, nevertheless may be a component of the normal urachus and that invocation of metaplasia or other processes to account for its presence and its neoplasms is probably unnecessary. It is important to bear in mind that the normal urachus is not always a smooth tube. As Begg noted and Schubert et al. illustrate, it often has small buds or ramifications branching from it in the wall of the urinary bladder and in the supravesical segment.[4,9]

MALFORMATIONS OF THE URACHUS

Patent urachus

In its complete form, patent urachus is a dramatically symptomatic lesion in which urine flows from the umbilical stump or umbilicus. Figure 5.9 illustrates a patent urachal canal in an umbilical cord. Cullen's review found 53 cases in the literature of the 18th and 19th centuries while an exhaustive review by Herbst found approximately 150 cases in the literature from 1550 to 1937.[12] In 1978, Bucchiere found that the literature included reports of 228 cases.[1] These reviews found a preponderance of males to females (2:1) and an age range from neonatal to old age. Often, the umbilicus was swollen and inflamed. In 1998, Jona described a girl with patent urachus which extended into the umbilical cord and terminated in a cyst within the umbilical cord.[13]

Although most of the patients had no other detectable developmental anomaly, Lattimer found that 11 of 22 children who had congenital deficiency of the abdominal musculature ('prune belly syndrome') also had a patent urachus.[14] Since 85% of these children had bladder outlet obstruction with dilatation of the bladder, hydroureter and hydronephrosis, he concluded that the elevated pressures caused the failure of urachal closure. In a group of eight children with complete patent urachus, Schreck and Campbell found only two had urinary outlet obstruction; both had urethral atresia.[15] Comparing the developmental sequence for anterior urethral strictures, bladder neck contractures and posterior urethral valves with the developmental sequence for the urachus, they concluded that the urachus would normally already be narrowed and its component of muscle well developed by the time that significant back pressure would arise. Thus, back pressure was not a satisfactory explanation for congenital patent urachus associated with outflow obstruction. Rather, they suggested that the association must be the result of either failure of the urachus to develop normally or errors in timing of the developmental sequences. The concept that pressure could cause reopening of the urachus after normal developmental narrowing was early offered to explain acquired urinary umbilical fistulas but Begg refuted this on the basis of his anatomic studies, concluding that such cases were almost always the result of malformations of the urinary bladder resulting in its apex remaining near the umbilicus.[4]

The incomplete forms of patent urachus are umbilicourachal sinus, vesicourachal sinus or diverticulum, and the blind variant in which the urachus is closed at both ends but remains patent in between. This classification was proposed by Vaughan in 1905.[16] In 1961, Hinman added the alternating urachal sinus to the classification in order to account for adults without histories of urinary drainage from the umbilicus in whom urachal infections drained both through the umbilicus and the bladder.[17] He distinguished this from complete patent urachus, in which the lumen from bladder to umbilicus is patent at birth, and concluded that in the alternating sinus the lumen was a potential one in which cellular debris accumulated and formed a focus for infection. In 1993, Groff described two girls in whom suprapubic dermoid sinus extended upward to the umbilicus, ending at the urachus.[18]

Rarely, calculi are formed in the cavities of urachal malformations.[19] In a case of vesicourachal sinus, the stone was similar to the usual vesical calculus and Vaughan described a case of complete patent urachus in which a ring-shaped calculus formed deep to the umbilicus.[16,20] Both of these were composed of salts

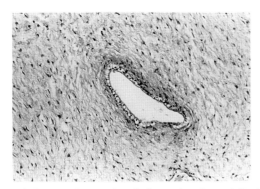

Fig. 5.9 Patent allantoic (urachal) canal in the umbilical cord. H&E ×63.

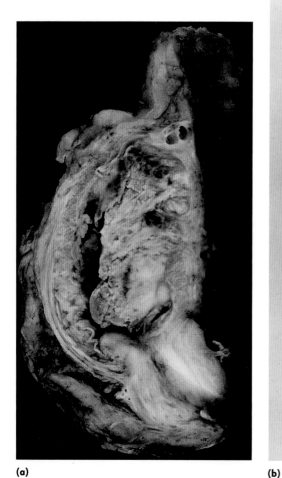

(a)

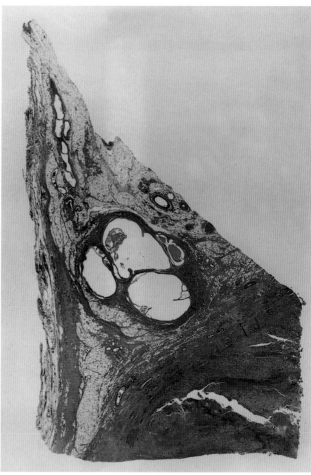

(b)

Fig. 5.10 **(a)** Multilocular cyst of the urachus found incidentally in a radical cystoprostatectomy specimen. The cyst is superior to the anterior superior portion of the wall of the urinary bladder. **(b)** Juxtavesical multilocular cyst of the urachus from Figure 2.17. H&E ×1.

similar to those making up vesical calculi. In the other malformations, where the calculi were not of urinary origin, the calculi were usually quite small and yellowish-brown or brown.[2]

Urachal cysts

Urachal cysts may occur at any level in the urachus and range from small incidental findings, such as the intramural multilocular cyst illustrated in Figure 5.10, to one described by Cullen which contained 50 liters of fluid.[2] Smaller cysts commonly are lined with urothelium or cuboidal cells. However, columnar epithelium may also form the lining (Fig. 5.11).[5,21] Larger cysts are usually lined by flattened, atrophic epithelium.

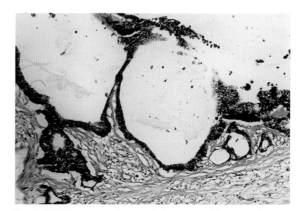

Fig. 5.11 Intramuscular urachal cyst lined by cuboidal and columnar epithelium. The small cysts branching off the larger ones are similar to the complexities seen in the type III variant of intramuscular urachus. H&E ×63.

INFECTIONS OF THE URACHUS

Bacterial infections of the urachus usually occur in the presence of a malformation or cyst.[22] Purulent bacterial infections related to umbilicourachal sinus, vesicourachal sinus, blind urachus or cyst, and alternating urachal sinus have been reported.[2,23–28] These infections often develop into abscesses and may drain spontaneously through the umbilicus or into the bladder. Rupture through the peritoneum is a serious complication. When the abscess is large and advanced, it may be difficult to determine the exact nature of the associated urachal anomaly. In some cases, abscesses may be confused with infiltrative bladder cancer.[29]

In Figure 5.12, the macroscopic appearance of a urachal abscess associated with vesicourachal sinus is

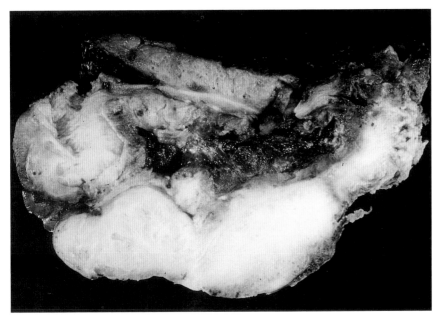

(a)

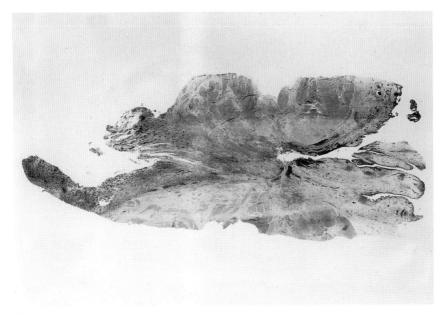

(b)

Fig. 5.12 Urachal abscess. (a) The whitish muscle of the urinary bladder is below, the urachal orifice in the bladder is to the left and the abscess is above. (b) The urachal canal in the specimen illustrated in (a) begins at the vesical mucosa to the right and extends to the abscess cavity at the left. H&E ×1.

shown. In this case, the urachus was resected with the adjoining cuff of urinary bladder. Treatment with antibiotics followed by prompt surgical removal of the infected cyst has been shown to be effective therapy.[30] More rarely, tuberculous, echinococcal, actinomycotic and tineal infections have been reported to involve the urachus.[1,31–33] The fetal, or type I, anatomic variant of urachal structure was found in 40 of 82 patients with chronic granulomatous omphalitis; 13 of the 40 had umbilical pilonidal disease. Steck and Helwig concluded that the urachal attachment produces umbilical dimples of greater depth than normal in these patients and thus predisposes them to pilonidal disease and granulomas.[34] Xanthogranulomatous inflammation has been reported.[35]

BENIGN NEOPLASMS OF THE URACHUS

Adenomas

Benign epithelial neoplasms of the urachus are rare, with fewer than 20 cases having been recorded.[36,37] The lesions are found most often in the lower third of the urachus but have been reported in all parts, including the supravesical segment near the umbilicus.[38] The reported sizes have ranged from less than a centimeter up to a lobulated mass $80 \times 80 \times 60$ mm which replaced the lower third of the urachus and involved the wall of the urinary bladder.[39] Macroscopically, these neoplasms are characteristically cavitary or cystic and may be multilocular. Often, the cavities are filled with mucus and Eble et al. noted that mucusuria is the most characteristic symptom, present in 7 of 11 symptomatic patients. In two cases, papillary fronds were seen to grow into the cavities (Fig. 5.13).[36,40] Microscopically, the epithelial component usually consists of tall columnar epithelium with a population of mucous goblet cells. The resemblance to rectal or enteric glandular epithelium may be striking (Fig. 5.14).

The epithelium may be arranged on papillary fronds (Fig. 5.15), or simply line the cyst cavities. Cuboidal epithelium and urothelium have also been found in some of these lesions and distinction between a multilocular urachal cyst and an adenoma may be difficult when the lesion is not complex and the epithelium is simple and without evidence of proliferative activity. Ultrastructurally, the columnar epithelium has long microvilli with prominent filamentous cores extending into the terminal webs.[36]

Surgical excision of the lesion was curative in all but one of the cases. The patient reported by de Korté died with numerous mucinous peritoneal implants 3 years after presentation.[41] There was no evidence of hematogenous or lymphatic metastasis in that case but it does appear that there is a risk of development of a condition similar to pseudomyxoma peritonei if spillage of neoplastic cells occurs during the resection. The case reported by Ng et al. evolved into adenocarcinoma.[37]

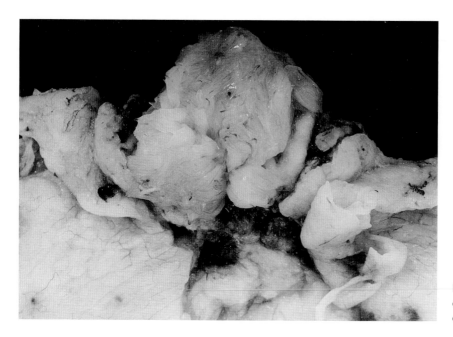

Fig. 5.13 Papillary extensions of a mucinous urachal adenoma.

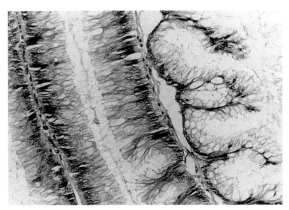

Fig. 5.14 The epithelium of urachal adenomas often closely resembles that of the intestinal mucosa. H&E ×100.

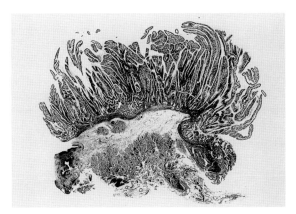

Fig. 5.15 Villous fronds covered by columnar epithelium with numerous mucous goblet cells make up this urachal adenoma. Trichrome ×1.

Benign mesenchymal and mixed neoplasms

Benign mesenchymal neoplasms of the urachus are very rare. Rankin and Parker described a case of a 5 cm fibroma of the upper urachus in a 45-year-old woman and Sonzini Astudillo reported a similar lesion in the supravesical urachus of an 80-year-old woman.[42,43] Both were treated successfully with surgical resection of the tumors. Bucchiere mentions two small leiomyomas found in the supravesical urachus and intramural urachus in a child and a 45-year-old woman, respectively.[1] Begg reported two cases of 'fibromyoma' of the supravesical urachus.[44] Dawson et al. described a 21 cm tumor composed of bland spindle cells without differentiation toward smooth muscle or nerve.[45]

Neoplasms composed of epithelial and mesenchymal elements have been reported as 'fibroadenomas' by Begg, Hagner, and Loening and Richardson[44,46,47] but the morphologic criteria for this diagnosis are not established, nor are the lesions well illustrated. In 1998, Defabiani et al. described a urachal tumor containing brain tissue, squamous epithelium, salivary glandular tissue, colonic and respiratory mucosa, smooth muscle and cartilage and concluded that it was a mature teratoma.[48]

MALIGNANT NEOPLASMS OF THE URACHUS

The report of Hue and Jacquin in 1863 of a colloid carcinoma arising in the region of the umbilicus and abdominal wall and invading the urinary bladder is generally regarded as the first report of urachal malignancy in the medical literature.[49] Since that time, urachal cancers have been reported as single cases and small series, aggregating to approximately 350 cases. Öhman et al., using data from the Swedish Cancer Registry, estimated the annual incidence of urachal cancer to be 1 case for every 5 million people; Cornil et al. found only 2 cases of urachal carcinoma in a survey of 17,688 patients hospitalized in Massachusetts and concluded that cancers of the urachus make up approximately 0.01% of malignancies.[50,51] Ghazizadeh et al. compared nine large series of urinary bladder carcinomas amounting in aggregate to more than 18,000 cases from North America, Europe and Asia.[52] They found that the incidence of urachal carcinoma ranged from 0.07 to 0.70% of bladder carcinomas in North America and Europe but from 0.55 to 1.2% of bladder carcinomas in Japan and concluded that this difference was significant.

Begg classified neoplasms of the urachus into seven groups, according to their locations and the developmental characteristics of the urachus and bladder:[44]

1. Intramucosal
2. Intramural
3. Supravesical
4. Of urachal rests between the urachal apex and umbilicus
5. Of an unformed or undescended urachus
6. Of the obliterated umbilical arteries
7. Of the apex of an ectopic bladder, the urachal anlage.

However, this classification is presently little used because advanced lesions often involve the anatomic zones of a number of categories and because examples fitting several of the categories are almost unknown. Figure 5.16 illustrates an adenocarcinoma of Begg's category 1, limited to the urachal mucosa. Most reports

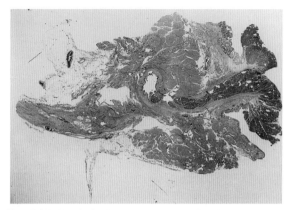

Fig. 5.16 Urachal adenocarcinoma confined to the urachal mucosa and protruding into the bladder lumen. Note that the muscular wall of the urachus parallels the lumen and consists of a homogeneous sheath distinct from the muscle of the urinary bladder. To the left, non-neoplastic urachal structures remain. H&E ×1.

attempt to categorize urachal neoplasms as arising in the wall of the bladder or in the supravesical segment and that suffices.

Since the great majority of urachal malignancies involve the urinary bladder, the most difficult problems of classification are those involved in distinguishing neoplasms of the urachus from neoplasms of the urinary bladder proper. Wheeler and Hill proposed criteria for determining that an adenocarcinoma of the urinary bladder is of urachal origin:[53]

- location in the dome of the bladder
- absence of cystitis cystica or cystitis glandularis
- predominant involvement of the muscularis rather than the submucosa, with an intact or ulcerated bladder epithelium
- demonstration of a urachal remnant connected with the neoplasm
- presence of a suprapubic neoplastic mass.

These criteria were accepted and amplified by Mostofi et al. who included location in the anterior wall of the bladder, sharp demarcation of the neoplasm from the surface epithelium, and extension to the space of Retzius or beyond to the umbilicus or anterior abdominal wall as confirmatory criteria.[54] All but the second criterion are also useful in evaluating other carcinomas and sarcomas with urinary bladder involvement for urachal origin. Recognizing that in many cases all of the criteria might not be met, Mostofi et al.[54] concluded that:

> A malignant epithelial tumor situated in the dome or anterior wall of the urinary bladder is urachal if the

tumor is mostly intramural, has deep ramifications in the bladder wall, and is demonstrated not to be secondary carcinoma.

While these criteria are helpful in many cases, advanced cancers in the dome of the urinary bladder cannot always be reliably classified as either of vesical mucosal or urachal origin. Indeed, urothelial and squamous carcinomas in this area are generally assumed to be of vesical mucosal origin unless the evidence of urachal origin is compelling and it has been the efforts to distinguish between the adenocarcinomas which have been the sources of these criteria. In cases of sarcomas of the dome of the bladder, the question is essentially moot and the recorded sarcomas of the urachus are almost invariably neoplasms which clearly are of supravesical origin.

These problems and conventions of classification have doubtless influenced the extent to which adenocarcinomas predominate among reported urachal neoplasms. In 1984, Sheldon et al. critically reviewed the literature in English on urachal malignancy and collected 117 acceptably documented cases while rejecting 43.[49] For purposes of comparison with the results of Sheldon et al., the author has collected 60 cases not included in that review and will also refer to other reviews including those of Ghazizadeh et al. and Petersen.[1,52,55,56]

Carcinomas

Urachal adenocarcinoma

Adenocarcinomas are by far the most common malignant neoplasms of the urachus. In their review, Sheldon et al. found that 99 of 117 cases were adenocarcinomas.[49] In his review, Petersen found 180 of 200 urachal malignancies to be adenocarcinomas while Bucchiere's review of urachal disease at the Mayo Clinic found that 18 of 21 malignancies were adenocarcinomas.[1,55] In Japan, Ghazizadeh et al. found 138 adenocarcinomas (88%) among 157 cases of carcinoma of the urachus.[52] This preponderance parallels the predominance of adenomatous lesions among the benign neoplasms of the urachus. Sheldon et al. found that more than two-thirds (68%) of urachal cancers arose in patients aged between 41 and 70 years; 73 of 99 adenocarcinomas were diagnosed in patients in that age range and they found only 19 reports of adenocarcinomas in patients aged 40 and under.[49] In the author's review, 36 of 53 patients (70%), for whom the age was reported, were in this age range; the mean age was 51 years and only 11 cases of adenocarcinoma arose in patients aged 40 and under.[1,56–70] In Japan, the mean age among 157 patients was 51 years and 26% were less than 40 years old.[52] For the 180 patients with adenocarcinoma included in Petersen's review, the mean age was 54.[55] Among patients with urachal cancer, there is a 3:1 predominance of men to women and when adenocarcinomas are considered separately, reviews find the male predominance to range from 2:1 to 3:1.[49,52,55–67,71,72]

In 66–75% of patients, the presenting symptom is hematuria.[49,52] Irritative voiding symptoms, a suprapubic mass and abdominal pain are also common but non-specific symptoms. Mucusuria, whether gross or microscopic, is a diagnostically helpful symptom which is seen in 25% of patients with adenocarcinoma.[49] In nearly 90% of the cases that present with hematuria, the tumor is visible at cystoscopy as a protrusion in the dome or anterior surface of the bladder, as a polypoid or papillary mass, or there is gelatinous or bloody discharge from the urachal orifice.[49] Transurethral biopsy is often helpful in establishing the diagnosis. Radiologically, the neoplasms are often seen as filling defects in the dome of the bladder. When stippled calcifications are present, they strongly suggest a neoplasm of urachal origin.[49]

Some adenocarcinomas present with symptoms and findings unrelated to the urinary bladder. Rarely, the neoplasm arises in the supravesical urachus and the symptoms may be umbilical, consisting of mass or discharge.[66] These lesions must be distinguished from Sister Mary Joseph's nodules, which are umbilical deposits of metastatic carcinoma from internal primary sites.[73]

Grossly, adenocarcinomas of the urachus are often extensively infiltrative of the surrounding muscle of the bladder wall and often extend superiorly toward the abdominal wall in the space of Retzius. Depending upon the extent to which they are mucinous, they may have a gelatinous appearance. The vesical mucosal surface of the lesions is often ulcerated and may be papillary. The tumors may be partially calcified.[74] In the absence of a generally accepted staging system for urachal cancer, Sheldon et al. have proposed that urachal carcinomas be staged using the system outlined in Table 5.1.[49]

Although not all reports have provided sufficient information to assign their cases to a precise stage or substage in this system, it is estimated that 83% of patients have presented in stage III.[49] The histogenesis of urachal adenocarcinomas has been debated because of the early concept that the normal epithelial lining of the urachus consisted solely of urothelium. Theories of

Table 5.1 Staging of urachal carcinoma

Stage	Clinical features
I	Carcinoma confined to the urachal mucosa
II	Invasion confined to the urachus
III	Local extension:
	— IIIA extension into urinary bladder
	— IIIB extension into abdominal wall
	— IIIC extension into the peritoneum
	— IIID extension into other viscera
IV	Metastasis:
	— IVA metastasis to regional lymph nodes
	— IVB metastasis to distant sites

After Sheldon CA, Clayman RV, Gonzalez R et al. Malignant urachal lesions. J Urol 1984; 131:1–8.[49]

metaplasia from urothelium and of embryonic rests of columnar epithelium have been invoked. More recent studies showing that mucus-secreting columnar epithelium is frequently found in otherwise normal urachal mucosa suggest that columnar epithelium is normal in the urachus and that other processes need not be invoked to account for the histogenesis of urachal adenocarcinomas.[8,9]

Microscopically, the appearance of urachal adenocarcinomas is varied. Sheldon et al. found that 83% of 99 adenocarcinomas were mucinous and 38 of 52 reports of adenocarcinomas in the author's review indicated mucinous features. The histologic spectrum ranges from well- or moderately differentiated mucinous or non-mucinous adenocarcinomas (Figs 5.17, 5.18), often resembling adenocarcinomas of the colon and rectum, through colloid carcinomas (Fig. 5.19) to signet-ring cell and poorly differentiated adenocarcinomas. A metastasis from colorectal adenocarcinoma must often be considered in the differential diagnosis but generally can be excluded on the basis of the clinical history and surgical observations. Tiltman and Maytom report that urachal adenocarcinomas differ histochemically from colorectal adenocarcinomas in that those of colorectal origin very frequently produce sulfated acid mucopolysaccharides, while those originating in the urachus and urinary bladder do not.[75] Immunohistochemistry is of limited value in distinguishing adenocarcinoma of the urachus from other adenocarcinomas of the urinary bladder.[76]

Signet-ring cell adenocarcinoma

Signet-ring cell adenocarcinomas have been considered a separate histopathologic group because of their

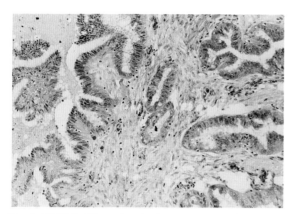

Fig. 5.17 Well-differentiated adenocarcinoma of the urachus consisting of tall columnar epithelium with prominent secretion. H&E ×63.

distinctive morphology (Fig. 5.20).[58,64,77–80] This group has included adenocarcinomas with a minority component of signet-ring cells as well as those composed purely of signet-ring cells. Three of the four cases reported by Johnson et al. were mixed, as was the case of Kondo et al.[62,64] The signet-ring cells are present as components of glandular structures or, perhaps more commonly, in the mucus lakes of colloid areas. Diffusely infiltrative patterns resembling linitis plastica have been observed.[62] Signet-ring cell morphology is rare, being reported in less than 10% of cases of urachal adenocarcinoma. In a review of 12 cases the ratio of males to females (3:1) was similar to that of urachal adenocarcinomas in general but the mean age[48] was somewhat lower than the mean for all adenocarcinomas.[55] In a study of 25 signet-ring carcinomas of the bladder, the nine cases of signet-ring carcinoma of the urachus had

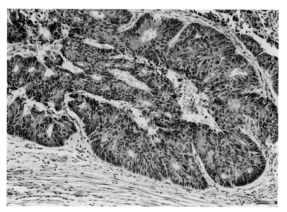

Fig. 5.18 Well-differentiated adenocarcinoma of the urachus without mucus secretion and localized within the urachus. H&E ×63.

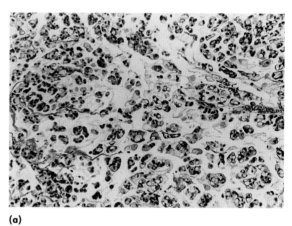

(a)

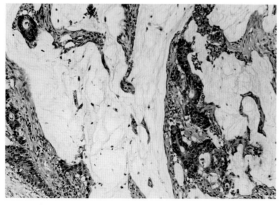

Fig. 5.19 Colloid carcinoma of the urachus. H&E ×63.

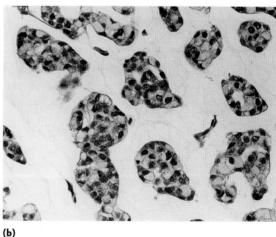

(b)

Fig. 5.20 Signet-ring cell carcinoma of the urachus: **(a)** with infiltration as small clusters of cells, H&E ×63; **(b)** with the cells forming clumps and glandular structures within a sea of mucus, H&E ×100.

a mean age of 54 years.[78] The prognosis for this group is poor, but, as discussed below, the prognosis is also poor for urachal adenocarcinomas in general. A study of 25 signet-ring carcinomas of the bladder found that those of the urachus had no excess mortality compared to other urachal carcinomas while the non-urachal signet-ring carcinomas of the bladder were more aggressive than other carcinomas of the urinary bladder.[78] In their series of 14 urachal carcinomas which included four with signet-ring cell morphology, Johnson et al. found no association between prognosis and the presence of signet-ring cells.[62] Mucin histochemistry does not appear to be of value in distinguishing between signet-ring carcinomas of the urinary bladder and those of urachal origin.[78]

Treatment of urachal adenocarcinoma

The consensus of surgeons is that en bloc resection of the involved segment of the bladder with the entire urachus, the umbilicus and the intervening abdominal wall (including the peritoneum) is essential to hope for a cure of urachal adenocarcinoma. Begg is credited with initiating this surgical approach and Lane's review 45 years later concurred in its value.[44,81] Sheldon et al. suggested that partial cystectomy is inadequate and that total cystectomy and pelvic lymphadenectomy should be added to the supravesical elements of the operation because 18% of patients treated with partial cystectomy suffered recurrences in the remaining parts of the urinary bladder.[49]

However, some studies have concluded that conservative surgery is appropriate in selected cases.[82–84] Although radiation therapy appears to have been effective in a few cases, most urachal carcinomas so treated have proved to be resistant to radiotherapy and Kakizoe et al. found the mean duration of radiation-induced remission to be only 18 months.[49,63] Chemotherapeutic trials have been very limited and the results are inconclusive with regard to their efficacy.

Prognosis of urachal adenocarcinoma

In general, the prognosis of urachal adenocarcinoma is poor. In a review of 75 cases, Whitehead and Tessler found a 2-year survival of only 31%, a 5-year survival of 9% and a 10-year survival of less than 3%.[85] Ghazizadeh et al. presented similar data on the survival of 66 Japanese patients: the 2-year survival was 22.7%, 5-year survival 6% and 10-year survival 1.5%.[52] Local recurrence occurs frequently in urachal cancer and distant metastasis without local recurrence is rare. Adenocarcinomas most frequently recur in the tissues of

the pelvis and urinary bladder and less frequently in the wound or abdominal wall.[49] In 81% of patients who develop local recurrence, this is apparent within 2 years. Metastasis is usually a late occurrence. In an analysis of 72 cases, Kakizoe et al. found the most common sites for metastasis to be (in descending order): lymph nodes, lung, peritoneum, omentum, mesentery, liver, bone and small intestine.[63]

Histology of urachal adenocarcinoma

Neuroendocrine cells may be seen in some urachal adenocarcinomas and can rarely give rise to malignant neoplasms in the urachus. Satake et al. demonstrated argyrophil cells in normal urachal epithelium and in a urachal adenocarcinoma.[67] These cells were observed on the basement membrane between columnar or cuboidal cells in the urachal epithelium of 8 of 14 normal adults and in the adenocarcinoma. Immunohistochemically, the argyrophil cells of the adenocarcinoma were found to contain carcinoembryonic antigen, glucagon and serotonin, whereas in those of the normal urachal epithelium, serotonin and secretin were observed. Ultrastructurally, the cells contained small and large electron-dense granules.

Abenoza et al. reported a case in which the cancer was a composite of adenocarcinoma of the colonic type and large-cell neuroendocrine carcinoma.[57] Immunohistochemical procedures showed reactivity for carcinoembryonic antigen, epithelial membrane antigen and cytokeratin in the well-differentiated adenocarcinoma, but no argyrophil cells. The neuroendocrine component was argyrophilic and immunohistochemical reactions demonstrated reactivity for chromogranin, serotonin, somatostatin, neuron-specific enolase and carcinoembryonic antigen. Ultrastructurally, the neuroendocrine component contained moderate numbers of membrane-bound dense-core granules in the size range 75–125 nm. A similar composite of adenocarcinoma and neuroendocrine carcinoma with cytoplasmic dense-core granules was reported by Melamed et al.[86] The series of Johnson et al. included one patient whose neoplasm consisted predominantly of oat cell carcinoma.[62] The patient reported by Abenoza et al. died with widespread metastases 30 months after diagnosis, while that of Johnson et al. was alive 6 years after treatment by partial cystectomy.

Squamous cell carcinoma of the urachus

Squamous cell carcinomas make up only 3–4% of cancers of the urachus and the sum of cases reported since 1870 is less than a dozen.[2,42,49,52,65,87–90] In the seven cases reviewed by Jimi et al. and the case reported by Mazzotti, the mean age was 50 years (range 27–77 years) and there were six men and two women.[65,87] Five cases were supravesical, while the rest were intramural. Four cases were associated with other lesions: two with cysts,[87,90] one with a vesicourachal diverticulum[88] and one with a vesical calculus.[89] Five of the patients died, one was free of disease for 9 months at the time of the report, and another was free of disease for an unspecified time;[65,87] the outcome was not reported for the last.

Histologically, these neoplasms are typical squamous carcinomas, similar to those that occur in the urinary bladder. Urothelial carcinomas of the urachus make up only about 3% of reported cases of urachal cancer.[49,52,55,91] These have occurred mainly in patients over the age of 40 and hematuria and pain have been the most common symptoms. Microscopically, they resemble urothelial carcinomas occurring elsewhere.[92] Kitami et al. have reported a case in which foci of adenocarcinoma and squamous carcinoma were found in a urothelial carcinoma.[93]

Urachal sarcoma

In their review of 117 urachal cancers, Sheldon et al. found nine cases of sarcoma reported in the English literature prior to 1983.[49] The author's review of cases of urachal malignancy not included in the review of Sheldon et al. found three more while Petersen's review found nine cases among 200 urachal malignancies.[1,55,94,95] Thus, sarcomas of the urachus make up approximately 5–10% of urachal cancers. Urachal sarcomas occur in a much younger population than the carcinomas. Petersen reports an age range from 4 months to 51 years with a mean age of only 22 years. The cases added by the author occurred in a 28-year-old man, a 2-month-old boy and 2-year-old boy.[1,94,95] In contrast to the male predominance in carcinomas, sarcomas occur nearly equally in males and females.

Urachal sarcomas frequently present with symptoms of pain, umbilical discharge or irritative bladder symptoms, but hematuria has not been reported. The principal therapy is surgical resection and Sheldon et al. noted that no recurrence has been reported in the remaining bladder after partial cystectomy and for that reason concluded that total cystectomy is not necessary in cases of urachal sarcoma.

Although specific diagnoses of fibrosarcoma, hemangiopericytoma, rhabdomyosarcoma and leiomyosarcoma have been made in some cases, often the neoplasms have been diagnosed as spindle cell sarcoma or merely as 'sarcoma' and the illustrations support no more specific diagnosis.[1,94,96–100] The case reported by Noyes and Vinson[94] illustrates the difficulties in establishing the urachal origin of a leiomyosarcoma arising in the dome of the urinary bladder. While it is reasonable to presume that an adenocarcinoma arising in the dome of the bladder and having extensive ramifications in the bladder muscle is of urachal origin, it is clear that the same reasoning cannot be applied to sarcomas. On the contrary, sarcomas primarily involving the wall of the urinary bladder are generally presumed not to be of urachal origin but rather of origin in the urinary bladder.

REFERENCES

1. Bucchiere JJ, Jr. Diseases of the Urachus. Unpublished Thesis, University of Minnesota. Minneapolis: 1978.
2. Cullen TS. Embryology, Anatomy and Diseases of the Umbilicus Together with Diseases of the Urachus. Philadelphia: W.B. Saunders, 1916.
3. Vio A, Battisti C, Torchi B. Patologia dell'Uraco. Parma: L'Ateneo Parmense, 1967.
4. Begg RC. The urachus: its anatomy, histology and development. J Anat 1930;64:170–182.
5. Trimingham HL, McDonald JR. Congenital anomalies in the region of the umbilicus. Surg Gynecol Obstet 1945;80:152–163.
6. Bauer SB, Retik AB. Urachal anomalies and related umbilical disorders. Urol Clin North Am 1978;5:195–211.
7. Hammond G, Yglesias L, Davis JE. The urachus, its anatomy and associated fasciae. Anat Rec 1941;80:271–287.
8. Blichert-Toft M, Koch F, Nielsen OV. Anatomic variants of the urachus related to clinical appearance and surgical treatment. Surg Gynecol Obstet 1973;137:51–54.
9. Schubert GE, Pavkovic MB, Bethke-Bedürftig BA. Tubular urachal remnants in adult bladders. J Urol 1982;127:40–42.
10. Wutz JB. Ueber Urachus und Urachuscysten. Virchows Arch Pathol Anat Physiol Klin Med 1883;92:387–423.
11. Tyler DE. Epithelium of intestinal type in the normal urachus: a new theory of vesical embryology. J Urol 1964;92:505–507.
12. Herbst WP. Patent urachus. South Med J 1937;30:711–719.
13. Jona JZ. Allantoic cyst and persistent urachal–allantoic communication: a rare umbilical anomaly. J Pediatr Surg 1998;33:1441–1442.
14. Lattimer JK. Congenital deficiency of the abdominal musculature and associated genitourinary anomalies: a report of 22 cases. J Urol 1958;79:343–352.
15. Schreck WR, Campbell WA, III. The relation of bladder outlet obstruction to urinary–umbilical fistula. J Urol 1972;108:641–643.

16. Vaughan GT. Patent urachus. Review of the cases reported. Operation on a case complicated with stones in the kidneys. A note on tumors and cysts of the urachus. Trans Am Surg Assoc 1905;23:273–294.

17. Hinman F, Jr. Urologic aspects of the alternating urachal sinus. Am J Surg 1961;102:339–342.

18. Groff DB. Suprapubic dermoid sinus. J Pediatr Surg 1993;28:242–243.

19. Nargund VH, Donaldson RA. Urachal calculi: a case report and review of the literature. Int Urol Nephrol 1994;26:409–411.

20. Nair KPN. Mucous metaplasia and rupture of urachal cyst as a rare cause of acute abdomen. Br J Urol 1987;59:281–282.

21. Dreyfuss ML, Fliess MM. Patent urachus with stone formation. J Urol 1941;47:77–81.

22. Iuchtman M, Rahav S, Zer M, et al. Management of urachal anomalies in children and adults. Urology 1993;42:426–430.

23. Brodie N. Infected urachal cysts. Am J Surg 1945;69:243–248.

24. MacMillan RW, Schullinger JN, Santulli TV. Pyourachus: an unusual surgical problem. J Pediatr Surg 1973;8:387–389.

25. Hinman F, Jr. Surgical disorders of the bladder and umbilicus of urachal origin. Surg Gynecol Obstet 1961;113:605–614.

26. Berman SM, Tolia BM, Laor E, et al. Urachal remnants in adults. Urology 1988;31:17–21.

27. MacNeily AE, Koleilat N, Kiruluta HG, Homsy YL. Urachal abscesses: protean manifestations, their recognition, and management. Urology 1992;40:530–535.

28. Lees VC, Doyle PT. Urachal cyst presenting with abscess formation. J R Soc Med 1991;84:367–368.

29. Chen W-J, Hsieh H-H, Wan Y-L. Abscess of urachal remnant mimicking urinary bladder neoplasm. Br J Urol 1992;69:510–512.

30. Newman BM, Karp MP, Jewett TC, Cooney DR. Advances in the management of infected urachal cysts. J Pediatr Surg 1986;21:1051–1054.

31. Nagy V, Sokol L, Baca M, et al. Actinomycosis of the urachus persistens penetrating into the ileum. Int Urol Nephrol 1997;29:627–631.

32. Micheli E, Hurle R, Losa A, et al. Primary actinomycosis of the urachus. BJU Int 1999;83:144–145.

33. Thompson NP, Stoker DL, Springall RG. Urachal abscess as a complication of tinea corporis. Br J Urol 1994;73:319.

34. Steck WD, Helwig EB. Umbilical granulomas, pilonidal disease, and the urachus. Surg Gynecol Obstet 1965;120:1043–1057.

35. Carrere W, Gutiérrez R, Umbert B, et al. Urachal xanthogranulomatous disease. Br J Urol 1996;77:612–613.

36. Eble JN, Hull MT, Rowland RG, Hostetter M. Villous adenoma of the urachus with mucusuria: a light and electron microscopic study. J Urol 1986;135:1240–1244.

37. Ng KJ, Newman P, Price-Thomas JM. Carcinoma of the urachus associated with urachal adenoma. Br J Urol 1991;67:215–216.

38. Boscaino N, Gambardella P. Contributo allo studio dei tumori primitivi dell'area ombelicale (neoplasie derivanti dal complesso onfalo-uraco-allantoideo). Chir Ital 1968;20:439–451.

39. Hamm FC. Benign cystadenoma of the bladder, probably of urachal origin. J Urol 1940;44:227–233.

40. Maar K, Wegner KW, Krüger R. Mucourie bei Urachusadenom. Urologe [A] 1975;14:240–242.

41. de Korté WE. An adenoma of the bladder. J Pathol Bacteriol 1918;22:319–323.

42. Rankin FW, Parker B. Tumors of the urachus, with report of seven cases. Surg Gynecol Obstet 1926;42:19–27.

43. Sonzini Astudillo C. Fibroma uraquico. Prensa Med Argent 1962;49:526.

44. Begg RC. The colloid adenocarcinoma of the bladder vault arising from the epithelium of the urachal canal: with a critical survey of the tumours of the urachus. Br J Surg 1931;18:422–466.

45. Dawson JS, Crisp AJ, Boyd SM, Broderick NJ. Case report: benign urachal neoplasm. Br J Radiol 1994;67:1132–1133.

46. Hagner FR. Report of a case of fibroadenoma in the bladder wall, occurring in fundus of bladder. Am J Urol 1907;3:414–415.

47. Loening S, Richardson JR, Jr. Fibroadenoma of the urachus. J Urol 1974;112:759–761.

48. Defabiani N, Iselin CE, Khan HG, et al. Benign teratoma of the urachus. Br J Urol 1998;81:760–761.

49. Sheldon CA, Clayman RV, Gonzalez R, et al. Malignant urachal lesions. J Urol 1984;131:1–8.

50. Öhman U, von Garrelts B, Moberg A. Carcinoma of the urachus, review of the literature and report of two cases. Scand J Urol Nephrol 1971;5:91–95.

51. Cornil C, Reynolds CT, Kickham CJE. Carcinoma of the urachus. J Urol 1967;98:93–95.

52. Ghazizadeh M, Yamamoto S, Kurokawa K. Clinical features of urachal carcinoma in Japan: review of 157 patients. Urol Res 1983;11:235–238.

53. Wheeler JD, Hill WT. Adenocarcinoma involving the urinary bladder. Cancer 1954;7:119–135.

54. Mostofi FK, Thomson RV, Dean AL, Jr. Mucous adenocarcinoma of the urinary bladder. Cancer 1955;8:741–758.

55. Petersen RO. Urologic Pathology. Philadelphia: J.B. Lippincott Company, 1986.

56. Taylor GD, McRae CU. Carcinoma of the urachus: report of four cases and review of the literature. N Z Med J 1978;87:384–386.

57. Abenoza P, Manivel C, Sibley RK. Adenocarcinoma with neuroendocrine differentiation of the urinary bladder, clinicopathologic, immunohistochemical, and ultrastructural study. Arch Pathol Lab Med 1986;110:1062–1066.

58. Alonso-Gorrea M, Mompo-Sanchis JA, Jorda-Cuevas M, et al. Signet ring cell adenocarcinoma of the urachus. Eur Urol 1985;11:282–284.

59. Bennett JK, Trulock TS, Finnerty DP. Urachal adenocarcinoma presenting as vesicoenteric fistula. Urology 1985;25:297–299.

60. Giglioli O. Il carcinoma dell'uraco. Arch de Vecchi Anat Patol 1961;34:901–925.

61. Hayman J. Carcinoma of the urachus. Pathology 1984;16:167–171.

62. Johnson DE, Hodge GB, Abdul-Karim FW, Ayala AG. Urachal carcinoma. Urology 1985;26:218–221.

63. Kakizoe T, Matsumoto K, Andoh M, et al. Adenocarcinoma of urachus, report of 7 cases and review of literature. Urology 1983;21:360–366.

64. Kondo A, Ogisu B-I, Mitsuya H. Signet ring cell carcinoma involving the urinary bladder, report of a case and review of 21 cases. Urol Int 1981;36:373–379.

65. Mazzotti G. Epitelioma in diverticolo dell'uraco. Urologia (Treviso) 1947;14:250–254.

66. Ross JE, Hill RB, Jr. Primary umbilical adenocarcinoma, a case report and review of the literature. Arch Pathol 1975;99:327–329.

67. Satake T, Takeda A, Matsuyama M. Argyrophil cells in the urachal epithelium and urachal adenocarcinoma. Acta Pathol Jpn 1984;34:1193–1199.

68. Mattelaer P, Wolff JM, Jung P, et al. Adenocarcinoma of the urachus: 3 case reports and a review of the literature. Acta Urol Belg 1997;65:63–67.

69. Michielsen D, Hoekx L, Dewilde L, Wyndaele JJ. Carcinoma of the urachus. Acta Urol Belg 1995;63:33–35.

70. Young RH. Urachal adenocarcinoma metastatic to the ovary simulating primary mucinous cystadenocarcinoma of the ovary: report of a case. Virchows Arch 1995;426:529–532.

71. Lurie A, Eisenkraft S, Shotland Y, Lurie M. Mucin-producing adenocarcinoma of the bladder of urachal origin, case report. Urol Int 1983;38:12–15.

72. Marcorelli E, Giuliani A, Menici M, Biagini C. Adenocarcinoma dell'uraco, presentazione di un caso e revisione della letteratura. Minerva Urol 1983;35:217–220.

73. Issa M, Feeley M, Kerin M, et al. Umbilical deposits from internal malignancy: Sister Mary Joseph's nodule. Ir Med J 1987;80:152–153.

74. Yu HHY, Leong CH. Carcinoma of the urachus: report of one case and a review of the literature. Surgery 1975;77:726–729.

75. Tiltman AJ, Maytom PAN. Adenocarcinoma of the urinary bladder, histochemical distinction between urachal and metastatic carcinomas. S Afr Med J 1977;51:74–75.

76. Torenbeek R, Lagendijk JH, Van Diest PJ, et al. Value of a panel of antibodies to identify the primary origin of adenocarcinomas presenting as bladder carcinoma. Histopathology 1998;32:20–27.

77. Jakse G, Schneider H-M, Jacobi GH. Urachal signet-ring cell carcinoma, a rare variant of vesical adenocarcinoma: incidence and pathological criteria. J Urol 1978;120:764–766.

78. Grignon DJ, Ro JY, Ayala AG, Johnson DE. Primary signet-ring cell carcinoma of the urinary bladder. Am J Clin Pathol 1991;95:13–20.

79. Fiter L, Gimeno F, Martin L, Gómez Tejeda L. Signet-ring cell adenocarcinoma of bladder. Urology 1993;41:30–33.

80. Loggie BW, Fleming RA, Hosseinian AA. Peritoneal carcinomatosis with urachal signet-cell adenocarcinoma. Urology 1997;50:446–448.

81. Lane V. Prognosis in carcinoma of the urachus. Eur Urol 1976;2:282–283.

82. Henly DR, Farrow GM, Zincke H. Urachal cancer: role of conservative surgery. Urology 1993;42:635–639.

83. Santucci RA, True LD, Lange PH. Is partial cystectomy the treatment of choice for mucinous adenocarcinoma of the urachus? Urology 1997;49:536–540.

84. D'Addessi A, Racioppi M, Fanasca A, et al. Adenocarcinoma of the urachus: radical or conservative surgery? A report of a case and a review of the literature. Eur J Surg Oncol 1998;24:131–133.

85. Whitehead ED, Tessler AN. Carcinoma of the urachus. Br J Urol 1971;43:468–476.

86. Melamed MR, Farrow GM, Haggitt RC. Case 19 in 'Urologic Neoplasms', Proceedings of the 50th Annual Anatomic Slide Seminar of the American Society of Clinical Pathologists. ASCP 98–103, 1987.

87. Jimi A, Munaoka H, Sato S-I, Iwata Y. Squamous cell carcinoma of the urachus, a case report and review of the literature. Acta Pathol Jpn 1986;36:945–952.

88. Lin R-Y, Rappoport AE, Deppisch LM, et al. Squamous cell carcinoma of the urachus. J Urol 1977;118:1066–1067.

89. Pujari BD, Phansopkar M, Deodhare SG. Squamous cell carcinoma of the urachus with vesical calculus. Br J Urol 1977;49:292.

90. Shaw RE. Squamous-cell carcinoma in a cyst of the urachus. Br J Urol 1958;30:87–89.

91. Satake I, Nakagomi K, Tari K, Kishi K. Metachronous transitional cell carcinoma of the urachus and bladder. Br J Urol 1995;75:244.

92. Fisher ER. Transitional cell carcinoma of the urachal apex. Cancer 1958;11:245–249.

93. Kitami K, Masuda N, Chiba K, Kumagi H. Carcinoma of the urachus with variable pathological findings: report of a case and review of the literature. Acta Urol Jpn 1987;33:1459–1464.

94. Noyes D, Vinson RK. Urachal leiomyosarcoma. Urology 1981;17:279–280.

95. Yokoyama S, Hayashida Y, Nagahama J, et al. Rhabdomyosarcoma of the urachus, a case report. Acta Cytol 1997;41:1293–1298.

96. Baglio CM, Crowson CN. Hemangiopericytoma of urachus: report of a case. J Urol 1964;91:660–662.

97. Butler DB, Rosenberg HS. Sarcoma of the urachus. Arch Surg 1959;79:724–728.

98. Powley PH. Sarcoma of the urachus. Br J Surg 1961;48:649–650.

99. Shaw RE. Sarcoma of the urachus, report of a case and brief review of the subject. Br J Surg 1949;37:95–98.

100. Herbut PA. Urological Pathology. Philadelphia: Lea & Febiger, 1952.

6

PATHOLOGY OF THE INFANTILE AND HETEROTOPIC BLADDER

George Kokai

EMBRYOLOGY OF THE URINARY BLADDER

In morphologic and functional terms, the fully mature/adult urinary bladder is a rather simple organ of saccular shape which receives, stores and expels urine. The development of the urinary bladder is, however, a very complex sequence of events, and results from a well-orchestrated interaction and differentiation of various structures during embryogenesis, including the urogenital sinus, cloacal membrane, Wolffian ducts, urachus and urogenital mesenchyme.

In a simplified way, the properly developed bladder is a result of three subtly coordinated embryological events:

- growth and fusion of excretory ducts which form the *trigone*
- closure of the infraumbilical portion of the anterior abdominal wall – a process which creates the *anterior wall*
- development of the urorectal septum which results in formation of the *posterior wall* and *dome* of the bladder.[1]

Excretory ducts represent the caudal portion of the mesonephric ducts distal to ureteral buds, which, after the fourth week of gestation, become incorporated into the urogenital sinus, while fusion of their epithelium towards the midline forms a triangular area (the future trigone), which receives the most distal segment of the developing ureters.[2] The closure of the anterior abdominal wall and the appropriate induction and differentiation of mesenchymal tissue, which will eventually create the anterior wall of the bladder, are preceded by caudal migration of the cloacal membrane.

The cloaca itself is divided in the frontal plane by a gradually descending urorectal septum, which fuses with proctodeum during the seventh week of gestation, separating the rectum from the portion of the urogenital sinus. This important 'septation' process will also contribute to creation of the posterior wall and dome of the urinary bladder, as well as the inferior urinary structures and their derivates.

The bulk of the bladder is therefore derived from the rostral portion of the urogenital sinus, which is in continuity with the embryonic allantois and urachus, although neither of these is regarded as a component of the human bladder, due to complete regression of the former and transformation into a cord of the latter.

CONGENITAL ANOMALIES

Grossly abnormal or even slightly disturbed development of any of the above listed structures/components of the bladder almost always affects maturation of others. It is, therefore, understandable that congenital anomalies of the bladder occur very rarely as an isolated defect, but usually as a part of a complex, with multiple anomalies involving the lower abdominal wall, pelvic girdle, penis/clitoris and other pelvic organs.[3] The malformed bladder is usually a part of multiple anomalies, which may represent a syndrome (e.g. prune belly), a sequence (e.g. Potter), an association (e.g. VATER – **v**ertebral anomalies, **a**nal atresia, **t**racheo-**e**sophageal fistula, **r**adial anomalies) or a complex (e.g. OEIS – **o**mphalocele–**e**xstrophy–**i**mperforate anus–**s**pinal defects).[4] Although these complicated congenital anomalies are rare, they are usually lethal or incompatible with long survival despite the remarkable achievements of both pediatric and reconstructive surgery. Congenital anomalies of the bladder, quite exceptionally, constitute a part of genetic disorders with a known pattern of inheritance, such as genito-palato-cardiac syndrome (autosomal recessive), caudal dysplasia syndrome and laryngeal cleft syndrome (sporadic).

Agenesis and hypoplasia

Agenesis/congenital absence of the urinary bladder is an extremely rare anomaly. The majority of affected infants are stillborn or have other associated urogenital anomalies[5] or anomalies of other organ systems.[6] In very few reported cases of bladder agenesis in girls the urethra was found to be blind and both ureters were draining into the vagina[7,8] while in a case of a male infant both ureters were inserted into the rectum.[9]

Bladder hypoplasia is extremely rare as an isolated anomaly[10] and is much more frequently seen in association with bilateral renal agenesis or other severe congenital abnormalities of the kidneys, which do not produce urine in utero. The hypoplastic bladder is usually very small with a thin wall and poorly developed detrusor musculature.

Persistent cloaca

Persistent cloaca (cloacogenic bladder) is a very rare condition in which abnormal differentiation of the urogenital sinus results in failure of separation of the intestines and the bladder by the urorectal septum.

Congenital division

This term denotes some sort of 'compartmentalization' of the bladder, i.e. the presence of two or more separate vesical lumina caused by duplication of the organ by abnormal sagittal or transverse septa. According to Abrahamson, bladder duplications are classified as complete or incomplete.[11]

- In *complete duplication* two separate bladders lie side by side in a common adventitial sheath and each has a separate urethra (and penis in males); duplication of the anus, rectum and internal and external genitalia, in addition to the caudal end of vertebral column, is almost always present.[12]
- *Incomplete duplication* of bladder is when two bladders lie side by side but share a common bladder neck and urethra.

The most common type of otherwise very rare *septation of bladder* is when a single complete sagittal septum divides the bladder into two halves. Externally, the bladder appears normal or bilobed. Histologically, the septum consists of two outer layers of mucosa with an intervening layer of connective tissue and variable components of smooth muscle. In septated bladder only one half drains to a single urethra; the other half would be dilated, with a kidney on that side being hydronephrotic and dysplastic.[13] In extreme situations the obstructed half of the bladder becomes hugely dilated and may displace (and occasionally cause hydronephrosis on) the functional side. A rare case of a multiseptate bladder with complete obstruction of both upper tracts in an infant dying from uremia has been reported.[14] Quite rarely a caudal duplication defect may be associated, but much less frequently than with bladder duplication. Incomplete sagittal septation is less common than the complete form and does not cause obstruction. Its significance lies in the other coexisting anomalies quite frequently present.

The *hourglass bladder* is an extremely rare anomaly in which a circular band of smooth muscle or fibrotic tissue divides or constricts the bladder horizontally into an upper and a lower portion, the latter receiving the ureters.[15]

MEGACYSTIS

The name of this descriptive entity means massively dilated bladder with markedly thinned and untrabeculated wall, and dilated and tortuous ureters allowing free vesicoureteral reflux associated with hydronephrotic or dysplastic kidneys.[13] The pathogenesis of this condition is unclear and there is no obvious anatomic obstruction of the bladder neck or urethra, as has been thought incorrectly in the past.[16]

Functionally, the bladder is able to contract and empty properly, although the constantly increasing amount of recycling urine between the massively dilated upper urinary tract and the bladder causes a gradual increase in the bladder volume, which is very difficult to correct surgically.[15] Rarely, megacystis is associated with intestinal pseudo-obstruction in the so-called 'megacystis–microcolon–intestinal hypoperistalsis syndrome'. The colon is abnormally short and narrow with some degree of vacuolization of the smooth muscle cells and a varying degree of fibrosis of the muscularis propria, suggesting that the condition is a form of hollow visceral myopathy.[17]

There are a few reports of familial occurrence and it is known to be ten times more common in females than in males.[13]

Urachus and its anomalies

The urachus is a solid cord that arises from the anterior bladder wall and extends from the apex of the bladder to the umbilicus. During early fetal life, the urachus is a tubular structure that connects the ventral cloaca with the allantoic duct. Subsequent development of the urachus is described in detail in Chapter 5.

Congenital anomalies of the urachus represent an arrest of the normal involutory process, resulting in defective closure. Anomalies of the urachus are rare events; they usually occur as an isolated defect and are not associated with other syndromes (with the exception of prune belly syndrome and bladder outlet

obstruction). They present primarily in early childhood (sometimes remaining silent into adult life) and occur in about 1 in 4000 pediatric autopsies with a male to female ratio of 2:1.[13] Four anomalies of urachal development have been described:

- *Patent urachus*: Complete failure of normal closure of the urachal tube/duct results in a fistula between the bladder and umbilicus, through which leakage of urine occurs, sometimes associated with umbilical granulation (Fig. 6.1).
- *Urachal cyst*: Incomplete closure of the urachal duct can produce a fluid-filled cyst at any level between bladder and umbilicus (most frequently in its lower half). The cyst may be infected and subsequently rupture into the bladder, the umbilicus or, rarely, the peritoneal space. In one case, a calcified urachal cyst was the cause of suprapubic pain in a 32-year-old man.[18]
- *Urachal sinus*: A sinus tract connecting the urachal rudiment to the skin, or less commonly to the bladder. This structure is probably formed by dissection from a chronically infected urachal cyst.
- *Vesicourachal diverticulum*: This develops by the persistence of the distal, incompletely obliterated urachus near to the apical dome of the bladder. When small, these diverticula are asymptomatic, but if large they may be infected or contain stone. Diverticula are commonly seen in prune belly syndrome and have also been associated with bladder outlet obstruction.

Although the urachal canal is usually lined by transitional epithelium, intestinal-type mucosa or

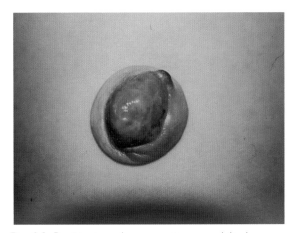

Fig. 6.1 Persistent urachus presenting as umbilical 'polyp/granulation'. (Courtesy of Dr Jean W. Keeling, Consultant Pediatric Pathologist, Edinburgh, UK.)

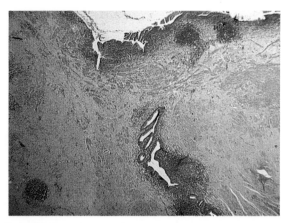

Fig. 6.2 Patent lumen of persistent urachus (central lower part of the image) lined by transitional epithelium. The underlying submucosa is edematous and contains lymphoid aggregates; the muscle layer is also obvious. The surface of the 'polyp/granulation' is also covered by transitional epithelium.

cuboidal cell layer is sometimes also found, with underlying submucosa and outer smooth muscle layer (Fig. 6.2).

Defects of the cloacal membrane: exstrophy–epispadiasis complex

The failure of mesodermal elements of the anterior abdominal wall below the umbilicus to fuse results in congenital anomalies. All defects of this nature fall into a group of anomalies called exstrophy. This term describes a group of congenital anomalies of which a malformed urinary bladder is the most prominent and is regularly associated with other abnormalities. Depending on the extent of this developmental defect, the spectrum of anomalies ranges from a minor degree of epispadiasis, through ectopia vesicae (bladder exstrophy) to the most severe cloacal exstrophy – also called exstrophy–epispadiasis complex.[19] Within the spectrum of exstrophies, classical bladder exstrophy occurs in 60% of cases, epispadiasis in 30% and cloacal exstrophy with variants of the exstrophy complex in 10%.

The difference between bladder exstrophy and cloacal exstrophy is the time of rupture of the cloacal membrane: if the urorectal septum has reached the cloacal membrane before the membrane's rupture, *bladder exstrophy* results. However, if the cloacal membrane ruptures before the division of the cloaca by the urorectal septum, a strip of intestine flanked by the

two hemibladders results, characteristic of *cloacal exstrophy*.[20]

Although the primary defect is not completely understood as yet, it is believed that the basic defect in all types of exstrophy is a failure of the primitive streak mesoderm to invade the anterior part of the cloacal membrane during the fourth week of gestation. Consequently, the ectoderm and endoderm in the developing lower abdominal wall are brought into direct contact, without intervening mesoderm, which results in weakness and ultimate breakdown of the infra-umbilical portion of the abdominal wall (along with the rest of the cloacal membrane as a part of the normal developmental process).[13] Thus, the abnormally extensive cloacal membrane holds apart the developing structures of the lower abdominal wall, causing separation of the pubic bones and often exomphalos. Not infrequently, duplication of the penis (in males) and of Müllerian derivate (in females) may also be present.

Exstrophy of bladder

This severe anomaly is very rare and occurs about once in every 10,000–40,000 births with a male to female ratio of 2–3:1,[21] although a ratio as high as 7:1 has been reported.[3] In bladder exstrophy, as a result of the absent anterior abdominal and bladder walls, the entire posterior wall of the bladder is exposed externally, re-placing the lower part of the anterior abdominal wall.[19]

The list of defects in classical bladder exstrophy regularly includes:

- absence of the lower anterior abdominal wall (infraumbilical portion) and ventral bladder wall with full externalization of the mucosa of the posterior bladder wall and trigone
- divergence of the rectus abdominis muscles
- epispadiasis
- cleft gland penis and short phallus (in males)
- bifid clitoris (in females)
- absence of symphysis pubis with externally rotated pelvic girdle
- low-set, elongated umbilicus.

Frequent coexisting abnormalities include bilateral inguinal hernias, undescended testes (males), stenosis of vaginal orifice and bicornuate uterus (females), patulous anus and rectal prolapse.[19] Less frequently, spina bifida, cleft palate and anal atresia have been found.[22] Upper urinary tract and/or scrotal anomalies are not usually associated with bladder exstrophy.

An established pattern of inheritance of this anomaly is, as yet, unknown. Although the defect is not familial, occurrence in siblings and twins has been reported.[23] In a follow-up of 26 females born with exstrophy and who became mothers, none of the offspring had the deformity.[23] The overall calculation, based on several comprehensive surveys performed during the past two decades, established a 400-fold increase in risk of exstrophy inheritance over the general population.[19,24]

Pathology of bladder exstrophy Gross appearances of the exstrophic bladder depend on the size of the defect, which in a typical case is visible as a slightly prominent area of reddened, glistening, edematous mucosa, which replaces the anterior abdominal wall between a low-set umbilicus and pubic region (Fig. 6.3), invariably associated with epispadiasis. Most often the trigone with orifices of otherwise normal ureters are apparent. If untreated for a long period of time, the exposed mucosa becomes infected, eroded, thickened and often has polypoid structures. Due to associated fibrosis, the underlying submucosa and detrusor musculature also become thickened, giving the appearance of a hardened, rigid, plaque-like structure.

Histologically, the lining mucosa of the exstrophic bladder is regularly covered by normal urothelium, consisting of transitional epithelium that almost invariably contains some kind of non-specific mucosal changes, unrelated to the duration of the defect. The lesions are mainly inflammatory or metaplastic in na-ture. Among the most frequent inflammatory changes are acute and/or chronic cellular infiltrate, erosions and ulcerations of the lining mucosa and follicular cystitis. Less frequently, cystic and glandular cystitis and fibrosis of the submucosa and muscular wall can be found. Among the metaplastic lesions, squamous type (with keratinization) is equally frequent, as is presence of intestinal (glandular) epithelial changes (rarely with Paneth cells in colonic glands if present)[3] (Fig. 6.4). Primary/genuine abnormality of the wall musculature has not been proven, and significant disorganization of muscle fibers has been found in only a very few cases.[25] Rather surprisingly and contrary to common belief, malignant epithelial tumors arise in exstrophied bladder no more frequently than in normally formed bladder (frequency rate does not exceed 8%). Among malignancies, adenocarcinoma is the predominant histological type, but squamous and transitional cell carcinoma have also been reported in some cases.[3]

Exstrophy of cloaca

Cloacal exstrophy is an exceedingly rare anomaly, found in approximately 1 in 40,000 births; no sex predominance is known.[15] In cloacal exstrophy the exstrophied bladder is in two halves, each with a ureteral orifice. The two hemibladders are separated by the interposed and exstrophied bowel that has two openings, the upper communicating with the terminal ileum (which frequently prolapses to form a sausage-shaped tube

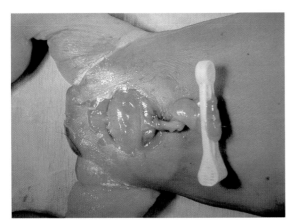

Fig. 6.3 Bladder exstrophy in a female infant. Defect of the lower abdominal wall exposing the trigone and the posterior wall of bladder which is covered by edematous and reddened mucosa. Note the low-set umbilicus with a segment of clamped cord. The pubic area is broadened. (Courtesy of Dr Jean W. Keeling, Consultant Pediatric Pathologist, Edinburgh, UK.)

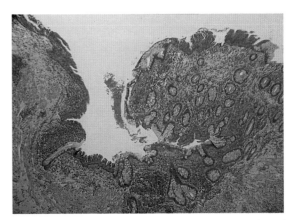

Fig. 6.4 Histology of a wall of exstrophic bladder. Polypoid appearances of the surface with intermittent segments of urothelium and colonic type of mucosa with chronic inflammation and focal superficial erosions. The submucosa and muscle layer are edematous.

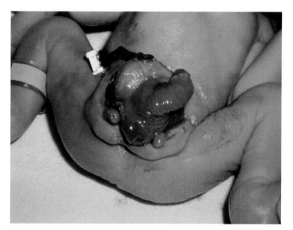

Fig. 6.5 Cloacal exstrophy in a male infant. Extensive defect of the entire lower abdominal wall with a prominent hemibladder next to the right margin of the defect and a red, hemorrhagic, sausage-shaped interposed terminal ileum. The broader structure below is consistent with atretic colon. The left-sided hemibladder is not visible. Two small nodules on each side of the lower margin of the defect represent the left- and right-sided penis, respectively. Two semi-lunar structures along each side of the lower margin of the defect are scrotal sacs containing no testicles. There is an atretic anus. Note the necrotic segment of umbilical cord (clipped) at the top of the defect. (Courtesy of Dr Jean W. Keeling, Consultant Pediatric Pathologist, Edinburgh, UK.)

covered by mucosa), while the lower orifice communicates with a blind-ending segment of colon (Fig. 6.5). The anus is imperforate and there may be a separate appendicular orifice, or sometimes two orifices, since the appendix is frequently duplicated. Half of the patients have upper urinary tract anomaly and 50% have spina bifida or meningomyelocele. Usually a large exomphalos (omphalocele) is associated and this often contains liver as well as intestine. In males the epispadiac penis is invariable and often duplicated, while the scrotum is absent and the testes are undescended. In females the vagina is septate, the uterus duplicated and the external genitalia are absent.[13]

The present understanding of the embryology of cloacal exstrophy postulates that the anomaly develops if the cloacal membrane ruptures *before* the eighth gestational week, prior to the process of complete descent of the urorectal septum, and as a result of a migration failure of the lateral mesodermal folds of the infraumbilical anterior abdominal wall, which results in an enlarged and weak/unstable persistent cloacal membrane composed exclusively of endoderm and ectoderm.[26] According to this theory, cloacal division

normally takes place between the sixth and seventh embryonic weeks and the cloacal membrane is believed to rupture during or after the eighth week of gestation.

However, this widely accepted sequence of embryological events (and the consequent explanation for genesis of cloacal exstrophy) has been challenged in the past by sporadically published papers[20] which reported on the birth of several infants with cloacal exstrophy who had intact cloacal membrane on ultrasound examination performed at the 18th gestational week and which ruptured before the subsequent ultrasound examination at 24 weeks (causing resolution of associated symptoms of bilateral hydronephrosis and reduced volume of amniotic fluid, identified during previous ultrasound). The finding of an intact cloacal membrane *at* and *after* the eighth week of gestation sheds new light on the embryogenesis of cloacal exstrophy and challenges the conventional embryological explanation for development of cloacal exstrophy, suggesting that cloacal exstrophy may develop even when the cloacal membrane ruptures much *later* than the proposed cut-off point of the eighth week of gestation (practically at any time during fetal development).[20]

There is no known pattern of inheritance for cloacal exstrophy in the literature. Collating data from the literature clearly shows that there have been only seven cases of cloacal exstrophy in twin gestations, all in monozygotic twins. In three sets of twins, cloacal exstrophy was present in both twins, while in the other four sets (two of which were conjoined) only one twin had the malformation. On the other hand, only one case of cloacal exstrophy in non-twin siblings has been reported. The degree of genetic and environmental influence on the development of cloacal exstrophy remains a mystery. The occurrence in one group of non-twin siblings suggests some degree of genetic influence, whereas the occurrence in monozygotic twins with varying concordance strongly supports the contribution of an environmental event.[20] A similar proposal has been put forward regarding the etiology of cloacal exstrophy (as a constant and most important feature of the OEIS complex) by other authors,[4] who argue that the sporadic occurrence of this rare complex suggests etiologic heterogeneity with a possible role for both environmental and genetic causes. The author, however, emphasises that developmental field defects involving the intraembryonic mesoderm favor the possible etiological role for homeobox genes, such as HLXB9 with mutations, resulting in anorectal and other abnormalities, or retinoic acid receptors.

Covered exstrophy

This term describes delayed closure of the abdominal wall defect after formation of an exstrophy. However, the abdominal wall is paper thin, the umbilicus is low set, and epispadiasis is usual along with some degree of pubic separation.[13]

REFERENCES

1. Maizels M. Normal development of urinary tract. In: Walsh PC, Gittes RF, Perlmutter AS, Stamey TA (eds) Campbell's Urology, 5th edn. Philadelphia: W.B. Saunders, 1986, pp 1638–1664.

2. Hanna MK, Jeffs RD, Sturgess JM, Barkin M. Ureteral structure and ultrastructure. Part I. The normal human ureter. J Urol 1976;116:718–724.

3. Murphy WM (ed.) Disease of the urinary bladder, urethra, ureters and renal pelves. In: Urological Pathology. Philadelphia: W.B. Saunders, 1989, pp 34–42.

4. Keppler-Noreuil KM. OEIS complex (omphalocele–exstrophy–imperforate anus–spinal defects): review of 14 cases. Am J Med Genet 2001;99:271–279.

5. Ducket JW, Caldamore AA. Bladder and urachus. In: Kelalis PP, King LR, Belman AB (eds) Clinical Pediatric Urology. Philadelphia: W.B. Saunders, 1985, pp 726–751.

6. Tortora FL Jr, Lusey DT, Fried FA, Mandell J. Absence of the bladder. J Urol 1983;129:1235–1237.

7. Glen JF. Agenesis of the bladder. JAMA 1959;169:2016.

8. Miller HL. Agenesis of the urinary bladder and urethra. J Urol 1948;59:1156.

9. Lepoutre C. Sur un cas d'absence congenital de la vessie (persistence du cloaque). J Urol Med Chir 1939; 40;48:334.

10. Perlmutter AD, Retik AB, Bauer SB. Anomalies of the upper urinary tract. In: Walsh PC, Gittes RF, Perlmutter AS, Stamey TA (eds) Campbell's Urology, 5th edn. Philadelphia: W.B. Saunders, 1986, p 1665.

11. Abrahamson J. Double bladder and related anomalies: clinical and embryological aspects and a case report. Br J Urol 1961;33:195–214.

12. Fouda-Neel K, Ahmed S, Borghol M. Complete bladder duplication with exstrophy of 1 moiety in a male infant. J Urol 1996;156:1468.

13. Bernstein J, Risdon RA, Gilbert-Barness E. Renal system. In: Gilbert-Barness E (ed.) Potter's Pathology of the Fetus and Infant. St Louis: Mosby, 1997, pp 903–909.

14. Kohler HH. Septate bladder. J Urol 1940;44:63.

15. Caldamone AA. Anomalies of the bladder and cloaca. In: Gillenwater JY, Grayhack JT, Howards SS, Ducket JW (eds) Adult and Pediatric Urology. Chicago: Year Book Medical Publishers, 1998, pp 1809–1835.

16. Williams DI. Congenital bladder-neck obstruction and megaureters: clinical observations. Br J Urol 1957;29:389–392.

17. Schuffler MD, Pagon RA, Shwartz R, Bill AH. Visceral myopathy of the gastrointestinal and genitourinary tracts in infants. Gastroenterology 1988;94:892–898.

18. Leyson JFJ. Calcified urachal cyst. Br J Urol 1984;54:438.

19. Muecke EC. Exstrophy, epispadiasis and other anomalies of the bladder. In: Walsh PC, Gittes RF, Perlmutter AS, Stamey TA (eds) Campbell's Urology, 5th edn. Philadelphia: W.B. Saunders, 1986, p 1856.

20. Bruch SW, Adzick NS, Goldstein RB, Harrison MR. Challenging the embryogenesis of cloacal exstrophy. J Pediatr Surg 1996;316:768–770.

21. Behrmann RE, Kliegman RM, Arvin AM (eds) Nelson's Textbook of Pediatrics, 15th edn. Philadelphia: W.B. Saunders, 1996, p 1638.

22. Herbut PA. Urological Pathology. Philadelphia: Lea & Febiger, 1952, pp 161–187.

23. Marshal VF, Muecke EC. Variations in exstrophy of the bladder. J Urol 1962;88:766.

24. Shapiro E, Lepor H, Jeffs RD. The inheritance of the exstrophy–epispadiasis complex. J Urol 1984;132:308–310.

25. Culp DA. The histology of the exstrophied bladder. J Urol 1964;91:538.

26. Parrott TS, Skandalakis JE, Gray SW. The bladder and urethra. In: Skandalakis JC, Gray SW (eds) Embryology for Surgeons: the embryonic basis for treatment of congenital anomalies. Baltimore: Williams & Wilkins, 1994, pp 693–694.

7

URINARY CYTOLOGY
Jonathan H. Hughes and Michael B. Cohen

INTRODUCTION

While urinary samples are used for a wide variety of diagnostic tests in clinical medicine, the principal function of urinary cytology is to detect primary and recurrent neoplasms of the urinary tract. The first account of the application of urinary cytology to the detection of urinary tract cancer is generally credited to Sanders, who in 1865 reported the detection of malignant cells in a patient with transitional cell carcinoma of the bladder.[1] However, the technique did not garner much interest until 1945, when Papanicolaou and Marshall published a series of 83 cases of urine cytology and demonstrated that cytologic examination of the urine could predict underlying urinary tract malignancy in a significant number of cases.[2]

Although urinary tract cytology is a discipline that is approximately 135 years old, its acceptance as a useful clinical tool has been slow. Moreover, it is a subject that engenders significant apprehension among pathologists, even specialty trained cytopathologists. Urinary tract specimens – particularly voided urine specimens – are inherently poorly preserved. Additionally, many of the cytologic features of low-grade urothelial malignancies are subtle and difficult to distinguish from reactive or degenerative processes.

In spite of its rather slow acceptance by the urology community and some of its inherent limitations, urinary cytology has become a mainstay technique for detecting urothelial malignancies. Urologists are increasingly dependent on expertise in urinary cytology for detecting primary and recurrent malignancies.

COLLECTION AND PROCESSING OF URINARY CYTOLOGY SAMPLES

In patients who do not require catheterization for some other reason, fresh, randomly voided urine is the most appropriate specimen for cytologic examination.[3] In general, patients should not be catheterized for the sole reason of obtaining diagnostic urothelial cells. While 24-hour urines and early morning specimens are more cellular than randomly voided samples, they are to be avoided because of the degenerative changes which frequently obscure cytologic detail in these specimens. In patients undergoing cystoscopy, bladder washing should be performed with 50–75 ml of saline.[3,4]

Most of the degenerative changes in urinary cytology specimens occur in the relatively hostile environment of the urinary bladder, prior to the collection of the specimen. Further degenerative changes can be prevented for several hours after collection of the specimen, provided that the specimen is refrigerated. Thus, unless the time to specimen processing is prolonged, in most cases the addition of preservatives can be avoided and specimen refrigeration will suffice. If longer storage times are needed, urine and bladder washing specimens can be preserved by adding an equal volume of 50% alcohol to the specimen, although this too results in its own set of morphologic alterations that may hinder diagnostic interpretation.[3,4]

Table 7.1 lists the different types of urinary tract specimens that may be submitted for cytologic examination, and summarizes the advantages and disadvantages of each technique.

A number of different methods of urinary sample preparation are available, including filter preparations, the so-called Saccomano blending technique, routine cytocentrifugation (e.g. Cytospin™) and liquid-based technologies (e.g. Surepath™ and Thin-Prep™).[5] In the authors' experience, cytocentrifugation is the easiest method and yields satisfactory results, obtained via the routine preparation of between two and four cytocentrifugation slides per specimen, although there is

Table 7.1 Types of urinary cytology specimens

Specimen type	Indications	Advantages	Disadvantages	Comment
Voided urine	Routine screening	Non-invasive; inexpensive; easily repeated	Low cellularity; prominent degenerative changes	Should be collected about 3 hours after patient's previous void; refrigerate or fix immediately
Catheterized urine	Routine screening; not usually justified unless indicated for some other reason	Greater cellularity than voided urine specimens	Increased risk of infection; instrumentation artifact; degenerative changes similar to voided urine	High cellularity and papillary-like groups can lead to overdiagnosis of UC
Urine obtained by cystoscopy	Performed in patients undergoing cystoscopic evaluation	Similar to catheterized urine	Similar to catheterized urine	Similar to catheterized urine
Bladder washing	Workup for suspected/recurrent bladder cancer	High cellularity; good cellular preservation; less contamination	None	Higher sensitivity than voided urine cytology, due to better cellularity and preservation
Ileal conduit urine	Monitoring for recurrent UC	Non-invasive: inexpensive; easily repeated	Obscuring crystals, inflammatory cells, intestinal epithelium	None
Upper tract brushing	Directed sampling of suspected upper tract lesion	Permits precise localization of lesion	Invasive; pathologists are frequently inexperienced with these specimens	High cellularity and papillary clusters can lead to overdiagnosis of UC

UC, urothelial carcinoma.

evidence that a single cytospin will suffice.[6] Urine and bladder washing specimens seldom contain adequate material for the preparation of a cell block, and this technique should be employed only in exceptional cases in which visible tissue fragments are present.

HISTOLOGY OF THE NORMAL URINARY TRACT

For the most part, the goal of urinary tract cytology is to detect neoplasms of the urothelium. Also known as transitional cell epithelium because its histologic appearance is between that of non-keratinizing squamous epithelium and pseudostratified columnar epithelium, urothelium is a specialized type of epithelium which lines the renal pelves, ureters, bladder and proximal urethra. The thickness of the urothelium varies with the anatomic site and the degree of distension. In the contracted bladder, it is usually six to seven cell layers thick, and in the ureter three to five cell layers thick.

Urothelium is composed of three different epithelial cell types: superficial, intermediate and basal.

- The *superficial* (also known as cap, dome or umbrella) cells are in contact with the urinary space. They are large, round to elliptical cells that have a 'fried-egg' morphology with abundant amphophilic cytoplasm. Superficial cells are frequently binucleated and lie on top of the smaller intermediate cells.
- The *intermediate* cell layer is typically three to five cell layers thick in the contracted bladder. The intermediate cells (also known as pyramidal cells) are oriented with their long axis perpendicular to the basement membrane. Their nuclei are smaller than superficial cell nuclei, and their cytoplasmic volume is less.
- The *basal* cell layer is in contact with the basement membrane and is typically only one cell layer thick. The basal cells are small cuboidal cells with small nuclei but higher nuclear/cytoplasmic (N/C) ratios than the overlying superficial and intermediate cells.[3–5,7,8]

NORMAL URINARY CYTOLOGY

All three types of transitional epithelial cell may be found in urinary cytology specimens, although basal cells are uncommon (Fig. 7.1). They may occur singly or

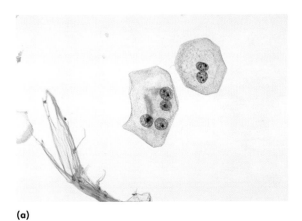

(a)

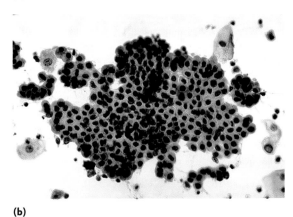

(b)

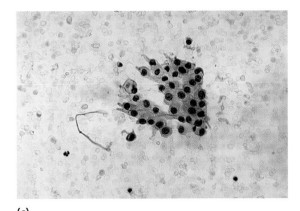

(c)

Fig. 7.1 Normal urothelium. (a) Superficial cells; (b, c) intermediate cells.

in loosely cohesive clusters. The basal cells are the smallest cells and are characterized by dense, basophilic cytoplasm and a single small nucleus. The intermediate cells are approximately three times larger and have an oval shape with a single nucleus. The superficial cells are approximately twice as large as the intermediate cells, and approximately 20% of superficial cells are binucleated.[3–5,7,8] It is important to remember that normal superficial cells can show a wide range in nuclear size, and that increased nuclear size in superficial cells should not be interpreted as evidence of a neoplastic process.

In addition to urothelial cells, a number of other cell types are routinely encountered in 'normal' urinary cytology specimens. Intermediate and superficial squamous cells are commonly seen, particularly in women, as a result of physiologic metaplasia in the urinary bladder as well as from vaginal and perineal contamination in voided urine specimens. Small numbers of neutrophils and histiocytes are also routinely seen in urinary cytology specimens and should be considered a normal finding. Spermatozoa are not uncommonly seen. Renal tubular epithelial cells may occasionally be observed, but their presence usually indicates renal parenchymal disease and should prompt further workup. These cells bear some resemblance to transitional cells, but can be recognized due to the fact that their cytoplasm is more granular than the dense cytoplasm of normal transitional cells.[4]

PATHOLOGY OF UROTHELIAL CARCINOMA

Urothelial (transitional cell) carcinoma is a relatively common disease, with approximately 50,000 new cases diagnosed annually in the United States; the national death rate is approximately 10,000 persons per annum.[4,9] Urothelial carcinoma (UC) is two to three times more common in men than in women. One of the most important risk factors for UC in the United States is smoking. Although tumors may arise anywhere along the course of the urothelial mucosa (including the ureters, renal pelvis and urethra), approximately 95% of UCs occur in the bladder. Moreover, approximately 95% of the malignant tumors that occur in the urinary bladder are UC.[7,10] Current theory suggests that UC may occur as one of two distinct disease processes, each of which has a distinct cytologic appearance and distinct clinical course: low-grade UC and high-grade UC.[4]

The majority of UCs are low-grade tumors; they have a papillary growth pattern and infrequently invade or metastasize. As a consequence, they are biologically indolent and are associated with long patient survivals. Cytologically, most papillary UCs are low-grade and may be difficult to distinguish from normal or reactive urothelial cells in voided urine specimens or bladder washings. High-grade UCs exhibit a sessile or nodular growth pattern with a high likelihood of invasion and metastasis. Not surprisingly, these tumors are associated with poor patient survival. The cytology of these tumors is almost always high-grade.[3,4,11–14]

Because the overwhelming majority of lower urinary cancers in the United States are UCs, and because the cytologic diagnosis of UC is the most problematic aspect of urinary tract cytology, this chapter will focus on developing a practical, criteria-based approach to the diagnosis of UC. While the cytologic features of other neoplastic, infectious and reactive processes of the lower urinary tract will be discussed, our scope will largely be limited to those lesions that enter the differential diagnosis of low- or high-grade UC.

CYTOLOGY OF UROTHELIAL CARCINOMA

Most cases of high-grade UC can be diagnosed accurately by the practicing pathologist. These lesions are characterized by malignant cells with pleomorphic, angulated nuclei, markedly increased N/C ratios, and coarse chromatin. There is good interobserver concordance among pathologists for diagnosing high-grade UC, and the sensitivity and specificity of urine cytology for high-grade UC are approximately 95% and 100%, respectively.[3,11–14]

The cytologic diagnosis of low-grade UC is more problematic. These tumors exhibit subtle cytomorphologic alterations that are difficult to distinguish from benign or reactive processes (Table 7.2). This unfortunate circumstance is confounded by the fact that low-grade lesions do not shed cells as readily as high-grade lesions, thereby resulting in a small amount of material upon which the pathologist must base a diagnosis.[3,11–15] The difficulty that pathologists have in diagnosing low-grade UC is reflected by the wide variation in diagnostic

Table 7.2 Characteristics of urothelial carcinomas

Superficial	Invasive
Approx. 66% of tumors	Approx. 25% of tumors
Papillary	Sessile
Low grade	High grade
Low stage	High stage
High recurrence rate	N/A
Low progression rate	High progression rate
Low mortality	High mortality

accuracy reported in the published literature, with a sensitivity ranging between 0 and 73%.[3,11–14,16–22]

Part of this wide range in diagnostic accuracy is due to disagreement among authors about which cytologic criteria are most important for establishing a diagnosis of UC. Reported features indicative of malignancy include nuclear enlargement, eccentrically placed nuclei, granular nuclear chromatin, irregular nuclear borders, homogeneous cytoplasm, absence of nucleoli, irregular papillary fragments, atypical single cells, and cell clusters with peripheral palisading.[3,4,7,11–14,16,17,22–28] While most of these studies attempt to assign a relative importance to each criterion, there have been few rigorous statistical analyses to assess the utility of these criteria for diagnosing UC. It is important to recognize the contributions of others in this area who have toiled before us. Two, in particular, are noteworthy: Kern and Murphy. In a seminal paper published in 1975, Kern reported on qualitative and quantitative features of UC as identified in cytologic specimens.[11] Murphy's 1984 paper articulating the cellular features of UC (particularly low-grade UC) should also be viewed as a landmark in this field.[13] Our contribution has merely refined their work.

Cytologic features of low-grade UC

As a result of our frustration in identifying the salient cytologic criteria, in 1994 we published a study which employed a stepwise logistic regression analysis to determine which cytologic features are most useful for separating low-grade UC from benign processes.[29] Eighty-two bladder wash specimens (33 low-grade UCs and 49 non-neoplastic lesions) were reviewed retrospec-

tively. The cases were reviewed by two cytopathologists who had no knowledge of the original cytologic or corresponding histologic diagnoses and were scored for the presence or absence of 20 cytomorphologic criteria, as outlined in Table 7.3. These features have been described as useful in the separation of low-grade UC from benign urothelium, including reactive and reparative conditions ('atypical').

The presence of individual cells was the only cytologic feature that was present in more than 90% of the patients with malignant disease. Only three cytologic features (nuclear molding, necrosis and anisonucleosis) were seen exclusively in patients with malignant disease. However, in most of the patients with malignant disease, these features were not present. Using a stepwise logistic regression analysis, three cytologic features were identified as useful in discriminating between low-grade UC and non-neoplastic lesions: increased N/C ratios, irregular nuclear borders and cytoplasmic homogeneity[30,31] (Figs 7.2–7.4).

The numbers of patients with benign and malignant disease in whom these criteria were observed are shown in Table 7.4. Fifteen (45%) of the patients with malignant disease had all three cytologic criteria, and 27 (82%) had at least two of the criteria. The contingency sensitivity, specificity, positive predictive value and negative predictive value for the diagnosis of low-grade UC using the three combined cytologic criteria were 45%, 98%, 94% and 73%, respectively (Table 7.5). The contingency table sensitivity, specificity, positive predictive value and negative predictive value using at least two of the three cytologic criteria for the diagnosis of low-grade UC were 85%, 96%, 93%, and 90%, respectively (Table 7.6).

Table 7.3 Cytomorphologic criteria for the diagnosis of low-grade urothelial carcinoma

- The presence of cell clusters or groups of five or more cells
- Individual cells other than superficial cells present in significant numbers to be observed in most high-power fields
- High cellularity, i.e. cells present in most high-power fields
- Acute inflammation
- Increased nuclear/cytoplasmic ratios, i.e. greater than 1:3 to 1:4 (normal, approximately 1:5), in cells other than superficial cells
- Nucleoli
- Granular nuclear chromatin

- Hyperchromatic nuclear chromatin
- Open nuclear chromatin
- Irregular nuclear borders
- Nuclear molding
- Nuclear eccentricity
- Elongated nuclei or spindle-shape nuclei
- Necrosis
- Anisonucleosis
- Cytoplasmic homogeneity
- Prominent nucleoli
- Irregular border fragments of cell clusters
- Absent cytoplasmic collars
- Peripheral palisading in cell clusters

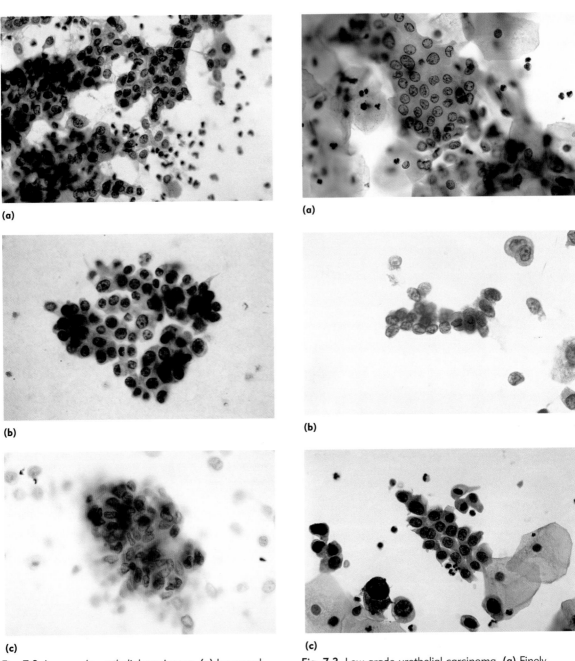

(a)

(b)

(c)

Fig. 7.2 Low-grade urothelial carcinoma. **(a)** Increased nuclear/cytoplasmic ratio; **(b)** cytoplasmic homogeneity, eccentrically placed nuclei; **(c)** cytoplasmic homogeneity, irregularity of nuclear borders, finely granular chromatin.

(a)

(b)

(c)

Fig. 7.3 Low-grade urothelial carcinoma. **(a)** Finely granular chromatin, irregularity of nuclear borders; **(b)** increased nuclear/cytoplasmic ratio, finely granular chromatin, irregularity of nuclear borders, eccentrically placed nuclei; **(c)** increased nuclear/cytoplasmic ratio, cytoplasmic homogeneity, irregularity of nuclear borders.

The results of our statistical analysis suggest that the diagnosis of low-grade UC should be based more upon individual cell morphology than upon architectural aberrations. Features such as increased cell clusters with peripheral cellular palisading and irregular border fragments, although suggested by other authors as indicative of malignancy, were not statistically significant in this study.[17,26] The three key cytologic criteria, if used in combination, resulted in a relatively low diagnostic

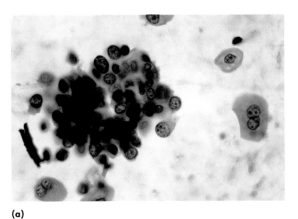

(a)

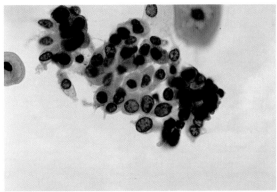

(b)

(c)

Fig. 7.4 Low-grade urothelial carcinoma. (a) Filter preparation; (b) Cytospin™ preparation; (c) SurePath™ preparation.

Table 7.4 Probability of low-grade urothelial carcinoma based on three cytologic features

Cytologic criteria			No. of patients		
Increased N/C ratio	Irregular nuclear borders	Cytoplasmic homogeneity	Probability of tumor (%)	Transitional cell carcinoma	Benign
+	+	+	94	15	1
+	+	−	88	8	1
+	−	+	100	4	0
−	+	+	100	1	0
+	−	−	0	0	3
−	+	−	22	2	7
−	−	+	29	2	5
−	−	−	3	1	32
Total				33	49

N/C, nuclear/cytoplasmic; +, presence of cytologic feature; −, absence of cytologic feature.

sensitivity (45%), reflecting the overlap of cytologic findings in benign and malignant conditions. If at least two of the key criteria were present, the sensitivity for detecting low-grade UC was 85%. This approach allowed for a significant increase in sensitivity, with only

a slight decrease in specificity (98% with three criteria and 96% with at least two criteria).

In addition, a couple of secondary criteria were also identified which were culled from the analysis after exclusion of the primary criteria (see Figs 7.2–7.4).

Table 7.5 Number of patients with low-grade urothelial carcinoma predicted by three cytologic criteria and observed by histology

All three cytologic features present?	Histology		
	Transitional cell carcinoma	Benign	Total
Yes	15	1	16
No	18	48	66
Total	33	49	82

Sensitivity, 45%; specificity, 98%; positive predictive value, 94%; negative predictive value, 73%.

Table 7.6 Number of patients with low-grade urothelial carcinoma predicted by at least two of three cytologic criteria and observed by histology

At least two cytologic features present?	Histology		
	Transitional cell carcinoma	Benign	Total
Yes	28	2	30
No	5	47	52
Total	33	49	82

Sensitivity, 85%; specificity, 96%; positive predictive value, 93%; negative predictive value, 90%.

These are: eccentrically placed nuclei and finely granular nuclear chromatin (hypochromasia). These additional criteria are of particular value when only two or one of the primary criteria are present. As noted, the ability to identify the criteria as well as their frequency is somewhat variable from case to case. Thus, from a pragmatic standpoint we have used the primary and secondary criteria in combination when evaluating specimens. It is worth recognizing that these criteria are essentially the same as those identified by Murphy a decade earlier when evaluating filter preparations. Thus, we believe that these criteria are evaluable in urinary specimens prepared by different methods, including filter preparations and cytospins, as done in our laboratory. These criteria are also identifiable with a liquid-based technology (Autocyte), although hypochromasia may be more difficult to appreciate.

Our statistical analysis demonstrated that low-grade UC can be diagnosed with a high degree of accuracy when key cytologic criteria are applied. Moreover, in a subsequent study in which these same criteria were applied prospectively to a new set of urine specimens by a panel of pathologists with varying degrees of experience, it was demonstrated that these key cytologic criteria can be learned and effectively applied with high accuracy.[32] However, our studies and those of others also demonstrate that, because of the cytologic overlap between low-grade UC and reactive processes, the sensitivity of cytology for detecting low-grade UC is less than 100%. This fact suggests that, in a small proportion of cases, cellular morphology alone may not be predictive of malignant behavior.

Cytologic features of high-grade UC

Fortunately, high-grade UC is much easier to diagnose than low-grade UC (Fig. 7.5). Urinary cytology specimens collected from patients with high-grade UC tend to be quite cellular, and the cells show obviously abnormal nuclear features.[4,11,13,17] The nuclei of high-grade UC are usually more than twice the size of normal urothelial cell nuclei, and they exhibit a coarse, hyperchromatic chromatin pattern with prominent nuclear pleomorphism, nucleoli and eccentric nuclei. Mitotic figures are usually present and may be atypical but are rarely appreciated in cytologic specimens. Another

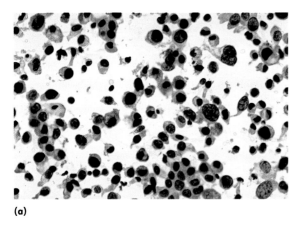

(a)

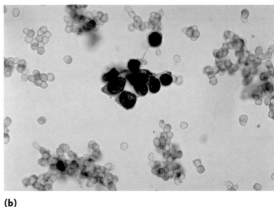

(b)

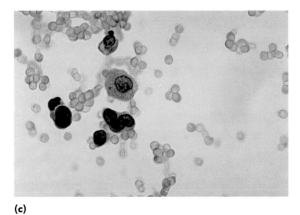

(c)

Fig. 7.5 High-grade urothelial carcinoma. (a–c) Individual cells or loosely cohesive clusters with cells displaying increased nuclear/cytoplasmic ratios, eccentrically placed nuclei, hyperchromasia and nucleoli.

important feature of high-grade UC, and one that distinguishes it from low-grade UC, is the presence of vacuolated cytoplasm.

Because of their overtly malignant cytologic features and high cellularity in urinary cytology specimens, most cases of high-grade UC can be diagnosed with a high degree of sensitivity and specificity. With few exceptions, the cytologic features of high-grade papillary UC and high-grade flat UC (so-called carcinoma in situ, CIS) are the same. Thus, the absence of a papillary lesion in a patient with a cytologic diagnosis of high-grade UC should suggest the possibility of flat CIS. On a similar note, the cytologic features of non-invasive high-grade UC and invasive high-grade UC are also very similar. The presence of inflammation and necrosis should suggest the possibility of an invasive process, although definitive assessment of invasion is usually made on the basis of surgical biopsy material that includes muscular tissue.

Table 7.7 summarizes the key cytologic features of reactive urothelial cells, low-grade UC and high-grade UC.

OTHER HISTOLOGIC TYPES OF URINARY TRACT MALIGNANCIES

While UC accounts for the overwhelming majority of urinary tract malignancies in the United States,[9,10] other histologic types of urothelial neoplasms do occur. Because of their rarity, an in-depth treatment of these lesions is beyond the scope and practicality of this chapter. However, two lesions – squamous cell carcinoma and adenocarcinoma – deserve brief mention.

Squamous cell carcinoma

Although squamous differentiation is frequently seen in UCs, particularly high-grade UCs, pure squamous cell carcinomas (SCCs) of the urinary tract are rare in the United States. They are thought to represent less than 5% of urinary bladder cancers in the US.[10] Most cases arise in the anterior bladder wall. Current theory suggests that these lesions arise out of a background of chronic cystitis with squamous metaplasia, which

Table 7.7 Cytologic features of reactive urothelial cells, low-grade UC and high-grade UC

Cytologic feature	Reactive	Low-grade UC	High-grade UC
Cell arrangement	Papillary aggregates	Papillary and loose clusters	Isolated cells and loose clusters
Cell size	Increased	Increased and uniform	Increased and pleomorphic
Cell number	Variable	Often numerous	Usually numerous
Cytoplasm	Vacuolated	Homogeneous	Vacuolated
N/C ratio	Normal/increased	Increased	Increased
Position of nucleus	Eccentric	Eccentric	Eccentric
Nuclear size	Uniform	Enlarged	Variable
Nuclear contour	Smooth	Irregular, notches and grooves	Markedly irregular
Nuclear chromatin	Fine, regular	Fine, irregular	Coarse, irregular
Nucleoli	Often large	Small/absent	Variable

N/C, nuclear/cytoplasmic; UC, urothelial carcinoma. Modified from Murphy et al.[13]

probably accounts for the high incidence of the disease in countries such as Egypt, where schistosomiasis of the bladder is common. The prognosis is generally poor.

Poorly differentiated SCCs are usually easy to diagnose, as they yield large numbers of overtly malignant squamous cells. The cytologic features are similar to poorly differentiated SCCs at other body sites. Well-differentiated SCCs, however, are more problematic. They may yield only anucleate squamous cells or squamous cells with minimal nuclear abnormalities. While keratinizing SCCs usually exhibit obvious squamous differentiation, non-keratinizing SCCs may be difficult to distinguish from high-grade UC.

The differential diagnosis of SCC includes leukoplakia/squamous metaplasia, UC with squamous differentiation, and metastatic SCC from some other body site.[4,33]

Adenocarcinoma

Primary adenocarcinoma of the lower urinary tract is also very rare, accounting for less than 2% of primary urinary bladder cancers in the United States. Similar to SCC, most adenocarcinomas develop from changes associated with chronic inflammation, such as cystitis glandularis, and most are mucin-producing. Adenocarcinomatous differentiation within a high-grade UC is far more common than a pure adenocarcinoma. The most common type of lower urinary tract adenocarcinoma is the so-called 'colonic' type. The cytology of this tumor is similar to that of colonic adenocarcinoma and is characterized by clusters of tumor cells with elongated, spindled nuclei and vacuolated cytoplasm. Signet-ring cell adenocarcinomas represent about 10% of primary bladder adenocarcinomas and have a

morphology similar to that of signet-ring cell carcinomas arising at other body sites, such as stomach.

The differential diagnosis of adenocarcinoma includes high-grade UC with glandular differentiation, cystitis glandularis, nephrogenic adenoma, upper tract adenocarcinomas such as renal cell carcinoma, and metastatic adenocarcinomas from other sites.[4,33]

CAUSES OF FALSE-POSITIVE DIAGNOSES IN URINARY CYTOLOGY

A number of benign conditions can cause false-positive diagnoses in urinary cytology, particularly when interpreted by inexperienced cytopathologists (Table 7.8). The most important sources of false-positive diagnoses are stone disease, drugs and irradiation, inflammatory/infectious processes and instrumentation artifacts.

Urinary tract calculi

Stone disease is perhaps the most important source of false-positive diagnoses, because it induces cytologic

Table 7.8 Non-neoplastic lesions that may be confused with transitional cell carcinoma

- Urolithiasis
- Bladder instrumentation/catheter(ization)
- Immunotherapy
- Chemotherapy – topical and systemic
- Radiation
- Renal epithelial fragments
- Diversions and conduits

changes in urothelium that mimic high-grade UC.[4,34,35] Confounding this fact is the unfortunate circumstance that the history of the urinary tract may be unknown to the pathologist and even to the urologist who submits the specimen for cytologic examination. Further, the history may not be of practical value. For example, the key differential diagnoses of a filling defect in the upper urinary tract are urothelial neoplasia and lithiasis. Stones can result in a spectrum of atypical cells that may overlap with neoplastic lesions. Inflammation, blood and necrotic debris may be present in the background and be misinterpreted as tumor diathesis. For obvious reasons, stone-induced reactive changes should be considered in every case that at first glance appears to represent high-grade UC. In many cases it may not be possible to distinguish between stone disease and high-grade UC. In these instances follow-up samples should be obtained for cytologic examination. If the atypical cytologic features persist for several weeks after passing a stone, the patient should be aggressively worked up for an underlying high-grade lesion. Conversely, if the urine cytology reverts to normal, then malignancy is excluded.

Chemotherapy and radiotherapy

Many chemotherapeutic and radiotherapeutic agents induce cytologic changes in urothelial cells that may mimic malignancy.[4,5,36–38] Some of the most common culprits include cyclophosphamide (Cyotxan) and busulfan (Myleran), which are systemic chemotherapeutic agents and are concentrated in the urine, and thiotepa and mitomycin C, which are intravesical chemotherapeutic agents used for the treatment of UC. In general, these agents produce varying degrees of nuclear and cytoplasmic enlargement that may lead to a false-positive diagnosis of high-grade UC. Unlike stone disease, in which the history may be unknown, chemotherapeutic and radiotherapeutic changes are usually suggested by the clinical history. None the less, false-positive diagnoses do occur. A useful clue is that chemotherapeutic and radiotherapeutic agents often produce cytologic changes that are more bizarre than those typically observed even in high-grade UC. This is especially true in the case of cyclophosphamide and busulfan. Another helpful clue is that therapy-induced atypia is often accompanied by more degenerative changes than is UC.

Radiation changes in urothelial cells are similar to radiation changes at other body sites. There is usually generalized cytomegaly and extreme multinucleation. The overall N/C ratio tends to be normal, and there is often cytoplasmic vacuolization and polychromasia. While normal superficial cells frequently contain two and sometimes three nuclei, the presence of many cells with three or more nuclei should raise the possibility of radiation change.[4,5,38]

Human polyoma virus

A variety of infectious processes can produce cytologic changes in urothelial cells that mimic urothelial carcinoma. As in the case of stone disease and chemo/radiotherapeutic changes, these potential pitfalls can usually be avoided if the cytologist is experienced and appropriately wary. Cytomegalovirus, herpes virus, human papilloma virus, fungi and parasites (e.g. schistosomes) can all be detected, albeit very rarely, in urine specimens and can lead to atypical cytologic features such as nuclear enlargement, irregular nuclear contours, prominent nucleoli and cytoplasmic vacuolization. The infectious agent most likely to cause a false-positive diagnosis of UC, however, is human polyoma virus.[39,40]

Also known as BK virus, human polyoma virus is a member of the papovavirus family. It is often found in immunocompromised patients, including transplant patients and patients with AIDS, diabetes mellitus or autoimmune diseases. However, it can also be found in persons who are less obviously recognized as immunocompromised, such as children, the elderly and pregnant women. It has even been detected in apparently immunologically competent persons. Infected urothelial cells contain a large homogeneous intranuclear inclusion that results in a markedly hyperchromatic nucleus with a disrupted nuclear membrane. At first inspection the viral cytopathic changes may be mistaken for high-grade UC. However, the polyoma virus-infected cells exhibit a more smudgy nucleus than cancer cells, and the viral intranuclear inclusion results in a glassy, empty appearance rather than the coarse chromatin pattern that characterizes high-grade UC. Another very useful clue is that polyoma virus-infected cells almost always occur singly, whereas the cells of high-grade UC are typically seen singly and in clusters.

Instrumentation artifact

During the course of the routine urologic workup, many patients undergo instrumentation of the urinary tract. Procedures such as catheterization, cystoscopy and retrograde studies all serve useful diagnostic functions, but they can also complicate the workup because they can dislodge large fragments of urothelial cells and produce urinary tract specimens that are alarmingly cellular and contain papillary groups.[4,5] Most often, these reactive changes are mild and are unlikely to lead to an erroneous diagnosis of high-grade UC. They can, however, be mistaken for low-grade UC. These cellular changes can persist for weeks after instrumentation. For this reason, in any case that raises the diagnostic consideration of low-grade UC, the possibility of instrumentation artifact should be considered and ruled out. It is worth noting that the inclusion in the report that there is instrumentation artifact present is of little value to the clinician. Therefore, we have chosen not to include such an observation in our reports.

It is clear from the preceding discussion that there are a number of pitfalls that can lead to false-positive diagnoses in urinary cytology specimens. It follows that good communication and close collaboration between the urologist and cytologist are necessary in order to prevent diagnostic errors. To this end, the requisition form for urinary cytology specimens should be filled out completely by the submitting physician and, in addition to the usual patient demographic data, should include the following information:

- History of previous urinary tract disease (including stones)
- History of chemotherapy/radiotherapy
- History of recent urinary tract instrumentation and surgery
- Type of specimen (voided urine, bladder washing, etc.) and location (bladder, ureter, etc.) of specimen.

THE WHO/ISUP CONSENSUS CLASSIFICATION

Before ending this discussion of the cytologic features of urinary tract lesions, it important to relate it to the current classification scheme being utilized by surgical pathologists for the histologic diagnosis of urothelial biopsies. The consensus classification of the World Health Organization/International Society of Urologic Pathology (WHO/ISUP) was published in 1998 (see Table 7.9).[41] The principal aim of this classification system was to provide a framework for the reproducible categorization of bladder neoplasia that could be used effectively by pathologists, urologists and oncologists. The WHO/ISUP classification recognizes the existence of

Table 7.9 The WHO/ISUP consensus classification

- Normal
  - normal
- Hyperplasia
  - flat hyperplasia
  - papillary hyperplasia
- Flat lesions with atypia
  - reactive (inflammatory) atypia
  - atypia of unknown significance
  - dysplasia (low-grade squamous intraurothelial neoplasia)
  - carcinoma in situ (high-grade squamous intraurothelial neoplasia)
- Papillary neoplasms
  - papilloma
  - inverted papilloma
  - papillary neoplasm of low malignant potential
  - papillary carcinoma, low-grade
  - papillary carcinoma, high-grade
- Invasive neoplasms
  - lamina propria invasion
  - muscularis propria (detrusor muscle) invasion

five general diagnostic categories for lower urinary tract biopsies:

1. normal
2. hyperplastic lesions
3. flat lesions with atypia
4. papillary neoplasms
5. invasive neoplasms.

Within each of these general categories, there are multiple specific diagnostic entities. For example, the general category of 'papillary neoplasms' includes papilloma, inverted papilloma, papillary neoplasm of low malignant potential, low-grade papillary carcinoma, and high-grade papillary carcinoma.

The WHO/ISUP classification scheme is a histologic classification system for biopsy specimens and therefore utilizes both cytologic and architectural criteria for subclassification of urothelial lesions. For this reason, many of the diagnostic entities in the WHO/ISUP system cannot be diagnosed in urinary tract cytology specimens. For example, 'flat hyperplasia', papilloma, and even papillary neoplasm of low malignant potential are difficult if not impossible to diagnose in cytology specimens because their cytologic features are very similar to those of normal urothelium. On the other hand, most cases classified by the WHO/ISUP scheme as low- and high-grade UC will yield diagnostic cells in urinary cytology specimens. These, of course, are the most clinically important lesions, and the WHO/ISUP committee recognizes the importance of urinary cytology for screening and monitoring patients for UC. Whenever possible, the cytologic diagnosis should be related to the corresponding diagnostic term in the WHO/ISUP system in order to foster uniform terminology and improve communication between pathologists and urologists. To the best of our knowledge, no publication has been reported utilizing this classification scheme in the evaluation of cytologic specimens. We predict that this will be more problematic than applying the Bethesda System for cervicovaginal cytology to histologic specimens.

FLOW CYTOMETRY AND OTHER ANCILLARY TECHNIQUES

In an effort to improve the diagnostic sensitivity for detecting UC, there has been considerable interest in developing new techniques to augment or replace urine cytology as a screening test (see chapter 22). These techniques, such as image analysis flow cytometry, interphase cytogenetics, immunocytochemistry and fluorescence in situ hybridization, among others, are generally costly and often not readily available in most laboratories.[42,43] Nevertheless, many hold promise as complementary tests to improve the accuracy of urine cytology. Many of these ancillary tests are best regarded as investigational at this time. Two categories of emerging technologies, however, deserve special mention, because they appear to have a greater likelihood of achieving widespread use: flow cytometry and exfoliated tumor markers.

Flow cytometry

Of all the ancillary techniques currently being utilized or investigated, flow cytometry has gained the most acceptance and is clearly becoming an important diagnostic tool in urinary cytology. The technique is based upon the detection of an aneuploid cell population or an increased number of cells in the S phase of the cell cycle. It is well established that flow cytometry can be a valuable tool for the detection and management of bladder cancer.[42,44,45] A major drawback of flow cytometry is that it is more costly and complex than urine cytology and requires bladder washings rather than voided urine.

Exfoliated tumor markers

Recently, another category of clinical tests has emerged which may improve the diagnostic accuracy of urine cytology, or perhaps replace urine cytology altogether.[46-54] This class of tests is based upon the detection of polypeptides or other macromolecules which are exfoliated into the urine by tumor cells. In theory, tests based upon the detection of exfoliated tumor markers afford several advantages over conventional cytology. Because tumor markers can be measured by immunologically based assay systems, these tests have the potential to provide an objective, quantitative result for the clinician and eliminate the subjectivity inherent with a cytologic examination. This quantitative result could be followed over time to monitor the patient's response to therapy or to detect tumor recurrence.

These immunoassays are easily automated and can be performed either in the urologist's office at the time of clinical testing or on a large scale in the clinical laboratory, thereby making them potentially less time-consuming and less expensive than cytologic examination. Because all of these new tests are non-invasive, they may also allow a significant reduction in the frequency of cystoscopic examinations for patients undergoing surveillance for recurrent UC. Currently, four different immunoassays based upon the detection of tumor markers in the urine have been approved by the US Food and Drug Administration (FDA): Polymedco's BTA™ (bladder tumor antigen), AuraTek's FDP™ (fibrin degradation product) and Matritech's NMP22™ (nuclear matrix protein). The fourth test, DAKO's ImmunoCyt™ test, is based on a related principle and involves staining of urinary cytology specimens with three different bladder-cancer-specific monoclonal antibodies and examining the cells under an immunofluorescence microscope (Table 7.10). The reader is referred to the bibliography and to our recent reviews of this subject for more details about the scientific basis for these tests.[54-65] Although these assays have not yet gained widespread acceptance, their relative ease of use and cost effectiveness may lead to greater utilization of these tests as diagnostic adjuncts to urinary cytology.

CONCLUSION

In this chapter we have attempted to set forth our approach to the accurate diagnosis of urothelial neoplasms in urinary cytology specimens. It is our belief that much of the apprehension associated with urinary

Table 7.10 Food and Drug Administration (FDA)-approved bladder tumor marker tests

Test	Substance measured	Type of assay
BTA™*	Basement membrane complexes	Latex agglutination (qualitative result)
AuraTek FDP™†	Fibrin/fibrinogen degradation products	Dipstick (qualitative result)
Matritech NMP22™‡	Nuclear mitotic apparatus protein	Enzyme immunoassay (quantitative result)
DAKO ImmunoCyt™§	Three different bladder-cancer specific tumor markers	Immunofluorescence microscopy

* Polymedco, Cortlandt Manor, NY.
† AuraTek (PerImmune, Rockville, MD, and Organon Teknika, Dublin, Ireland): FDP.
‡ Matritech (Newton, MA): NMP22.
§ DAKO (Carpinteria, CA): ImmunoCyt.

cytology can be eliminated if the cytopathologist uses a practical, clinically useful, diagnostic algorithm. Fortunately, most cases of high-grade UC can be diagnosed with a high degree of sensitivity and specificity. The most important sources of false-positive diagnoses of high-grade UC are stone disease and radiation/chemotherapy. Once these potential pitfalls have been ruled out by the patient history and/or repeat cytologic examinations following passing of a stone or cessation of therapy, a diagnosis of high-grade UC can usually be made with confidence and accuracy.

There is no question that the diagnosis of low-grade UC is more difficult than the diagnosis of high-grade UC. None the less, we believe that a systematic approach to the specimen will lead to a high diagnostic accuracy. In the cytologic evaluation of urinary specimens for low-grade UC we have found key criteria, both primary and secondary, which appear to be useful prospectively. However, we believe a few additional points are important. It is worth noting that most of our experience is based on the evaluation of bladder wash specimens. While these criteria also have merit in voided urine samples, such specimens are often hypocellular and admixed with large numbers of inflammatory cells, which can obscure cellular details. It is also important to point out that our experience is based on the use of Cytospin preparations, and more recently Autocyte (see Fig. 7.4).

Just as it is important for the cytopathologist to use a systematic, criteria-based approach to urinary cytology specimens, it is equally important that the cytology report itself be concise and convey meaningful information to the treating physician. Over the years we have tried to make a concerted effort to make a definitive diagnosis, and to limit the number of diagnostic categories. Whilst fully recognizing that not all specimens are appropriately categorized as either benign or malignant,

we do try to be as black and white as possible. In this vein, cells which are reactive, reparative, degenerative, etc. have, by and large, been categorized as benign, or, in our terminology: 'No tumor cells identified'. Generally, we have consciously tried to avoid diagnosing such samples as 'atypical'. In our opinion, the term 'atypical' is vague and undermines the clinician's confidence in the test results and, sometimes, in the cytopathologist. Thus, we have typically diagnosed cells as benign (including reactive processes such as stones), suspicious for low-grade UC, low-grade UC, and high-grade UC. It is very important always to specify the grade of the (suspected) tumor, since the clinical implications are dramatically different. For example, the identification of cells that suggest a high-grade tumor(s) will elicit a different algorithm by the urologist in the context of cystoscopically visible papillary tumors than a sessile tumor. Similarly, the concern for a cytologic diagnosis of low-grade tumor will be viewed differently depending on the additional information available to the urologist. Therefore, we feel strongly that all reports should indicate clearly the grade, or suspected grade, of the tumor.

With respect to microscopic evaluation, a few final points are noteworthy:

- Superficial (cap, umbrella, dome) cells are not part of the neoplastic process. Consequently, we have tended to ignore this cell type when evaluating the specimens.
- As stated previously, the key criteria for diagnosing low-grade UC are based on cytologic detail and not architectural features. Therefore, we have generally not found it useful to evaluate urothelial clusters for the presence or absence of specific criteria. Rather, the evaluation of criteria in single cells or small clusters of cells has been most useful.

- These criteria can be learned but do require attention to cytologic details.

It is our hope that the criteria we have identified and found useful prospectively will be of value to others in the microscopic evaluation for low-grade UC and increase their accuracy.

REFERENCES

1. Sanders WR. Cancer of the bladder: fragments forming urethral plugs discharged in urine. Edinburgh Med J 1865;10:273–274.
2. Papanicolaou GN, Marshall VF. Urine sediment smears as a diagnostic procedure in cancer of the urinary tract. Science 1945;101:519.
3. Murphy WM. Urinary cytology in diagnostic pathology. Diagn Cytopathol 1985;1:173–175.
4. Yazdi HM. Genitourinary cytology. Clin Lab Med 1991;11:369–401.
5. Kern WH. Urinary tract. In: Bibbo M (ed.) Comprehensive Cytopathology. Philadelphia: W.B. Saunders, 1997, pp 445–476.
6. Burton JL, Goepel JR, Lee JA. Demand management in urine cytology: a single cytospin slide is sufficient. J Clin Pathol 2000;53:718–719.
7. Friedell GH, Bell JR, Burney SW, et al. Histopathology and classification of urinary bladder carcinoma. Urol Clin North Am 1976;3:53–70.
8. Murphy WM. Urothelial neoplasia. Monogr Pathol 1992;77–111.
9. Greenlee RT, Murray T, Bolden S, Wingo PA. Cancer statistics, 2000. CA Cancer J Clin 2000;50:7–33.
10. Lynch CF, Cohen MB. Urinary system. Cancer 1995;75:316–329.
11. Kern WH. The cytology of transitional cell carcinoma of the urinary bladder. Acta Cytol 1975;19:420–428.
12. Murphy WM. Current status of urinary cytology in the evaluation of bladder neoplasms. Hum Pathol 1990;21:886–896.
13. Murphy WM, Soloway MS, Jukkola AF, et al. Urinary cytology and bladder cancer. The cellular features of transitional cell neoplasms. Cancer 1984;53:1555–1565.
14. Murphy WM. Current topics in the pathology of bladder cancer. Pathol Annu 1983;18:1–25.
15. Maier U, Simak R, Heuhold N. The clinical value of urinary cytology: 12 years of experience with 615 patients. J Clin Pathol 1995;48:314–317.
16. Esposito PLZJ. Grading of transitional cell neoplasms of the urinary bladder from smears of bladder washings: a critical review of 326 tumors. Acta Cytol 1972;16:529–537.
17. Koss LG, Deitch D, Ramanathan R, Sherman AB. Diagnostic value of cytology of voided urine. Acta Cytol 1985;29:810–816.
18. Murphy WM. ASCP survey on anatomic pathology examination of the urinary bladder. Am J Clin Pathol 1994;102:715–723.
19. Murphy WM, Crabtree WN, Jukkola AF, Soloway MS. The diagnostic value of urine versus bladder washing in patients with bladder cancer. J Urol 1981;126:320–322.
20. Renshaw AA, Nappi D, Weinberg DS. Cytology of grade 1 papillary transitional cell carcinoma. A comparison of cytologic, architectural and morphometric criteria in cystoscopically obtained urine. Acta Cytol 1996;40:676–682.
21. Rife CC, Farrow GM, Utz DC. Urine cytology of transitional cell neoplasms. Urol Clin North Am 1979;6:599–612.
22. Shenoy UA, Colby TV, Schumann GB. Reliability of urinary cytodiagnosis in urothelial neoplasms. Cancer 1985;56:2041–2045.
23. Badalament RA, Gay H, Cibas ES, et al. Monitoring endoscopic treatment of superficial bladder carcinoma by postoperative urinary cytology. J Urol 1987;138:760–762.
24. El-Bolkainy MN. Cytology of bladder carcinoma. J Urol 1980;124:20–22.
25. Jordan AM, Weingarten J, Murphy WM. Transitional cell neoplasms of the urinary bladder. Can biologic potential be predicted from histologic grading? Cancer 1987;60:2766–2774 [published erratum appears in Cancer 1988;61:1385].
26. Kannan V, Bose S. Low grade transitional cell carcinoma and instrument artifact: a challenge in urinary cytology. Acta Cytol 1993;37:899–902.
27. Schwalb DM, Herr HW, Fair WR. The management of clinically unconfirmed positive urinary cytology. J Urol 1993;150:1751–1756.
28. Umiker W. Accuracy of cytologic diagnosis of cancer of the urinary tract. Symp Diagn Accur Cytolog Tech 1964;8:186–193.
29. Raab SS, Lenel JC, Cohen MB. Low grade transitional cell carcinoma of the bladder: cytologic diagnosis by key features as identified by logistic regression analysis. Cancer 1994;74:1621–1626.
30. Cohen MB, Egerter DP, Holly EA, et al. Pancreatic adenocarcinoma: regression analysis to identify improved cytologic criteria. Diagn Cytopathol 1991;7:341–345.
31. Prentice RL. Use of the logistic model in retrospective studies. Biometrics 1976;32:599–606.
32. Raab SS, Slagel DD, Jensen CS, et al. Low-grade transitional cell carcinoma of the urinary bladder: application of select cytologic criteria to improve diagnostic accuracy. Mod Pathol 1996;9:225–232.
33. Young RH, Eble JN. Unusual forms of carcinoma of the urinary bladder. Hum Pathol 1991;22:948–965.
34. Highman W, Wilson E. Urine cytology in patients with calculi. J Clin Pathol 1982;35:350–356.
35. Rubben H, Hering F, Dahm HH, Lutzeyer W. Value of exfoliative cytology for differentiation between uric acid stone and tumor of upper urinary tract. Urology 1982;22:571–573.
36. Stella F, Troccoli R, Stella C. Urinary cytologic abnormalities in bone marrow transplant recipients of cyclosporin. Acta Cytol 1987;31:615–619.
37. Stella F, Battistelli S, Marcheggiani F. Urothelial cell changes due to busulfan and cyclophosphamide treatment in bone marrow transplantation. Acta Cytol 2000;34:885–890.

38. Loveless KJ. The effects of radiation upon the cytology of benign and malignant bladder epithelium. Acta Cytol 1973;17:355–360.

39. Coleman DV, Gardner SD, Field AM. Human polyomavirus infection in renal allograft recipients. BMJ 1973;3:371–375.

40. Coleman DV. The cytodiagnosis of human polyomavirus infection. Acta Cytol 1975;19:93–96.

41. Epstein JI, Amin MB, Reuter VR, Mostofi FK. The World Health Organization/International Society of Urological Pathology consensus classification of urothelial (transitional cell) neoplasms of the urinary bladder. Am J Surg Pathol 1998;22:1435–1448.

42. Badalament RA, Kimmel M, Gay H, et al. The sensitivity of flow cytometry compared with conventional cytology in the detection of superficial bladder carcinoma. Cancer 1987;59:2078–2085.

43. Cajulis RS, Haines GK, Frias-Hidvegi D, et al. Cytology, flow cytometry, image analysis, and interphase cytogenetics by fluorescence in situ hybridization in the diagnosis of transitional cell carcinoma in bladder washes: a comparative study. Diagn Cytopathol 1995;13:214–224.

44. Aamoldt RL, Coon JS, Deitch A. Flow cytometric evaluation of bladder cancer: recommendations of the NCI flow cytometry network for bladder cancer. World J Urol 1992;10:63–67.

45. Badalament RA, Hermansen DK, Kimmel M. The sensitivity of bladder wash flow cytometry, bladder wash cytology and voided cytology in the detection of bladder carcinoma. Cancer 1987;60:1423–1427.

46. Casella R, Huber P, Blochlinger A, et al. Urinary level of nuclear matrix protein 22 in the diagnosis of bladder cancer: experience with 130 patients with biopsy confirmed tumor. J Urol 2000;164:1926–1928.

47. Casetta G, Gontero P, Zitella A, et al. BTA quantitative assay and NMP22 testing compared with urine cytology in the detection of transitional cell carcinoma of the bladder. Urol Int 2000;65:100–105.

48. Droller MJ. Improved detection of recurrent bladder cancer using the Bard BTA stat test. J Urol 1998;159:601–602.

49. Ellis WJ, Blumenstein BA, Ishak LM, Enfield DL. Clinical evaluation of the BTA TRAK assay and comparison to voided urine cytology and the Bard BTA test in patients with recurrent bladder tumors. The Multi Center Study Group. Urology 1997;50:882–887.

50. Giannopoulos A, Manousakas T, Mitropoulos D, et al. Comparative evaluation of the BTA stat test, NMP22, and voided urine cytology in the detection of primary and recurrent bladder tumors. Urology 2000;55:871–875.

51. Grocela JA, McDougal WS. Utility of nuclear matrix protein (NMP22) in the detection of recurrent bladder cancer. Urol Clin North Am 2000;27:47–51, viii.

52. Halachmi S, Linn JF, Amiel GE, et al. Urine cytology, tumour markers and bladder cancer. Br J Urol 1998;82:647–654.

53. Heino A, Aaltomaa S, Ala-Opas M. BTA test is superior to voided urine cytology in detecting malignant bladder tumours. Ann Chir Gynaecol 1999;88:304–307.

54. Hughes JH, Katz RL, Rodriguez-Villanueva J, et al. Urinary nuclear matrix protein 22 (NMP22): a diagnostic adjunct to urine cytologic examination for the detection of recurrent transitional-cell carcinoma of the bladder. Diagn Cytopathol 1999;20:285–290.

55. Johnston B, Morales A, Emerson L, Lundie M. Rapid detection of bladder cancer: a comparative study of point of care tests. J Urol 1997;158:2098–2101.

56. Leyh H, Marberger M, Conort P, et al. Comparison of the BTA stat test with voided urine cytology and bladder wash cytology in the diagnosis and monitoring of bladder cancer. Eur Urol 1999;35:52–56.

57. Menendez V, Filella X, Alcover JA, et al. Usefulness of urinary nuclear matrix protein 22 (NMP22) as a marker for transitional cell carcinoma of the bladder. Anticancer Res 2000;20:1169–1172.

58. Miyanaga N, Akaza H, Ishikawa S, et al. Clinical evaluation of nuclear matrix protein 22 (NMP22) in urine as a novel marker for urothelial cancer. Eur Urol 1997;31:163–168.

59. Sarosdy MF, DeVere White RW, Soloway MS, et al. Results of a multicenter trial using the BTA test to monitor for and diagnose recurrent bladder cancer. J Urol 1995;154:379–384.

60. Schamhart DH, de Reijke TM, van der Poel HG, et al. The Bard BTA test: its mode of action, sensitivity and specificity, compared to cytology of voided urine, in the diagnosis of superficial bladder cancer. Eur Urol 1998;34:99–106.

61. Serretta V, Pomara G, Rizzo I, Esposito E. Urinary BTA-stat, BTA-trak and NMP22 in surveillance after TUR of recurrent superficial transitional cell carcinoma of the bladder. Eur Urol 2000;38:419–425.

62. Sozen S, Biri H, Sinik Z, et al. Comparison of the nuclear matrix protein 22 with voided urine cytology and BTA stat test in the diagnosis of transitional cell carcinoma of the bladder. Eur Urol 1999;36:225–229.

63. Mian C, Pycha A, Wiener H, et al. Immunocyt: a new tool for detecting transitional cell carcinoma of the urinary tract. J Urol 1999;161:1486–1489.

64. Hughes JH, Raab SR, Cohen MB. The cytologic diagnosis of low-grade transitional cell carcinoma. Am J Clin Pathol 2000;114:59–67.

65. Ross, JS, Cohen MB. Biomarkers for the detection of bladder cancer. Adv Anat Pathol 2001;8:37–45.

8

INTERSTITIAL CYSTITIS

Sonny L. Johansson, Magnus Fall and Ralph Peeker

PATHOLOGY OF INTERSTITIAL CYSTITIS

Interstitial cystitis (IC) as a descriptive term was first used by A.J. Skene in 1887.[1] However, the ulcer present in the classic subtype was first recognized and described by Guy L. Hunner some 30 years later. Hunner also described the histologic changes of specimens removed from some of his patients as presenting a uniform picture.[2]

A separation of interstitial cystitis into two categories – classic or ulcer type, and non-ulcer or early type – was first done by Messing and Stamey in 1978.[3] The clinical symptoms (which include urgency, frequency and bladder-associated pain with sterile urine) are virtually identical in both groups but display a different cystoscopic picture. When patients are subjected to cystoscopy with bladder distension with a pressure of up to 70–80 cm of H_2O, ulcer patients show single or multiple reddened mucosal areas with small vessels radiating towards a central scar, fibrin deposit or coagulum. This site ruptures with increasing bladder distension, causing petechial oozing of blood from the ulcer and the mucosal margins. Another rather typical finding is slightly bullous edema developing after the distension. In contrast, a non-ulcer patient shows normal bladder mucosa at the initial cystoscopy and, upon the second distension, develops multiple superficial, petechial, strawberry-like hemorrhages generally referred to as glomerulations. Some patients also develop multiple confluent superficial mucosal cracks during the distension.[4,5] It is important to recognize that generally the trigone is not involved in IC.

In 1988, Gillenwater et al. published a summary of the National Institute of Diabetes and Digestive and Kidney Diseases Workshop on Interstitial Cystitis criteria for interstitial cystitis.[6] A number of automatic exclusions are given, as outlined in Table 8.1. Automatic

Table 8.1 Automatic exclusions to the diagnosis of interstitial cystitis

- Less than 18 years old
- Bladder tumor
- Radiation cystitis
- Tuberculous cystitis
- Bacterial cystitis
- Vaginitis
- Cyclophosphamide cystitis
- Symptomatic urethral diverticulum
- Uterine, cervical, vaginal or urethral cancer
- Active herpesvirus infection
- Bladder or lower ureteral calculi
- Waking frequency less than five times in 12 hours
- Nocturia less than two times
- Symptoms relieved by antibiotics, urinary antiseptics or urinary analgesics
- Duration less than 12 months
- Involuntary bladder contractions
- Functional capacities larger than 400 ml
- Absence of sensory urgency

Data from Gillenwater et al.[6]

inclusions include Hunner's ulcer. Positive factors include:

- pain on bladder filling relieved by emptying
- pain (suprapubic, pelvic, ureteral, vaginal or perineal)
- glomerulations on endoscopy
- decreased compliance on cystometrogram.

The true prevalence of IC is unknown but estimates range from 37 to 67 cases per 100,000 individuals. It is a chronic disease with 90% of the patients being female. No current treatments have a significant impact on symptoms with time.[7]

The value of histopathologic examination of biopsies from patients with IC remains somewhat controversial. Some individuals state that histopathologic findings are completely non-specific and of limited value except to rule out carcinoma in situ.[8] Others, including Lynes et al. and ourselves, suggest that histopathologic changes may play a supportive role in the diagnosis. Such changes are helpful in excluding other inflammatory conditions such as eosinophilic cystitis and tuberculous cystitis as well as carcinoma in situ, all of which may have symptoms identical to IC.[5,9] An older, often quoted

study from the Armed Forces Institute of Pathology (AFIP), comprising 28 cases, is of limited value because criteria for inclusion were based on histologic findings and not on clinical and cystoscopic findings. Furthermore, the majority of patients were men and 12 of 14 patients undergoing urine culture showed positive findings. Thus, it is likely that many of the patients suffered from conditions other than IC.[10]

DEMOGRAPHIC AND CLINICAL DESCRIPTIONS OF A SERIES OF PATIENTS WITH IC EXAMINED HISTOLOGICALLY

All patients with IC or verified IC treated at Sahlgrenska University Hospital in Göteborg, Sweden, from 1976 to 1988 were included. The patients were diagnosed according to the National Institutes of Health/National Institute of Diabetes and Digestive and Kidney Diseases (NIH/NIDDK) criteria. Patients diagnosed between 1976 and 1988 were subsequently reassessed to conform to the NIDDK framework.

A total of 210 patients were clinically and cystoscopically evaluated by one of the authors (MF). Evaluation included cystoscopy with bladder distension with a pressure of up to 70 cm of H_2O. All patients underwent cystoscopy with biopsies. The biopsy procedure was usually transurethral resection of the bladder (TURB). Besides resecting the ulcers, biopsies were often taken from normal-appearing bladder mucosa and areas showing glomerulations and/or mucosal cracks. In addition, nine patients with classic disease as well as one non-ulcer patient underwent partial or total cystectomy. Of the 210 patients in the study, 64 had non-ulcer disease and 146 had ulcer-type IC. The ratio of 11 men (6 ulcer and 5 non-ulcer) to 199 women confirms the characteristic female prevalence of this condition. The median age of the patients with classic IC was 57 years (range 27–84 years), whereas the mean age of the 64 patients with the non-ulcer type of IC was 38 years (range 19–71 years). The high number of patients with classic disease is partly related to referral patterns and the fact that the non-ulcer IC condition was not recognized until the early 1980s. In the present Swedish patient population, the ratio between classic and non-ulcer disease is approximately 1:1. This is different from the experience in the US where the majority (approximately 90% of the patients) are reported to be non-ulcer patients.

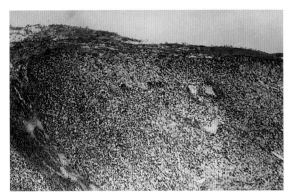

Fig. 8.1 Classic interstitial cystitis with denuded mucosa covered with blood and fibrinous debris. Note the marked inflammatory infiltrate.

Light microscopic findings

Patients with classic IC display striking histologic changes dominated by ulcerations which are often covered by fibrin mixed with inflammatory cells – in particular, neutrophils. The ulcerations are often wedge shaped and involve the superficial part of the lamina propria, sometimes extending to the level of the muscularis mucosa (Fig. 8.1). Underlying granulation tissue is present in almost 90% of the patients (Fig. 8.2, Table 8.2).[11] Interestingly, Hunner described similar findings with regard to the ulcer and granulation tissue formation but he also reported chronic inflammation involving all coats of the bladder.[2] In our experience, that is not usually the case in either the classic or the non-ulcer type of IC. The classic type of IC displays findings similar to ulcerative colitis, i.e. inflammatory changes involving mucosa and lamina propria (submucosa) with little or no change in the detrusor muscle with the exception of perineural infiltrates of lymphocytes (Fig. 8.3) (see also below).

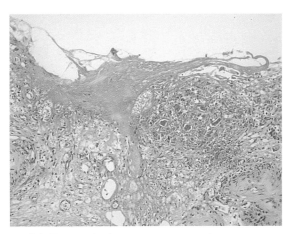

Fig. 8.2 Transurethral resection specimen from a patient with classic interstitial cystitis. Note the wedge-shaped ulceration and completely denuded mucosa covered with fibrinous debris with underlying granulation tissue.

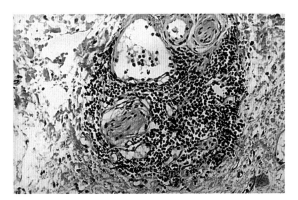

Fig. 8.3 Perineural mononuclear inflammatory infiltrate in a patient with classic interstitial cystitis.

Table 8.2 Histopathologic findings in interstitial cystitis patients

Patient category	Ulcer	Granulation tissue	Mucosal hemorrhage	Mucosal rupture	Mononuclear infiltrate (+)	+	++	+++	Perineural infiltrate
Ulcer (classic; 146 patients)	140 (96%)	130 (89%)	126 (86%)	0	0	16 (11%)	70 (48%)	60 (41%)	118 (81%)
Non-ulcer (early; 64 patients)	0	0	57 (89%)	53 (83%)	49 (77%)	9 (14%)	6 (9%)	0	0

From Johansson SL, Fall M. Pathology of interstitial cystitis. Urol Clin North Am 1994; 21: 55–62.

Hemorrhage and granulation tissue

There is often relatively marked hemorrhage in the lamina propria. The granulation tissue present in approximately 90% of the patients is likely to be caused by rupture of the mucosa during normal filling. There is probably a locus minoris resistentie which ruptures. One study indicates abnormal microvascularity in the lamina propria, especially a reduction of suburothelial blood vessels.[12] More sparsely spaced capillaries may not accommodate bladder distension, resulting in petechial hemorrhage or glomerulations of patients with IC, and possibly also ulceration as a result of ischemia.[12] There is no evidence that the granulation tissue is a result of previous surgical manipulations to the bladder, such as transurethral resection or bladder biopsies. These procedures generally cause non-specific inflammatory changes, collagenous scar or foreign body granuloma, or necrotizing granuloma of the rheumatoid type or pseudosarcoma, the last often referred to as postoperative spindle-cell nodule or inflammatory pseudotumor. Classic IC generally has marked inflammatory changes involving the lamina propria, dominated by lymphocytes, plasma cells, mast cells and neutrophils, especially in association with the ulcer. Eosinophils are absent or very rare. Germinal center formation is frequently seen.

Perineural inflammatory lymphocytic infiltrate

Another prominent finding is the presence of perineural inflammatory lymphocytic infiltrates which can be seen in the deep lamina propria or in the detrusor muscle or fat. This is the main exception to the statement that the inflammatory changes mainly involve the lamina propria in a way similar to ulcerative colitis, which has previously been pointed out by Hand[13] and Bohne et al.[14] Approximately 10% of the classic IC cases had significant fibrosis of the detrusor muscle. We have been unable to confirm the findings of Larsen et al. who described fibrosis with collagen distribution in a characteristic fashion inside the muscle fascicles of the detrusor muscle.[15]

Mucosal denudation, mucosal cracks and glomerulations

Biopsies taken from cystoscopically normal-looking areas often showed mucosal denudation with urothelium floating detached over the surfaces (Fig. 8.4). Frequently there was mucosal denudation even in areas that looked relatively normal endoscopically, a fact that was also pointed out by Hunner in his 1918 paper.[2]

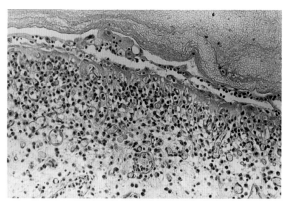

Fig. 8.4 Biopsy of endoscopically normal-appearing bladder mucosa in a patient with classic interstitial cystitis showing detached urothelial cells 'floating' above the surface. Note the marked inflammatory infiltrate in the lamina propria.

Mucosal detachment and denudation are typical findings in classic IC. In non-ulcer patients, mucosal denudation is almost never seen. However, dense mucosal cracks are abundant in non-ulcer disease. Mucosal cracks are very rare in control patients. Lynes et al. proposed that denudation is probably a result of instrumentation; however, the urothelium in IC patients seems to detach very easily and may be less cohesive than normal urothelium.[9]

In spite of the fact that classic IC patients and non-ulcer-type IC patients have virtually identical clinical symptoms (including urgency, frequency and pain), the light microscopic findings in non-ulcer patients are quite meager. The majority of patients display suburothelial hemorrhages corresponding to glomerulations (Fig. 8.5). In most cases, hemorrhages are relatively subtle although occasionally they can be more marked. However, in a recent paper, Waxman et al. reported that glomerulations are, in fact, as common in control patients as in non-ulcer patients.[16] Another frequently seen finding was mucosal ruptures or mucosal cracks present in more than 80% of the patients (Fig. 8.6). These mucosal cracks were generally very superficial with involvement of the upper part of the lamina propria. They were not associated with increased inflammatory infiltrate and, overall, inflammatory changes in patients with a non-ulcer disease are mild or absent. We are convinced that the mucosal cracks are real and not artifacts since we have not detected these lesions in 30 carefully studied control patients subjected to the same treatment as the IC patients. Most likely the cracks develop as a result of a weakness in the urothelial lining.

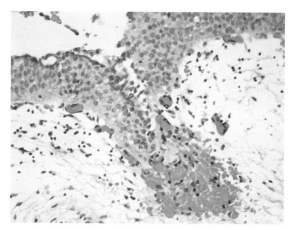

Fig. 8.5 Biopsy from a non-ulcer interstitial cystitis patient with suburothelial hemorrhage corresponding to glomerulation. Note the early mucosal crack and mild chronic inflammation.

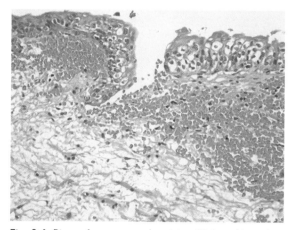

Fig. 8.6 Biopsy from a non-ulcer interstitial cystitis patient with mucosal crack and associated suburothelial hemorrhage (corresponding to glomerulation).

Increased vascularity and dilatation of the vasculature of the lamina propria is a frequent finding, both in classic IC patients and in non-ulcer-type IC patients, but can also be seen in some control patients: this may possibly be related to the instrumentation procedure as suggested by Lynes et al.[9]

IC subtypes and their differences

Some 18 years ago, the subdivision of patients into classic and non-ulcer IC seldom occurred whereas during the last 14 years, the literature is generously endowed with articles on IC, where this subdivision is recognized. The differences between the two subtypes include clinical presentation and age distribution and

this has been demonstrated in several series.[4,17] There has been no single report by any author on progression from IC without ulcer to classic IC, a fact which has been emphasized by several authors.[18] Besides expressing different histopathologic, immunologic and neurobiologic features, the two subtypes also respond differently to a variety of treatments.[19–23]

Diagnostic investigation of IC

TURB has been performed on almost all the Swedish patients with IC and is resulting in excellent diagnostic material. In many countries, including the United States, most patients with suspected IC are subjected to forceps or cold cup biopsies. During the past 10 years, biopsy material from 97 patients with a suspected or established diagnosis of IC has been evaluated at the University of Nebraska Medical Center by one of the authors (SLJ). The patients were either seen at the university and biopsied there, or were seen elsewhere and the histopathologic material sent in consultation. Of the 97 patients, 86 underwent cold cup or forceps biopsies, 8 partial or total cystectomy and 3 patients underwent TURB. Material was obtained from 49 individuals with a diagnosis of non-ulcer IC (46 women and 3 men, mean age 39 years, range 19–73), 24 patients with classic IC (20 women and 4 men, mean age 59 years, range 22–86) and 24 patients either without diagnostic abnormality or where another diagnosis was identified (19 women and 5 men, mean age 57 years, range 22–81). Eleven of these patients had no diagnostic abnormality in the bladder biopsies and those patients with normal findings may or may not have had a non-ulcer IC. Interestingly, these patients had a 10-year higher mean age than the patients with both clinical cystoscopic and microscopic findings of non-ulcer IC.

The main differential diagnosis seemed to be eosinophilic cystitis which was diagnosed in 8 patients (4 men and 4 women). They had a mean age of 60 years, similar to patients with the classic type of IC. Clinically, the symptoms may be indistinguishable from those of IC. However, the bladder is often thickened due to the fact that eosinophilic cystitis is a true pancystitis, with inflammatory changes often extending into the perivesicular fat. Detrusor muscle necrosis is frequently present and, as the name implies, there are a significant number of eosinophils present.[24,25] Of the remaining 5 patients in whom another diagnosis was identified, 2 had bacterial cystitis, 1 had carcinoma in situ and 1 had been treated with intravesical chemotherapy for bladder cancer and developed marked fibrosis of the lamina propria. The final patient with a clinical suspicion of IC was found to have cystitis glandularis. Tuberculosis of the urinary bladder is an additional condition that can clinically simulate IC.

Ultrastructural studies

Few ultrastructural studies have been performed on IC patients. Collan et al., in a transmission electron microscopic study, were unable to find any morphologic abnormalities.[26] Eldrup and colleagues reported on differences in the permeability of the urothelium between IC patients and controls, possibly related to defects in the tight junctions.[27] Dixon et al. reported on variations in the thickness of the glycosaminoglycan layer (glycocalyx). The difference appeared to be related to the surface topography of the luminal cells and there were no differences in the variability between IC patients and controls.[28] Following their transmission electron microscopy study, Said et al. reported widening of the intercellular spaces between the urothelial cells in all layers of the epithelium.[29] They also reported on the presence of microvilli.

Using scanning electron microscopy, we studied 13 classic IC patients and 9 control patients and found that the proportion of cells covered by round, uniform and pleomorphic microvilli was higher in the IC patients than in the controls. The IC patients also had a reduced mucin layer.[30] The presence of microvilli, which initially was thought to be associated with neoplasia or pre-neoplasia, is now considered to be a response that develops in conditions with increased cell turnover, for example inflammatory conditions such as catheter-associated polypoid cystitis.[31]

In contrast to what is previously stated about lack of diagnostic positive histopathologic signs in non-ulcer IC, Elbadawi and Light concluded that ultrastructural changes appear to be sufficiently distinctive to be diagnostic in specimens submitted for pathologic confirmation of non-ulcer IC. In their detailed ultrastructural study on patients with non-ulcer IC, a distinctive combination of peculiar muscle cell profiles, injury of intrinsic vessels and nerves in muscularis and suburothelium, and discohesive urothelium was observed in lesional and less markedly in non-lesional samples of all specimens. Marked edema of various tissue elements and cells appeared to be a common denominator of many observed changes. Urothelial changes disrupted the true permeability barrier. Neural changes included a combination of degenerative and regenerative features.[32]

Uroplakins

Specific urothelial proteins named uroplakins have been isolated from the asymmetric unit membrane (AUM) of bovine urothelium. Distinct proteins (uroplakin 1a, 1b, 2 and 3) have been characterized. Monospecific polyclonal antibodies to these proteins have demonstrated that all of them are associated with AUM.[33] AUM is typical of the mammalian bladder and is considered to be important in strengthening the cohesiveness of the urothelial surface areas and preventing the urothelial cells from separating during bladder distension. We performed a preliminary study and evaluated 16 classic IC patients (mean age 61 years, range 32–77), 11 non-ulcer patients (mean age 36 years, range 20–29) and 6 controls (mean age 44 years, range 26–52) by immune histochemical examination. The antibody used has been shown to react strongly with uroplakin 3, moderately with uroplakins 1a and 1b and weakly with uroplakin 2. The classic IC patients were generally negative, with the exception of a few positive urothelial cells which were found floating above the surface. It is possible that the negative findings could be associated with ulceration and mucosal denudation. However, even when there was some urothelium present, the staining was generally negative.

We cannot exclude the possibility that the reduced uroplakin expression in classic IC patients could be related to the higher age of these patients. AUM becomes reduced in number with increasing age. The non-ulcer patients all had positive staining of their urothelium with one exception. The staining was discontinuous, which may be due to detachment of some superficial cells or as a result of focal breakdown of AUM (Fig. 8.7). The possibility of changes as a result of artifacts cannot be completely ruled out and additional studies are needed. Interestingly, all six control patients had a continuous positive staining (Fig. 8.8).

Mast cells

The etiology of IC remains elusive. Allergic type 1 reactions and drug hypersensitivity were previously reported in IC patients.[13,34] The presence of detrusor mastocytosis is suggestive of an activation of the mast cell system in IC.[14,35] Evidence of mast cell secretion is supported by electron microscopic studies as well as from the findings of histamine and mast cell proteinase tryptase in bladder washings and voided urine from such patients.[36–38] Using histochemical methods, we have found increased mast cells in IC and evidence of

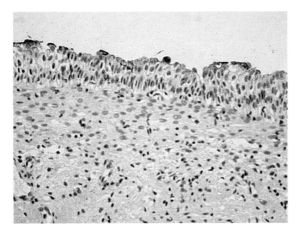

Fig. 8.7 Discontinuous superficial uroplakin staining in a 37-year-old non-ulcer patient. (From Johansson SL, Ogawa K, Fall M: The pathology of interstitial cystitis. In: Interstitial Cystitis, Sant G (ed.). Lippincott Raven, New York, 1997; 143–151.)

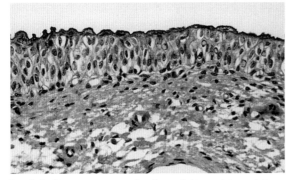

Fig. 8.8 Continuous superficial uroplakin staining of the umbrella cells in a 46-year-old control patient. (From Johansson SL, Ogawa K, Fall M. The pathology of intersitial cystitis. In: Interstitial Cystitis, Sant G (ed). Lippincott Raven, New York, 1997; 143–151.)

mast cell heterogeneity. Mast cells with a typical appearance of connective tissue mast cells were increased in number in the detrusor muscle while mucosal mast cells were increased in the lamina propria.[5,35] In a recent study, classic IC patients displayed a six- to ten-fold increase in mast cells identified by their proteinase content, whereas in non-ulcer IC patients there were twice as many mast cells as in control patients.[39] In contrast to non-ulcer IC controls, classic IC patients had an abundance of intraepithelial mast cells.

Classic IC patients co-expressed stem cell factor and interleukin-6 (IL-6) in the urothelium and displayed numerous stem cell factor and IL-6 positive cells in the detrusor muscle, many of which were mast cells.

Redistribution of mast cells in the urothelium and a high bladder wall mast cell density distinguished classic IC from non-ulcer IC. These findings suggest a stem cell factor and IL-6-driven mast cell response in IC and a downregulation of the stem cell factor.[40] A similar mast cell response has been described in nephrogenic metaplasia.[41]

Although many of the symptoms and findings in classic IC (e.g. pain, frequency, edema and fibrosis) could be explained by an increased number of mast cells, release of mast cell-derived factors and the cause of increased mast cell numbers remain unclear. In particular, in non-ulcer IC, damage to the peripheral nerve supply to the urinary bladder and possibly subsequent reinnervation is a potential pathogenetic mechanism. Sprouting of nerve fibers has been described and, in particular, an increase in the sympathetic outflow of patients with IC.[42,43] Furthermore, altered levels of S-100 protein were found in non-ulcer IC patients as compared to controls, and this is consistent with an altered pattern of innervation of the bladder.[44]

In a recent study, we found a prominent increase in tyrosine hydroxylase (the rate-limiting enzyme in catecholamine synthesis) in bladder tissue from patients with classic as well as non-ulcer IC as compared to controls.[45] This finding is interesting in the light of a recent report on increased tyrosine hydroxylase immune reactivity in the locus coeruleus of cats with IC.[46] This may be interpreted as a sign of a general increase in sympathetic outflow.

Mast cell recruitment and maturation may possibly be induced by different mechanisms in the two subtypes of IC. Thus, the non-ulcer type may be associated with neurally induced recruitment and maturation while the classic subtype may be associated with an inflammatory or autoimmune mast cell process. These findings also support the premise that IC is a syndrome rather than a specific disease. Thus, although mast cells are increased in both types of IC, specific staining and counting of mast cells are not needed in the routine evaluation of bladder biopsies from IC patients.

An additional theory is that the pathogenesis of IC involves an alteration of the mucin coat of the bladder lining which affects its permeability. The mucin is, in part, composed of glycosaminoglycans (GAG layer). An alteration in this mucin coat would allow noxious solutes present in the urine to irritate the bladder wall.[47] A specific protein, GP51, has been isolated from bladder mucosa and seems to be associated with antibacterial effects in the bladder. Immunohistochemical examination of bladder biopsies from IC patients and controls revealed decreased expression in some IC patients.[48] In a recent study of 36 patients with IC and 23 controls, low GP51 levels were identified in the IC patients as compared with controls: this is the strongest evidence so far reported that a specific molecular deficiency in the GAG layer exists in patients with IC.[49]

Autoimmunity and IC

IC is a chronic condition that is often associated with exacerbations, remissions and relapses which, in combination with the fact that the patients are predominantly women, has championed the idea that an immune mechanism (especially autoimmunity) is involved in the etiology. Thus, there are numerous reports on antibodies in patients with IC.[34,50–54] In a study of 47 IC patients, Mattila et al. found immune deposits in the vessel walls of 33 patients.[55] In a subsequent study, electron microscopy evidence of endothelial injury was found in 14 of 20 IC patients.[56]

Independent studies of autoantibodies in IC have shown that they mainly consist of antinuclear antibodies and these findings are similar to the autoantibody profiles in some systemic diseases such as systemic lupus erythematosus and Sjögren's syndrome, both of which are known to be of autoimmune origin.[51,53,56,57] Thus, the role of autoimmunity in IC is controversial and there is no evidence to support the theory that this disease is caused by a direct autoimmune attack on the bladder. It seems likely that some of the autoimmune reactions and pathologic findings in IC occur as a secondary result of bladder tissue destruction and inflammation from other (as yet unknown) causes. In addition, classic IC symptoms generally disappear after urinary diversion without cystectomy, whereas this is not always the case in non-ulcer disease, a condition with few immunologic changes but rather demonstrable alterations in the nervous system consistent with the notion of a primary neurogenic etiology. This, in conjunction with a report of occurrence of IC-like changes following colocystoplasty, mitigates an immune mechanism as a sole explanation.[58]

The fact that there is a chronic inflammatory response in IC makes the possibility of cell-mediated autoimmune response possible. We studied 24 classic IC patients, 9 non-ulcer patients and 10 controls. The classic IC patients displayed aggregates of T cells as well as B-cell nodules with focal germinal centers. There was a decreased or normal helper/suppressor ratio and suppressor cytotoxic cells were present in the germinal center. The non-ulcer group, in contrast, had only slightly increased numbers of lymphoid cells dominated by T-helper cells with occasional T-cell aggregates. No B-cell nodules were identified and plasma cells were rare. Interestingly, the non-ulcer patients did not differ significantly from the control group. We also studied the peripheral blood flow cytometry and found an increased number of secretory IgM+ B cells and activated lymphocytes in the non-ulcer group within a mildly abnormal kappa/lambda ratio. Activated lymphocytes were identified in the ulcer group.[59] The control group displayed no such changes, and thus there is some evidence for the role of an immunologic mechanism in the physiology of interstitial cystitis.

Pathogenetic complexity

In recent years, several reports have indicated that the etiology of IC is probably more complex than has previously been anticipated. In fact, it has been proposed that IC is a neuroimmunoendocrine disorder and Theoharides et al. have shown that activation of mast cells in close proximity to nerve terminals can be influenced by estradiol as well as corticotropin-releasing hormone.[60] Moreover, Okragly et al. found elevated levels of tryptase, nerve growth factor, neurotrophin-3 and glial cell line-derived neurotrophic factor in IC as compared to controls.[61] These findings indicate that the pathogenesis in IC may include interactions between the peripheral nervous system, the immune system and hormone release from different endocrine systems at varying levels.

As previously mentioned, we proposed that the distribution of mast cells into the epithelium in classic IC could be explained by the epithelial co-expression of stem cell factor and IL-6.[39,40] What could possibly cause an IL-6 overexpression in IC epithelium? Abdel-Mageed et al. have previously demonstrated an increased expression of p65, a nuclear factor-kappa B (NF-κB) subunit, in patients with IC.[62] Interestingly, these authors have also detected a five-fold increase in the expression of the gene for IL-6 after NF-κB activation, indicating that intricate systems on cytokine gene expression level may be operating in IC.[63]

Nitric oxide and interstitial cystitis

Nitric oxide (NO) is a free radical gas synthesized from L-arginine by a family of isoenzymes called nitric oxide synthase (NOS). NO is an important biological mediator and cell signalling molecule that plays various roles in physiology and pathophysiology and, furthermore, functions as a mediator in smooth muscle relaxation as well as in neurotransmission and vasodilatation.[64] Evidence has accumulated that nitric oxide plays an important role in the regulation of micturition[65] and, moreover, regulation of urinary nitric oxide synthase activity has been proposed to be of importance for immunologic responses in IC.[66,67]

In a recent paper, comprising 17 IC patients, all patients with classic IC had high or very high levels of NO whereas none of the nonulcer patients had any significant increase in NO levels in their bladder. The NO level in classic IC patients was not in relation to the symptoms but rather to the assignment to this specific subgroup of IC. However, the stage of the disease seemed to influence the NO levels. On the other hand, the level of efficacy of different treatments like DMSO or transurethral resection did not seem to have any correlation to the NO levels. Thus, in patients free of symptoms NO levels were still elevated. The highest levels of NO were found in patients in the initial phase of classic IC.[68]

It has been advocated that cystoscopy is crucial for adequate subtyping of IC patients. Perhaps, NO-measurements may be a sufficient substitute for cystoscopy. Catheterization is a less invasive and less bothersome diagnostic procedure than cystoscopy, which in this group of patients requires general anesthesia to be conclusive. Even if cystoscopy is performed, classic disease may be overlooked due to inability to recognize the so called Hunner's ulcer, a lesion that may be more or less prominent, in the latter case sometimes requiring a lot of experience to identify. NO-measurements, however, could easily be performed in a standardized fashion by any clinician, allowing for correct subtyping of IC patients.

CONCLUSION

More than 30 years ago, Hanash and Pool wrote the following about IC: 'The cause is unknown, the diagnosis is difficult and the treatment is temporary and palliative', a statement which, to a significant degree, is still accurate today.[64] We can, from cystoscopic and histopathologic findings, identify classic and non-ulcer disease but the data indicate that we are dealing with a syndrome rather than a specific disease and additional research to clarify etiology and pathogenesis is needed.

The cystoscopic findings are crucial to the assignment to the different categories and the use of the NIH/NIDDK guidelines is helpful in excluding IC-like conditions with different etiologies such as carcinoma in situ, bacterial or radiation-induced cystitis. Recent observations suggest a different pathogenesis for the two subtypes of IC and, hence, it appears to be of the utmost importance to separate the two entities, both when formulating therapeutic strategies and when analyzing and comparing scientific materials.

REFERENCES

1. Skene AJC. Diseases of Bladder and Urethra in Women. New York: Wm Wood, 1887, p 167.
2. Hunner GL. Elusive ulcer of the bladder: further notes on a rare type of bladder ulcer, with a report of twenty-five cases. Am J Obstet 1918;78:374–395.
3. Messing EM, Stamey TA. Interstitial cystitis: early diagnosis, pathology and treatment. Urology 1978;12:381–392.
4. Fall M, Johansson SL, Aldenborg F. Chronic interstitial cystitis: a heterogeneous syndrome. J Urol 1987;137(1):35–38.
5. Johansson SL, Fall M. Clinical features and spectrum of light microscopic changes in interstitial cystitis. J Urol 1990;143:1118–1124.
6. Gillenwater JY, Wein AJ. Summary of the National Institute of Diabetes and Digestive and Kidney Diseases Workshop on Interstitial Cystitis, National Institutes of Health, Bethesda, Maryland; August 28–29, 1987. J Urol 1988;140:203–206.
7. Propert KJ, Schaeffer AL, Brensinger CM, et al. A prospective study of interstitial cystitis: results of longitudinal follow-up of the interstitial cystitis database cohort. J Urol 2000;163:1434–1439.
8. Messing EM. The diagnosis of interstitial cystitis. Urology 1987;(Suppl.):4–7.
9. Lynes WL, Flynn SD, Shortliffe LD, et al. The histology of interstitial cystitis. Am J Surg Pathol 1990;14:969–976.
10. Smith B, Dehner LP. Chronic ulcerating interstitial cystitis. A study of 28 cases. Arch Pathol 1972;93:76–81.
11. Johansson SL, Ogawa K, Fall M. The pathology of interstitial cystitis. In: Sant G (ed.) Interstitial Cystitis. Philadelphia: Lippincott Raven, 1997, pp 143–151.
12. Rosamilia A, Cann L, Dwyer P, et al. Bladder microvascularity in women with interstitial cystitis. J Urol 1999;161:1865–1870.
13. Hand JR. Interstitial cystitis. Report of 223 cases (204 women and 19 men). J Urol 1949;61:291–310.
14. Bohne AW, Hodson JM, Rebuck JW, et al. An abnormal leukocyte response in interstitial cystitis. J Urol 1962;88:387–391.
15. Larsen S, Thompson SA, Hald T, et al. Mast cells in interstitial cystitis. Br J Urol 1982;54:283–286.
16. Waxman JA, Sulak PJ, Kuehl TJ. Cystoscopic findings consistent with interstitial cystitis in normal women undergoing tubal ligation. J Urol 1998;160(5):1663–1667.
17. Koziol JA, Adams HP, Frutos A. Discrimination between the ulcerous and the non-ulcerous forms of interstitial cystitis by non-invasive findings. J Urol 1996;155(1):87–90.

18. Lechevallier E. Interstitial cystitis. Prog Urol 1995;5(1):21–30.

19. Fall M. Conservative management of chronic interstitial cystitis: transcutaneous electrical nerve stimulation and transurethral resection. J Urol 1985;133:774–778.

20. Fall M, Lindström S. Transcutaneous electrical nerve stimulation in classic and non-ulcer interstitial cystitis. Urol Clin North Am 1994;21(1):131–139.

21. Fritjofsson A, Fall M, Juhlin R, et al. Treatment of ulcer and non-ulcer interstitial cystitis with sodium pentosanpolysulfate. A multicenter trial. J Urol 1987;138(3):508–512.

22. Hanno PM. Amitriptyline in the treatment of interstitial cystitis. Urol Clin North Am 1994;21(1):89–91.

23. Peeker R, Aldenborg F, Fall M. The treatment of interstitial cystitis with supratrigonal cystectomy and ileocystoplasty: difference in outcome between classic and non-ulcer disease. J Urol 1998;159(5):1479–1482.

24. Hellstrom HR, Davis BK, Shonnard JW. Eosinophilic cystitis. A study of 15 cases. Am J Clin Pathol 1979;72:777–784.

25. Johansson SL, Smout MS, Taylor RJ. Eosinophilic cystitis associated with symptomatic ureteral involvement. A report of two cases. J Urol Pathol 1993;1:69–71.

26. Collan Y, Alfthan O, Kivilaakso E, Oravisto KJ. Electron microscopic and histological findings on urinary bladder epithelium in interstitial cystitis. Eur Urol 1976;2:242–247.

27. Eldrup J, Thorup J, Nielsen SL, et al. Permeability and ultrastructure of human bladder epithelium. Br J Urol 1983;55:488–492.

28. Dixon JS, Holm-Bentzen M, Gilpin CJ, et al. Electron microscopic investigation of the bladder urothelium and glycocalyx in patients with interstitial cystitis. J Urol 1986;135:621–625.

29. Said JW, Van De Velde R, Gillespie L. Immunopathology of interstitial cystitis. Mod Pathol 1989;2:593–602.

30. Anderström C, Fall M, Johansson SL. Scanning electronmicroscopy in interstitial cystitis. Br J Urol 1989;63:270–275.

31. Anderström C, Ekelund P, Hansson HA, Johansson SL. Scanning electron microscopy of polypoid cystitis, a reversible lesion of the human urinary bladder. J Urol 1984;131:242–246.

32. Elbadawi A, Light JK. Distinctive ultrastructural pathology of non-ulcerative interstitial cystitis. Urol Int 1996;56:137–162.

33. Wu X-R, Lin JH, Walz T. Mammalian uroplakins, a group of highly conserved urothelial differentiation-related membrane proteins. J Biol Chem 1994;269:13716–13724.

34. Oravisto KJ. Interstitial cystitis as an autoimmune disease. A review. Eur Urol 1980;6:10–13.

35. Kastrup J, Hald J, Larsen L. Histamine content and mast cell count of detrusor muscle in patients with interstitial cystitis. Br J Urol 1983;5:495–500.

36. Aldenborg F, Fall M, Enerbäck L. Proliferation and transepithelial migration of mucosal mast cells in interstitial cystitis. Immunology 1986;8:411–416.

37. Letourneau R, Pang X, Sant GR, Theoharides TC. Intragranular activation of bladder mast cells and their association with nerve processes in interstitial cystitis. Br J Urol 1996;77:41–54.

38. Boucher W, el-Mansoury M, Pang X, et al. Elevated mast cell tryptase in the urine of patients with interstitial cystitis. Br J Urol 1995;76:94–100.

39. Lundeberg T, Liedberg H, Norling L, et al. Interstitial cystitis: correlation with nerve fibres, mast cells and histamine. Br J Urol 1993;71:427–429.

40. Peeker R, Enerbäck L, Fall M, Aldenborg F. Recruitment, distribution and phenotypes of mast cells in interstitial cystitis. J Urol 2000;163:1009–1015.

41. Aldenborg F, Peeker R, Fall M, et al. Metaplastic transformation of urinary bladder epithelium. Effect on mast cell recruitment, distribution and phenotype expression. Am J Pathol 1998;153:149–157.

42. Christmas TJ, Rode J, Chapple CR, et al. Nerve fibre proliferation in interstitial cystitis. Virchows Arch [A] Pathol Anat 1990;416:447–451.

43. Hohenfeller M, Nunes L, Schmidt RA, et al. Interstitial cystitis: increased sympathetic innervation and related neuropeptide synthesis. J Urol 1992;147:587–591.

44. Peeker R, Aldenborg F, Haglid K, et al. Decreased levels of S-100 protein in nonulcer interstitial cystitis. Scand J Urol Nephrol 1998;32:395–398.

45. Peeker R, Aldenborg F, Johansson SL, et al. Increased tyrosine hydroxylase immunoreactivity in bladder tissue from patients with classic and nonulcer interstitial cystitis. J Urol 2000;163:112–115.

46. Reche A, Buffington CA. Increased tyrosine hydroxylase immunoreactivity in the locus coeruleus of cats with interstitial cystitis. J Urol 1998;159:1045–1048.

47. Parsons CL, Lilly J, Stein P. Epithelial dysfunction in non-bacterial cystitis (interstitial cystitis). J Urol 1991;145:732–735.

48. Moskowitz MO, Shupp Byrne D, Callahan HJ, et al. Decreased expression of a glycoprotein component of bladder surface mucin (GP51) in interstitial cystitis. J Urol 1994;151:343–347.

49. Shupp Byrne D, Sedor JF, Estojak J, et al. The urinary glycoprotein GP51 as a clinical marker for interstitial cystitis. J Urol 1999;161:1786–1799.

50. Silk MR. Bladder antibodies in interstitial cystitis. J Urol 1970;103:307–309.

51. Jokinen EJ, Alfthan OS, Oravisto KJ. Antitissue antibodies in interstitial cystitis. Clin Exp Immunol 1972;11:333–339.

52. Anderson JB, Parivar F, Lee G, et al. The enigma of interstitial cystitis – an autoimmune disease? Br J Urol 1989;63:58–63.

53. Ochs RL, Stein F Jr, Peebles CL, et al. Autoantibodies in interstitial cystitis. J Urol 1994;151:587–592.

54. Mattila J. Vascular immunopathology in interstitial cystitis. Clin Immunol Immunopathol 1982;23:648–655.

55. Mattila J, Pitkanen R, Vaalasti T. Fine-structural evidence for vascular injury in patients with interstitial cystitis. Virchows Arch 1983;398:347–355.

56. Tan EM. Antinuclear antibodies: diagnostic markers for autoimmune diseases and probes for cell biology. Adv Immunol 1989;44:93–151.

57. Von Mühlen CA, Tan EM. Autoantibodies in the diagnosis of systemic rheumatic diseases. Semin Arthritis Rheum 1995;24:323–358.

58. McGuire ES, Lytton B, Carnog SL. Interstitial cystitis following colocystoplasty. Urology 1973;2:28–29.

59. Harrington DS, Johansson SL, Fall M. Interstitial cystitis: an immune histological and cytofluorimetric analysis of bladder mucosa and peripheral blood. J Urol 1990;44:868–871.

60. Theoharides TC, Pang X, Letourneau R, Sant GR. Interstitial cystitis: a neuroimmunoendocrine disorder. Ann N Y Acad Sci 1998;840:619–634.

61. Okragly AJ, Niles AL, Saban R, et al. Elevated tryptase, nerve growth factor, neurotrophin-3 and glial cell line-derived neurotrophic factor levels in the urine of interstitial cystitis and bladder cancer patients. J Urol 1999;161(2):438–441, discussion 441–442.

62. Abdel-Mageed AB, Ghoniem GM. Potential role of Rel/nuclear factor-kappa B in the pathogenesis of interstitial cystitis. J Urol 1998;160(6 Pt 1):2000–2003.

63. Abdel-Mageed AB, Ghoniem G, Human L, Agrawal KC. Induction of proinflammatory cytokine gene expression by NF-kappa B in human bladder epithelial (t-24) cells: possible mechanism for interstitial cystitis. J Urol 1999;161 (Suppl. 4):26.

64. Moncada S, Higgs A. The L-arginine-nitric oxide pathway. N Engl J Med 1993;329:2002–2012.

65. Andersson KE. Neurotransmitters and neuroreceptors in the lower urinary tract. Curr Opin Obstet Gynecol 1996;8:361–365.

66. Smith SD, Wheeler MA, Foster H, Jr. et al. Urinary nitric oxide synthase activity and cyclic GMP levels are decreased with interstitial cystitis and increased with urinary tract infections. J Urol 1996;155:1432–1435.

67. Lundberg JO, Ehren L, Jansson O, et al. Elevated nitric oxide in the urinary bladder in infectious and noninfectious cystitis. Urology 1996;48:700–702.

68. Logadottir Y, Ehren I, Fall M, et al. Intravesical nitric oxide production discriminates between classic and nonulcer interstitial cystitis. J Urol 2004;171(3):1148–1150.

69. Hanash KA, Pool TL. Interstitial cystitis in men. J Urol 1969;102:427–428.

9

AN INTRODUCTION TO THE WHO/ISUP CONSENSUS CLASSIFICATION OF UROTHELIAL LESIONS OF THE URINARY BLADDER

Stephen J. Cina, Rolando A. Milord and Jonathan I. Epstein

INTRODUCTION

For decades the terminology applied to the various reactive, pre-neoplastic and neoplastic lesions of the urinary bladder has been confusing. A single slide depicting flat urothelium with mild hyperchromasia, increased nuclear size and architectural unrest could be sent to several experts resulting in a smorgasbord of diagnoses including 'dysplasia', 'reactive atypia', 'mild urothelial atypia' and 'carcinoma in situ, grade I'. Similarly, a papillary lesion which might be considered a papilloma in the classification schemes promulgated by Murphy[1] and Bergkvist et al.[2] could have been diagnosed as a papillary transitional cell carcinoma, grade I/III, in the previous World Health Organization (WHO) grading system[3] or as a papillary carcinoma grade I/IV in the Broders/Ash classification.[4,5] The impact on practicing pathologists, oncologists and urologists was obvious and disconcerting. In the best of circumstances, clinicians could feel comfortable with the diagnoses rendered by their own hospital pathologists. In other instances, however, under- or overtreatment could result from actions based on the wording employed by a pathologist at an outside institution.

In addition to the potential for problems with clinical management, disparity in the nomenclature of bladder lesions rendered interinstitutional research problematic, made collection of accurate cancer statistics difficult, and caused difficulties in interpreting the urological literature at the local level. As the evidence mounted linking the grade of flat and papillary urothelial lesions with prognosis, it became apparent that a consensus classification scheme for the reactive, pre-neoplastic and neoplastic lesions of the bladder was becoming a necessity.

The initial steps toward a revised classification system were taken in October 1997 when Dr F.K. Mostofi assembled a group of pathologists, oncologists, urologists and basic scientists sharing a common interest in bladder neoplasia. The attendees were tasked with reviewing currently employed terminology for bladder neoplasia and making recommendations to the WHO Committee on urothelial tumors. Several months later, at the 1998 meeting of the United States and Canadian Academy of Pathologists, a second group, composed predominantly of members of the International Society of Urologic Pathologists (ISUP), further debated the existing terminology and eventually arrived at a consensus statement. The WHO/ISUP consensus classification of urothelial (transitional cell) neoplasms of the urinary bladder was published in a leading pathology journal in late 1998 (Table 9.1).[6] Since then, efforts have been made to propagate this system in order to establish a single language that may be spoken by urologists, pathologists, oncologists and basic scientists throughout the medical world.

DESCRIPTION OF ENTITIES

The WHO/ISUP classification scheme favors the use of 'urothelial' over 'transitional' in describing the epithelium lining the bladder. Since so-called 'transitional' mucosa may be seen in several anatomic sites including the female genital tract, sinonasal region and anorectal zone, it was felt that 'urothelial' was a more specific descriptor for lesions of the lower urinary tract. It is acceptable, however, to use 'transitional' in lieu of 'urothelial' within this system. As always, it is of paramount importance that the pathologist chooses the modifier that will be best understood by the local community. Further, for this reason, when introducing the WHO/ISUP system to a new community, it may be advisable either to discuss the diagnosis with the referring urologist or to include a comment that will roughly equate the diagnosis with a previously employed system (Table 9.2). It should be emphasized that exact translation between WHO/ISUP diagnoses and diagnoses from prior systems is neither intended nor entirely accurate.

Normal urothelium

By virtue of the normal physiologic role of the kidneys and the nature of the contents stored by the urinary bladder, it is readily apparent that the urothelium is routinely exposed to a variety of toxins and other inhospitable substances. Thus, it should be no surprise that a slight degree of architectural unrest falls within the spectrum of 'normal' (Fig. 9.1). For years there has been a tendency to diagnose 'dysplasia' in urothelium showing even the slightest disorder; this may result in desensitization on the part of the urologist with a subsequent muted response to a truly worrisome preneoplastic diagnosis. The consensus group, therefore, determined that urothelium with mild architectural disorder but benign cytologic features should be diagnosed as 'benign urothelium' rather than mild dysplasia. A recent study demonstrated a negligible proliferative index and essentially no p53 positivity in most benign urothelium.[7] In one case, however, 29% of benign urothelial cells overexpressed p53; interestingly, there was concurrent high-grade intraurothelial neoplasia (carcinoma in situ (CIS), see below) elsewhere in the bladder.

Table 9.1 WHO/ISUP consensus classification system

- Normal
  - normal*
- Hyperplasia
  - flat hyperplasia
  - papillary hyperplasia
- Flat lesions with atypia
  - reactive (inflammatory) atypia
  - atypia of unknown significance
  - dysplasia (low-grade squamous intraurothelial neoplasia)
  - carcinoma in situ (high-grade squamous intraurothelial neoplasia)†
- Papillary neoplasms
  - papilloma
  - papillary neoplasm of low malignant potential
  - papillary carcinoma, low-grade
  - papillary carcinoma, high-grade
- Invasive neoplasms
  - lamina propria invasion
  - muscularis propria (detrusor muscle) invasion

* Includes cases formerly diagnosed as 'mild dysplasia'.
† Includes cases formerly diagnosed as 'severe dysplasia' .
Reproduced with permission from Epstein et al.[6]

Table 9.2 Comparison of WHO/ISUP diagnoses of papillary urothelial lesions with other systems

WHO/ISUP	Previous WHO	Murphy[1]	Broders[5]/Ash[4]
Papilloma	Papilloma	Papilloma	Some carcinoma, grade I/IV
LMP	Most grade I/III	Some papilloma	Most carcinoma, grade I/IV
		Some carcinoma, low grade	Some grade II/IV
PAP CA LG	Some grade I/III	Most carcinoma, low grade	Most grade II/IV
	Most grade II/III		Some carcinoma, grade III/IV
PAP CA HG	Carcinoma, grade III/III	Carcinoma, high grade	Most grade III/IV
	Some carcinoma, grade II/III		Carcinoma, grade IV/IV

LMP, papillary neoplasm of low malignant potential; PAP CA HG, papillary urothelial carcinoma, high grade; PAP CA LG, papillary urothelial carcinoma, low grade.

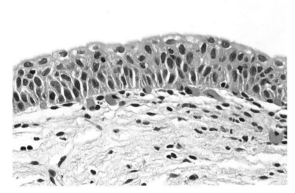

Fig. 9.1 Normal urothelium. Note that slight nuclear irregularity still falls within the spectrum of normal urothelium.

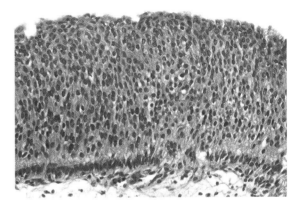

Fig. 9.2 Flat urothelial hyperplasia.

Flat urothelial hyperplasia

This entity is defined as markedly thickened mucosa without cytologic atypia (Fig. 9.2). Unlike a previous publication, which required the urothelium to exceed seven cell layers in thickness,[8] the consensus system simply requires obvious thickening of the urothelium that cannot be explained by tangential sectioning. While there are no data to support that this lesion is pre-neoplastic, it may be seen in mucosa adjacent to low-grade papillary urothelial lesions.

Papillary urothelial hyperplasia

This asymptomatic lesion is most often detected on routine follow-up cystoscopy for papillary urothelial carcinoma.[9] Histologically, it is characterized by cytologically bland urothelium of varying thickness that has assumed a 'tenting' or undulating configuration (Figs 9.3, 9.4). While one to a few dilated capillaries

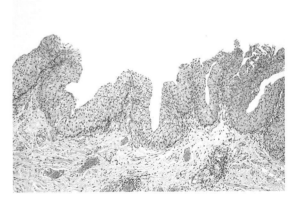

Fig. 9.3 Papillary urothelial hyperplasia without atypia.

may be found at the base of the 'tents', true fibrovascular cores are lacking. In some cases, it may be difficult to determine whether a lesion represents a florid example of papillary hyperplasia or a rather stubby papillary urothelial neoplasm of low malignant potential (see below). The presence of a single papillary lesion

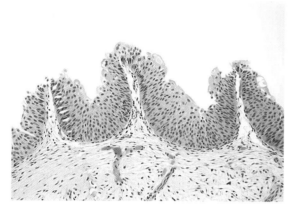

Fig. 9.4 Papillary urothelial hyperplasia without atypia. Nuclear architecture and cytologic arrangement appear normal.

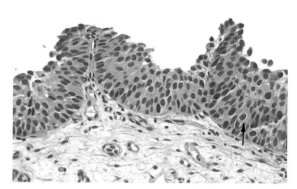

Fig. 9.5 Atypical papillary urothelial hyperplasia. Papillary urothelial hyperplasia is lined by cells with marked pleomorphism (arrow) similar to those seen in carcinoma in situ.

favors a neoplastic process whereas multiple, contiguous short papillary projections may be more consistent with hyperplasia. In select cases, immunohistochemical staining for p53 and Ki-67 may be helpful in discriminating between the two lesions (Table 9.3).[7]

A de novo diagnosis of papillary urothelial hyperplasia does not necessarily place a patient at risk for developing carcinoma; however, cystoscopic follow-up is recommended. If this diagnosis is made in a patient with a history of papillary tumors of the bladder, however, there is an association with an increased risk of recurrence of papillary neoplasms. Recently, we have studied cases of low- and high-grade intraurothelial neoplasia superimposed on papillary urothelial hyperplasia, which we have termed 'atypical papillary hyperplasia' (Fig. 9.5).

Atypical papillary hyperplasia is most frequently associated with CIS and high-grade papillary cancer.

This suggests that, in some cases, flat CIS or dysplasia may evolve into atypical papillary hyperplasia, with further progression to high-grade papillary cancer. This process is analogous to ordinary papillary hyperplasia progressing to low-grade papillary urothelial neoplasms.

Reactive atypia

Reactive atypia represents a response of benign urothelium to inflammation. An inflammatory infiltrate or a history of intravesical therapy, instrumentation or urolithiasis often accompanies epithelial changes. This lesion is characterized by a mild increase in nuclear size (2–2.5 times the size of a lymphocyte) and central prominent nucleoli within a vesicular nucleus (Fig. 9.6). Significant nuclear hyperchromasia, pleomorphism or

Table 9.3 Ki-67 and p53 staining characteristics of lesions in the WHO/ISUP system

Entity	p53			Ki-67		
	Mean	Median	Range	Mean	Median	Range
Benign	1.1	0	0–29	0.6	0	0–5.5
LGIUN	3.2	0	0–22.5	3.3	1	0–30
HGIUN	5.9	0.25	0–70	11.6	9.2	0–36
PH	0	0	0–0	1.1	1.2	0–2
Papilloma	0	0	0–0	4.3	4	1–8
LMP	0.4	0	0–2	2.5	1	0.5–15
LG cancer	2.9	1	0–20.5	7.3	3.7	0.5–38.5
HG cancer	25.7	8.5	0–100	15.7	11	1–65

HG, high grade; HGIUN, high-grade intraurothelial neoplasia; LG, low grade; LGIUN, low-grade intraurothelial neoplasia; LMP, papillary neoplasm of low malignant potential; PH, papillary hyperplasia. Modified with permission from Cina et al.[7]

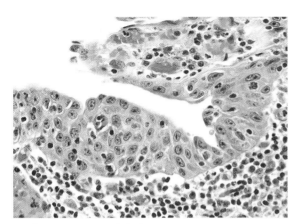

Fig. 9.6 Reactive urothelial atypia.

chromatin irregularity should not be evident, although mitotic figures may be frequent.

Atypia of unknown significance

In some cases it may be difficult to determine whether mild urothelial atypia represents a reactive or neoplastic process. There may be nuclear hyperchromasia and/or mild pleomorphism that seem out of proportion to the background inflammatory infiltrate. In these instances where dysplasia cannot be ruled out with certainty, it may be prudent to employ the term 'atypia of unknown significance' (AUS). For the time being, this diagnosis should initiate close follow-up with possible re-biopsy after treatment. However, a recent retrospective study presented at the 2000 United States and Canadian Academy of Pathologists meeting suggested that AUS behaves in a fashion identical to reactive atypia and is not associated with an increased risk of progression to carcinoma. This group further states that AUS should be dropped from future iterations of the WHO/ISUP system.[10]

Although the validity and longevity of this entity remain in question, it should be remembered that a similar diagnosis, 'atypical squamous cells of undetermined significance', has become an accepted part of the practice of cytology. Perhaps the diagnosis of AUS will eventually require a modifier such as 'favor reactive' or 'favor dysplasia'.

Low-grade intraurothelial neoplasia

The term 'dysplasia' has been applied in the past to lesions ranging from reactive atypia to CIS. The WHO/ISUP definition of low-grade intraurothelial neoplasia (LGIUN, dysplasia) is applied to urothelium showing considerable cytologic atypia and architectural disorder but which falls short of meeting criteria for high-grade intraurothelial neoplasia (HGIUN, CIS, see below). As such, LGIUN is characterized by increased nuclear size (3–5 times the size of a lymphocyte), nuclear hyperchromasia, some anisonucleosis, increased nuclear/cytoplasmic (N/C) ratio and mild-to-moderate architectural disorder (Fig. 9.7).

Since umbrella cells may show some degree of atypia due to the chemical milieu of the bladder, care should be taken to evaluate the lower and mid levels of the bladder epithelium when making a diagnosis of LGIUN. Given the lack of reproducibility of this diagnosis in the medical literature to date,[11] the natural history of LGIUN is poorly understood. Even with these vagaries, however, it is clear that well-established urothelial dysplasia is a precursor lesion to invasive carcinoma in at least a cohort of cases. The frequent observation of concurrent dysplasia and carcinoma, the lack of dysplasia in bladders not involved by a neoplastic process, and the genetic similarities shared by LGIUN and HGIUN support this contention.[12–15]

High-grade intraurothelial neoplasia

HGIUN (CIS) is a flat urothelial lesion which is characterized by the presence of cells with marked nuclear enlargement (> 3–5 times the size of a lymphocyte), hyperchromasia, nuclear membrane irregularities and architectural disarray (Fig. 9.8). Whereas enlarged hyperchromatic nuclei without visible nucleoli are typical, some examples of CIS demonstrate prominent nucleoli (Fig. 9.9). Mitotic figures are frequently noted, as is overexpression of p53

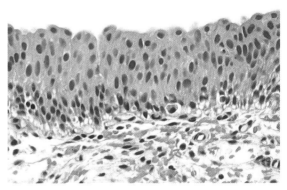

Fig. 9.7 Urothelial dysplasia.

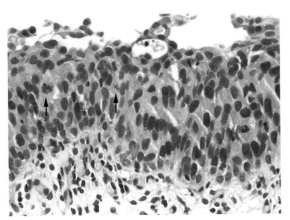

Fig. 9.8 Classic carcinoma in situ with hyperchromatic nuclei and numerous mitotic figures (arrows).

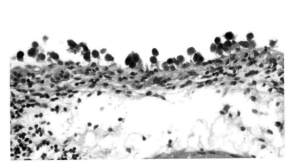

Fig. 9.10 Carcinoma in situ (CIS) with hyperchromatic enlarged nuclei tenuously clinging to the basement membrane. The remaining CIS cells have denuded off into the lumen.

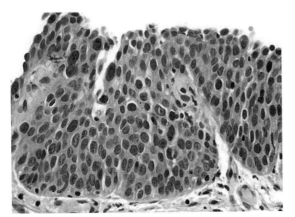

Fig. 9.9 Carcinoma in situ with prominent nucleoli.

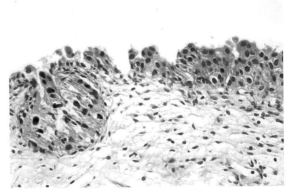

Fig. 9.11 Carcinoma in situ (CIS) involving von Brunn's nests. Often the surface urothelium is entirely denuded of CIS cells leaving pockets of CIS within von Brunn's nests.

gene product and increased proliferation as measured by immunoreactivity to Ki-67.[7] In previous systems these lesions have been termed 'marked atypia', 'severe dysplasia', 'moderate dysplasia' and 'carcinoma in situ, grade III'. This entity is clearly a precursor lesion to and frequent companion of invasive urothelial carcinoma. Despite the clinical significance of this lesion, it has often been underdiagnosed for a variety of reasons:

- The cells of HGIUN are easily disassociated from the mucosa, resulting in predominantly denuded epithelium with rare markedly atypical cells (so-called 'denuding cystitis' or 'clinging CIS') on biopsy specimens; this same tendency, however, results in relatively easy detection of HGIUN cells in bladder barbotage cytology specimens (Figs 9.10, 9.11). In the only study specifically to address the significance of denudation in urothelium, we found that in bladder biopsies removed by hot wire loop,

denudation most likely results from thermal injury where there is a low risk of subsequent CIS. Where the denuded biopsy has been taken by cold cup biopsy, in particular with a history of CIS, most cases represent denudation of neoplastic cells and a high risk of subsequent CIS.[16] Although it is reasonable to make a diagnosis of HGIUN in a biopsy specimen that is predominantly denuded, the pathologist may wish to examine additional levels or employ immunohistochemical stains in equivocal cases.

- Full thickness atypia is not required to make the diagnosis of HGIUN (Fig. 9.12). In some cases an intact, unremarkable umbrella cell layer will overlie diagnostic CIS. A variation on this theme is pagetoid HGIUN, in which occasional neoplastic cells are

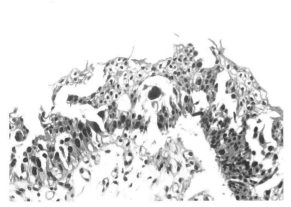

Fig. 9.12 Carcinoma in situ with scattered markedly hyperchromatic enlarged nuclei in otherwise normal urothelium.

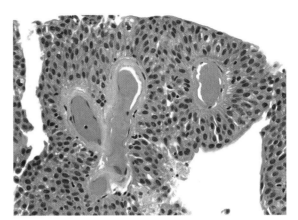

Fig. 9.14 Benign urothelial papilloma.

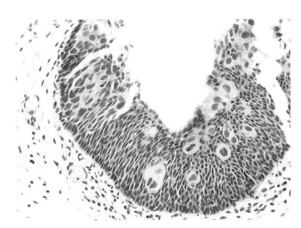

Fig. 9.13 Pagetoid carcinoma in situ.

dispersed in a 'buckshot' fashion throughout the urothelium (Fig. 9.13).

• There is frequently a spectrum of cytologic atypia in cases of HGIUN. Although the N/C ratio will be high in some cells, this feature may not be apparent in others.

In making the diagnosis of HGIUN on a urothelial biopsy, as in a cytology specimen, nuclear features are of paramount importance.

Urothelial papilloma

This diagnosis describes an exophytic papillary neoplasm comprised of a fibrovascular core lined by urothelium of normal thickness with no cytologic atypia (Fig. 9.14). It usually occurs as a solitary growth and is characteristically found in a younger population than the urothelial carcinomas. This benign neoplasm may recur but has not been shown to progress or be associated with an increased risk of carcinoma. In the only study using the WHO/ISUP system, none of the papillomas recurred.[17]

Employing the strict histologic criteria described above, this lesion should be quite rare. A comparison of the histologic features of the papillary neoplasms of the WHO/ISUP system is included in Table 9.4.

Papillary urothelial neoplasm of low malignant potential

This lesion may be discriminated from papilloma by virtue of the urothelial thickening and/or nuclear enlargement exhibited by low malignant potential (LMP) tumors (Figs 9.15, 9.16). In contrast to low-grade papillary carcinoma, there is no nuclear disorder, pleomorphism or hyperchromasia. Mitotic figures are unusual in LMP tumors and should be limited to the basal cell layer. Fusion of adjacent papillae is more common in carcinoma than tumors of LMP. A urothelial lesion meeting the criteria for LMP should not be invasive and should rarely metastasize. Nevertheless, this indolent lesion should serve as a marker for an increased risk of developing recurrent or subsequent papillary tumors that may be of higher grade.

In several studies analyzing the prognosis of LMP tumors, they have had lower recurrence rates than low-grade papillary cancers[17–19] (Table 9.5). With the exception of the study by Cheng et al., studies have not found LMP tumors to progress.[17–20] However, despite its claim, the Cheng study does not really use the WHO/ISUP classification. An abstract was submitted to the

Table 9.4 Histologic features of papillary urothelial lesions in the WHO/ISUP system

	Papilloma	Papillary neoplasm of low malignant potential	Low-grade papillary carcinoma	High-grade papillary carcinoma
Architecture				
Papillae	Delicate	Delicate; occasionally fused	Fused, branching and delicate	Fused, branching and delicate
Organization of cells	Identical to normal	Polarity identical to normal; any thickness; cohesive	Predominantly ordered, yet minimal crowding and minimal loss of polarity; any thickness; cohesive	Predominantly disordered with frequent loss of polarity; any thickness; often discohesive
Cytology				
Nuclear size	Identical to normal	May be uniformly enlarged	Enlarged with variation in size	Enlarged with variation in size
Nuclear shape	Identical to normal	Elongated, round–oval, uniform	Round–oval; slight variation in shape and contour	Moderately marked pleomorphism
Nuclear chromatin	Fine	Fine	Mild variation within and between cells	Moderately marked variation both within and between cells with hyperchromasia
Nucleoli	Absent	Absent to inconspicuous	Usually inconspicuous*	Multiple prominent nucleoli may be present
Mitoses	Absent	Rare, basal	Occasional, at any level	Usually frequent, at any level
Umbrella cells	Uniformly present	Present	Usually present	May be absent

* If present, small and regular and not accompanied by other features of high-grade carcinoma.
Reproduced with permission from Epstein et al.[6]

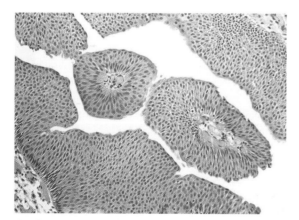

Fig. 9.15 Plain view of papillary urothelial neoplasm of low malignant potential.

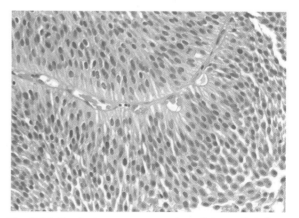

Fig. 9.16 Cytologic appearances of papillary urothelial neoplasm of low malignant potential.

Table 9.5 Prognosis of papillary urothelial lesions in the WHO/ISUP system

	Author	Papilloma (%)	LMP (%)	Low-grade cancer (%)	High-grade cancer (%)
Recurrence					
	Alsheikh et al.[18]		25	48	
	Desai et al.[17]	0	33.3	64.1	56.4
	Holmang et al.[19]		35	71	
Progression*					
	Alsheikh et al.[18]†		0	10.3	
	Desai et al.[17]	0	0	7.9	18.8
	Holmang et al.[19]		0	2.4	

* Progression defined as muscularis propria invasion, metastases or death from bladder cancer.

† Unable to determine if progression also includes lamina propria invasion.

LMP, papillary neoplasm of low malignant potential.

USCAP meeting from Cheng et al. before the classification system was published with its definitional images. As the authors admit, they have merely equated prior WHO grade I cancers with LMP tumors. As shown in Table 9.2, some WHO grade I cancers without any atypia except nuclear enlargement are WHO/ISUP LMP tumors and other WHO grade I cancers with some more atypia are WHO/ISUP low-grade cancers.

Papillary urothelial carcinoma, low grade

This lesion is characterized by a neoplastic proliferation comprised of fibrovascular cores lined by easily recognized, disordered, cytologically atypical urothelium (Figs 9.17, 9.18). Mitotic figures are infrequent but may be seen at any level of the urothelium (though they are usually seen in the lower half). The cytologic features commonly found in this urothelial neoplasm include variation in nuclear size, shape and chromatin texture and somewhat disordered cell polarity. Much like the relationship of LGIUN to HGIUN, the architectural and cytologic atypia of low-grade carcinoma falls short of meeting diagnostic criteria for high-grade urothelial carcinoma. It is important to evaluate only well-oriented fibrovascular cores (i.e. those that are sectioned perpendicularly to the long axis of the core) as tangential sectioning can lead to an overestimate of the degree of atypia present. Fusion of adjacent papillae may be seen in low-grade carcinomas, though it is more commonly seen in high-grade lesions.

The histologic differences of low-grade papillary carcinoma and urothelial neoplasms of low malignant potential can be subtle. If the nuclear changes of a

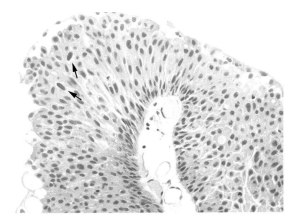

Fig. 9.17 Low-grade papillary urothelial carcinoma. Note that even at low magnification there is slight but definite nuclear pleomorphism with scattered nuclei that are more hyperchromatic and enlarged (arrows) relative to surrounding nuclei.

papillary urothelial lesion consist of anything more atypical than modest nuclear enlargement, a diagnosis of carcinoma is probably warranted. Low-grade cancers frequently recur (more so than LMP tumors), yet have a low risk of progression[17-19] (see Table 9.5). Some of the old WHO grade II tumors (on the low-grade side) would be classified as WHO/ISUP low-grade, as would some of the old WHO grade I tumors with some atypia.

Papillary urothelial carcinoma, high grade

These aggressive tumors may often be diagnosed at low power due to the obvious architectural disorder of the

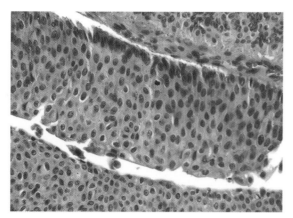

Fig. 9.18 Low-grade papillary urothelial carcinoma. Although there is slight nuclear pleomorphism and disarray in the architecture, the overall appearance is much more ordered and there is less nuclear atypia than seen in high-grade papillary urothelial carcinoma.

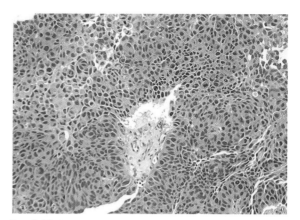

Fig. 9.20 High-grade papillary urothelial carcinoma with marked architectural disorder.

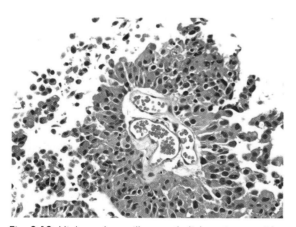

Fig. 9.19 High-grade papillary urothelial carcinoma with cells similar to carcinoma in situ lining papillary fronds. Note cellular discohesion with individual cells shedding off from papillae.

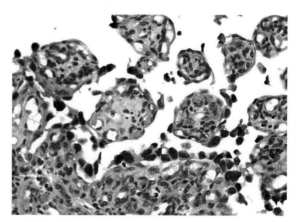

Fig. 9.21 High-grade papillary urothelial carcinoma where many of the cells have shed off from papillae leaving 'naked' papillae.

urothelium. The epithelium often shows full thickness disorder, abnormal cell clustering, abundant mitotic figures and fusion of papillae (Figs 9.19, 9.20). Just as CIS cells may show prominent denudation, high-grade papillary carcinomas may lose their epithelium, resulting in 'naked' papillae (Fig. 9.21). Moderate to marked nuclear pleomorphism, abnormal mitotic figures, clumped chromatin and nucleolar prominence all favor high-grade over low-grade carcinoma. In some tumors, a spectrum of cytologic atypia and architectural disorder ranging from low- to high-grade carcinoma will be noted. In tumors with admixed histologic features, the carcinoma should be graded according to

the highest grade present. If, however, the high-grade component represents a miniscule portion of an otherwise low-grade carcinoma, the lesion should be considered low-grade.

Studies are currently being undertaken to determine how significant a focal high-grade component must be in order to impact upon prognosis. A recent study examining 52 stage Ta papillary urothelial lesions with mixed histologic grades assigned scores of 1, 2, and 3 to LMP tumors, low-grade carcinoma and high-grade carcinoma, respectively.[20] These authors found that a composite grade could be obtained by adding the score for the primary grade and the secondary grade (defined as accounting for at least 5% of the neoplasm). In this study, there were significantly different survival rates, 68% and 40%, noted between composite scores 5 and 6, respectively. The current WHO/ISUP system, however, does not employ composite grading. Regardless, the presence of significant high-grade carcinoma is associated with a higher risk of disease progression and is often associated with invasive disease at the time of presentation[17–20] (see Table 9.5). Papillary urothelial carcinoma may also be distinguished from the other papillary lesions by virtue of its overexpression of p53 and high proliferative index (see Table 9.3). Some old WHO grade II cancers (on the high end) and all WHO grade III cancers would be classified as WHO/ISUP high-grade cancer.

DEPTH OF INVASION

Confusion in terminology is not limited to the diagnostic entities in the various classification schemes, as it also exists for the descriptive terminology applied to invasive urothelial lesions. Vagaries in this arena include 'superficial muscle invasion', 'deep muscle invasion', 'muscle invasion (not otherwise specified)' and 'superficial bladder cancer'. The last term is particularly confusing as it could be applied to HGIUN, non-invasive papillary neoplasms or truly invasive urothelial carcinoma. Due to the variations in treatment and the prognostic significance related to the depth of invasion of bladder tumors, the WHO/ISUP consensus group developed several recommendations to provide clinicians with this essential information in an unambiguous manner.

Invasion of the lamina propria is characterized by nests, clusters or single urothelial cells which have breached the epithelial basement membrane. In contrast to von Brunn's nests, nests of invasive carcinoma are often smaller and more irregular (Fig. 9.22). If rounded nests of atypical urothelium are present in the lamina propria, the diagnosis of non-invasive, low-grade papillary carcinoma with an inverted growth pattern should be considered. The leading edge of invasive urothelial carcinoma will often show 'paradoxical maturation' – an increase in cytoplasmic eosinophilia, similar to that seen in invasive squamous carcinoma of the uterine cervix.

Another useful feature in identifying invasion is the presence of marked retraction artifact around the infiltrating cellular clusters. This may be so pronounced as to mimic closely lymphovascular space invasion. Since vascular invasion is uncommon in urothelial carcinomas limited to the lamina propria, care should be taken not to overinterpret this artifact. Immunohistochemical confirmation of the presence of endothelium

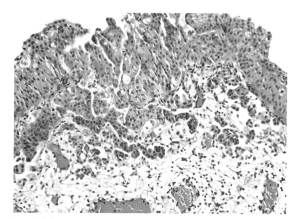

Fig. 9.22 Lamina propria invasion with small irregular nests extending into underlying connective tissue.

(e.g. factor VIII, CD31, CD34) may be of utility in cases in which this diagnosis is considered.

As invasion extends into the mid-level of the lamina propria, carcinoma will eventually infiltrate into wispy smooth muscle bundles, the muscularis mucosae. Although several studies have shown that the depth of lamina propria invasion with respect to the muscularis mucosae has prognostic significance, the consensus committee chose to make substaging of lamina propria invasion optional. Pathologists are encouraged, however, to assess the extent of invasion (i.e. focal versus extensive) to help guide urologists to an appropriate treatment plan.

The distinction between invasion of the muscularis mucosae and muscularis propria is critical but may be difficult (Figs 9.23, 9.24). The presence of numerous blood vessels admixed with small bundles of smooth

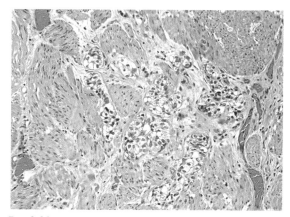

Fig. 9.23 Muscularis propria invasion with tumor extending between thick muscle bundles.

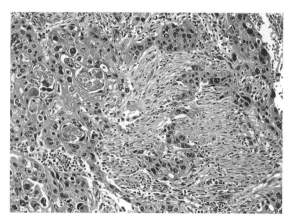

Fig. 9.24 Extensive high-grade infiltrating urothelial carcinoma situated between smaller bundles of smooth muscle. Given the extensive high-grade nature of the carcinoma along with the extensive nature of disrupted muscle bundles, this case would be considered by many as muscularis propria invasion even though thick muscle bundles are not identified.

muscles favors muscularis mucosae whereas dense bundles of smooth muscle characterize the muscularis propria. In some specimens, particularly cauterized tissue from transurethral resection of bladder tumor, it may be difficult to determine the derivation of residual smooth muscle fibers within extensive tumor. In these cases, a Masson's trichrome stain or immunohisto-chemical staining for smooth muscle actin may help to quantify the amount and distribution of the remaining muscle. It is recognized that the depth of invasion cannot be accurately determined in all instances. In these equivocal biopsies, the pathologist should convey any uncertainty to the urologist, who will likely initiate a restaging procedure.

Three final comments on depth of invasion are warranted:

- The pathologist has done his job if he can discri-minate between invasion of the muscularis mucosae and muscularis propria on a bladder biopsy speci-men. Attempts at substaging the depth of invasion of the muscularis propria on a biopsy specimen are neither required nor expected. Definitive assessment of the depth of invasion should be reserved for the final resection specimen.
- The presence of adipose tissue admixed with tumor on a biopsy specimen is not necessarily indicative of extravesical spread of tumor. In fact, fat may be present at any level of the bladder, including both the lamina propria and muscularis propria.

- The consensus committee recommends mentioning the presence or absence of muscularis propria in all bladder biopsy specimens as this provides useful feedback to the urologist regarding biopsy technique and adequacy.

URINARY CYTOLOGY

This topic is covered in greater detail elsewhere in this text. Cytologic evaluation of voided urine and bladder barbotage ('wash') specimens may be a useful screening and surveillance tool for lesions of the lower urinary tract. In routine bladder cytology specimens, it will be very difficult to distinguish the bland epithelial clusters of papilloma and papillary neoplasms of low malignant potential from reactive urothelium. Depending on the degree of atypia present, low-grade papillary carcinomas may exfoliate cells that are either suspicious for or diag-nostic of malignancy. Urinary cytology is most useful at identifying the markedly atypical cells sloughed from high-grade papillary carcinomas or HGIUN. The pre-sence of urothelial cells with nuclear enlargement, high N/C ratios and coarsely granular chromatin most likely indicate the presence of a high-grade lesion and should prompt cystoscopy. It has yet to be seen whether the heightened nuclear detail seen in thin-preparation urine specimens will facilitate discrimination of reactive/neoplastic bladder lesions at the lower end of the cytologic spectrum.

CONCLUSION

The 1998 WHO/ISUP consensus classification is a first step toward developing a nomenclature for urothelial lesions of the urinary bladder that can be understood and used by pathologists, urologists, oncologists and scientists regardless of where they practice or where they trained. It is a system designed to reduce ambiguity in diagnoses, facilitate communication between clini-cians and pathologists, and promote interinstitutional research and data collection. Being an initial effort, it is likely that this system will be revised over time. Early studies, however, show that the entities described herein represent a set of lesions that show a progressive spec-trum from benignancy to malignancy as evidenced by prognosis, p53 expression and proliferative index.[7,17–20] This system is easily learned and applied in daily practice; additional familiarity with the WHO/ISUP system can be acquired from a web-based tutorial located at http://162.129.103.34/bladder/.

REFERENCES

1. Murphy WM (ed.) Diseases of the urinary bladder, urethra, ureters, and renal pelves. In: Urological Pathology. Philadelphia: W.B. Saunders, 1989, pp 64–96.

2. Bergkvist A, Ljungqvist A, Moberger G. Classification of bladder tumors based on the cellular pattern. Acta Chir Scand 1965;130:371–378.

3. Mostofi FK, Sobin LH, Torloni H. Histological typing of urinary bladder tumors. International histological classification of tumours, No. 10. Geneva: World Health Organization, 1973.

4. Broders AC. Epithelium of the genito-urinary organs. Ann Surg 1922;75:574–604.

5. Ash JE. Epithelial tumors of the bladder. J Urol 1940;44:135–145.

6. Epstein JI, Amin MB, Reuter VR, et al. and the Bladder Consensus Conference Committee. The WHO/ISUP classification of urothelial (transitional cell) neoplasms of the urinary bladder. Am J Surg Pathol 1998;22:1435–1448.

7. Cina S, Lancaster K, Lecksell K, et al. Correlation of Ki-67 and p53 with the new WHO/ISOP classification scheme for urothelial neoplasia. Arch Pathol Lab Med 2001;125:646–651.

8. Mostofi FK, Sesterhann IAH, Davis CJ Jr. Dysplasia versus atypia versus carcinoma in situ of the bladder. In: McCullough DL (ed.) Difficult Diagnoses in Urology. New York: Churchill Livingstone, 1988.

9. Taylor DC, Bhagavan BS, Larsen MP, et al. Papillary urothelial hyperplasia. A precursor to papillary neoplasms. Am J Surg Pathol 1996;20:1481–1488.

10. Cheng L, Cheville JC, Neumann RM, et al. Flat intaepithelial lesions of the urinary bladder. Cancer 2000;88:625–631.

11. Robertson AJ, Swanson Beck J, Burnett RA, et al. Observer variability in histopathological reporting of transitional cell carcinoma and epithelial dysplasia in bladders. J Clin Pathol 1990;43:17–21.

12. Farrow GM, Utz DC, Rife CC. Morphological and clinical observations of patients with early bladder cancer treated with total cystectomy. Cancer Res 1976;36:2495–2501.

13. Koss LG. Mapping of the urinary bladder: its impact on the concepts of bladder cancer. Hum Pathol 1979;10:533–548.

14. Rubben H, Lutzeyer W, Fischer N, et al. Natural history and treatment of low and high risk superficial bladder tumors. J Urol 1988;139:283–285.

15. Hofstader F, Delgado R, Jakse G, et al. Urothelial dysplasia and carcinoma in situ of the bladder. Cancer 1986;57:356–361.

16. Levi AW, Potter SR, Schoenberg MP, et al. Denuded urothelium in bladder biopsies. J Urol 2001;166:457–460.

17. Desai S, Lim SD, Jimenez RE, et al. Relationship of cytokeratin 20 and CD44 protein expression with WHO/ISUP grade in pTa and PT1 papillary urothelial neoplasia. Mod Pathol 2000;13;1315–1323.

18. Alsheikh A, Mohamedali Z, Jones E, et al. Comparison of the WHO/ISUP classification and cytokeratin 20 expression in predicting the behavior of low-grade papillary urothelial tumors. Mod Pathol 2001;14;267–272.

19. Holmang S, Hedelin H, Anderstrom C, et al. Recurrence and progression in low grade papillary urothelial tumors. J Urol 1999;162:702–707.

20. Cheng L, Neumann RM, Bostwick DG. Papillary urothelial neoplasms of low malignant potential. Clinical and biologic implications. Cancer 1999;86:2102–2108.

carcinomas.[8] The authors noted that these tumors were mostly high-stage and high-grade. They also reported a higher frequency (50%) of synchronous or metachronous non-urothelial carcinomas, most arising in the colon, prostate or cervix.[8]

It is important to distinguish cystic change in urothelial carcinoma from benign and malignant mimics. This pattern may be confused with benign proliferations such as cystitis cystica, cystitis glandularis and nephrogenic adenoma.[3] The presence of significant nuclear atypia at least focally and areas of typical invasive urothelial carcinoma allow for accurate distinction. More problematic is the separation between this variant of urothelial carcinoma and adenocarcinoma. As indicated, the diagnosis of adenocarcinoma should be restricted to pure tumors with true gland formation. In microcystic urothelial carcinoma, the lining cells are urothelial in origin and the spaces are pseudoglandular, not true glands.[8]

NESTED VARIANT

In 1992, Murphy and Deana described four cases of invasive urothelial carcinoma with a distinctive growth pattern of small nests composed of benign-appearing urothelial cells, infiltrating the lamina propria (Fig. 10.5), closely resembling von Brunn's nests.[9] Since then more than 40 cases have been reported, emphasizing the aggressive clinical behavior of this type of tumor, contrasting with its innocuous histologic appearance.[10–18]

The estimated incidence of this variant is less than 0.3% of all invasive bladder tumors.[10] Most of the patients are men with a mean age of 68 years. The

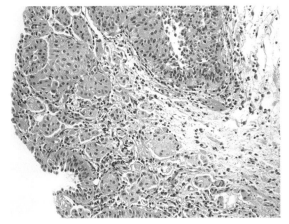

Fig. 10.5 Nested variant. Nests of neoplastic cells invading the lamina propria.

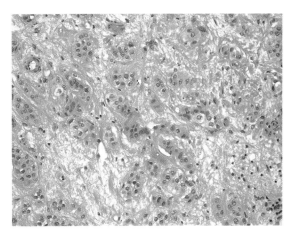

Fig. 10.6 Nested variant. The nests of bland-looking neoplastic cells are irregularly distributed within the lamina propria.

presenting symptoms are similar to those of typical urothelial carcinoma, with hematuria representing the most frequent symptom, followed by hydronephrosis. The latter is likely to result from the fact that 50% of the cases with this variant occur in the periureteral orifice. In the cases where follow-up was available, approximately one-third of the patients died of the disease or of treatment complications.

Histologically, the tumor is formed by small nests of urothelial cells; tubular structures may be seen. The cells show minimal cytologic atypia and rare mitosis. The cytoplasm is clear to pale eosinophilic. The nests are irregularly distributed within the lamina propria and invade the muscularis propria in some cases (Fig. 10.6). A tendency for increasing cellular anaplasia is noted in the deeper aspects of the lesion.[9] The tumor seems to arise de novo without a preceding superficial stage.[17,18]

The differential diagnosis of the nested variant of urothelial carcinoma includes prominent von Brunn's nests, cystitis cystica, cystitis glandularis, inverted papilloma, nephrogenic adenoma, paraganglionic tissue and paragangliomas.[3] Useful features in recognizing the nested variant of urothelial carcinoma as malignant are the infiltrative nature of the lesion, the presence of muscle invasion and the presence of marked cytologic atypia in its deeper portion.

Nephrogenic adenoma typically has a papillary component and prominent tubular growth pattern. The prominent vascular network of paraganglioma which surrounds individual nests is typical, as is the constant expression of neuroendocrine markers and absence of reactivity for cytokeratin.

UROTHELIAL CARCINOMA WITH INVERTED GROWTH PATTERN

This variant of urothelial carcinoma is characterized by an endophytic growth pattern (Fig. 10.7) mimicking inverted papilloma. However, it has, by definition, significant nuclear pleomorphism (Fig. 10.8) and mitotic figures, and lacks the orderly maturation and the peripheral palisading typically present in inverted papilloma.[1,19] Moreover, an exophytic papillary or a conventional invasive component is often associated with the inverted elements.[19] For some authors, the presence of keratinization should raise the suspicion for urothelial carcinoma since this is a rare finding in inverted papilloma.[19]

This variant was first described in 1976 by Cameron and Lupton[20] in a report of two cases. Amin et al.

described a series of 18 patients with this variant and emphasized the problems with interpretation of invasion in these cases.[19] Most patients were men with a mean age of 68 years. The small number of patients and the limited follow-up do not permit the evaluation of the impact of the endophytic growth pattern on outcome.

UROTHELIAL CARCINOMA WITH TROPHOBLASTS

Choriocarcinoma of the urinary bladder was first described in 1904 by Djewitzki.[21] Since then more than 30 cases have been reported in the literature.[21-47] Like its counterpart in the female genital tract, choriocarcinoma in the urinary bladder is defined by the presence of cytotrophoblastic and syncytiotrophoblastic elements (Fig. 10.9). Most tumors are mixed with typical invasive urothelial carcinoma, but they can also be present in a pure form.[32]

These tumors occur most commonly in men, with a mean age of 63 years. The trigone is the most common location in the bladder. In all the cases, the patients presented with hematuria, and a characteristic clinical finding was the presence of gynecomastia secondary to high serum levels of human chorionic gonadotropin (hCG), as demonstrated in nine cases.[23,24,26,27,30,33,35,40,46]

The presence of a trophoblastic component (Fig. 10.10) confers to the tumor a bad prognosis.[48] Surgical therapy is mandatory at an early stage. Chemotherapy is the treatment of choice. However, rapid recurrence usually occurs. Metastases are also common and occur early in the course of the disease.[46]

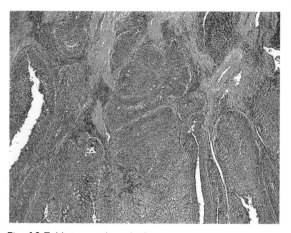

Fig. 10.7 Variant with endophytic growth pattern. Broad-front endophytic growth with smooth borders; no desmoplasia is noted.

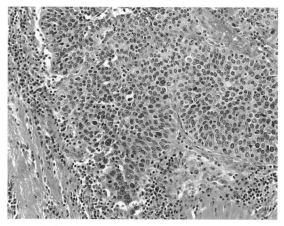

Fig. 10.8 The base of the tumor shows cellular pleomorphism and mitosis.

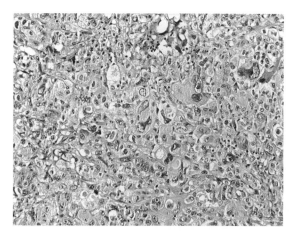

Fig. 10.9 Urothelial carcinoma with trophoblasts. The tumor is formed by two types of cells: cytotrophoblasts and syncytiotrophoblasts.

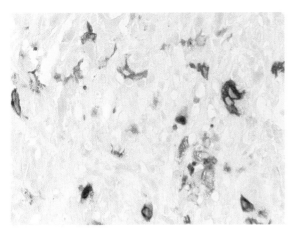

Fig. 10.10 Urothelial carcinoma with trophoblasts. Immunohistochemical stain for β-human chorionic gonadotropin showing positivity in the trophoblastic cells within the tumor.

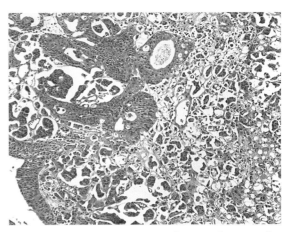

Fig. 10.11 Micropapillary variant. Clusters of tumor cells within clear spaces present in a loose stroma; the tumor invades the lamina propria.

It is important to distinguish this variant from invasive urothelial carcinomas with positive immunohistochemical staining for hCG. This positivity was detected in 11.5–46.2% of urothelial carcinoma cases[49,50] and was strongly correlated with grade and stage. This finding, however, has no prognostic implications.

MICROPAPILLARY VARIANT

The occurrence of this distinctive morphologic variant of urothelial carcinoma in the urinary bladder was first presented in detail by Amin et al.[51] in 1994 in a description of 18 cases. Johansson et al. reported recently on 20 additional cases,[52] describing an incidence of 0.7% of all bladder carcinomas.

The tumor is composed of cytologically malignant cells arranged in small papillary clusters floating free in empty spaces (Fig. 10.11). Although initially thought to represent vascular spaces, factor VIII and CD31 immunostaining revealed that the majority of these lacunae were not vascular but represent tissue retraction artifacts.[51–53] Some authors believe that the micropapillary carcinoma is a variant of adenocarcinoma.[52]

Morphologically, the tumor bears a striking resemblance to serous papillary carcinoma of the ovary (Fig. 10.12), a differential diagnosis which may require clinical correlation for exclusion in female patients. It is often associated with overlying in situ or invasive conventional urothelial carcinoma.

The tumor has no distinctive epidemiologic features. However, it is known for its aggressive clinical course

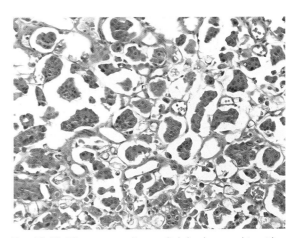

Fig. 10.12 The tumor cells are slightly pleomorphic with eosinophilic cytoplasm.

and propensity for extensive and deep invasion.[51,52] Therefore, when seen in biopsy specimens, rebiopsy of the area is indicated if muscle invasion is not demonstrable in the original material. Optimal treatment for this tumor is not well determined due to its rarity.

LYMPHOEPITHELIOMA-LIKE VARIANT

This variant of urothelial carcinoma resembles lymphoepithelioma or undifferentiated carcinoma of the nasopharynx (Fig. 10.13). It is characterized histologically by poorly differentiated epithelial cells with indistinct cytoplasmic borders and a syncytial growth pattern, densely infiltrated by lymphoid cells and sometimes

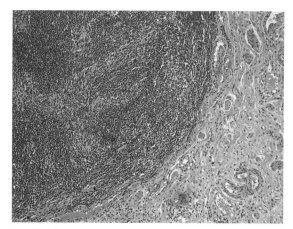

Fig. 10.13 Lymphoepithelioma-like variant. The tumor is invading the lamina propria with a pushing border.

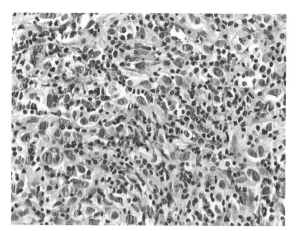

Fig. 10.14 Lymphoepithelioma-like variant. Syncytial growth pattern of the tumor cells, mixed with inflammatory cells, predominantly lymphocytes. The inflammatory cells obscure the neoplastic urothelial cells.

plasma cells, histiocytes, neutrophils and eosinophils (Fig. 10.14). Histologically, this variant may be pure or mixed with typical urothelial carcinoma, the latter being focal and inconspicuous in some instances. Glandular and squamous differentiation can be seen.[3] The tumor usually involves the dome, posterior wall or trigone with a sessile growth pattern. Most of the tumors are muscle invasive at the time of diagnosis.[54–60]

Few series and case reports of this variant involving the urinary bladder are reported in the literature.[54–60] These tumors occur more commonly in men and most frequently in late adulthood. Most patients present with hematuria.[59,60]

Histologically similar tumors have been described in other sites where a relation with Epstein–Barr virus (EBV) infection was found in some cases. However, no association with EBV was identified in bladder tumors.[59–61]

The major differential diagnostic consideration is lymphoma. Another diagnostic consideration is chronic cystitis. The presence of a syncytial pattern of large malignant cells with a dense polymorphous lymphoid background are important clues. Immunohistochemistry shows cytokeratin in the malignant cells, confirming their epithelial nature (Fig. 10.15).

Lymphoepithelioma-like carcinoma is believed to be a variant with a favorable prognosis. Patients with a predominant or a pure pattern seemed to do better than patients having a focal component.[57,59,60] This is possibly due to the host response to the tumor, mainly composed of T lymphocytes.[57] This type of tumor appears to be sensitive to multiagent chemotherapy;[54,57] the low numbers of cases, however, preclude a definite conclusion.

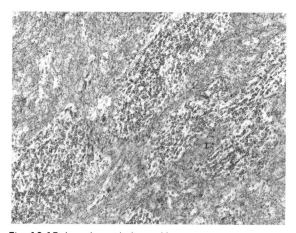

Fig. 10.15 Lymphoepithelioma-like variant. Immunohistochemical stain for cytokeratin confirming the epithelial nature of the tumor.

PLASMACYTOID VARIANT

Zukerberg et al. described two cases of bladder carcinoma diffusely invading the bladder wall (Fig. 10.16) and composed of cells with a monotonous appearance mimicking lymphoma.[55] A tumor with similar morphology was reported by Sahin et al., where the patient initially presented with multiple lytic bone metastases and was diagnosed with multiple myeloma.[62] In fact, in the three cases, the tumor cells had an eosinophilic cytoplasm with an eccentric nucleus producing a plasmacytoid appearance (Fig. 10.17). On immunohistochemical staining, these cells

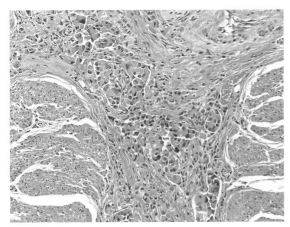

Fig. 10.16 Plasmacytoid variant. The neoplastic cells invade the muscularis propria.

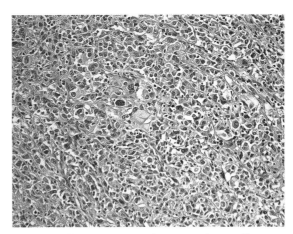

Fig. 10.18 Giant cell variant. Large neoplastic cells, poorly cohesive, growing in sheets.

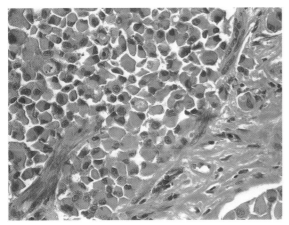

Fig. 10.17 Plasmacytoid variant. The cells have plasmacytoid features.

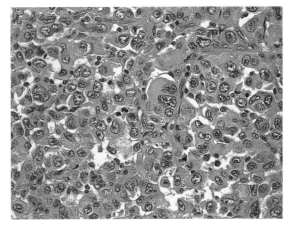

Fig. 10.19 Giant cell variant. The cells have abundant eosinophilic cytoplasm.

were positive for cytokeratin and negative for plasma cell and lymphocytic markers, thus confirming the diagnosis of carcinoma. Only one tumor was associated with a typical urothelial carcinoma.

The differential diagnostic considerations are plasmacytoma/multiple myeloma or lymphoma. Identification of a typical urothelial component confirms the diagnosis, but immunohistochemistry may be necessary to confirm the histologic impression in some cases.

GIANT CELL VARIANT

Morphologically, the tumor resembles giant cell carcinoma as seen typically in lung or other organs. It is formed by poorly cohesive large pleomorphic cells (Fig. 10.18) with abundant amphophilic to eosinophilic cytoplasm and multiple nuclei (Fig. 10.19). Cells stain positively for cytokeratin. This tumor has a very poor prognosis.[1]

This variant should be distinguished from urothelial carcinoma with trophoblastic differentiation in which staining for hCG is positive. It should also be distinguished from tumors containing osteoclast-like giant cells in the stroma.[1,63] Giant cells can also be seen in association with urothelial carcinoma in patients who have received bacille Calmette–Guérin (BCG) therapy, or in patients who have undergone prior resection or biopsy. In these two conditions the giant cells are benign and form granulomas.

SARCOMATOID VARIANT

This is an uncommon variant of urothelial carcinoma showing both carcinomatous and sarcomatous components. Various terms have been used for these neoplasms, including carcinosarcoma, sarcomatoid carcinoma, malignant mesodermal mixed tumor, spindle cell and giant cell carcinoma. Some authors include all such tumors under the term 'sarcomatoid carcinoma' or 'carcinosarcoma', while others prefer to use 'sarcomatoid carcinoma' for those cases without heterologous elements in the spindle cell component and 'carcinosarcoma' for cases with heterologous elements.[64,65] They both have similar clinical characteristics (patient age, sex, presentation and outcome) regardless of their histologic features.[3]

Sarcomatoid variant of urothelial carcinoma is more common in males than in females[66–71] and tends to occur in patients at the end of their seventh decade.[66,70,72] The most frequent presenting sign is hematuria, although irritative and obstructive symptoms can occur.[66,68,73,74] A role of radiation therapy or cyclophosphamide therapy, although minor, was suggested in carcinosarcoma. Sarcomatoid carcinoma classically arises in a background of recurrent urothelial carcinoma as well as irritative lesions, recurrent cystitis, diabetes, neurogenic bladder and bladder diverticulum.[75]

Grossly, sarcomatoid carcinoma is usually largely exophytic, often with a polypoid growth pattern, ulceration and hemorrhage, and invading deep into the bladder wall.[66,70,75] In fact, patients usually present with high stage disease.[66,71,75–77]

Histologically, the epithelial component is urothelial in 85% of cases, with squamous carcinoma being the next most frequent; adenocarcinoma and small cell carcinoma can also occur.[66] In some cases, the epithelial component consists only of carcinoma in situ, while in others the epithelial component cannot be recognized histologically, and special studies are required to prove the epithelial nature of the spindle cells.[72,75]

In most cases, the sarcomatous component consists of neoplastic spindle cells (Fig. 10.20) forming fascicles or growing with no particular arrangement. The merging of the epithelial and spindle cell components is helpful in the diagnosis (Figs 10.21, 10.22). Heterologous differentiation, when present, usually consists of chondrosarcoma (47%), osteosarcoma (31%) or rhabdomyosarcoma (24%).[3] The sarcoma is almost always high-grade.

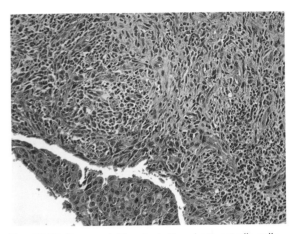

Fig. 10.20 Sarcomatoid variant. Neoplastic spindle cells arising from the surface epithelium showing carcinoma in situ.

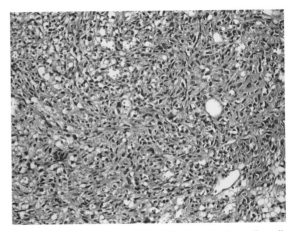

Fig. 10.21 Sarcomatoid variant. Sarcomatoid spindle cell carcinoma with highly pleomorphic cells.

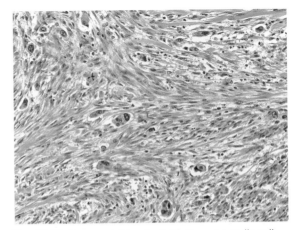

Fig. 10.22 Sarcomatoid variant. Malignant spindle cells are mixed with nests of epithelioid cells.

Several immunohistochemical studies of this variant have been reported. In most reports, the spindle cell elements have been found to express cytokeratin at least focally, although in some cases cytokeratin has not been demonstrable.[78] Other epithelial markers, such as epithelial membrane antigen, may also be expressed, although even less consistently. Co-expression of vimentin in the spindle cell component is usual. Occasionally, the spindle cells express muscle-specific actin or desmin.[79] Heterologous elements express markers appropriate to the type of differentiation.

The differential diagnoses to be considered are urothelial carcinoma with a pseudosarcomatous stroma.[80–82] Sarcomatoid carcinoma with heterologous elements should be differentiated from osseous metaplasia that is present in some cases of urothelial carcinoma.[83–93] The giant cells of giant cell cystitis should not be confused with sarcomatoid carcinoma. These cells typically have several small, round, uniform nuclei and scant cytoplasm. In cases without obvious carcinoma, the main differential diagnostic consideration is sarcoma. Because of the rarity of primary bladder sarcoma, a malignant spindle cell tumor in the urinary bladder of an adult should be considered sarcomatoid carcinoma until proven otherwise. Extensive sectioning of the tumor and surrounding mucosa may reveal an in situ or invasive epithelial component. Immunohistochemical studies with antibodies to low molecular weight cytokeratin may give evidence of epithelial differentiation; ultrastructural studies may also be helpful.

Surgical resection, either cystectomy or transurethral, followed by radiation therapy is the treatment of choice.[66] The value of chemotherapy is controversial.[66,72] Even with optimal treatment, survival is 25% at 2 years.[3]

UROTHELIAL CARCINOMA WITH UNUSUAL STROMAL REACTIONS

Pseudosarcomatous stroma

In rare cases the stroma of the urothelial carcinoma shows sufficient cellularity and atypia to raise a serious concern of sarcomatoid carcinoma.[80–82] The stroma varies from myxoid with stellate or multinucleated cells (similar to those seen in giant cell cystitis) to cellular and spindled with fascicle formation (Fig. 10.23). They differ from the malignant cells in sarcomatoid carcinoma by the degenerated appearance of the nuclei and

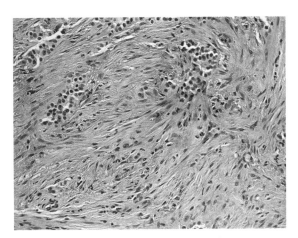

Fig. 10.23 Urothelial carcinoma with pseudosarcomatous stroma. The tumor grows in a cellular desmoplastic stroma with myxoid changes. There is no evidence of significant atypia in the stromal cells.

lack of atypical mitosis. Immunohistochemically the stromal cells of pseudosarcoma show fibroblastic and myofibroblastic differentiation and invariably lack cytokeratin.[80,81]

Osseous or cartilaginous metaplasia

Osseous metaplasia is present in some cases of urothelial carcinoma,[83–93] and this should be differentiated from an osteosarcoma component. This finding has also been described in metastatic urothelial carcinoma. The metaplastic bone is histologically benign, with a normal lamellar pattern. The tumor is usually found adjacent to areas of hemorrhage. The cells in the adjacent stroma are cytologically benign.

Osteoclast-type giant cells

Zukerberg et al. described the presence of osteoclast-like giant cells in two cases of invasive high-grade urothelial carcinoma (Fig. 10.24), both of which had a sarcomatoid spindle cell component.[63] The giant cells had abundant eosinophilic cytoplasm and numerous small, round, regular nuclei and stained positively for vimentin and tartrate-resistant acid phosphatase but not for epithelial markers. Similar tumors have been described by other authors as giant cell reparative granuloma[94] and giant cell tumor.[95] The osteoclast-type giant cells probably reflect a stromal response to the tumor. There is no evidence that osteoclast-like giant cells in urothelial carcinoma indicate increased aggressiveness (Fig. 10.25).

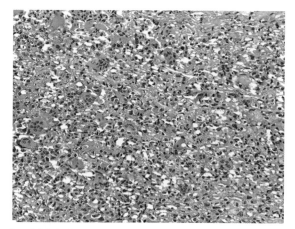

Fig. 10.24 Urothelial carcinoma with osteoclast-type giant cells. Osteoclast-type giant cells are interspersed among neoplastic urothelial cells.

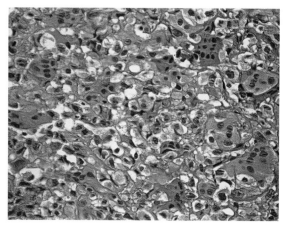

Fig. 10.25 Urothelial carcinoma with osteoclast-type giant cells. The giant cells do not show atypical features.

REFERENCES

1. Eble JN, Young RH. Carcinoma of the urinary bladder: a review of its diverse morphology. Semin Diagn Pathol 1997;14(2):98–108.

2. Donhuijsen K, Schmidt U, Richter HJ, et al. Mucoid cytoplasmic inclusions in urothelial carcinomas. Hum Pathol 1992;23:860–864.

3. Grignon DJ. Neoplasms of the urinary bladder. In: Bostwick DG, Eble JN (eds) Urologic Surgical Pathology. St Louis: Mosby Year-Book, 1997, pp 214–305.

4. Ayala AG, Ro JY. Premalignant lesions of the urothelium and transitional cell tumors. In: Young RH (ed.) Pathology of the Urinary Bladder. New York: Churchill Livingstone, 1989, pp 65–101.

5. Martin JE, Jenkins BJ, Zuk RJ, et al. Clinical importance of squamous metaplasia in invasive transitional cell carcinoma of the bladder. J Clin Pathol 1989;42:250–253.

6. Young RH, Oliva E. Transitional cell carcinomas of the urinary bladder that may be underdiagnosed: a report of four cases exemplifying the homology between neoplastic and non-neoplastic transitional cell lesions. Am J Surg Pathol 1996;20:1448–1454.

7. Young RH, Zukerberg LR. Microcystic transitional cell carcinoma of the urinary bladder: a report of four cases. Am J Clin Pathol 1991;96:635–639.

8. Paz A, Rath-Wolfson L, Lask D, et al. The clinical and histological features of transitional cell carcinoma of the bladder with microcysts: analysis of 12 cases. Br J Urol 1997;79:722–725.

9. Murphy WM, Deana DG. The nested variant of transitional cell carcinoma: a neoplasm resembling proliferation of Brunn's nests. Mod Pathol 1992;5:240–243.

10. Holmang S, Johansson SL. The nested variant of transitional cell carcinoma – a rare neoplasm with poor prognosis. Scand J Urol Nephrol 2001;35:102–105.

11. Badoual C, Bergemer-Fouquet AM, Renjard L, et al. An unusual variant of urothelial carcinoma: the nested variant of urothelial carcinoma. Report of two cases. Ann Pathol 1999;19:119–123.

12. Drew PA, Furman J, Civantos F, et al. The nested variant of transitional cell carcinoma: an aggressive neoplasm with innocuous histology. Mod Pathol 1996;9:989–994.

13. Ozdemir BH, Ozdemir G, Sertcelik A. The nested variant of transitional cell bladder carcinoma: a case report and review of the literature. Int Urol Nephrol 2000;32:257–258.

14. Auriault ML, Comoz F, Bottet P, et al. A diagnostic pitfall in the pathology of bladder tumors: the nested variant of urothelial carcinoma. Ann Pathol 2000;20:400–401.

15. Paik SS, Park MH. The nested variant of transitional cell carcinoma of the urinary bladder. Br J Urol 1996;78:793–794.

16. Tatsura H, Ogawa K, Sakata T, et al. A nested variant of transitional cell carcinoma of the urinary bladder: a case report. Jpn J Clin Oncol 2001;31:287–289.

17. Liedberg F, Chebil G, Davidsson T, et al. The nested variant of urothelial carcinoma: a rare but important bladder neoplasm with aggressive behavior. Three case reports and review of literature. Urol Oncol 2003;21:7–9.

18. Xiao GQ, Savage SJ, Gribetz ME, et al. The nested variant of urothelial carcinoma. Clinicopathology of 2 cases. Arch Pathol Lab Med 2003;127:e333–336.

19. Amin MB, Gomez JA, Young RH. Urothelial transitional cell carcinoma with endophytic growth patterns. Am J Surg Pathol 1997;21(9):1057–1068.

20. Cameron KM, Lupton, CH. Inverted papilloma of the lower urinary tract. Br J Urol 1976;48:567–577.

21. Djewitzki WS. Primary chorionepithelioma of the urinary bladder in a male: report of a case. Virchows Arch 1904;178:451–464.

22. Weinberg T. Primary chorionepithelioma of the urinary bladder in a male. Am J Pathol 1939;15:783–795.

23. Hyman A, Leiter HE. Extratesticular chorioepithelioma in a male probably primary in the urinary bladder. J Mt Sinai Hosp 1943;10:212–219.

24. Ainsworth RW, Gresham GA. Primary choriocarcinoma of the urinary bladder in a male. J Pathol Bacteriol 1906;79:185–192.

25. Civantos F, Rywlin AM. Carcinomas with trophoblastic differentiation and secretion of chorionic gonadotropins. Cancer 1906;29:789–798.

26. Kawamura J, Rhinsho K, Taki Y, et al. Choriocarcinoma and undifferentiated cell carcinoma of the bladder with gonadotropin secretion. J Urol 1979;121:684–686.

27. Hattori M, Yoshimoto Y, Matsukura S. Qualitative and quantitative analyses of human chorionic gonadotropin and its subunits produced by malignant tumours. Cancer 1980;46:355–361.

28. Obe JA, Rosen N, Koss LG. Primary choriocarcinoma of the urinary bladder: report of a case with probable epithelial origin. Cancer 1983;52:1405–1409.

29. Gallagher L, Lind R, Oyasu R. Primary choriocarcinoma of the urinary bladder in association with undifferentiated carcinoma. Hum Pathol 1984;15:793–795.

30. Dennis PM, Turner AG. Primary choriocarcinoma of the bladder evolving from a transitional cell carcinoma. J Clin Pathol 1984;37:503–505.

31. Burry AF, Munn SR, Arnold EP, et al. Trophoblastic metaplasia in urothelial carcinoma of the bladder. Br J Urol 1986;58:143–146.

32. Okamura T, Watase H, Watanabe H, et al. A case of chorio-carcinoma of the bladder. Jpn J Urol 1988;79:160–163.

33. Sone A, Furukawa Y, Nakatsuka S, et al. Primary choriocarcinoma of the bladder: a case report of autopsy. Jpn J Urol 1989;80:902–906.

34. Masui T, Asamoto M, Imaida K, et al. Primary choriocarcinoma of the urinary bladder. Jpn J Clin Oncol 1988;8:59–64.

35. Ishikawa J, Nishimura R, Maeda S, et al. Primary choriocarcinoma of the urinary bladder. Acta Pathol Jpn 1988;38:113–120.

36. Morton KD, Burnett RA. Choriocarcinoma arising in transitional cell carcinoma of the bladder: a case report. Histopathology 1988;12:325–328.

37. Abratt RB, Temple CRE, Pontin AR. Choriocarcinoma and transitional cell carcinoma of the bladder: a case report and review of the clinical evolution of disease in reported cases. Eur J Surg Oncol 1989;15:149–153.

38. Campo E, Algab F, Palacin A, et al. Placental proteins in high grade urothelial neoplasm. An immunohistochemical study of human chorionic gonadotropin, human placental lactogen, and pregnancy specific beta-1-glycoprotein. Cancer 1989;63:2947–2954.

39. Schmidt HP, Hering F, Torhorst J. Primary extragonadal choriocarcinoma of the urinary bladder, A case report with a review of 19 cases already reported. Urologe 1991;30:72–74.

40. Fowler AL, Hall E, Rees G. Choriocarcinoma arising in transitional cell carcinoma of the bladder. Br J Urol 1992;70:333–334.

41. Yokoyama S, Hayashida Y, Nagahama J, et al. Primary and metaplastic choriocarcinoma of the bladder: a report of two cases. Acta Cytol 1992;36:176–182.

42. Cho JH, Yu E, Kim KH, et al. Primary choriocarcinoma of the bladder: a case report. J Korean Med Sci 1992;7:369–372.

43. Puig RAM, Furio BY, Martin DF, et al. Primary choriocarcinoma of the bladder. A case report with immunohistochemical and ultrastructural study. Arch Esp Urol 1993;46:415–418.

44. Tinkler SD, Roberts JT, Robinson MC. Primary choriocarcinoma of the urinary bladder: a case report. Clin Oncol 1996;8:59–61.

45. McKendrick JJ, Theaker J, Mead GM. Nonseminomatous germ cell tumor with very high serum human chorionic gonadotropin. Cancer 1991;67:684–689.

46. Campbell PA, McKendrick J. Choriocarcinoma of the urinary bladder. Aust N Z J Surg 1999;69:533–537.

47. Sievert KD, Weber EA, Herwig R, et al. Pure primary choriocarcinoma of the urinary bladder with long-term survival. Urology 2000;56:856, vii–ix.

48. Dirnhofer S, Koessler P, Ensinger C, et al. Production of trophoblastic hormones by transitional cell carcinoma of the bladder: association to tumor stage and grade. Hum Pathol 1998;29:337–382.

49. Shah VM, Newman J, Crocker J, et al. Ectopic beta human chorionic gonadotropin production by bladder urothelial neoplasia. Arch Pathol Lab Med 1986;110:107–111.

50. Yamase HT, Wurich RS, Hich PI, et al. Immunohisto-chemical demonstration of human chorionic gonadotropin in tumors of the urinary bladder. Ann Clin Lab Sci 1985;15:414–417.

51. Amin MB, Ro JY, El-Sharkawy T, et al. Micropapillary variant of transitional cell carcinoma of the urinary bladder, Histologic pattern resembling ovarian papillary serous carcinoma. Am J Surg Pathol 1994;18(12):1224–1232.

52. Johansson SL, Borghede G, Holmang S. Micropapillary bladder carcinoma: a clinicopathological study of 20 cases. J Urol 1999;161:1798–1802.

53. Maranchie JK, Bouyounes BT, Zhang PL, et al. Clinical and pathological characteristics of micropapillary transitional cell carcinoma: a highly aggressive variant. J Urol 2000;163:748–751.

54. Dinney CPN, Ro JY, Babaian RJ, et al. Lymphoepithelioma of the bladder, A clinicopathological study of 3 cases. J Urol 1993;149:840–841.

55. Zukerberg LR, Harris NL, Young RH. Carcinoma of the urinary bladder simulating malignant lymphoma. Am J Surg Pathol 1991;15:569–576.

56. Young RH, Eble JN. Lymphoepithelioma-like carcinoma of the urinary bladder. J Urol Pathol 1993;1:63–67.

57. Amin BM, Ro JY, Lee KM, et al. Lymphoepithelioma-like carcinoma of the urinary bladder. Am J Surg Pathol 1994;18:466–473.

58. Bianchini E, Lisato L, Rimondi AP, et al. Lymphoepithelioma-like carcinoma of the urinary bladder. J Urol Pathol 1996;5:45–49.

59. Holmang S, Borghede G, Johansson S. Bladder carcinoma with lymphoepithelioma-like differentiation: a report of 9 cases. J Urol 1998;159:779–782.

60. Lopez-Beltran A, Luque RJ, Vicioso L, et al. Lymphoepithelioma-like carcinoma of the urinary bladder: a clinicopathologic study of 13 cases. Virchows Arch 2001;438:552–557.

61. Gulley ML, Amin MB, Nicholls JM, et al. Epstein–Barr virus is detected in undifferentiated nasopharyngeal carcinoma but not in lymphoepithelioma-like carcinoma of the urinary bladder. Hum Pathol 1995;26:1207–1214.

62. Sahin AA, Myhre M, Ro JY. Plasmacytoid transitional cell carcinoma: report of a case with initial presentation mimicking multiple myeloma. Acta Cytol 1991;35:277–280.

63. Zukerberg LR, Amin AR, Pisharodi L. Transitional cell carcinoma of the urinary bladder with osteoclast-type giant cells: a report of two cases and review of the literature. Histopathology 1990;17:407–411.

64. Reuter VE. Sarcomatoid lesions of the urogenital tract. Semin Diagn Pathol 1993;10:188–201.

65. Wick MR, Swanson PE. Carcinosarcomas: current perspectives and a historical review of nosological concepts. Semin Diagn Pathol 1993;10:118–127.

66. Lopez-Beltran A, Pacelli A, Rothenberg HJ, et al. Carcinosarcoma and sarcomatoid carcinoma of the bladder: a clinicopathological study of 41 cases. J Urol 1998;159:1497–1503.

67. Xu YM, Cai RX, Wu P, et al. Urethral carcinosarcoma following total cystectomy for bladder carcinoma. Urol Int 1993;50:104–107.

68. Sigal SH, Tomaszewski JE, Brooks JJ, et al. Carcinosarcoma of bladder following long-term cyclophosphamide therapy. Arch Pathol Lab Med 1991;115:1049–1051.

69. Nedergaard LP, Jacobsen GK. Simultaneous occurrence of carcinosarcoma of the bladder and seminoma of the testis. Scand J Urol Nephrol 1993;27:429–430.

70. Young RH. Carcinosarcoma of the urinary bladder. Cancer 1987;59:1333–1339.

71. Chen KT. Coexisting leiomyosarcoma and transitional cell carcinoma of the urinary bladder. J Surg Oncol 1986;33:36–37.

72. Torenbeek R, Blomjous CM, De Bruin PC, et al. Sarcomatoid carcinoma of the urinary bladder: clinicopathologic analysis of 18 cases with immunohistochemical and electron microscopy findings. Am J Surg Pathol 1994;18:241–249.

73. Young RH, Wick MR, Mills SE. Sarcomatoid carcinoma of the urinary bladder. Am J Clin Pathol 1988;90:653–661.

74. Serio G, Zampatti C, Ceppi M. Spindle and giant cell carcinoma of the urinary bladder: a clinicopathological light microscopic and immunohistochemical study. Br J Urol 1995;75:167–172.

75. Perret L, Chaubert P, Hessler D, et al. Primary heterologous carcinosarcoma (metaplastic carcinoma) of the urinary bladder, a clinicopathologic, immunohistochemical, and ultrastructural analysis of eight cases and a review of the literature. Cancer 1998;82:1535–1549.

76. Chen KT. Carcinosarcoma of the bladder. Letter to the editor. Arch Pathol Lab Med 1992;116:811.

77. Wick MR, Brown BA, Young RH, et al. Spindle cell proliferations of the urinary tract. An immunohisto-chemical study. Am J Surg Pathol 1988;12:379–389.

78. Jones EC, Young RH. Myxoid and sclerosing sarcomatoid transitional cell carcinoma of the urinary bladder: a clinicopathologic and immunohistochemical study of 25 cases. Mod Pathol 1997;10:908–916.

79. Ikegami H, Iwasaki H, Ohjimi Y, et al. Sarcomatoid carcinoma of the urinary bladder: a clinicopathologic and immunohistochemical analysis of 14 patients. Hum Pathol 2000; 31:332–340.

80. Young RH, Wick MR. Transitional cell carcinoma of the urinary bladder with pseudosarcomatous stroma. Am J Clin Pathol 1988;90:216–219.

81. Mahadevia PS, Alexander JE, Rojas-Corona R, et al. Pseudosarcomatous stromal reaction in primary and metastatic urothelial carcinoma: a source of diagnostic difficulty. Am J Surg Pathol 1989;13:782–790.

82. Young RH (ed.) Non-neoplastic epithelial abnormalities and tumor-like lesions. In: Pathology of the Urinary Bladder. New York: Churchill Livingstone, 1989, pp 1–63.

83. Pang LSC. Bony and cartilaginous tumours of the urinary bladder. J Pathol Bacteriol 1958;76:357–377.

84. Friedman NB, Ash JE. Atlas of Tumor Pathology (section 8, fascicle 31): Tumors of the Urinary Bladder. Washington, DC: Armed Forces Institute of Pathology, 1959, pp 25–33.

85. Collins DH, Curran RC. Pathological ossification and osseous metaplasia in man. In: Collins DH (ed.) Modern Trends in Pathology. London: Butterworth, 1959, pp 321–323.

86. Delides GS. Bone and cartilage in malignant tumors of the urinary bladder. Br J Urol 1972;44:571–581.

87. Yushita Y, Suzu H, Imamura A, et al. A case of primary vesical undifferentiated carcinoma with heterotopic ossification. Acta Urol Jpn 1982;28:1419–1426.

88. Toma H, Yamashita N, Nakazawa H, et al. Transitional cell carcinoma with osteoid metaplasia. Urology 1986;27:174–176.

89. Nakachi K, Miyamoto I, Kuroda J, et al. A case of transitional cell carcinoma of the bladder with heterotopic bone formation. Acta Urol Jpn 1988;34:1651–1655.

90. Eble JN, Young RH. Stromal osseous metaplasia in carcinoma of the urinary bladder. J Urol 1991;145:823–825.

91. Cornes, JS, Sussman T, Dawson IMP. Bone formation in metastasis from carcinoma of urinary bladder: report of a case with review of the literature. Br J Urol 1960;32:290–294.

92. Chinn D, Genant HK, Quivey JM, et al. Heterotopic-bone formation in metastatic tumor from transitional-cell carcinoma of the urinary bladder: a case report. J Bone Joint Surg 1976;58A:881–883.

93. Evison G, Pizey N, Roylance J. Bone formation associated with osseous metastases from bladder carcinoma. Clin Radiol 1981;32:303–309.

94. Lidgi S, Embon O, Turani H, et al. Giant cell reparative granuloma of the bladder associated with transitional cell carcinoma. J Urol 1989;142:120–122.

95. Kitazawa M, Kobayashi H, Ohnishi Y, et al. Giant cell tumor of the bladder associated with transitional cell carcinoma. J Urol 1985;133:472–475.

11

NON-TRANSITIONAL EPITHELIAL TUMORS

Gail Bentley and David Grignon

PRIMARY ADENOCARCINOMA

Adenocarcinoma may arise primarily from the urinary bladder; however, secondary involvement from tumors developing in adjacent organs is more common. A primary adenocarcinoma accounts for 0.5–2% of all malignant bladder tumors.[1-3] Petersen reviewed the literature in 1992 and found 321 reported cases.[4] The largest published series, with 72 and 185 cases respectively, were reported by Grignon et al.[5] and El-Mekresh et al.[6]

Traditionally, adenocarcinoma of the bladder has been divided into two major categories based on their site of origin:

- those arising in the bladder proper
- those arising from the urachal remnants.

Whether it is necessary to separate adenocarcinomas into urachal or non-urachal type is controversial. Most authors agree that both tumors have the same pathogenesis: metaplastic transformation to a glandular epithelium, leading to malignant transformation and to adenocarcinoma.[7] The separation of these two tumors is predominantly due to the treatment differences discussed below. For clinical and pathologic reasons, urachal and non-urachal adenocarcinoma will be addressed in separate sections. Specific variants of clinical significance (signet-ring cell carcinoma and clear cell adenocarcinoma) are dealt with individually.

URACHAL ADENOCARCINOMA

Diagnostic criteria

The histologic distinction in separating urachal from non-urachal adenocarcinoma may be difficult and requires correlation of clinical and pathologic findings. The clinicopathologic criteria for urachal origin have been well described. A sharp demarcation between normal surface epithelium and tumor, presence of a suprapelvic mass, primary involvement of muscle or deeper structures, tumor location in the bladder dome, tumor growth in the bladder wall extending into the space of Retzius, an intact or ulcerated epithelium, absence of cystitis cystica or glandularis elsewhere in the bladder, and documentation of the presence of urachal remnants, have all been applied.[8–10] The criteria of Johnson et al.[11] are perhaps the most practical: the tumor should be located anteriorly or in the dome, there should be a sharp demarcation between tumor and normal epithelium, and a primary, elsewhere, must be excluded. There are no specific pathologic features that distinguish urachal from non-urachal tumors. Immunohistochemistry has not been helpful in making this distinction.

Clinical features

Approximately one-third of primary bladder adeno-carcinomas arise in the urachus. The majority of cases occur in adulthood, during the fifth and sixth decades of life. The mean age is 51 years, approximately 10 years younger than the mean age for adenocarcinoma else-where in the bladder. The youngest case reported was that of a 15-year-old girl.[12] There is a predominance of men over women (ratio 1.8:1), which is lower than the 3:1 ratio for non-urachal adenocarcinoma.[1,5,6,8,9,13–15] The symptoms presented most frequently are hematuria (71%), pain (42%), irritative symptoms (40%), mucu-suria (25%) and umbilical discharge (2%).

The pathogenesis is controversial. Three theories have been offered to explain the source of glandular epi-thelium in the histogenesis of bladder adenocarcinomas.

- Pund et al.[16] proposed a theory of *cataplasia*, in which an epithelium that has lost its function reverts to a type it has passed through in previous development.
- Wright and McFarlane[17] proposed that, following the division of the cloaca, there may be *cloacal inclusions or rests of enteric tissue* remaining in the bladder.
- *Intestinal metaplasia* of the urachal epithelium is the favored mechanism accounting for the preponder-ance of adenocarcinomas of the urachus.[18,19]

Cases arising from villous adenoma of the urachus have been described.[20,21]

Pathologic features

The vast majority of urachal adenocarcinomas form discrete masses within the dome of the bladder. The tumor appears to have an epicenter in the wall of the bladder rather than being mucosally based, as is typical for non-urachal tumors. The bladder mucosa may be intact or ulcerated. The cut surface usually has a glistening mucoid appearance due to the abundant mucin secretion; however, the tumor less commonly appears solid. The tumor may extend along the urachal tract and be found within the abdominal wall.

Urachal adenocarcinoma has a variety of histologic appearances. The most frequent is mucinous (colloid) carcinoma, in which there are single cells, and, at times, nests of malignant cells floating within extracellular mucin (Fig. 11.1). The cells may have columnar or signet-ring morphology. The next most frequent pattern is enteric adenocarcinoma, with features typical of colorectal adenocarcinoma, which can include Paneth cells and argyrophil neuroendocrine cells.[22,23] An uncommon pattern is linitis plastica-like, signet-ring cell carcinoma (discussed below).[24] Histochemical stains reveal neutral and acid (sulfated and non-sulfated) mucin in these tumors.[5] Urachal adenocarcinoma expresses cytokeratin, carcinoembryonic antigen (CEA), Leu-M1 and epithelial membrane antigen (EMA).[5] A recent study showed CK20 positivity and consistent negativity for vimentin, OC125 and HER2/*neu*.[3] There have been conflicting reports concerning immuno-reactivity for prostate specific antigen (PSA) and prostatic acid phosphatase (PAP); in sum, PSA is nega-tive and occasionally may show focal PAP reactivity.[10,25]

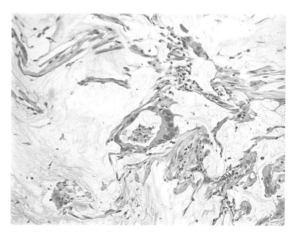

Fig. 11.1 Urachal adenocarcinoma with a malignant gland suspended in extravasated mucin in keeping with the mucinous (colloid) pattern.

Differential diagnosis

The major differential diagnostic considerations are non-urachal bladder adenocarcinoma and metastatic adenocarcinoma. As discussed above, these distinctions require clinicopathologic correlation. Torenbeek et al.[3] suggest that a histochemical profile may help in identifying metastatic adenocarcinomas from the prostate, female genital tract and colon. PSA enables the identification of prostatic origin in 90% of cases; prostatic specific acid phosphatase (PSAP) is less specific and more sensitive. Primary colonic neoplasms account for 20% of all secondary tumors involving the urinary bladder. Cervical and endometrial adenocarcinomas can extend to the urinary bladder, but this is rare.

Urachal adenocarcinoma should be distinguished from urachal villous adenoma.[26] This rare lesion is histologically identical to those found in the gastrointestinal tract, characterized by papillary and finger-like projections, with delicate fibrovascular stroma. The epithelial cells show nuclear stratification, loss of cellular polarity and nuclear hyperchromasia. The presence of invasion indicates malignancy.

Treatment and natural history

The treatment of urachal adenocarcinoma remains unsettled. Most authorities recommend segmental resection of the tumor, with en bloc resection of the urachus and umbilicus.[13,27,28] Partial cystectomy in the initial management of urachal cancer may be considered in selected cases, as this can enhance quality of life without reducing survival.[7] The role of adjuvant radiotherapy and chemotherapy is unclear at this time.

Urachal adenocarcinoma has been staged with the same systems used for urothelial bladder cancer.[5,9,14] Application of these systems is problematic in urachal carcinoma because, by virtue of their anatomic origin, all are 'muscle invasive'. Sheldon et al.[29] have proposed a system specific for urachal tumors:

- Stage I cancer is confined to the urachal mucosa
- Stage II cancer is invasive but is confined to the urachus
- Stage III cancer includes local extension to bladder (IIIA), abdominal wall (IIIB), peritoneum (IIIC) or viscera other than the bladder (IIID)
- Stage IV includes metastases to regional lymph nodes (IVA) or distant sites (IVB).

Nakanishi et al.[30] applied a modification of this system to 41 cases of urachal adenocarcinoma and found stage to be a significant predictor of outcome.

Dandekar et al.[7] also found that stage and grade at presentation were significant predictors of outcome.

The reported prognosis for these tumors also varies considerably. In a study of 72 cases, Grignon et al.[5] reported 5-year crude survival rates of 61%, and 31% for urachal and non-urachal adenocarcinoma, respectively ($p = 0.07$). The 10-year survival for urachal cases was 46%.[5] Survival curves, based on 71 patients reported in the literature, combined with raw data obtained from Grignon et al.,[5] revealed 5- and 10-year survival rates of 37% and 17%, respectively.[15] In this analysis, there was no significant difference in crude survival rates between adenocarcinoma of urachal and non-urachal origin. Dandekar et al.[7] reported a series of 48 patients, comprising 21 of urachal and 27 of non-urachal origin. The overall 5-year survival rates were reported as 45.7% and 29.9%, for urachal and non-urachal adenocarcinoma, respectively ($p = 0.14$). In a study limited to signet-ring cell adenocarcinoma of the bladder, Grignon et al.[24] reported significantly better survival rates for those originating in the urachus than elsewhere in the bladder.

NON-URACHAL ADENOCARCINOMA

Clinical features

Non-urachal adenocarcinoma accounts for 61–80% of primary bladder adenocarcinomas.[8,31] This tumor occurs over a wide age range, with a mean of 59 years; it is more common in males than in females (3:1).[1,5,8,9,13,14] Hematuria is the most common presentation (88%), followed by irritative symptoms (48%) and, rarely, mucusuria (2%).[5] The tumors are often advanced, with metastases in up to 40% of patients at the time of presentation.[5]

The histogenesis of primary non-urachal adenocarcinoma is controversial; however, most agree that it arises from metaplasia of the urothelium. There is strong evidence for the pluripotent metaplastic capacity of the normal urothelium due to the complex embryologic origin of the bladder. The dome and median regions are formed by the cloacal endoderm; the trigone is formed by the mesodermal Wolffian ducts. It is easy to see how the urothelium can undergo metaplastic and then dysplastic change. Support for this mechanism comes from cases arising in patients with longstanding diffuse intestinalization of the bladder mucosa, associated with a non-functioning bladder, chronic irritation, obstruction and cystocele. Cystitis glandularis is present in 14–67% of patients with non-urachal adenocarcinoma.[2,10]

Origin from metaplasia is also considered to be the mechanism in patients with exstrophy.[32,33] Most cancers arising in association with exstrophy are adeno-carcinomas, although occasional examples of squamous cell carcinoma and urothelial carcinoma have been described. The risk of adenocarcinoma in patients with exstrophy is in the range of 4.1–7.1%.[33,34] There is also an increased risk of adenocarcinoma in patients with pelvic lipomatosis; this is attributed to its association with cystitis glandularis.[35] Adenocarcinoma also arises in patients with *Schistosoma haematobium* infection.[6,36] Rare cases of adenocarcinoma[37,38] and adenosarcoma[39] have been described in association with endometriosis involving the bladder.

Pathologic features

Primary non-urachal adenocarcinoma can appear as an exophytic, papillary, solid, sessile, ulcerating or infiltra-tive mass. The signet-ring variant frequently shows diffuse thickening of the bladder wall, producing a linitis plastica-like appearance, and urothelial mucosal biopsies may be negative.

There has been some variability in defining adenocarcinoma in the literature. Most reports have excluded any case containing a recognizable urothelial carcinoma component, preferring to classify these as urothelial carcinoma with glandular differentiation.[5] Although others have included these cases as adeno-carcinoma if this pattern predominated,[8] the former approach is recommended. Grignon et al.[5] recognized six histologic variants of adenocarcinoma of the urinary bladder:

- *non-specific*, when the tumor did not resemble another recognized pattern (Fig. 11.2)
- *enteric*, when the cancer was composed of pseudo-stratified columnar cells forming glands, often with central necrosis typical of colonic adenocarcinoma (Fig. 11.3)
- *mucinous* (colloid), when the tumor cells were single or in nests floating in extracellular mucin
- *signet-ring*, when the tumor consisted of signet-ring cells diffusely infiltrating the bladder wall (Fig. 11.4)
- *clear cell*, when the tumor was composed of papillary and tubular structures with cytologic features identical to mesonephric adenocarcinoma
- *mixed*, when two or more of the described patterns were found (Fig. 11.5).

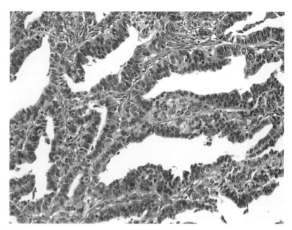

Fig. 11.2 Non-urachal adenocarcinoma with glands lined by a pseudostratified epithelium. This does not recapitulate any specific pattern of adenocarcinoma and so would be included in a not otherwise specified category.

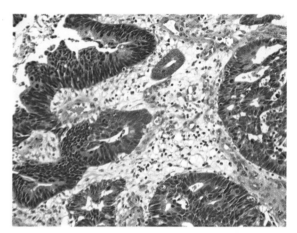

Fig. 11.3 Non-urachal adenocarcinoma having histologic features similar to usual enteric adenocarcinomas.

For non-urachal tumors, the non-specific and enteric types were the most common.

A uniform grading system has not been applied to adenocarcinoma of the bladder.[2,40] Anderstrom et al.[40] found grade to be a significant prognostic indicator, whereas Thomas et al.[2] did not find a correlation be-tween grade and outcome. In the former system, grade was assessed based on the degree of gland formation with two specific histologic subtypes (pure colloid and signet-ring) considered to be poorly differentiated. The histologic pattern did not correlate with outcome in the M.D. Anderson Cancer Center series, although the poor prognosis of the signet-ring variant was noted.[5]

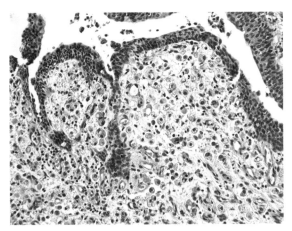

Fig. 11.4 Signet-ring cell carcinoma composed of dispersed cells in the bladder submucosa, the majority of which contain a single cytoplasmic mucin vacuole or have bubbly, finely vacuolated cytoplasm.

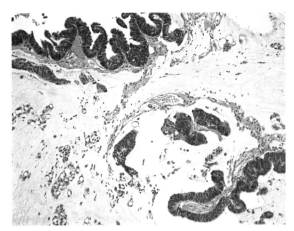

Fig. 11.5 Non-urachal adenocarcinoma with a mixed pattern including enteric and mucinous types.

Chan and Epstein reported 19 cases of what they termed 'adenocarcinoma in situ'.[41] In 17 cases these appear to represent urothelial carcinoma in situ (CIS) with glandular or pseudoglandular differentiation, a well-described pattern in urothelial CIS. In these cases the term adenocarcinoma in situ is not appropriate and potentially highly confusing. This term should be reserved for true cases of adenocarcinoma in situ with colonic-type epithelium having severe dysplastic change.

Differential diagnosis

The differential diagnosis of adenocarcinoma is extensive. First, benign mimics of adenocarcinoma need to be excluded. In some cases, cystitis cystica and cystitis glandularis may be florid, producing pseudopapillary or polypoid lesions, which may mimic a tumor. The benign cytology of the lining cells, and lack of invasion, are important features. In unusual cases, extracellular mucin is present, and careful evaluation for malignant cells is essential. Patients with longstanding intestinal metaplasia are at risk for the development of adenocarcinoma, and such cases should be carefully evaluated for early evidence of neoplastic transformation. Villous adenoma rarely occurs in the urinary bladder,[42] and shows the cytologic and architectural abnormalities of adenomatous epithelium without stromal invasion. Nephrogenic adenoma must be distinguished from adenocarcinoma, particularly the clear cell variant (see below).

Endometriosis often involves the bladder and should be considered in females of child-bearing age to distinguish it from adenocarcinoma. The histology is similar to endometriosis elsewhere, with variable amounts of endometrial glands, and stroma with hemosiderin-laden macrophages. Other Müllerian types of glandular tissue have been described in the urinary bladder under the terms Müllerianosis and endocervicosis.[43,44]

As for urachal adenocarcinoma, secondary involvement of the bladder must be excluded. Clinicopathologic correlation should always be obtained. Mucin histochemistry does not distinguish primary adenocarcinoma (urachal or non-urachal) from colorectal adenocarcinoma.[45] Immunohistochemistry has been reported to be of value in the distinction from colonic adenocarcinoma, with the latter being CK20 positive and CK7 negative in the majority of cases and with primary tumors being variably reactive to both CK7 and CK20.[3,46] Thrombomodulin is also reported to be positive in primary but not secondary tumors.[46]

Treatment and natural history

Surgery is the preferred therapy for primary adenocarcinoma of the bladder, with radical cystectomy or cystoprostatectomy with pelvic lymph node dissection. Non-urachal adenocarcinoma is staged using the standard AJCC-TNM or the Marshall modification of the Jewett staging system. Although stage is considered to be the most significant prognostic indicator in bladder adenocarcinoma, only three studies have confirmed this statistically; all found few long-term survivors in patients with transmural invasion.[5,7,40]

Prognosis for this tumor is poor. The overall 5- and 10-year survival rates for the 48 cases of non-urachal adenocarcinoma reported by Grignon et al.[5] were 31% and 28%, respectively. These data indicate that most patients who die of this tumor do so in the first 5 years, with uncommon late recurrences and deaths. The 5-year survival rate for patients with stage B (T2 and T3a) cancer was 76%, indicating the potential curability of earlier stages.[5] Dandekar et al.[7] reported that the overall 5-year survival rate for 27 cases was 29.9%. The survival rate, by stage, was 100% for stage A, 75% for stage B, 20.8% for stage C and 8.3% for stage D. The 5-year survival rate in patients treated with radical cystectomy was 35%. There were no long-term survivors in patients treated with radiotherapy and/or chemotherapy. Survival rate also showed a significant correlation to grade ($p = 0.003$).

SIGNET-RING CELL ADENOCARCINOMA

Primary signet-ring cell carcinoma of the urinary bladder is a rare tumor, with only 80 cases reported to date.[47] The first report of the signet-ring variant of bladder adenocarcinoma, as a distinct clinicopathologic entity, is attributed to Saphir in 1955.[48] In 1991, Grignon et al.[24] reported 12 cases and reviewed 56 cases from the literature. They provided a detailed analysis on their 12 cases, and on the 37 cases from the literature in which their criteria for diagnosis were met and sufficient clinical details were available. They required, at least, a focal component of diffuse, linitis plastica-like signet-ring cell adenocarcinoma, and no element of urothelial carcinoma. In 47% of cases, cystoscopy did not show a mucosal or mass lesion, with the mucosa most often being described as 'edematous' or 'bullous'.

Histologically, two variants have been identified. One type is composed of signet-ring cells floating in a pool of mucin and separated by cores of fibrous stroma. The second type features diffuse permeation by single signet-ring cells, some with single cytoplasmic vacuoles and others with a bubbly cytoplasm, associated with a scirrhous stroma identical to linitis plastica of the stomach (see Fig. 11.4).[47] In some cases, the cytoplasm was pale and eosinophilic with the nucleus pushed to one end, a pattern referred to as monocytoid (Fig. 11.6).[24,48] Mixtures of the two patterns have been reported.[47] Immunohistochemical staining results for the signet-ring cells show positive reactivity with pancytokeratin, Cam 5.2, CK20, EMA, CEA, 115D8 and OVTL 12/30.[49]

When diagnosing signet-ring cell carcinoma of the

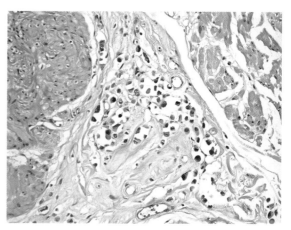

Fig. 11.6 Signet-ring cell carcinoma with individual cells having a monocytoid appearance infiltrating between muscle bundles. The cytoplasm in this case stained intensely positive for mucin.

bladder, care should be taken to exclude metastasis from a primary tumor at another site. The presence of a predominant signet-ring cell component in a urinary bladder tumor should prompt a thorough search to exclude a primary tumor in another area.[49] Patients with bladder involvement by metastasis usually present with extravesical symptoms, while patients with primary adenocarcinoma of the bladder commonly present with symptoms related to the bladder.[49] Prostatic adenocarcinoma may contain signet-ring cells, and it is important to eliminate the prostate as a primary source in male patients. Prostatic adenocarcinomas with signet-ring cells are usually not mucin-secreting, and are immunoreactive for PSA and PAP.

Since Grignon et al.[5] reported their series in 1991, there have been additional series of signet-ring cell carcinoma published. In 1996, Torenbeek et al.[49] reviewed 13 cases of primary signet-ring cell carcinoma of the bladder. The clinical presentation was similar to other bladder malignancies with the most common sign being hematuria. Mucinuria was not a feature. Patients were in their seventh or eighth decade of life, and there was a strong male predominance (11:2). These tumors followed an aggressive course, with 77% of all patients dead of the disease, with a mean survival of 20 months; the 2- and 5-year survival rates were 46% and 23%, respectively. Holmang et al.[47] reported their experience with 10 cases of signet-ring cell carcinoma of the bladder. In their series, survival was related to stage of disease at presentation. The disease was incurable when the margins were positive or when distant metastases were present. All patients with these features were dead of disease within 1 year. Similarly, Yamamato et al.[50] reported a very poor prognosis.

Convincing information regarding the effective management of signet-ring cell carcinoma is not available. In most cases, signet-ring carcinoma has a diffusely infiltrative growth pattern and radical cystectomy therefore appears prudent; however, outcome remains poor. These tumors are relatively radioresistant, and chemotherapy has not been shown to be effective.[47,49]

CLEAR CELL ADENOCARCINOMA

Primary clear cell adenocarcinoma of the urinary bladder is rare, with fewer than 25 well-documented cases in the English language literature.[37,51–54] Only a single case of clear cell carcinoma was included[40] in the four largest published series of bladder adenocarcinoma, totaling 232 cases. In contrast to the bladder, the urethra is a relatively frequent site for clear cell adenocarcinoma, particularly in females.[55]

The pathogenesis of clear cell adenocarcinoma in the bladder remains unresolved. Various hypotheses have been proposed. In early reports, the concept of origin from embryonic rests of mesoderm, from the mesonephric ducts, was generally accepted.[56] Frequent occurrence of clear cell adenocarcinomas in the trigone, bladder neck and urethra suggests an origin from mesonephric ducts; however, not all arise in these areas. Reported cases have occurred in the posterior wall and left lateral wall, in which mesodermal tissue derived from the mesonephric duct is not present. This suggests the possibility of malignant transformation of tissue originating from an aberrant Müllerian duct as an origin. There have also been three cases reported in the English literature in association with endometriosis, again suggesting Müllerian origin for at least some cases.[37,54,57] The hypothesis of a metaplastic origin from urothelium has recently been supported by Drew et al.[52] who studied six clear cell adenocarcinomas of the lower urinary tract (including four from the bladder) by histochemistry and immunohistochemistry; all six cases demonstrated positivity for Ca-125. Mai et al.[58] reported a case of multicentric clear cell adenocarcinoma arising in the urinary bladder and urethral diverticulum. This case had convincing evidence of Müllerian duct origin.

Grossly, the tumors are solid or papillary, and are most often located in the trigone or posterior wall.

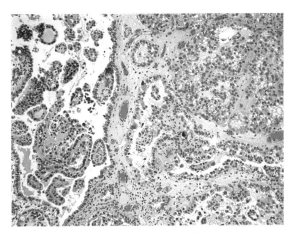

Fig. 11.7 Clear cell adenocarcinoma with papillary, alveolar and tubular architectures.

Histologically, the tumor cells proliferate in papillary, solid or tubular patterns (Fig. 11.7). The tubules may be cystically dilated. There are two distinct populations of cells:

- a papillary component consisting of cells having a distinct 'hobnail' appearance
- a second component consisting of clear cells in an alveolar or tubular pattern.

The cells have significant nuclear pleomorphism with frequent mitotic figures. Special stains demonstrate abundant cytoplasmic glycogen and, in most, focal cytoplasmic and luminal mucin.

The major differential diagnostic considerations are nephrogenic adenoma and metastatic clear cell carcinoma. Nephrogenic adenoma is typically small and has both papillary and tubular components that are lined by a single layer of flattened, cuboidal, low columnar or hobnail cells, with scant amphophilic cytoplasm. It lacks solid areas, shows minimal cytologic atypia and has no or rare mitotic figures.[59–61] Nephrogenic adenoma can infiltrate the muscular wall and the presence of this feature should not be used as a diagnostic criterion for malignancy.[59,60] A clinical history of trauma, infection, calculi, immunosuppressive therapy or instrumentation may be helpful. Gilcrease et al.[61] reported that MIB-1 positivity greater than 30/200 cells supports the diagnosis of clear cell carcinoma over nephrogenic adenoma. Alsanjari et al.[62] evaluated immunohistochemical markers in 10 nephrogenic adenomas and compared these to a clear cell carcinoma case. The nephrogenic adenomas were EMA-positive and CEA-negative, in contrast to the clear cell carcinoma that showed CEA positivity. Metastatic clear cell (mesonephric) carcinoma should be excluded in all female patients and requires clinical correlation. Renal cell carcinoma can metastasize to the bladder.[63] Recognition of the typical sinusoidal vascular pattern, lack of tubular differentiation and the absence of mucin, as well as relevant clinical features, should resolve this differential.

A standard treatment for clear cell adenocarcinoma has not yet been established. Transurethral resection appears to be an inadequate treatment in most cases; radical cystectomy may be the surgery of choice. There may be a role for neoadjuvant and adjuvant chemotherapy.[64]

HEPATOID ADENOCARCINOMA

Primary hepatoid adenocarcinoma of the urinary bladder is extremely rare, with only three cases reported in the literature, one in the renal pelvis and two in the bladder.[65] This adenocarcinoma is more common in the elderly population, and is reported to have an aggressive course and poor prognosis. Lymph node metastases are common. The hepatoid variant histologically features a pattern similar to that of hepatocellular carcinoma, with nests and trabecular structures of polygonal cells, with abundant granular eosinophilic cytoplasm, occasional hyaline globules, vesicular nuclei and prominent nucleoli. No bile pigment is present. Tumor nests diffusely infiltrate the muscular layer of the bladder. The tumor may be associated with areas of necrosis and hemorrhage. The original description of hepatoid adenocarcinoma was in the stomach and is the most common location. Other organs reported as being involved include ovary, lung, intestine, adrenal gland and, as we have mentioned, the urothelium.[65]

The tumor shows immunoreactivity for alpha-fetoprotein (AFP), α_1-antitrypsin (AAT), albumin and CAM (CK) 5.2. There is membrane reactivity to EMA. Interestingly, polyclonal CEA is expressed in a canalicular pattern, as is seen in hepatocellular carcinoma. Hepatocyte growth factor (HGF), and its receptor *c-met*, show strong positivity, with HGF staining being cytoplasmic and *c-met* expressed in a membrane pattern.[65]

A careful search should be made for a primary hepatocellular carcinoma before a diagnosis of hepatoid adenocarcinoma of the bladder is made. Although they are decidedly rare in the bladder, they should be included in the differential diagnosis of a poorly differentiated neoplasm.

SQUAMOUS CELL CARCINOMA

Clinical features

Squamous cell carcinoma of the urinary bladder is relatively rare in Western countries, representing only 3–5% of all bladder tumors.[66] However, the prevalence of squamous cell carcinoma in areas of Africa and the Middle East, where schistosomiasis is endemic, is much higher, with squamous cell carcinoma accounting for up to 80% of bladder cancers.[36,67] In the United States and Europe, the male to female ratio is 1.7:1, with an age range of 30–90 years (mean 65.5 years). Most patients present with hematuria and/or irritative symptoms. Rare cases with associated hypercalcemia have been described.[67]

The pathogenesis of squamous cell carcinoma of the urinary bladder not associated with bilharziasis is still unknown. There is evidence suggesting that these lesions may arise from extensive squamous differentiation of transitional cell carcinoma, or from direct malignant transformation from squamous metaplasia of the urinary bladder.[68] Most authorities would consider cases in the first instance to represent urothelial carcinomas with squamous differentiation rather than squamous cell carcinomas. Experimental studies by Kunze[69] in a rat model found that the histogenetic pathway exists by increasing atypia in metaplastic squamous epithelium, and ultimately a transition into invasive carcinoma. Kunze concluded that, in both rats and humans, squamous cell carcinomas arise in metaplastic areas from pre-existing squamous metaplasia. In support of the latter theory, it has been documented that many patients with squamous cell carcinoma have long histories of bladder irritation caused by infection,[70–72] stones,[70,72] indwelling catheters,[73] intermittent self-catheterization[73] or urinary retention.[72] This seems to support the notion of malignant transformation of squamous metaplasia, in which the chronic irritation led to a metaplastic process, which eventually became dysplastic and then malignant.

Keratinizing squamous metaplasia is an important risk factor for the development of squamous cell carcinoma.[68,74] In one series, 33 of 78 patients with keratinizing squamous metaplasia had simultaneous or subsequent carcinoma. In those who subsequently developed cancer, the tumor developed an average of 12 years after the diagnosis of metaplasia. Further study is needed in this area. It is also reported that many tumors arising in bladder diverticula are squamous cell carcinoma.[75] It is rare to find squamous cell carcinomas in tumors arising in bladder exstrophy or in the urachus.[29]

Many studies have established an etiologic role of human papilloma virus (HPV) in the development of cancer. Wilczynski et al.[76] identified HPV6 in a case of squamous cell carcinoma of the bladder. Oft et al.[77] has also reported a case in which HPV6 was present in squamous cell carcinoma of the bladder. Further study is needed to conclude whether HPV is a risk factor in squamous cell carcinoma of the bladder.

Schistosome infection is a worldwide medical problem[78,79] and its role in the pathogenesis of bladder cancer in endemic areas is of considerable interest. There are three major species pathogenic to humans: *S. mansoni*, *S. japonicum* and *S. haematobium*; only *S. haematobium* causes bladder cancer.[79] In a series of 1095 cases of bladder cancer from Egypt, schistosome eggs were identified in the bladder wall in 902 cases (82%).[36] Bladder infection by *S. haematobium* may result in polyposis, ulceration, urothelial hyperplasia and metaplasia, dysplasia or carcinoma.[80] Although squamous cell carcinoma is the most frequent type of cancer, a relatively high prevalence of adenocarcinoma (5.8%) is also seen.[36]

New markers are now available for the detection of squamous cell carcinoma. Psoriasin, a calcium-binding protein expressed by squamous epithelial cells, has been detected in the urine of patients with squamous cell carcinoma of the bladder.[66] Recent information suggests that the measurement of plasma, and tissue concentration of SCC-Ag, may assist in the diagnosis and follow-up of bladder squamous cell carcinoma.[66] Further studies are necessary to assess the clinical relevance of this antigen.

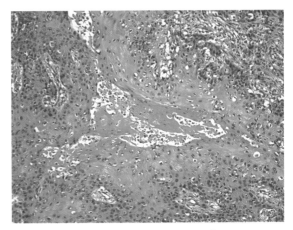

Fig. 11.8 Well-differentiated squamous cell carcinoma with abundant keratinization.

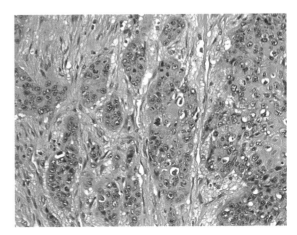

Fig. 11.9 Poorly differentiated squamous cell carcinoma without keratin formation.

Pathologic features

Grossly, most squamous cell carcinomas are bulky, polypoid, solid, necrotic masses, often filling the bladder lumen,[81] although some are predominantly flat and irregularly bordered[71] or ulcerated and infiltrating.[82] The presence of necrotic material and keratin debris on the surface is relatively constant.

The diagnosis of squamous cell carcinoma has been restricted by most authors to pure tumors.[70,72,81,83] The tumors may be well differentiated, in which histologically well-defined islands of squamous cells with keratinization, prominent intercellular bridges and minimal nuclear pleomorphism or atypia are found (Fig. 11.8). Poorly differentiated tumors exhibit marked nuclear pleomorphism with only focal evidence of squamous differentiation (Fig. 11.9). Squamous metaplasia is identifiable in the adjacent epithelium in 17–60% of cases from Europe and North America.[72] Squamous cell carcinoma of the bladder is graded according to the amount of keratinization present, as well as the degree of nuclear pleomorphism.[70,71,83] Histologic grade may correlate with stage and outcome,[70,84] although this has not been uniform.[71] Winkler et al.[83] found tumor grade correlated with DNA content, but not with survival. In the latter study, DNA ploidy was a powerful predictor of progression with 35, 45 and 92% of patients having diploid, tetraploid and aneuploid tumors progressing, respectively.

Differential diagnosis

The major differential diagnostic consideration for squamous cell carcinoma is urothelial carcinoma with squamous differentiation, which occurs in up to 20% of high-grade urothelial carcinomas.[85,86] In North America, Europe and other regions where primary squamous cell carcinoma is uncommon, such tumors should be carefully studied for a urothelial component. If an identifiable urothelial element (including urothelial carcinoma in situ) is found, the tumor should be classified as urothelial carcinoma with squamous differentiation.[86] The presence of keratinizing squamous metaplasia, especially if associated with dysplasia, favors a diagnosis of squamous cell carcinoma. Secondary invasion of the bladder by an adjacent primary, such as squamous cell carcinoma of the cervix or vagina, should always be considered and excluded clinically.

Treatment and natural history

A high proportion of patients have advanced cancer at the time of diagnosis.[66,81,83,84] The incidence of distant metastasis at the time of diagnosis is reported in the literature to be 10%.[66] Overall, the prognosis is poor and the majority of patients die after locoregional failure, which accounts for up to 90% of deaths in squamous cell carcinoma of the bladder.[66]

In the M.D. Anderson Cancer Center series, 5- and 10-year survival rates were only 13.5% and 5.3%, respectively.[82] Other studies have reported 5-year survival rates ranging from 7.4%[72] to 50%,[87] the latter in a small series of patients treated with preoperative radiation and radical cystectomy.[87] Jones et al.[88] reported an overall 5-year survival of 16%. In this series, patients that underwent radical radiotherapy had a 5-year survival of 36%, and of those patients that had neoadjuvant radiotherapy and cystectomy, none survived over 1 year. Tannenbaum[89] reported that 16% survived 2 years after cystectomy without adjuvant radiotherapy. Metastases show a striking predilection for bone.[72,81,90]

The treatment of choice for pure squamous cell carcinoma of the bladder has been radical cystectomy or cystoprostatectomy. Radiation therapy alone is not effective.[91] Recent reports suggest that preoperative radiation therapy, with[92] or without[87] neoadjuvant chemotherapy, may be useful. Clearly the role of radiotherapy needs further study. Tumor stage, by either the AJCC-TNM or Jewett (or Marshall modification of Jewett) staging system, is the most important prognostic indicator for squamous cell carcinoma.[70,81]

VERRUCOUS CARCINOMA

Rare cases of verrucous carcinoma of the urinary bladder have been described.[93–100] Most are in association with bilharzial cystitis, accounting for 3% of bladder cancers in one such series.[36] Only eight cases have been reported in the literature not associated with bilharzial infection.

Verrucous carcinoma derives its name from its gross appearance, which has been described as a wart-like, fungating, exophytic mass. Microscopically, there is well-differentiated hyperkeratotic squamous epithelium, extending down toward the submucosa in large, broad, bulbous projections that push the tissue rather than invade. There is minimal nuclear and architectural atypia. The criteria established by Ackerman[101] for the oral cavity include the following:

- It must be exophytic with multiple warty surface projections composed of well-differentiated squamous epithelium.
- It must lack features of anaplasia.
- The advancing margin must push, not infiltrate.

We would apply the same criteria in the urinary bladder.

Three cases in the urinary bladder were free of recurrence and progression after 3, 24 and 36 months.[93–95] One case in the urinary bladder developed in a patient with longstanding anogenital condyloma acuminata, suggesting a possible link with the bladder tumor.[95]

BASALOID SQUAMOUS CELL CARCINOMA

Basaloid squamous cell carcinoma is a recently described variant of squamous cell carcinoma. It arises predominantly in the upper aerodigestive tract. Vakar-Lopez and Abrams[102] have described a basaloid squamous cell carcinoma arising in the urinary bladder. Grossly, the mass was tan-brown, sessile and multilobulated, involving the posterior wall. Microscopically, the tumor was composed of nests of small basaloid cells with minimal cytoplasm. The nests featured peripheral palisading of the basaloid cells. Some of the larger nests showed central necrosis with the smaller nests having a pseudoglandular pattern in some areas. The tumor infiltrated in a desmoplastic stroma. Cytologically, the cells displayed a high nuclear/cytoplasmic ratio with dense hyperchromatic nuclei. Mitotic and apoptotic figures were numerous. Squamous differentiation and microscopic focus of transitional cell carcinoma were present. The remaining bladder had extensive squamous metaplasia with foci of dysplasia and squamous carcinoma in situ. This patient had a longstanding history of recurrent urinary tract infections, as well as multiple surgical procedures, which explain the extensive squamous metaplasia.[102]

The literature indicates that basaloid squamous carcinoma in other areas may have a more aggressive course, and a worse prognosis, than the usual squamous cell carcinoma. Given the rarity of this histology in the bladder, there is no information regarding behavior or optimal treatment.

SMALL CELL CARCINOMA

Clinical features

Small cell carcinoma of the urinary bladder is defined as histologically identical to that occurring in the lung. The first published case was in 1981 by Cramer et al.[103] and to date there are over 135 reported cases.[104] The largest series reported the outcome of 25 patients over a 27-year period. Angulo et al.[105] summarized 106 cases from the world literature, including two of their own.

The tumor has been estimated to represent 0.5–1% of bladder malignancies.[106,107] It develops much more frequently in men than in women (ratio 4:1) and is essentially a tumor of older patients (range 20–85 years, mean 66 years).[105] Hematuria is the most frequent presentation (90% of cases), with symptoms of bladder irritability or obstruction occurring less commonly. The patients often present with locally advanced or metastatic cancer. Paraneoplastic syndromes – including ectopic adrenocorticotropic hormone (ACTH) production,[108] hypercalcemia[106] and hypophosphatemia – rarely occur.[102,109] At least four cases have arisen in bladder diverticula, and one case in a patient following augmentation cystoplasty.

At least three theories have been proposed to account for these tumors in the bladder. The most often cited, and currently favored, is an origin from multipotential undifferentiated or stem cells present in the urothelium.[106,110] These cells have been demonstrated in the basal cell layer of the urothelium. The frequent association of this tumor with other histologic variants, such as urothelial carcinoma and adenocarcinoma, supports this theory.[111] A second hypothesis is origin from neuroendocrine cells within normal[112] or metaplastic urothelium.[102] A third hypothesis is origin from an undefined population of submucosal neuroendocrine cells.[113]

Pathologic features

There are no specific gross features separating small cell carcinoma from other carcinomas of the bladder. They are usually polypoid or solid lesions, frequently ulcerating, and range in size from 2 to 10 cm. They can develop at any location including the dome and within diverticula. They usually show diffuse infiltration into the bladder wall and occasional extension into the perivesical adipose tissue.

Microscopically, the tumor has two major patterns: it can show either an oat cell or intermediate cell pattern; both may be present in the same tumor. The oat cell type consists of a relatively uniform population of cells with scant cytoplasm, hyperchromatic nuclei with dispersed chromatin, and absent or inconspicuous nucleoli (Fig. 11.10). The intermediate cell type has more abundant cytoplasm, larger nuclei with less hyperchromasia, but with dispersed chromatin and absent or inconspicuous nucleoli. In some cases, the intermediate type of small cell carcinoma contains elongate or spindled cells (Fig. 11.11). Both types have extensive necrosis, prominent nuclear molding, frequent mitotic figures and may have DNA encrustation of blood vessel walls ('Azzopardi phenomenon'). A single case with a large cell neuroendocrine carcinoma phenotype has been described[114] and the presence of scattered cells with 'monstrous nuclei' has also been reported.[115]

Between 23%[115] and 67%[111] of cases are mixed with other histologic patterns. A urothelial carcinoma component (papillary or non-papillary) is most common, but glandular and squamous differentiation have been

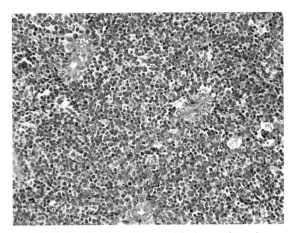

Fig. 11.10 Small cell carcinoma with sheets of poorly cohesive cells having uniform small nuclei, fine chromatin and inconspicuous nucleoli.

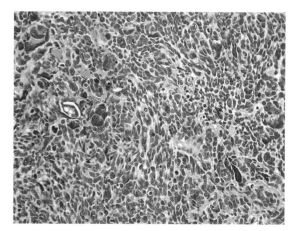

Fig. 11.11 Small cell carcinoma composed of intermediate cells, many of which are spindled and have bizarre nuclei. The chromatin is finely distributed with inconspicuous nucleoli.

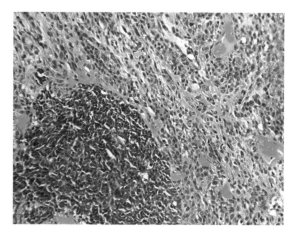

Fig. 11.12 Mixed small cell carcinoma with high-grade urothelial carcinoma. In this case, the small cell component has an intermediate cell type.

growth pattern is present, and tumor cells have more abundant cytoplasm. Too few cases, with limited follow-up, have been reported to allow for conclusions regarding treatment or clinical behavior of these rare tumors.

In most reported cases studied by electron microscopy, dense core neurosecretory granules have been found.[115,120] Other features such as cytoplasmic processes have also been noted. In the majority of cases, evidence of neuroendocrine differentiation can be found immunohistochemically, with neuron-specific enolase immunoreactivity being the most frequently expressed. Chromogranin A had a 97% specificity and synaptophysin had an 86% specificity in one report.[121] CD44v6 has been found to be negative in the majority of small cell carcinomas and positive in the majority of urothelial tumors. Although cytokeratin is present in most tumors, some are non-reactive, and this is significant in differential diagnosis. The presence of a 'dot-like' pattern for cytokeratin has been noted in some cases.[115,121]

Atkin et al.[122] have recently studied cytogenetics and flow cytometry in this tumor. They reported that small cell carcinoma of the bladder demonstrated numerous structural chromosomal changes and karyotypic variability. Teracciano et al.[123] found rearrangements of chromosomes 6, 9, 11, 13 and 18.

Differential diagnosis

The major differential diagnostic considerations are small cell carcinoma from another site and malignant lymphoma. Small cell carcinoma may arise in the prostate gland and in about 50% of cases there is a coexistent adenocarcinoma component; positive staining of this element for PSA and PAP would indicate prostatic origin. The small cell component is usually negative for these markers;[124] in pure cases, therefore, clinical correlation may be essential to separate prostate from bladder primaries. Metastases from other sites also need to be considered. Interestingly, symptomatic bladder metastasis from bronchogenic small cell carcinoma is a rare occurrence,[125] but clinical correlation is necessary to exclude this possibility. The identification of a urothelial component, including urothelial carcinoma in situ, would strongly support primary bladder origin.[115] Malignant lymphoma should be distinguishable in most cases on histologic grounds, but in difficult cases immunohistochemical staining for cytokeratin and leukocyte common antigen should readily distinguish the two.[115]

observed (Fig. 11.12). One case of small cell carcinoma arose in association with urachal adenocarcinoma.[116] In some cases, the adjacent urothelium has severe dysplasia or urothelial carcinoma in situ.[115] In contrast to urothelial carcinoma with squamous or glandular distinction, pure and mixed tumors are reported as small cell carcinoma with other histologic patterns, when present, indicated.

Rare examples of better differentiated neuroendocrine neoplasms, showing histologic features of carcinoid tumors, without associated urothelial carcinoma, have been described.[109,117–119] In these cases, an organoid

Treatment and natural history

The aggressive behavior of this tumor has been noted repeatedly; overall survival is poor. Recent reports suggest that patients may respond to aggressive combination therapy if given at the time of diagnosis.[106,113,115] In a series from the M.D. Anderson Cancer Center,[115] six patients were treated with cystectomy or cystoprostatectomy combined with adjuvant multiagent chemotherapy. All were alive at the time of the report, from 10 to 77 months after treatment, including three patients who had documented metastases at the time of diagnosis. In the review of Angulo et al.,[105] tumor stage and method of treatment were the most important predictors of outcome. Patients receiving adjuvant or neoadjuvant chemotherapy had a 5-year survival rate of 46%, while patients whose treatment did not include systemic therapy had a 5-year survival rate of 20%, despite the latter having an overall lower stage. This report, and others, underscores the importance of recognizing this distinct form of bladder cancer which may respond to aggressive therapy.[104–106,113,115,126–129]

REFERENCES

1. Jacobo E, Loening S, Schmidt JD, et al. Primary adenocarcinoma of the bladder: a retrospective study of 20 patients. J Urol 1977;117:54–56.
2. Thomas DG, Ward AM, Williams JL. A study of 52 cases of adenocarcinoma of the bladder. Br J Urol 1971;43:4–15.
3. Torenbeek R, Ladendijk JH, Van Diest PJ, et al. Value of a panel of antibodies to identify the primary origin of adenocarcinomas present as bladder carcinoma. Histopathology 1998;32:20–27.
4. Petersen RO. Urologic Pathology, 2nd edn. Philadelphia: J.B.Lippincott, 1992.
5. Grignon DJ, Ro JY, Ayala AG, et al. Primary adenocarcinoma of the urinary bladder: a clinicopathologic analysis of 72 cases. Cancer 1991;67:2165–2172.
6. El-Mekresh MM, el-Baz MA, Abol-Enein H, et al. Primary adenocarcinoma of the urinary bladder: a report of 185 cases. Br J Urol 1998;82:206–212.
7. Dandekar NP, Dalal AV, Tongaonkar HB, et al. Adenocarcinoma of bladder. Eur J Surg Oncol 1997;23:157–160.
8. Mostofi FK, Thomson RV, Dean AL Jr. Mucous adenocarcinoma of the urinary bladder. Cancer 1955;8:741–758.
9. Jones WA, Gibbons RP, Correa RJ Jr, et al. Primary adenocarcinoma of bladder. Urology 1980;15:119–122.
10. Abenoza P, Manivel C, Fraley EE. Primary adenocarcinoma of urinary bladder: clinicopathologic study of 16 cases. Urology 1987;29:9–14.
11. Johnson DE, Hogan JM, Ayala AG. Primary adenocarcinoma of the urinary bladder. South Med J 1972;65:527–530.
12. Cornil C, Reynolds CT, Kickham CJE. Carcinoma of the urachus. J Urol 1967;98:93–95.
13. Kamat MR, Kulkarni JN, Tongaonkar HB. Adenocarcinoma of the bladder: study of 14 cases and review of the literature. Br J Urol 1991;68:254–257.
14. Wilson TG, Pritchett TR, Lieskovsky G, et al. Primary adenocarcinoma of bladder. Urology 1991;38:223–226.
15. Grignon DJ. Neoplasms of the urinary bladder. In: Bostwick DG, Eble JN (eds) Urologic Surgical Pathology. Philadelphia: Mosby-Year Book, 1996.
16. Pund ER, Yount HA, Blumberg JM. Variations in morphology of urinary bladder epithelium. Special reference to cystitis glandularis and carcinomas. J Urol 1952;68:242.
17. Wright HB, McFarlane DJ. Carcinoma of the urachus. Am J Surg 1955;90:693.
18. Begg RC. The colloid adenocarcinoma of the bladder vault arising from the epithelium of the urachal canal: with a critical survey of the tumours of the urachus. Br J Surg 1931;18:422–464.
19. Pantuck AJ, Bancila E, Das KM, et al. Adenocarcinoma of the urachus and bladder expresses a unique colonic epithelial epitope: an immunohistochemical study. J Urol 1997;158:1722–1727.
20. Lucas DR, Lawrence WD, McDevitt WJ, et al. Mucinous papillary adenocarcinoma of the bladder arising within a villous adenoma of urachal remnants: an immunohistochemical and ultrastructural study. J Urol Pathol 1994;2:173–182.
21. Cheng L, Montironi R, Bostwick DG. Villous adenoma of the urinary tract: a report of 23 cases, including 8 with coexistent adenocarcinoma. Am J Surg Pathol 1999;23:764–771.
22. Pallesen G. Neoplastic Paneth cells in adenocarcinoma of the urinary bladder: a first case report. Cancer 1981;47:1834–1837.
23. Satake T, Matsuyama M. Neoplastic nature of argyrophil cells in urachal adenocarcinoma. Acta Pathol Jpn 1986;36:1587–1592.
24. Grignon DJ, Ro JY, Ayala AG, et al. Primary signet-ring cell carcinoma of the urinary bladder. Am J Clin Pathol 1991;95:13–20.
25. Epstein JI, Kuhajda FP, Lieberman PH, et al. Prostate specific acid phosphatase immunoreactivity in adenocarcinomas of the urinary bladder. Hum Pathol 1986;17:939–942.
26. Eble JN, Hull MT, Rowland RG, et al. Villous adenoma of the urachus with mucusuria: a light and electron microscopic study. J Urol 1986;135:1240–1244.
27. Johnson DE, Hodge GB, Abdul Karim FW, et al. Urachal carcinoma. Urology 1985;26:218–221.
28. Ravi R, Shrivastava BR, Chandrasekhar GM, et al. Adenocarcinoma of the urachus. J Surg Oncol 1992;50:201–203.
29. Sheldon CA, Clayman RV, Gonzalez R, et al. Malignant urachal lesions. J Urol 1984;131:1–8.

30. Nakanishi K, Kawai T, Suzuki M, et al. Prognostic factors in urachal adenocarcinoma: a study in 41 specimens of DNA status, proliferating cell–nuclear antigen immunostaining and argyrophilic nucleolar organizer region counts. Hum Pathol 1996;27:240–247.

31. Ohman U, von Garrelts B, Moberg A. Carcinoma of the urachus: review of the literature and report of two cases. Scand J Urol Nephrol 1971;5:91–95.

32. O'Kane HOJ, Megaw JMcI. Carcinoma in the exstrophic bladder. Br J Surg 1968;55:631–635.

33. Engel RM, Wilkinson HA. Bladder exstrophy. J Urol 1970;104:699–704.

34. Goyanna R, Emmett JL, McDonald JR. Exstrophy of the bladder complicated by adenocarcinoma. J Urol 1951;65:391–400.

35. Heyns CF, De Kock MLS, Kirsten PH, et al. Pelvic lipomatosis associated with cystitis glandularis and adenocarcinoma of the bladder. J Urol 1991;145:364–366.

36. El Bolkainy MN, Mokhtar NM, Ghoneim MA, et al. The impact of schistosomiasis on the pathology of bladder carcinoma. Cancer 1981;48:2643–2648.

37. Chor PJ, Gaum LD, Young RH. Clear cell adenocarcinoma of the urinary bladder: report of a case of probable mullerian origin. Mod Pathol 1993;6:225–228.

38. Yoshimura S, Ito Y. Malignant transformation of endometriosis of the urinary bladder: Case report. Gann 1951;42:2.

39. Vara AR, Ruzics EP, Moussabeck O, et al. Endometrioid adenosarcoma of the bladder arising from endometriosis. J Urol 1990;143:813–815.

40. Anderstrom C, Johansson SL, von Schultz L. Primary adenocarcinoma of the urinary bladder. A clinicopathologic and prognostic study. Cancer 1983;52:1273–1280.

41. Chan TY, Epstein JI. In situ adenocarcinoma of the bladder. Am J Surg Pathol 2001;25:892–899.

42. Saleh HA, Papas P, Khatib G. Villous adenoma of the urinary bladder presenting as gross hematuria: a morphologic, histochemical and immunohistochemical study. J Urol Pathol 1996;4:299–306.

43. Nazeer T, Ro JY, Tornos C, et al. Endocervical type glands in urinary bladder: a clinicopathologic study of six cases. Hum Pathol 1996;27:816–820.

44. Young RH, Clement PB. Mullerianosis of the urinary bladder. Mod Pathol 1996;9:731–737.

45. Nakanishi K, Tominaga S, Kawai T, et al. Mucin histochemistry in primary adenocarcinoma of the urinary bladder (of urachal or vesicular origin) and metastatic adenocarcinoma originating in the colorectum. Pathol Int 2000;50:297–303.

46. Wang HL, Lu DW, Yerian LM, et al. Immunohistochemical distinction between primary adenocarcinoma of the bladder and secondary colorectal adenocarcinoma. Am J Surg Pathol 2001;25:1380–1387.

47. Holmang S, Borghede G, Johansson SL. Primary signet-ring cell carcinoma of the bladder: a report on 10 cases. Scand J Urol Nephrol 1997; 31:145–148.

48. Saphir O. Signet-ring cell carcinoma of the urinary bladder. Am J Pathol 1955;31:223–231.

49. Torenbeek R, Koot RA, Blomjous CE, et al. Primary signet-ring cell caricnoma of the urinary bladder. Histopathology 1996;28:33–40.

50. Yamamoto S, Akiyama A, Miki M, et al. Primary signet-ring cell carcinoma of the urinary bladder inducing renal failure. Int J Urol 2001;8:190–193.

51. Young RH, Scully RE. Clear cell adenocarcinoma of the bladder and urethra: a report of three cases and review of the literature. Am J Surg Pathol 1985;9:816–826.

52. Drew PA, Murphy WM, Civantos F, et al. The histogenesis of clear cell adenocarcinoma of the lower urinary tract: case series and review of the literature. Hum Pathol 1996;27:248–252.

53. Honda N, Yamada Y, Nanaura H. Mesonephric adenocarcinoma of the urinary bladder: a case report. Acta Urol Jpn 2000;45:27–31.

54. Oliva E, Amin MB, Jiminez R, Young RH. Clear cell carcinoma of the urinary bladder: a report and comparison of four tumors of Mullerian origin and nine of probable urothelial origin with discussion of histogenesis and diagnostic problems. Am J Surg Pathol 2002;26:190–197.

55. Oliva E, Young RH. Clear cell adenocarcinoma of the urethra: a clinicopathologic analysis of 19 cases. Mod Pathol 1996;9:513–520.

56. Kanokogi M, Uematsu K, Kakudo K, et al. Mesonephric adenocarcinoma of the urinary bladder: an autopsy case. J Surg Oncol 1983;22:118–120.

57. Balat O, Kudelaka AP, Edwards CL, et al. Malignant transformation in endometriosis of the urinary bladder: case report of clear cell adenocarcinoma. Eur J Gynaecol Oncol 1996;17:13–16.

58. Mai KT, Yazdi HM, Perkins DG, et al. Multicentric clear cell adenocarcinoma in the urinary bladder and the urethral diverticulum: evidence of origin of clear cell adenocarcinoma of the female lower urinary tract from Mullerian duct remnants. Histopathology 2000;36:380–382.

59. Ford TF, Watson GM, Cameron KM. Adenomatous metaplasia (nephrogenic adenoma) of urothelium: an analysis of 70 cases. Br J Urol 1985;57:427–433.

60. Young RH, Scully RE. Nephrogenic adenoma. Am J Surg Pathol 1986;10:268–275.

61. Gilcrease MZ, Delgado R, Vuitch F, et al. Clear cell adenocarcinoma and nephrogenic adenoma of the urethra and urinary bladder: a histopathologic and immunohistochemical comparison. Hum Pathol 1998;29:1451–1456.

62. Alsanjari N, Lynch MJ, Fisher C, et al. Vesicle clear cell adenocarcinoma versus nephrogenic adenoma: a diagnostic problem. Histopathology 1995;27:43–49.

63. Goldstein AG. Metastatic carcinoma to the bladder. J Urol 1967;98:209–215.

64. Ito K, Yamanaka H, Ichinose Y, et al. A case of adenocarcinoma with clear cell carcinoma of the bladder. Acta Urol Jpn 1999;45:637–640.

65. Burgues O, Ferrer J, Navarro S, et al. Hepatoid adenocarcinoma of the urinary bladder. An unusual neoplasm. Virchows Arch 1999;435:72–75.

66. Serretta V, Pomara G, Piazza F, et al. Pure squamous cell carcinoma of the bladder in western countries. Report on 19 consecutive cases. Eur Urol 2000;37:85–89.

67. Desai PG, Ali Khan S, Jayachandran S, et al. Paraneoplastic syndrome in squamous cell carcinoma of urinary bladder. Urology 1987;30:262–264.

68. Celis JE, Celis P, Ostergaard M, et al. Proteomics and immunohistochemistry define some of the steps involved in the squamous differentiation of the bladder transitional epithelium: a novel strategy for identifying metaplastic lesions. Cancer Res 1999;59:3003–3009.

69. Kunze E. Histogenesis of nonurothelial carcinomas in the human and rat urinary bladder. Exp Toxic Pathol 1998;50:341–355.

70. Faysal MH. Squamous cell carcinoma of the bladder. J Urol 1981;126:598–599.

71. Newman DM, Brown JR, Jay AC, et al. Squamous cell carcinoma of the bladder. J Urol 1968;100:470–473.

72. Bessette PL, Abell MR, Herwig KR. A clinicopathologic study of squamous cell carcinoma of the bladder. J Urol 1974;112:66–67.

73. Kaye MC, Levin HS, Montague DK, et al. Squamous cell carcinoma of the bladder in a patient on intermittent self catheterization. Cleveland Clin Q 1992;59:645–646.

74. Roehrborn CG, Teigland CM, Spence HM. Progression of leukoplakia of the bladder to squamous cell carcinoma 19 years after complete urinary diversion. J Urol 1988;140:603–604.

75. Shirai T, Arai M, Sakata T, et al. Primary carcinomas of urinary bladder diverticula. Acta Pathol Jpn 1984;34:417–424.

76. Wilczynski SP, Oft M, Cook N, et al. Human papilloma-virus type 6 in squamous cell carcinoma of the bladder and cervix. Hum Pathol 1993;24:96–102.

77. Oft M, Bohm S, Wilczynski SP, et al. Expression of the different viral mRNAs of human papilloma virus 6 in a squamous-cell carcinoma of the bladder and the cervix. Int J Cancer 1993;53:924–931.

78. Warren KS. The relevance of schistosomiasis. N Engl J Med 1980;303:203–206.

79. Nash TE, Cheever AW, Ottesen EA, et al. Schistosome infections in humans: perspectives and recent findings. Ann Intern Med 1982;97:740–754.

80. Smith JH, Christie JD. The pathobiology of *Schistosoma haematobium* infection in humans. Hum Pathol 1986;17:333–345.

81. Sarma KP. Squamous cell carcinoma of the bladder. Int Surg 1970;53:313–318.

82. Johnson DE, Schoenwald MB, Ayala AG, et al. Squamous cell carcinoma of the bladder. J Urol 1976;115:542–544.

83. Winkler HZ, Nativ O, Hosaka Y, et al. Nuclear deoxyribonucleic acid ploidy in squamous cell bladder cancer. J Urol 1989;141:297–302.

84. Richie JP, Waisman J, Skinner DG, et al. Squamous carcinoma of the bladder: treatment by radical cystectomy. J Urol 1976;115:670–672.

85. Martin JE, Jenkins BJ, Zuk RJ, et al. Clinical importance of squamous metaplasia in invasive transitional cell carcinoma of the bladder. J Clin Pathol 1989;42:250–253.

86. Sakamoto N, Tsuneyoshi M, Enjoji M. Urinary bladder carcinoma with neoplastic squamous component: a mapping study of 31 cases. Histopathology 1992;21:135–141.

87. Swanson DA, Liles A, Zagars GK. Preoperative irradiation and radical cystectomy for stages T2 and T3 squamous cell carcinoma of the bladder. J Urol 1990;143:37–40.

88. Jones MA, Bloom HJF, Williams G, et al. The management of squamous cell carcinoma of the bladder. Br J Urol 1980;52:511.

89. Tannenbaum M. Inflammatory proliferative lesion of urinary bladder: squamous metaplasia. Urology 1976;7:428–429.

90. Sakkas JL. Clinical pattern and treatment of squamous cell carcinoma of the bladder. Int Surg 1966;45:71–76.

91. Rundle JSH, Hart AJL, McGeorge A, et al. Squamous cell carcinoma of bladder: a review of 114 patients. Br J Urol 1982;54:522–526.

92. Patterson JM, Ray EH Jr, Mendiondo OA, et al. A new treatment for invasive squamous cell bladder cancer: the NIGRO regimen. Preoperative chemotherapy and radiation therapy. J Urol 1988;140:379–380.

93. Wyatt JK, Craig I. Verrucous carcinoma of urinary bladder. Urology 1980;16:97–99.

94. Holck S, Jorgensen L. Verrucous carcinoma of urinary bladder. Urology 1983;22:435–437.

95. Walther M, O'Brien DP III, Birch HW. Condylomata acuminata and verrucous carcinoma of the bladder: case report and literature review. J Urol 1986;135:362–365.

96. Ellsworth PI, Schned AR, Heaney JA, et al. Surgical treatment of verrucous carcinoma of the bladder unassociated with bilharzial cystitis: case report and literature review. J Urol 1995;153:411–414.

97. Wiedemann A, Diekmann WP, Holtmann G, et al. Report of a case with giant condyloma (Buschke–Lowenstein tumor) localized in the bladder. J Urol 1995;153:1222–1224.

98. Blackmore CC, Ratcliffe NR, Harris RD. Verrucous carcinoma of the bladder. Abdom Imaging 1995;20:480–482.

99. Mahran MR, el-Baz M. Verrucous carcinoma of the bilharzial bladder. Impact of invasiveness on survival. Scand J Urol Nephrol 1993;27:189–192.

100. Oida Y, Yasuda M, Kajiwara H, et al. Double squamous cell carcinomas, verrucous type and poorly differentiated type, of the urinary bladder unassociated with bilharzial infection. Pathol Int 1997;47:651–654.

101. Ackerman LV. Verrucous carcinoma of the oral cavity. Surgery 1948;23:670–678.

102. Vakar-Lopez F, Abrams J. Basaloid squamous cell carcinoma occurring in the urinary bladder. Arch Pathol Lab Med 2000;124:455–459.

103. Cramer SF, Aikawa M, Cebelin M. Neurosecretory granules in small cell invasive carcinoma of the urinary bladder. Cancer 1981;47:724–730.

104. Trias I, Algaba F, Condom E, et al. Small cell carcinoma of the urinary bladder: presentation of 23 cases and review of 134 published cases. Eur Urol 2001;39:85–90.

105. Angulo JC, Lopez JI, Sanchez Chapado M, et al. Small cell carcinoma of the urinary bladder: a report of two cases with complete remission and a comprehensive literature review with emphasis on therapeutic decisions. J Urol Pathol 1996;5:1–19.

106. Blomjous CEM, Vos W, De Voogt HJ, et al. Small cell carcinoma of the urinary bladder: a clinicopathologic, morphometric, immunohistochemical, and ultrastructural study of 18 cases. Cancer 1989;64:1347–1357.

107. Lohrish C, Murray N, Pickles T, et al. Small cell carcinoma of the bladder: long term outcome with integrated chemoradiation. Cancer 1999;86:2346–2352.

108. Partanen S, Asikainen U. Oat cell carcinoma of the urinary bladder with ectopic adrenocorticotropic hormone production. Hum Pathol 1985;16:313–315.

109. Ali SZ, Reuter VE, Zakowski MV. Small cell neuroendocrine carcinoma of the urinary bladder. A clinicopathologic study with emphasis on cytologic features. Cancer 1997;79:356–361.

110. Podesta AH, True LD. Small cell carcinoma of the bladder: report of five cases with immunohistochemistry and review of the literature with evaluation of prognosis according to stage. Cancer 1989;64:710–714.

111. Mills SE, Wolfe JT III, Weiss MA, et al. Small cell undifferentiated carcinoma of the urinary bladder: a light microscopic, immunocytochemical, and ultrastructural study of 12 cases. Am J Surg Pathol 1987;11:606–617.

112. Sen SE, Malek RS, Farrow GM, et al. Sarcoma and carcinosarcoma of the bladder in adults. J Urol 1985;133:29–30.

113. Oesterling JE, Brendler CB, Burgers JK, et al. Advanced small cell carcinoma of the bladder: successful treatment with combined radical cystoprostatectomy and adjuvant methotrexate, vinblastine, doxorubicin and cisplatin chemotherapy. Cancer 1990;65:1928–1936.

114. Abenoza P, Manivel C, Sibley RK. Adenocarcinoma with neuroendocrine differentiation of the urinary bladder: clinicopathologic, immunohistochemical and ultrastructural study. Arch Pathol Lab Med 1986;110:1062–1066.

115. Grignon DJ, Ro JY, Ayala AG, et al. Small cell carcinoma of the urinary bladder: a clinicopathologic analysis of 22 cases. Cancer 1992;69:527–536.

116. DeMay RM, Grathwohl MA. Signet-ring cell (colloid) carcinoma of the urinary bladder: cytologic, histologic and ultrastructural findings in one case. Acta Cytol 1985;29:132–136.

117. Colby TV. Carcinoid tumor of the bladder. Arch Pathol Lab Med 1980;104:199–200.

118. Walker BF, Someren A, Kennedy JC, et al. Primary carcinoid tumor of the urinary bladder. Arch Pathol Lab Med 1992;116:1217–1220.

119. Stanfield BL, Grimes MM, Kay S. Primary carcinoid tumor of the bladder arising beneath an inverted papilloma. Arch Pathol Lab Med 1994;118:666–667.

120. van Hoeven KH, Artymyshyn RL. Cytology of small cell carcinoma of the urinary bladder. Diagn Cytopathol 1996;14:292–297.

121. Iczkowski KA, Shands JH, Allsbrook WV, et al. Small cell carcinoma of urinary bladder is differentiated from urothelial carcinoma by chromogranin expression, absence of CD44 variant 6 expression, a unique pattern of cytokeratin expression, and more intense γ-enolase expression. Histopathology 1999;35:150–156.

122. Atkin NB, Baker MC, Wilson D. Chromosome abnormalities and p53 expression in a small cell carcinoma of the bladder. Eur Urol 1999;35:323–326.

123. Terracciano L, Richter J, Tornillo L, et al. Chromosomal imbalances in small cell carcinomas of the urinary bladder. J Pathol 1999;189:230–235.

124. Tetu B, Ro JY, Ayala AG, et al. Small cell carcinoma of the prostate. Part I. A clinicopathologic study of 20 cases. Cancer 1987;59:1803–1809.

125. Coltart RS, Stewart S, Brown CH. Small cell carcinoma of the bronchus: a rare cause of haematuria from a metastasis in the urinary bladder. J R Soc Med 1985;78:1053–1054.

126. Davis MP, Murthy MSN, Simon J, et al. Successful management of small cell carcinoma of the bladder with cisplatin and etoposide. J Urol 1989;142:817.

127. Holmang S, Borghede G, Johansson SL. Primary small cell carcinoma of the bladder: a report of 25 cases. J Urol 1995;153:1820–1822.

128. Nejat RJ, Purohit R, Gtoluboff ET, et al. Cure of undifferentiated small cell carcinoma of the urinary bladder with M-VAC chemotherapy. Urol Oncol 2001;6:53–55.

129. Matsui Y, Fujikawa K, Iwamura H, et al. Durable control of small cell carcinoma of the urinary bladder by gemcitabine and paclitaxel. Int J Urol 2002;9:122–124.

12

MESENCHYMAL TUMORS OF THE URINARY BLADDER

Pheroze Tamboli and Jae Y. Ro

INTRODUCTION

Mesenchymal tumors make up 1% (or less) of the tumors arising in the urinary bladder. It is difficult to estimate the true incidence of these tumors as most have been reported as single case reports. In 1955 Melicow[1] reported an incidence of 4% (40/954) in patients with primary tumors of the urinary bladder. In a series of 30 primary mesenchymal tumors of the urinary bladder from two institutions, Kunze et al.[2] reported an incidence of 1% of all bladder tumors at one center (1980–1991) and 0.32% at the other (1982–1991).

Some benign and malignant mesenchymal tumors originate from cell types normally found in the bladder. Other tumors, such as osteosarcomas and chondrosarcomas, arise from cell types that are not normally present there. Tumor-like lesions (e.g. postoperative spindle cell nodule) arising in the urinary bladder are of particular interest to the surgical pathologist as they present as a mass and may be misdiagnosed as more serious tumors.

BENIGN MESENCHYMAL TUMORS

Almost the entire spectrum of benign mesenchymal neoplasms seen in soft tissues and other viscera also arise in the urinary bladder. These tumors generally do not pose a diagnostic problem for the surgical pathologist. However, because of their rarity, pathologists need to be aware of the existence of these tumors in the urinary bladder, as they may rarely mimic more serious tumors.

Leiomyoma

Leiomyoma is the most common benign mesenchymal tumor occurring within the urinary bladder. Leiomyomas have been variously referred to as fibroids, fibromyomas and fibroma in the past. Most of these tumors have been reported as single case reports, or small series.[2–6] The largest series from one institution consisted of 23 leiomyomas of the urinary bladder and urethra, which attests to the uncommon nature of this tumor, as these patients were treated between 1940 and 1995.[7]

Most of these tumors have been reported in women.[5,7] Leiomyomas may affect patients of all ages, including children. These patients usually present with urinary symptoms such as hematuria, dysuria and increased frequency of urination. Some patients have presented with urinary obstruction[7] and some with discomfort due to the presence of a pelvic mass. A number of cases have also been detected incidentally during cystoscopy or surgery for incidental reasons.[5,7]

Leiomyomas can arise from the smooth muscle of the muscularis mucosae or the muscularis propria. Depending on the location of the tumor, they may be pedunculated and project into the lumen of the urinary bladder. Some tumors have been reported to project from the mucosa surface, where they may act as an intermittent or 'ball-valve' obstruction, although this is rare and of interest as a medical curiosity. Tumor size can vary from less than 1 cm to several centimeters in diameter. The largest vesical leiomyoma was $25 \times 22 \times 15$ cm; however, the weight of this tumor was not reported.[3] The second largest leiomyoma was 23 cm in greatest dimension and weighed 3500 grams. Although the vast majority of patients only have a single tumor, there are reports of multiple leiomyomas.[6] Grossly, these tumors are firm, well circumscribed and whorled, resembling leiomyomas of the uterus.

Microscopically, they show features typical of leiomyoma, including smooth muscle cells arranged in interlacing bundles (Fig. 12.1). The vast majority of leiomyomas are composed of spindle cells with ovoid blunt-ended nuclei. Mild nuclear atypia may be present in some tumors. Leiomyomas with epithelioid cells have also been reported.[8] The periphery of the tumor is well circumscribed and tumor cells do not invade the adjacent tissue. Some tumors may be more cellular than the usual leiomyoma. Most leiomyomas lack mitoses; however, up to 2 mitoses per 10 high power fields (hpf) may be present,[4] which is permissible within the definition of benign stromal tumors. Most importantly, bladder leiomyomas do not have foci of tumor necrosis.

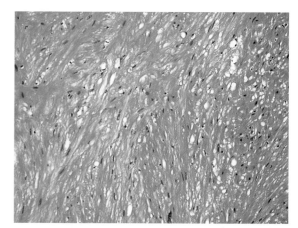

Fig. 12.1 Leiomyoma of the urinary bladder composed of interlacing bundles of uniform spindle cells lacking atypia.

As expected, the tumor cells stain positive for smooth muscle actin (SMA), muscle-specific actin (MSA), desmin and vimentin (Table 12.1). Immunohistochemical expression of estrogen and progesterone receptors has been reported in rare cases. Martin et al.[5] also reported positive staining for CD34 in three of eight leiomyomas they examined, and lack of staining for c-kit (CD117) in all nine. One of these leiomyomas was DNA aneuploid, two were near-diploid and five were diploid.[5]

It may be difficult to distinguish some leiomyomas from low-grade leiomyosarcomas. Tumors lacking circumscription, those with > 3 mitoses per 10 hpf, and those with significant nuclear atypia and necrosis should be considered leiomyosarcomas.[5,9] Most leiomyomas are treated by transurethral resection, enucleation or partial cystectomy, and rarely by cystectomy. All reported cases were benign; none has been reported to undergo malignant transformation.[5]

Hemangioma

More than 100 cases of urinary bladder hemangioma have been reported,[2,10,11] most of which were single case reports. The largest series of 19 cases spans 67 years (1932–1998).[11] Many hemangiomas are thought to be congenital in origin, as most patients with these tumors have been less than 20 years of age. However, vesical hemangiomas have also been reported in older patients. Hemangiomas are slightly more common in males than in females. Vesical hemangiomas can be associated with other cutaneous hemangiomas, or may be part of Sturge–Weber or Klippel–Trenaunay syndrome. In 1900, Klippel and Trenaunay first described the

Table 12.1 Reported immunohistochemical profiles of some mesenchymal tumors of the urinary bladder

Tumor type	Reference	Year	Cytokeratin	EMA	Desmin	MSA	SMA	S-100	Vimentin
Leiomyoma	Kunze et al.[2]	1994	0/5	ND	5/5	5/5	ND	3/5 f	5/5
	Martin et al.[5]	2002	0/9	ND	9/9	9/9	9/9	0/9	9/9
Leiomyosarcoma	Wick et al.[41]	1988	0/4	0/4	3/4	3/4	ND	0/4	4/4
	Mills et al.[9]	1989	0/12	0/12	8/12	12/12	ND	0/12	12/12
	Kunze et al.[2]	1994	1/7	ND	5/7	7/7	ND	4/7 f	5/7
	Iczkowski et al.[33]	2001	3/8	1/8	0/8	1/5	3/7	0/2	7/7
	Martin et al.[5]	2002	0/18	ND	7/18	14/18	12/18	0/18	17/18
PSCN	Wick et al.[41]	1988	2/2	0/2	2/2	2/2	ND	0/2	2/2
	Iczkowski et al.[33]	2001	2/4	1/3	2/3	2/3	2/4	0/3	4/4
IMT	Albores-Saavedra et al.[73]	1990	2/6	0/6	2/6	6/6	ND	0/6	6/6
	Ro et al.[70]	1993	0/8	ND	0/8	ND	8/8	0/8	8/8
	Jones et al.[69]	1993	2/10	2/8	2/9	10/10	3/8	0/10	10/10
	Lundgren et al.[72]	1994	5/12	0/12	0/12	6/12	6/12	0/12	12/12
	Hojo et al.[71]	1995	6/9	0/9	8/8	7/8	8/8	0/9	9/9
	Iczkowski et al.[33]	2001	5/14	4/8	3/11	5/9	5/8	0/4	10/10

EMA, epithelial membrane antigen; f, focal; IMT, inflammatory myofibroblastic tumor; MSA, muscle specific actin; ND, not done; PSCN, postoperative spindle cell nodule; SMA, smooth muscle actin.

syndrome triad, which consists of cutaneous port-wine hemangiomas, varicose veins and hemihypertrophy of soft tissue and bone. This syndrome is thought to represent a vascular malformation syndrome involving the capillary, lymphatic and venous channels, which do not behave like usual hemangiomas. Fewer than 30 cases of this syndrome affecting the urinary bladder have been reported.[12] These vascular malformations are generally also present on the skin of the lower abdomen and pelvis, and the external genitalia; there may be malformations within the pelvis itself, including malformations of other genitourinary structures.[12]

Most patients with hemangiomas present with painless gross hematuria. Rarely, obstructive symptoms and pain are also reported. Hemangiomas can be single or multiple and on cystoscopy appear as small (usually < 3 cm in diameter), red–blue, sessile lesions. They may also be pedunculated, lobulated or flat. They are most commonly located in the dome of the urinary bladder or in the posterior wall and trigone. Tumor diameters have been reported from less than a centimeter up to 10 cm.

The morphologic features of vesical hemangiomas are typical of hemangiomas seen in the skin and other organs. Cavernous hemangiomas are more common than capillary and arteriovenous hemangiomas, and tend to affect children. Of the 19 cases of bladder hemangioma reported by Cheng et al.,[11] 15 were cavernous hemangiomas, 2 were capillary hemangiomas, and 2 were arteriovenous hemangiomas.

Many different therapeutic options have been used to treat these patients. The treatments include biopsy and fulguration, partial or radical cystectomy, injection of sclerosing agents, radiation therapy and laser therapy. Imaging studies prior to planning therapy are helpful in defining the extent and location of the tumor, as some of these tumors may extend into the perivesical adipose tissue and only the 'tip' of the tumor is visible on cystoscopy as a submucosal lesion.

Paraganglioma

Paraganglioma (also known as pheochromocytoma) is thought to arise from remnants of paraganglionic tissue that migrates into the urinary bladder wall during development. Paragangliomas have been reported in almost all age groups and are equally common in both sexes. About two-thirds of these tumors may be hormonally active, most commonly causing hypertension and tachycardia.[13,14] Other symptoms related to catecholamine release include palpitations, headaches, blurred vision and profuse sweating. Patients with submucosal masses may present with hematuria. Catecholamine assays and the I-MIBG scintigraphy scan are used to diagnose and localize these tumors.

Most bladder paragangliomas form intramural masses, most commonly in the dome and trigone of the urinary bladder. The tumor may also extend into the perivesical adipose tissue. Most tumors are less than 4 cm in diameter (range < 1 cm up to 15 cm). Microscopically, the tumors have the characteristic morphologic features of paraganglioma, including the 'zenballen' appearance of nests of cells separated by a prominent vascular network (Fig. 12.2). The cells have moderate to abundant pale eosinophilic or clear cytoplasm with uniform round or oval nuclei. As in adrenal pheochromocytoma, large bizarre nuclei may be present. Mitoses are uncommon. Immunohistochemical markers for neuroendocrine differentiation, such as chromogranin, synaptophysin and CD56, are positive in the tumor cells. Stain for S-100 protein is positive in the sustentacular cells. Cytokeratin, epithelial membrane antigen (EMA) and carcinoembryonic antigen (CEA) are negative. Neurosecretory granules are also visible by electron microscopy.

The differential diagnosis of these tumors includes the nested variant of urothelial carcinoma, which has a rather bland appearance, and metastases to the bladder. Use of immunohistochemical stains easily resolves these dilemmas.

The presence of metastasis is the most reliable indicator of malignancy. Histologic criteria for distinguishing benign from malignant paraganglioma have not been well defined.[14] However, tumors with necrosis, mitoses and vascular invasion may behave more aggressively. DNA ploidy analysis, p53 status and

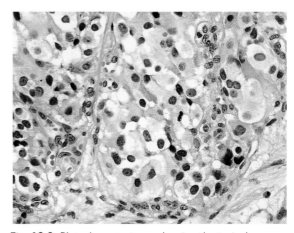

Fig. 12.2 Pheochromocytoma showing the typical 'zenballen' appearance. A rare mitosis is present.

proliferative indices are not predictive of malignant potential.[13,14]

Neurofibroma

Neurofibromas affecting the urinary bladder generally occur in conjunction with neurofibromatosis (von Recklinghausen's disease).[15–17] The urinary bladder is the most common site of genitourinary tract involvement in neurofibromatosis, but only about 50 cases have been reported.[16] The typical patient is a young male with type 1 neurofibromatosis. A number of these patients present early in childhood with urinary symptoms such as dysuria, increased frequency, incontinence or hematuria. A few cases have also been reported in adults.[16]

Grossly, neurofibromas form plexiform submucosal masses that can project into the lumen. These masses can extensively involve the bladder wall, making cystectomy the only treatment option. Bladder neurofibromas have the typical features of neurofibroma, being composed of spindle cells with wavy eosinophilic cytoplasm and elongated cigar-shaped nuclei without nucleoli. There are no mitoses or rare mitotic figures. In a few cases, cells with large pleomorphic nuclei and prominent nucleoli have been reported. These are similar to cellular neurofibromas and may be confused with sarcoma. Transformation into malignant peripheral nerve sheath tumor (MPNST) has also been reported.[16]

Schwannoma

Schwannoma (neurilemmoma) of the urinary bladder has been reported in a handful of patients without any evidence of neurofibromatosis.[18,19] These tumors include one case of epithelioid schwannoma[19] and one case of giant ancient schwannoma. Bladder schwannomas are solitary and morphologically resemble schwannomas seen elsewhere in the body.

Lipoma

Bladder lipomas are rare, although there can be adipose tissue in all layers of the urinary bladder, including in the lamina propria. Only five cases of lipoma of the urinary bladder have been reported and, of those reports, only two recent cases were in the English language literature.[20,21] The latter two patients were both 53-year-old men. The first patient presented with microscopic hematuria, and microscopic hematuria was detected in the second patient while he was being evaluated for sexual dysfunction. A CT scan showed that the first patient had a 1.3×1.2 cm, round, fat density, filling defect in the urinary bladder.[20] The tumor in the other patient was only seen on cystoscopy and measured 0.7 cm in diameter.[21] Cystoscopy of both patients revealed smooth, symmetric, rounded masses on the posterior wall of the bladder. Microscopic examination revealed that both tumors were typical lipomas.[20,21]

Other benign tumors

- *Granular cell tumors* originating in the urinary bladder have been reported in fewer than 10 patients. Morphologic features of these tumors are similar to those of granular cell tumors at other sites.[22]
- Only three well-documented cases of *lymphangioma* have been reported.[23–25] Two of these three cases were described as hemangiolymphangiomas occurring in children with associated cutaneous hemangiomas of the external genitalia.[23,24] The third case was a lymphangioma in a 13-year-old who presented with gross painless hematuria.[25] All three cases had the typical microscopic features of lymphangioma, including cystic spaces lined by flattened cells with proteinaceous fluid in the lumens.
- Three cases of *benign fibrous histiocytoma* have been reported, in three men aged 33, 63 and 82.[2,26,27] One man presented with painless gross hematuria and one with acute urinary retention and hematuria. Clinical presentation was not reported for the third patient. All three tumors were submucosal in location, measuring 0.5 cm, 5 cm and 10 cm in greatest dimension. These tumors were described as having typical morphologic features of benign fibrous histiocytoma, but histiocytic cells were noted in only one tumor.
- Two cases of *ganglioneuroma* of the urinary bladder have been reported.[28,29] The first case was reported in a 17-year-old boy with no stigmata of neurofibromatosis.[28] The second case was reported to be a calcified tumor in a patient with neurofibromatosis.[29]
- A case of *rhabdomyoma* was described in an 8-year-old boy, the tumor measuring 8 cm in maximum dimension.[2] The tumor was composed of cells with abundant eosinophilic cytoplasm, with small peripherally located nuclei. However, there were no cross-striations visible. Mitoses were also absent. The tumor was vimentin, desmin and MSA positive.[2]

• In 2000, Lasota et al.[30] reported a single case of a tumor that was phenotypically and genotypically similar to *gastrointestinal stromal tumor* (GIST). The patient was a 52-year-old woman with a 5 cm tumor grossly and microscopically resembling leiomyoma, located on the external aspect of the urinary bladder. However, unlike leiomyoma, the tumor cells were positive for *c-kit* (CD117) and CD34, and negative for SMA and desmin. Furthermore, analysis of exon 11 of the *c-kit* gene revealed a point mutation in the region commonly mutated in GISTs. The patient was alive without evidence of disease 36 months after surgery.

MALIGNANT MESENCHYMAL TUMORS

Primary sarcomas arising in the urinary bladder are rare and involve the entire spectrum of mesenchymal tissues. Part of the difficulty in studying these tumors is their rarity and the fact that most have been reported either as single case reports or small case series. Further confusing the picture is the nomenclature used for these tumors, especially before the era of immunohistochemistry, which makes it difficult to determine accurately the total number of reported cases.

Another hurdle has been clinical studies in which all sarcomas of the genitourinary tract are reported as a group,[31,32] which makes it difficult to precisely identify the clinicopathologic features of urinary bladder sarcomas that impact on diagnosis and prognosis. Notwithstanding these difficulties, there have been a few studies in the past decade that have focused on the clinicopathologic features of urinary bladder sarcomas.[2,5,9,33]

Leiomyosarcoma

Clinical features

Leiomyosarcoma is the most common sarcoma arising in the urinary bladder. Most patients with leiomyosarcomas are in the fifth to seventh decades of life, but they have been reported to occur in a wide age range, including in children.[2,5,9,31,33–37] Leiomyosarcomas affect men more frequently than women.

Treatment with cyclophosphamide has been associated with vesical leiomyosarcomas in a few cases.[38] Rare cases of vesical leiomyosarcoma have also been reported in patients with a history of hereditary retinoblastoma.[39] Some of these patients were treated

with chemotherapy including cyclophosphamide, but a few patients did not receive any form of chemotherapy.[40]

Most patients present with gross hematuria; the largest series reported hematuria in more than 80% of patients.[5,9,31,33,34] Other urinary symptoms may be present, or there may be symptoms related to the presence of a pelvic mass.

Histologic features

Most leiomyosarcomas are reported to be larger than 5 cm in diameter (range 0.5–10 cm).[2,5,9,33,34] The following are average sizes and size ranges reported by the largest series:

• 5.1 cm (1–10 cm) by Mills et al.[9]
• 8.4 cm (2–16 cm) by Kunze et al.[2]
• 4.0 cm (0.5–7 cm) by Iczkowski et al.[33]
• 7.1 cm (3–15 cm) by Martin et al.[5]
• 4.2 cm (1.5–9.0 cm) by Rosser et al.[34]

The tumor can involve any part of the urinary bladder wall. There may be a polypoid intraluminal component. The cut surfaces of the tumors are generally soft and fleshy with an infiltrative growth pattern. Foci of necrosis, hemorrhage and myxoid change may be grossly evident. The mucosal surface overlying the tumor is usually ulcerated (Fig. 12.3), which often leads to the gross hematuria so commonly reported in leiomyosarcomas.

Leiomyosarcomas of the urinary bladder have morphologic features similar to those seen in other sites. The typical microscopic feature is interlacing fascicles of malignant spindle cells (see Fig. 12.3). Some tumors

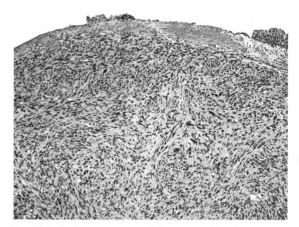

Fig. 12.3 Leiomyosarcoma of the urinary bladder forming a polypoid submucosal mass with ulceration of overlying urothelium.

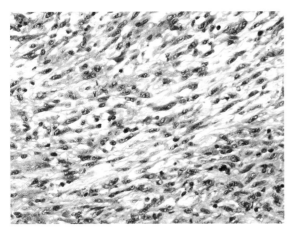

Fig. 12.4 Leiomyosarcoma of the urinary bladder with myxoid features. This tumor superficially resembles an inflammatory myofibroblastic tumor; however, the cells have a greater degree of nuclear pleomorphism.

have a prominent myxoid stroma (Fig. 12.4) and have been called myxoid leiomyosarcomas.[2,9] Typical tumor cells have eosinophilic cytoplasm and hyperchromatic pleomorphic nuclei with one or more nucleoli. Leiomyosarcomas composed predominantly of epithelioid cells have also been reported.[2]

Mitoses are commonly present, but the mitotic count may be variable. Mills et al.[9] reported mitotic counts ranging from 0 to 15 per 10 hpf. Iczkowski et al.[33] reported 1–16 mitoses per 10 hpf in high-grade leiomyosarcomas and 0–3 mitoses per 10 hpf in low-grade leiomyosarcomas. Martin et al.[5] reported 1–42 mitoses per 10 hpf (mean 12 per 10 hpf), with < 5 mitoses per 10 hpf in low-grade leiomyosarcomas and 3–42 mitoses per 10 hpf in high-grade leiomyosarcomas. Tumor necrosis is present in most cases; Martin et al.[5] reported necrosis in 14 of 18 (78%) leiomyosarcomas, Iczkowski et al.[33] in all of 13 tumors, and Mills et al.[9] in only 3 of 15 leiomyosarcomas.

Leiomyosarcomas stain positive with antibodies to MSA, SMA and sometimes desmin[2,5,9,41] (see Table 12.1). Cytokeratin and EMA are generally negative.[2,5,9,41] However, cytokeratin staining has been reported positive in up to 30% of non-vesical leiomyosarcomas. Iczkowski et al.[33] reported cytokeratin positivity in three of eight leiomyosarcomas and EMA positivity in one of eight. Martin et al.[5] also reported positive staining for CD34 and *c-kit* (CD117) in two and three tumors, respectively. Both Martin et al.[5] and Iczkowski et al.[33] measured p53 immunohistochemically. Iczkowski et al.[33] reported positive staining in 9 of 11 leiomyosarcomas, with moderate to strong staining of up to

40% of cells in five low-grade leiomyosarcomas and up to 70% of cells in four high-grade leiomyosarcomas. Martin et al.[5] reported p53 staining ranging from 0.1 to 70.8% (median 9.7%) in all of 18 leiomyosarcomas studied: three DNA diploid, seven aneuploid and eight tetraploid leiomyosarcomas. However, DNA content did not correlate with grade, as 1 of 12 high-grade leiomyosarcomas was diploid, compared with two of six low-grade tumors. Proliferative index (using MIB-1) ranged from 0.1 to 51.4% (median 9.1%) for all the 18 leiomyosarcomas, with a median of 4.2% in low-grade leiomyosarcomas and 26.1% in high-grade tumors.[5]

Differential diagnosis

The main differential diagnostic consideration for high-grade leiomyosarcomas is sarcomatoid urothelial carcinoma. The latter has a distinct malignant epithelial component. Cytokeratin and EMA stains may help in distinguishing between these two entities. Low-grade leiomyosarcomas need to be distinguished from leiomyomas and inflammatory myofibroblastic tumors. Unlike leiomyomas, low-grade leiomyosarcomas have cytologic atypia, mitoses and necrosis, and are not well circumscribed. Most importantly, tumors that have an invasive growth pattern, necrosis and significant nuclear pleomorphism should be characterized as leiomyosarcomas. The mitotic count is also important; however, caution is recommended as Martin et al.[5] reported two patients who died of metastatic disease from low-grade leiomyosarcomas with only 1 mitosis per 10 hpf.

Staging system

There is no universally accepted grading or staging system for vesical leiomyosarcomas. Iczkowski et al.[33] reported seven low-grade and six high-grade leiomyosarcomas, but did not provide any information on the criteria used for grading these tumors. Martin et al.[5] described leiomyosarcomas with mild to moderate nuclear atypia, < 5 mitoses per 10 hpf and < 25% tumor necrosis as low-grade, and leiomyosarcomas with moderate to severe nuclear atypia, > 5 mitoses per 10 hpf and/or > 25% tumor necrosis as high-grade. Russo et al.[31] and others[32,34] have used a modification of the Memorial Sloan-Kettering Cancer Center (MSKCC) staging system for soft-tissue sarcomas, which is based on tumor grade, tumor size, depth of invasion and presence or absence of metastasis. Rosser et al.[34] found that patients with higher MSKCC stage tumors had significantly lower disease-specific survival rates at 3 years and 5 years, and that on multivariate analysis only the

MSKCC stage was a significant predictor of disease-specific survival. Russo et al.[31] and Froehner et al.[32] also used this staging system; however, as both these studies combined all the sarcomas of the genitourinary tract, it is difficult to discern the precise impact of this staging system on bladder leiomyosarcomas.

Patient outcome

Reported outcomes of patients with urinary bladder leiomyosarcomas have varied widely. Moreover, it is difficult to compare these studies, as the patients were treated with different regimens. Three of five (60%) patients reported by Sen et al.[35] died of disease at 16, 18 and 46 months. Six of 10 (60%) patients reported by Swartz et al.[36] also died of disease, with survival times of 6 weeks, 3 months, 9 months, 2 years, 4 years and 10 years. Six of seven patients reported by Ahlering et al.[37] were alive with no evidence of disease with 4–97 months of follow-up; one patient was lost to follow-up. Mills et al.[9] reported that of 15 patients, only two (13%) died of disease, at 3 months and 6 years. One of three (33%) patients reported by Froehner et al.[32] died of disease, at 10 months. Iczkowski et al.[33] also reported death of 2 of 13 (15%) patients (one each with low-grade and high-grade leiomyosarcomas), both patients surviving 3 months. Eight of 18 patients (44%) reported by Martin et al.[5] died of disease, and three were alive with disease. The patients who died of disease included two of six patients with low-grade leiomyosarcoma (who had survival times of 61 and 68 months) and 6 of 12 patients with high-grade leiomyosarcoma (who had a mean survival time of 7 months). Based on these findings Martin et al.[5] concluded that high-grade leiomyosarcomas are more aggressive than low-grade tumors. Rosser et al.[34] reported 1-year, 3-year and 5-year disease-specific survival rates of 88.6%, 62.0% and 62.0%, respectively, for their 36 patients. Finally, Grignon[42] estimated 2-year and 5-year crude survival rates of 81% and 67%, respectively, based on a review of 62 cases reported between 1962 and 1993. These 62 cases include the patients reported by Swartz et al.,[36] Ahlering et al.[37] and Mills et al.[9]

Rhabdomyosarcoma

Rhabdomyosarcoma most commonly affects the urinary bladder in children, with a few cases also reported in adults.[31,35,37,43] Most large studies on bladder rhabdomyosarcomas are from the cooperative groups such as the Intergroup Rhabdomyosarcoma Study (IRS)[44,45] and the International Rhabdomyosarcoma Workshop[46]

which combine information from the cooperative groups in Europe and the United States. Most of these studies have grouped together urinary bladder and prostate rhabdomyosarcomas, as it is frequently difficult to distinguish the primary site, especially in patients with large tumors.[44] The latest classification system of rhabdomyosarcoma – the International Classification for Rhabdomyosarcoma – was proposed after a review of 800 cases by 16 pathologists from 8 cooperative groups.[47] There are few large studies on the pathology of vesical rhabdomyosarcomas. One of the largest studies by Leuschner et al.[48] from the German cooperative group reported the pathologic features of 51 rhabdomyosarcomas of the urinary bladder alone, excluding tumors of the prostate gland.

Clinical features

Rhabdomyosarcoma is the most common bladder tumor in children and has been reported in children of all ages, including those less than 1 year of age.[45] Boys are affected more often than girls.[45] Hematuria is the most common presenting symptom and may be accompanied by other urinary symptoms such as frequency and dysuria. Urinary obstruction has also been reported infrequently. Cystoscopic examination usually reveals a polypoid mass, sometimes filling the urinary bladder.

Histologic features

On gross examination most rhabdomyosarcomas in children are polypoid, usually of the botryoid type. Some tumors in adults may also be polypoid. The cut surfaces of the tumors are generally soft and fleshy, with necrosis and sometimes foci of hemorrhage. The overlying urothelial surface is usually ulcerated.

All types of rhabdomyosarcoma occur in the urinary bladder. In the IRS I–III studies, 90% of bladder/prostate rhabdomyosarcomas were embryonal type, with about a third of those being of the botryoid subtype.[44] Of the 51 rhabdomyosarcomas reported by Leuschner et al.,[48] 28 were classic embryonal type, 15 were botryoid, 5 were alveolar rhabdomyosarcomas and 3 were spindle cell embryonal rhabdomyosarcomas. In 16 of these 51 cases, the tumor formed a polypoid structure covered by urothelium or squamous epithelium, whereas 37 had a diffuse growth pattern.[48] Rhabdomyosarcoma cells are typically spindled or stellate, and form a cambium layer in the botryoid subtype (Fig. 12.5). Typical rhabdomyoblasts with eosinophilic cytoplasm and cytoplasmic cross-striations are present. Rhabdomyoblasts are most common in the botryoid subtype and least common in the spindle cell type.

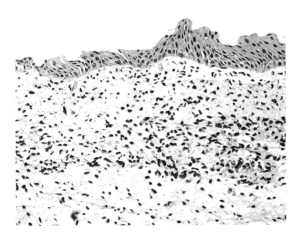

Fig. 12.5 Botryoid subtype of embryonal rhabdomyosarcoma composed of malignant cells within a loose myxoid stroma underlying intact urothelium. A condensation of rhabdomyoblasts forming the cambium layer is also visible.

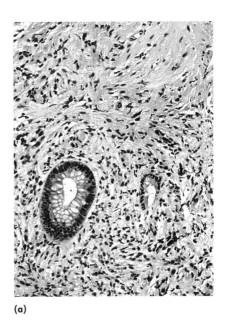

(a)

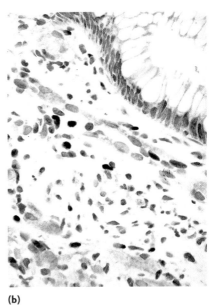

(b)

Fig. 12.6 Recurrence of rhabdomyosarcoma in the neobladder of a child treated with cystectomy. **(a)** Malignant spindle cells and rhabdomyoblasts infiltrate in between colonic glands; **(b)** Myo-D1 highlights the nuclei of malignant cells.

Alveolar rhabdomyosarcomas may lack rhabdomyoblasts, myotubes and cross-striations. Mitotic count is generally highest in classic embryonal rhabdomyosarcomas, followed by alveolar, botryoid, and spindle cell subtypes.[48]

An important morphologic finding in patients treated with chemotherapy is the presence of well-differentiated rhabdomyoblasts that may persist for a long time. These rhabdomyoblasts often have a large, smooth, single nucleus without significant pleomorphism or atypia, and, most importantly, there is no mitotic activity.[49] This cytodifferentiation is most common in embryonal rhabdomyosarcomas (both botryoid and classic) and should not be confused with persistent tumor.[50] Leuschner et al.[48] also studied the histology of 15 recurrent tumors: nine patients had the same histologic tumor type in both the primary and recurrent tumor; in six cases there was a different type in the recurrence.

Rhabdomyosarcomas stain positive for desmin, MSA, sarcomeric myosin, myoglobin, myogenin and myo-D1. Myogenin and myo-D1 are muscle transcription factors that are the most sensitive and specific proteins useful in immunohistochemical diagnosis and classification of rhabdomyosarcoma.[51] Non-specific cytoplasmic staining may be present, but only nuclear staining is considered to be positive (Fig. 12.6). Strong diffuse staining is commonly seen in alveolar rhabdomyosarcoma, whereas a heterogeneous pattern is more typical of embryonal rhabdomyosarcoma.[51]

Patient outcome

Outcome is best in patients with botryoid embryonal rhabdomyosarcoma, even in those patients who relapse.[48] For children with bladder/prostate non-metastatic rhabdomyosarcoma, the 3-year failure-free survival rates were 75% in IRS-III and 79% in IRS-IV, for all subtypes.[52] Leuschner et al.[48] reported an overall 91% 10-year survival rate for botryoid embryonal rhabdomyosarcoma compared to 73% for classic embryonal rhabdomyosarcoma. Patients who relapsed had a 65% 5-year survival rate for the botryoid subtype, compared with 26% for the embryonal type and 5% for the alveolar type.

Interestingly, the growth pattern of the tumors also had a statistically significant effect on survival: 92% 10-year survival in patients with polypoid intraluminal tumors, compared to 68% 10-year survival in patients with diffuse growth patterns.[48] This difference, it is speculated, is probably due to less aggressive invasion into the organ wall by the tumors with a polypoid growth pattern.

Outcome in adults is worse than in children. Two of three patients reported by Sen et al.[35] died of disease at 1 month and 8 months; the third patient was free of disease at 12 months. One patient reported by Ahlering et al.[37] died of disease at 18 months. All three patients reported by Russo et al.[31] were alive for more than 6 years. Ferrari et al.[43] reported 40% overall 5-year survival and 28% 5-year event-free survival for all adult rhabdomyosarcomas; they did not report results of each site individually.

Osteosarcoma

Primary osteosarcoma of the urinary bladder is uncommon; only about 30 cases have been reported.[53,54] Osteosarcoma affects men more often than women. Patients have been reported to range in age from 25 to 86 years. One patient received radiation therapy 27 years before the development of osteosarcoma. Most patients complain of gross hematuria.

Grossly, these tumors are large, polypoid and deeply invasive. Trigone of the bladder is the most common site involved. Microscopic features are typical of osteosarcoma with a malignant spindle or epithelioid cell component separated by pale, eosinophilic, lace-like osteoid (Fig. 12.7). A rare case with scant osteoid has also been reported.[54]

The most important differential diagnostic consideration in these cases is sarcomatoid urothelial carcinoma with an osteosarcoma component (carcinosarcoma). Urothelial carcinoma with osseous metaplasia has also been reported.[55] Both these types of tumor should have a clear-cut neoplastic epithelial component, which may be minimal in some cases, and sometimes an in situ carcinoma component is also pre-

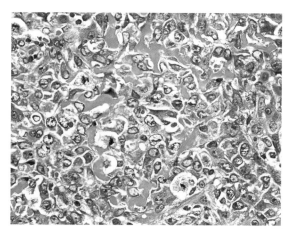

Fig. 12.7 Osteosarcoma of the urinary bladder. Malignant cells are separated by eosinophilic lace-like osteoid.

sent. Therefore, to exclude the possibility of sarcomatoid carcinoma with a heterologous osteosarcoma component and to make a diagnosis of primary osteosarcoma of the urinary bladder, one should thoroughly examine the specimen for malignant epithelium. Immunohistochemical stain for cytokeratin may help in this differential diagnosis. Osteosarcomas of the urinary bladder are highly aggressive and most patients succumb to this disease.[53]

Malignant fibrous histiocytoma

Malignant fibrous histiocytoma (MFH) of the urinary bladder is uncommon. Although a number of cases have been reported, probably only a small number are truly MFH.[2,32,56] Many of these reports are from before the immunohistochemistry era, and may be other types of sarcoma or sarcomatoid carcinoma. The largest series included eight cases, which Kunze et al.[2] reported along with other primary mesenchymal tumors of the urinary bladder. Most cases have been reported in men.

Kunze et al.[2] reported tumors ranging from 1 to 15 cm in diameter. A number of these tumors were large hemorrhagic necrotic masses that occupied most of the urinary bladder. Microscopically, they had the typical morphologic characteristics of MFH. All the morphologic variants of MFH have been reported, including the myxoid type.[2,56]

The most important differential diagnostic consideration is sarcomatoid urothelial carcinoma, which needs to be excluded before a diagnosis of MFH can be rendered. Most patients with vesical MFH have a poor outcome.

Angiosarcoma

Angiosarcoma has only been reported in 10 patients (7 men, 3 women).[57] Three patients had received radiation therapy to the pelvic region: two women for gynecologic malignancy and one man for prostate cancer.[58] One of these 10 patients may actually be considered to be a primary penile angiosarcoma that extended locally into the urinary bladder. Two patients were reported to have hemangiomas adjacent to their angiosarcomas, but these may in fact have been well-differentiated areas of the angiosarcoma rather than a true malignant transformation of the hemangioma.

Microscopically, tumors were in the lamina propria and/or muscularis propria and consisted of irregular, anastomosing vascular spaces lined by neoplastic cells with hyperchromatic nuclei and scant cytoplasm, typical of angiosarcoma (Fig. 12.8). Five of these 10 patients died of disease.[57]

Malignant peripheral nerve sheath tumor

At least 10 cases of malignant peripheral nerve sheath tumor (MPNST) have been reported.[2,17,32,59,60] Most patients with MPNST are adults with a history of neurofibromatosis, with one case reported in a child.[17] Two cases of epithelioid MPNST have also been reported; neither patient had a history of neurofibromatosis.[2,60] One of these patients was a 39-year-old paraplegic man,[60] the other was a 76-year-old woman.[2]

Morphologic features are similar to those of MPNST affecting the soft tissue. S-100 protein stain is frequently positive, but staining may be focal and limited to a small number of cells.

Chondrosarcoma

Chondrosarcoma of the urinary bladder is extremely rare; only four cases have been reported,[61,62] all of whom were adults aged 65, 66, 73, and 81 years (three men and one woman). One of these tumors was originally reported as a fibrosarcoma with foci of cartilage, but in retrospect has been considered to be a chondrosarcoma.[61] One tumor had the morphologic features typical of a myxoid chondrosarcoma, and the other two had features more typical of dedifferentiated chondrosarcoma, with small areas of neoplastic cartilage surrounded by pleomorphic spindle cells. Only cytogenetic findings were reported on the fourth case.[62]

As with osteosarcoma, a chondrosarcoma component is more frequently seen in sarcomatoid carcinomas of the urinary bladder. Therefore, to render a diagnosis of primary chondrosarcoma, sarcomatoid carcinoma with a chondrosarcoma component has to be excluded.

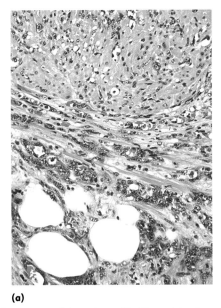
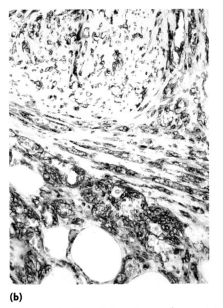

(a)   (b)

Fig. 12.8 Angiosarcoma of the urinary bladder, arising in a patient treated with radiation therapy for prostate cancer. (a) Tumor infiltrates in between the muscularis propria and perivesical adipose tissue, and is composed of irregular, anastomosing vascular spaces lined by neoplastic cells with scant cytoplasm and hyperchromatic nuclei; (b) CD31 immunohistochemical stain confirms the vascular nature of this sarcoma.

Assorted sarcomas of the urinary bladder

- *Fibrosarcoma* has rarely been reported.[63] Most tumors described as fibrosarcomas in the past were probably leiomyosarcomas or sarcomatoid carcinomas.
- At least three cases of *rhabdoid tumor* have been reported.[64] The latest report describes a 'pure' rhabdoid tumor.[64] Rhabdoid change has also been reported in sarcomatoid urothelial carcinoma and in malignant fibrous histiocytoma.
- Other rare sarcomas of the urinary bladder include *malignant mesenchymoma,*[31] *liposarcoma*[2] including the myxoid type, *hemangiopericytoma,*[65] *Kaposi's sarcoma*[66] and *malignant paraganglioma* (see paraganglioma).[13,14]

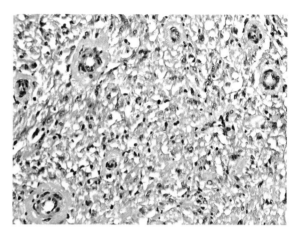

Fig. 12.9 Postoperative spindle cell nodule composed of spindle cells within an edematous stroma with prominent small blood vessels and scattered inflammatory cells.

MYOFIBROBLASTIC LESIONS

Postoperative spindle cell nodule (PSCN) and inflammatory myofibroblastic tumor are two lesions that have similar morphologic features, characterized by the presence of myofibroblasts. The term postoperative spindle cell nodule, first coined by Proppe et al.,[67] is used for lesions associated with a history of prior surgery. Tumors arising de novo, i.e. without a history of prior instrumentation, are referred to as inflammatory myofibroblastic tumor (inflammatory pseudotumor). The term inflammatory myofibroblastic tumor has not been used in the past for these tumors arising in the urinary bladder, but we use this term here because it is the currently favored term for this type of tumor.

Postoperative spindle cell nodule

The PSCN is a proliferation of spindle cells occurring at the site of surgery or trauma.[33,67,68] Grossly, these lesions form nodular masses at the site of a prior surgical intervention. Reported sizes have ranged from 0.4 to 3.0 cm, with most being less than 1.0 cm in greatest dimension.

Microscopically, the lesions consist of spindle cells arranged in interlacing fascicles set within an edematous or myxoid stroma with delicate small blood vessels and a smattering of inflammatory cells (Fig. 12.9). Numerous mitoses may be present. However, there is no or minimal nuclear pleomorphism and atypia. More proliferative areas may be present that can resemble low-grade leiomyosarcoma. Most PSCNs resolve spontaneously. They may have an infiltrative pattern and

interdigitate between the bundles of the muscularis propria. Wick et al.[41] and Iczkowski et al.[33] reported positive staining for cytokeratin, SMA, MSA, and desmin (see Table 12.1). Conservative surgery and close follow-up are is recommended in all these cases.

The differential diagnosis from leiomyosarcoma (especially low-grade leiomyosarcoma) may prove difficult. However, the presence of multiple small blood vessels is not common in leiomyosarcoma. Although the mitotic count may be similar, atypical mitoses are not present in PSCN. The presence of atypical mitoses in a highly cellular spindle cell tumor precludes a diagnosis of PSCN. Clinical history may be important in such cases; however, vigilance is essential as the discovery of a history of prior trauma or therapy (e.g. instrumentation) may lead to the discovery of a leiomyosarcoma. There are no good immunohistochemical stains to differentiate between these two lesions. Cytokeratin stain is positive in the spindle cells of PSCN, but leiomyosarcoma may also occasionally be positive for cytokeratin.[33] Muscle markers, of course, are positive in both.[33,41]

Inflammatory myofibroblastic tumor

Inflammatory myofibroblastic tumor (IMT) or inflammatory pseudotumor, is a proliferation of myofibroblasts, fibroblasts and inflammatory cells. This tumor was first described in the lung, and since has been recognized to involve numerous other organs and soft tissues. In the urinary bladder this tumor has been variously called inflammatory pseudotumor,[33,69] pseudosarcomatous fibromyxoid tumor,[70] pseudosarcomatous myofibroblastic tumor,[71] pseudomalignant spindle cell proliferation,[72] pseudosarcomatous myofibroblastic proliferation,[73] atypical myofibroblastic tumor, atypical fibromyxoid tumor, nodular fasciitis and plasma cell granuloma.

Most inflammatory myofibroblastic tumors (IMTs) have been reported in adults or young adults, but there are some reports of these also occurring in children.[71,73] Among adults, IMTs are slightly more common in women. Some patients present with hematuria and/or other urinary symptoms.

These lesions have been reported to range from small nodules or ulcerated masses in the mucosa to large pedunculated masses protruding into the lumen of the urinary bladder. Most of these tumors are 2–5 cm in diameter. Some lesions have been reported to be sessile and may deeply infiltrate the muscularis propria. The cut surface is generally soft, and may be myxoid.

Microscopically, IMTs are typically composed of spindle cells arranged in a haphazard pattern within a myxoid stroma (Fig. 12.10). Some areas may have a more cellular pattern with the spindle cells arranged in fascicles (Fig. 12.11). The less cellular areas may resemble granulation tissue. The tumor cells may have an infiltrative pattern, splitting the bundles of muscularis propria (Fig. 12.11), and sometimes even extending into the perivesical adipose tissue. The spindle cells may have eosinophilic or amphophilic cytoplasm (Fig. 12.12). Stellate and polygonal cells may also be present, especially in the myxoid areas. Occasional cells may be strap shaped or tadpole-like with eosinophilic cytoplasm. The nuclei may be large but do not have sig-nificant pleomorphism or hyperchromasia (Fig. 12.12), except in rare cases. Single or multiple small nucleoli or prominent nucleoli may be present.

Most tumors have 1–3 mitoses per 10 hpf. Albores-Saavedra et al.[73] reported 2 (of 10) cases with 5 mitoses per 10 hpf; Ro et al.[70] reported < 3 mitoses per 10 hpf in all 8 cases; Jones et al.[69] reported < 2 mitoses per 10 hpf in 12 tumors and 4 mitoses per 10 hpf in one tumor; Hojo et al.[71] reported 0–3.2 (mean 1) mitoses per 10 hpf in their 11 cases, and Iczkowski et al.[33] reported 0–1 mitoses per 10 hpf in all 4 cases. Most importantly, atypical mitoses were not reported in any of these studies.[33,69–73] Therefore, the presence of atypical mitoses should lead to a critical re-evaluation of the lesion.

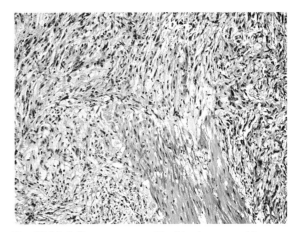

Fig. 12.11 Inflammatory myofibroblastic tumor with more cellular area showing fascicles of spindle cells infiltrating in between bundles of muscularis propria.

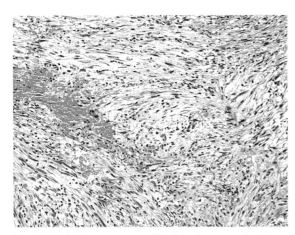

Fig. 12.10 Inflammatory myofibroblastic tumor showing typical features of spindle cells arranged in a haphazard pattern within a myxoid stroma with inflammatory cells and microscopic foci of hemorrhage.

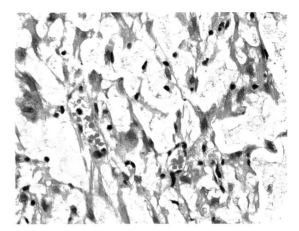

Fig. 12.12 Inflammatory myofibroblastic tumor, high-power view, showing cells with minimal atypia set within a myxoid stroma.

The stroma is generally myxoid and rich in non-sulfated acid mucopolysaccharides, which is highlighted by alcian blue staining at pH 2.7.[70] There is a prominent meshwork of small capillary-like blood vessels, with dilated or slit-like blood vessels in some foci. Numerous red blood cells may be present within the myxoid stroma and may form microscopic foci of hemorrhage (see Fig. 12.10). An inflammatory infiltrate composed predominantly of lymphocytes and plasma cells is present. Eosinophils may also be present. Iczkowski et al.[33] reported a mean of 153 (range 41–412) chronic inflammatory cells per hpf.

The myofibroblastic nature of this tumor is evident on positive staining for MSA, SMA (Fig. 12.13a) and desmin (Fig. 12.13b) (see Table 12.1). Cytokeratin is also positive in a number of these tumors (Fig. 12.14) (see Table 12.1). At the ultrastructural level tumor cells have a well-developed, rough endoplasmic reticulum, prominent Golgi apparatus and lysosomes. Some of the cells exhibit myofibroblastic differentiation with cytoplasmic microfilaments and associated dense bodies. All cases studied for DNA content have shown a lack of aneuploidy; almost all cases have a diploid DNA content with a low S-phase fraction.[33,70,72] A recent report on the cytogenetic analysis of one case revealed an unbalanced translocation between chromosomes 12 and 20, with a 46XY,der(20)t(12;20)(q13~q15;q13) karyotype in 5 of 20 metaphases examined.[74] This type of structural chromosomal change may be indicative of its neoplastic and clonal evolution. Interestingly, the q13~q15 region of chromosome 12 has been shown to be associated with numerous benign mesenchymal neoplasms.

IMTs in the urinary bladder are thought to be benign. However, tumors that have not been adequately resected may recur.[33] IMTs of the urinary bladder have not been reported to metastasize, however there are a few reports of this type of tumor undergoing malignant transformation in other organs.

DIFFERENTIAL DIAGNOSIS OF SPINDLE CELL TUMORS OF THE URINARY BLADDER

Sarcomatoid urothelial carcinoma may closely resemble sarcoma (Fig. 12.15) and should be considered in the differential diagnosis of any malignant mesenchymal lesion, especially in limited tissue samples. Because sarcomatoid carcinomas are much more common than sarcomas affecting the bladder, sarcomatoid carcinoma should be excluded by generous sampling of the tumor and immunohistochemical and/or electron microscopic analysis, before establishing a diagnosis of sarcoma. Also, as with any rare tumor, a metastasis to the urinary bladder needs to be excluded before a diagnosis of primary sarcoma can be made.

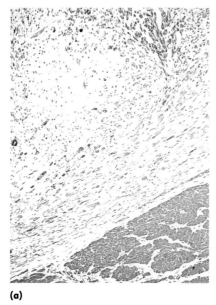
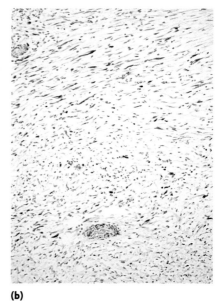

(a)   **(b)**

Fig. 12.13 Inflammatory myofibroblastic tumor: **(a)** showing patchy staining for smooth muscle actin, compared to uniform strong staining in adjacent bundles of muscularis propria; **(b)** staining for desmin is also patchy.

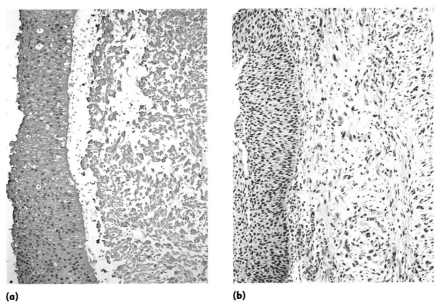

Fig. 12.14 Inflammatory myofibroblastic tumor: **(a)** exhibiting strong positive staining for cytokeratin in the spindle cells and overlying urothelium; **(b)** corresponding area on H&E stain.

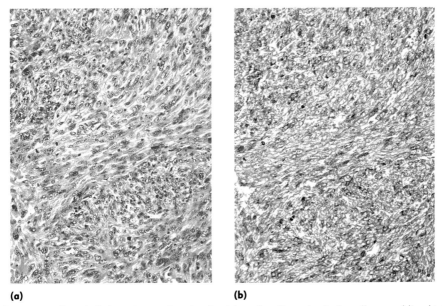

Fig. 12.15 (a) Sarcomatoid urothelial carcinoma forming fascicles of malignant spindle cells resembling high-grade leiomyosarcoma; **(b)** intense positive staining for cytokeratin is indicative of this tumor's epithelial origin.

A well-circumscribed neoplasm consisting of relatively uniform spindle cells with minimal atypia and mitoses, with expression of smooth muscle markers, should be considered a leiomyoma. Tumors with an infiltrative pattern may be PSCN, IMT or leiomyosarcoma. Clinical history of prior therapy or trauma

may help in distinguishing PSCN from the other two entities. PSCNs may have a high mitotic count but do not have significant nuclear pleomorphism or atypia, unlike leiomyosarcomas.

Distinguishing low-grade leiomyosarcoma from IMT may be extremely difficult. Tumors with a myxoid appearance may be either leiomyosarcoma or IMT. In myxoid leiomyosarcomas, most of the tumor has a relatively uniform appearance and consists of neoplastic cells with hyperchromasia and marked atypia, and has atypical mitoses. In IMTs, the myxoid areas typical of this lesion are interspersed with more cellular areas. IMTs may be mitotically active; however, they do not have atypical mitoses.

Immunohistochemical stains can help in this differential diagnosis, but caution is advised as myofibroblastic tumors may have a similar profile. Therefore, when faced with a spindle myxoid tumor with unusual histologic features where it is difficult to decide whether the lesion is benign or malignant, a diagnosis of a spindle cell tumor of uncertain malignant potential should be made and close clinical follow-up should be recommended.

CONCLUSION

Mesenchymal tumors of the urinary bladder are uncommon and infrequently pose diagnostic dilemmas for the surgical pathologist. Nevertheless, the clinicopathologic presentation, appearance and behavior of these lesions strongly suggest that current morphologic classifications do not fully represent the biological origins, genotype and phenotype of these lesions. While immunohistochemistry, with the small number of antibodies presently available, has provided some assistance in their differential diagnosis, these lesions require molecular genetic analysis to allow their classification to be brought into contemporary understanding of the type that is now common for soft tissue tumors elsewhere beyond the urinary bladder.[75] Through such an approach, which is likely to become commonplace within the near future, the obtained information will provide understanding of these lesions and their place in the overall spectrum of soft tissue dysplasia-neoplasia.

REFERENCES

1. Melicow MM. Tumors of the urinary bladder: a clinicopathological analysis of over 2500 specimens and biopsies. J Urol 1955;74:728–731.
2. Kunze E, Theuring F, Kruger G. Primary mesenchymal tumors of the urinary bladder. A histological and immunohistochemical study of 30 cases. Pathol Res Pract 1994;190:311–332.
3. Bramwell SP, Pitts J, Goudie SE, Abel BJ. Giant leiomyoma of the bladder. Br J Urol 1987;60:178.
4. Knoll LD, Segura JW, Scheithauer BW. Leiomyoma of the bladder. J Urol 1986;136:906–908.
5. Martin SA, Sears DL, Sebo TJ, et al. Smooth muscle neoplasms of the urinary bladder: a clinicopathologic comparison of leiomyoma and leiomyosarcoma. Am J Surg Pathol 2002;26:292–300.
6. Larsson G. Multiple leiomyomata of the urinary bladder in a hysterectomized woman. Acta Obstet Gynecol Scand 1994;73:78–80.
7. Cornella JL, Larson TR, Lee RA, et al. Leiomyoma of the female urethra and bladder: report of twenty-three patients and review of the literature. Am J Obstet Gynecol 1997;176:1278–1285.
8. Soloway D, Simon MA, Milikowski C, Soloway MS. Epithelioid leiomyoma of the bladder: an unusual cause of voiding symptoms. Urology 1998;51:1037–1039.
9. Mills SE, Bova GS, Wick MR, Young RH. Leiomyosarcoma of the urinary bladder. A clinicopathologic and immunohistochemical study of 15 cases. Am J Surg Pathol 1989;13:480–489.
10. Jahn H, Nissen HM. Haemangioma of the urinary tract: review of the literature. Br J Urol 1991;68:113–117.
11. Cheng L, Nascimento AG, Neumann RM, et al. Hemangioma of the urinary bladder. Cancer 1999;86:498–504.
12. Furness PD III, Barqawi AZ, Bisignani G, Decter RM. Klippel–Trenaunay syndrome: 2 case reports and a review of genitourinary manifestations. J Urol 2001;166:1418–1420.
13. Grignon DJ, Ro JY, Mackay B, et al. Paraganglioma of the urinary bladder: immunohistochemical, ultrastructural, and DNA flow cytometric studies. Hum Pathol 1991;22:1162–1169.
14. Cheng L, Leibovich BC, Cheville JC, et al. Paraganglioma of the urinary bladder: can biologic potential be predicted? Cancer 2000;88:844–852.
15. Kaefer M, Adams MC, Rink RC, Keating MA. Principles in management of complex pediatric genitourinary plexiform neurofibroma. Urology 1997;49:936–940.
16. Cheng L, Scheithauer BW, Leibovich BC, et al. Neurofibroma of the urinary bladder. Cancer 1999;86:505–513.
17. Blatt J, Jaffe R, Deutsch M, Adkins JC. Neurofibromatosis and childhood tumors. Cancer 1986;57:1225–1229.
18. Cummings JM, Wehry MA, Parra RO, Levy BK. Schwannoma of the urinary bladder: a case report. Int J Urol 1998;5:496–497.
19. Kindblom LG, Meis-Kindblom JM, Havel G, Busch C. Benign epithelioid schwannoma. Am J Surg Pathol 1998;22:762–770.
20. Eggener SE, Hairston J, Rubenstein JN, Gonzalez CM. Bladder lipoma. J Urol 2001;166:1395.
21. Meraj S, Narasimhan G, Gerber E, Nagler HM. Bladder wall lipoma. Urology 2002;60:164.
22. Fletcher MS, Aker M, Hill JT, et al. Granular cell myoblastoma of the bladder. Br J Urol 1985;57:109–110.
23. Stanley KE Jr. Hemangioma–lymphangioma of the bladder in a child: report of a case with associated hemangiomas of the external genitalia. J Urol 1966;96:51–54.

24. Chandna S, Bhatnagar V, Mitra DK, Upadhyaya P. Hemangiolymphangioma of the urinary bladder in a child. J Pediatr Surg 1987;22:1051–1052.

25. Bolkier M, Ginesin Y, Lichtig C, Levin DR. Lymphangioma of bladder. J Urol 1983;129:1049–1050.

26. Stearns MM, Mitchell AD, Powell NE, et al. Fibrous histiocytoma of the bladder. J Urol 1976;115:114–115.

27. Karol JB, Eason AA, Tanagho EA. Fibrous histiocytoma of bladder. Urology 1977;10:593–595.

28. Wyman HE, Chappell BS, Jones WRJ. Ganglioneuroma of bladder: report of a case. J Urol 1950;63:526.

29. Graham RT, Herschorn S, Srigley J. Calcified ganglioneuroma of the bladder. Urol Radiol 1987;9:177–180.

30. Lasota J, Carlson JA, Miettinen M. Spindle cell tumor of urinary bladder serosa with phenotypic and genotypic features of gastrointestinal stromal tumor. Arch Pathol Lab Med 2000;124:894–897.

31. Russo P, Brady MS, Conlon K, et al. Adult urological sarcoma. J Urol 1992;147:1032–1036.

32. Froehner M, Lossnitzer A, Manseck A, et al. Favorable long-term outcome in adult genitourinary low-grade sarcoma. Urology 2000;56:373–377.

33. Iczkowski KA, Shanks JH, Gadaleanu V, et al. Inflammatory pseudotumor and sarcoma of urinary bladder: differential diagnosis and outcome in thirty-eight spindle cell neoplasms. Mod Pathol 2001;14:1043–1051.

34. Rosser CJ, Slaton JW, Izawa JI, et al. Clinical presentation and outcome of high-grade urinary bladder leiomyosarcoma in adults. Urology 2003;61:1151–1155.

35. Sen SE, Malek RS, Farrow GM, Lieber MM. Sarcoma and carcinosarcoma of the bladder in adults. J Urol 1985;133:29–30.

36. Swartz DA, Johnson DE, Ayala AG, Watkins DL. Bladder leiomyosarcoma: a review of 10 cases with 5-year followup. J Urol 1985;133:200–202.

37. Ahlering TE, Weintraub P, Skinner DG. Management of adult sarcomas of the bladder and prostate. J Urol 1988;140:1397–1399.

38. Rowland RG, Eble JN. Bladder leiomyosarcoma and pelvic fibroblastic tumor following cyclophosphamide therapy. J Urol 1983;130:344–346.

39. Parekh DJ, Jung C, O'Conner J, et al. Leiomyosarcoma in urinary bladder after cyclophosphamide therapy for retinoblastoma and review of bladder sarcomas. Urology 2002;60:164.

40. Liang SX, Lakshmanan Y, Woda BA, Jiang Z. A high-grade primary leiomyosarcoma of the bladder in a survivor of retinoblastoma. Arch Pathol Lab Med 2001;125:1231–1234.

41. Wick MR, Brown BA, Young RH, Mills SE. Spindle-cell proliferations of the urinary tract. An immunohistochemical study. Am J Surg Pathol 1988;12:379–389.

42. Grignon DJ. Neoplasms of the urinary bladder. In: Bostwick DG, Eble JN (eds) Urologic Surgical Pathology. St. Louis: Mosby-Year Book, 1997, pp 277–279.

43. Ferrari A, Dileo P, Casanova M, et al. Rhabdomyosarcoma in adults. A retrospective analysis of 171 patients treated at a single institution. Cancer 2003;98:571–580.

44. Hays DM. Bladder/prostate rhabdomyosarcoma: results of the multi-institutional trials of the Intergroup Rhabdomyosarcoma Study. Semin Surg Oncol 1993;9:520–523.

45. Raney B Jr, Heyn R, Hays DM, et al. Sequelae of treatment in 109 patients followed for 5 to 15 years after diagnosis of sarcoma of the bladder and prostate. A report from the Intergroup Rhabdomyosarcoma Study Committee. Cancer 1993;71:2387–2394.

46. Rodary C, Gehan EA, Flamant F, et al. Prognostic factors in 951 nonmetastatic rhabdomyosarcoma in children: a report from the International Rhabdomyosarcoma Workshop. Med Pediatr Oncol 1991;19:89–95.

47. Newton WA Jr, Gehan EA, Webber BL, et al. Classification of rhabdomyosarcomas and related sarcomas. Pathologic aspects and proposal for a new classification – an Intergroup Rhabdomyosarcoma Study. Cancer 1995;76:1073–1085.

48. Leuschner I, Harms D, Mattke A, et al. Rhabdomyosarcoma of the urinary bladder and vagina: a clinicopathologic study with emphasis on recurrent disease: a report from the Kiel Pediatric Tumor Registry and the German CWS Study. Am J Surg Pathol 2001;25:856–864.

49. Ortega JA, Rowland J, Monforte H, et al. Presence of well-differentiated rhabdomyoblasts at the end of therapy for pelvic rhabdomyosarcoma: implications for the outcome. J Pediatr Hematol Oncol 2000;22:106–111.

50. Coffin CM, Rulon J, Smith L, et al. Pathologic features of rhabdomyosarcoma before and after treatment: a clinicopathologic and immunohistochemical analysis. Mod Pathol 1997;10:1175–1187.

51. Cessna MH, Zhou H, Perkins SL, et al. Are myogenin and myoD1 expression specific for rhabdomyosarcoma? A study of 150 cases, with emphasis on spindle cell mimics. Am J Surg Pathol 2001;25:1150–1157.

52. Crist WM, Anderson JR, Meza JL, et al. Intergroup rhabdomyosarcoma study IV: results for patients with nonmetastatic disease. J Clin Oncol 2001;19:3091–3102.

53. Ghalayini IF, Bani-Hani IH, Almasri NM. Osteosarcoma of the urinary bladder occurring simultaneously with prostate and bowel carcinomas: report of a case and review of the literature. Arch Pathol Lab Med 2001;125:793–795.

54. Young RH, Rosenberg AE. Osteosarcoma of the urinary bladder. Report of a case and review of the literature. Cancer 1987;59:174–178.

55. Eble JN, Young RH. Stromal osseous metaplasia in carcinoma of the bladder. J Urol 1991;145:823–825.

56. Oesterling JE, Epstein JI, Brendler CB. Myxoid malignant fibrous histiocytoma of the bladder. Cancer 1990;66:1836–1842.

57. Engel JD, Kuzel TM, Moceanu MC, et al. Angiosarcoma of the bladder: a review. Urology 1998;52:778–784.

58. Navon JD, Rahimzadeh M, Wong AK, et al. Angiosarcoma of the bladder after therapeutic irradiation for prostate cancer. J Urol 1997;157:1359–1360.

59. Rober PE, Smith JB, Sakr W, Pierce JM Jr. Malignant peripheral nerve sheath tumor (malignant schwannoma) of urinary bladder in von Recklinghausen neurofibromatosis. Urology 1991;38:473–476.

60. Eltoum IA, Moore RJ III, Cook W, et al. Epithelioid variant of malignant peripheral nerve sheath tumor (malignant schwannoma) of the urinary bladder. Ann Diagn Pathol 1999;3:304–308.

61. Torenbeek R, Blomjous CE, Meijer CJ. Chondrosarcoma of the urinary bladder: report of a case with immunohistochemical and ultrastructural findings and review of the literature. Eur Urol 1993;23:502–505.

62. Kingsley KL, Peier AM, Meloni-Ehrig AM, et al. Cytogenetic findings in a bladder chondrosarcoma. Cancer Genet Cytogenet 1997;96:183–184.

63. Keenan RA, Buchanan JD. Fibrosarcoma of bladder exhibiting endocrine characteristics of phaeochromocytoma. J R Soc Med 1979;72:618–620.

64. Duvdevani M, Nass D, Neumann Y, et al. Pure rhabdoid tumor of the bladder. J Urol 2001;166:2337.

65. Prout MN, Davis HL Jr. Hemangiopericytoma of the bladder after polyvinyl alcohol exposure. Cancer 1977;39:1328–1330.

66. Rha SE, Byun JY, Kim HH, et al. Kaposi's sarcoma involving a transplanted kidney, ureter and urinary bladder: ultrasound and CT findings. Br J Radiol 2000;73:1221–1223.

67. Proppe KH, Scully RE, Rosai J. Postoperative spindle cell nodules of genitourinary tract resembling sarcomas. A report of eight cases. Am J Surg Pathol 1984;8:101–108.

68. Huang WL, Ro JY, Grignon DJ, et al. Postoperative spindle cell nodule of the prostate and bladder. J Urol 1990;143:824–826.

69. Jones EC, Clement PB, Young RH. Inflammatory pseudotumor of the urinary bladder. A clinicopathological, immunohistochemical, ultrastructural, and flow cytometric study of 13 cases. Am J Surg Pathol 1993;17:264–274.

70. Ro JY, el-Naggar AK, Amin MB, et al. Pseudosarcomatous fibromyxoid tumor of the urinary bladder and prostate: immunohistochemical, ultrastructural, and DNA flow cytometric analyses of nine cases. Hum Pathol 1993;24:1203–1210.

71. Hojo H, Newton WA Jr, Hamoudi AB, et al. Pseudosarcomatous myofibroblastic tumor of the urinary bladder in children: a study of 11 cases with review of the literature. An Intergroup Rhabdomyosarcoma Study. Am J Surg Pathol 1995;19:1224–1236.

72. Lundgren L, Aldenborg F, Angervall L, Kindblom LG. Pseudomalignant spindle cell proliferations of the urinary bladder. Hum Pathol 1994;25:181–191.

73. Albores-Saavedra J, Manivel JC, Essenfeld H, et al. Pseudosarcomatous myofibroblastic proliferations in the urinary bladder of children. Cancer 1990;66:1234–1241.

74. Fadl-Elmula I, Gorunova L, Mandahl N, Heim S. Chromosomal abnormalities in inflammatory pseudotumor of the urinary bladder. Cancer Genet Cytogenet 2003;143:169–171.

75. Sandberg AA, Bridge JA. Updates on the cytogenetics and molecular genetics of bone and soft tissue tumors: chondrosarcoma and other cartilaginous neoplasms. Cancer Genet Cytogenet 2003;143:1–31.

13

DIAGNOSIS AND PROGNOSIS OF BLADDER NEOPLASMS BY ANALYTICAL AND QUANTITATIVE TECHNIQUES

Christer Busch and Rodolfo Montironi

INTRODUCTION

Diagnosis in pathology is either nominal or ordinal, the former giving names or qualitative labels to diseases, whereas the latter represents grading of the severity of the condition. In spite of the fact that it is subjective, microscopic nominal diagnosis is a relatively reproducible exercise, which may be arrived at by a rather quick recognition of a set of features that together characterize the condition. Grading of the severity of a disease usually depends on subclassification along a more or less continuous scale. Grading of atypia, dysplasia and degree of malignancy are examples of ordinal diagnoses. These often suffer from poor reproducibility, and numerous attempts to apply more objective, quantitative methods (e.g. by computer-assisted image analysis) have been made over the last few decades. Bladder cancer provides an interesting model for such efforts. This carcinoma is relatively pure in the sense that stroma is relatively scarce and the complexity is mainly the result of disorganization of architecture and cellular features of the epithelial compartment as a consequence of the malignancy itself.

Analytical and quantitative methods, such as image analysis and flow cytometry, are useful for the study of bladder neoplasia in histologic sections[1–6] as well as in specimens prepared for cytologic analysis.[7,8] The diagnostic and prognostic utility of these methods have been observed in several studies, and have been based both on object-related and texture- or contexture-based features (Figs 13.1–13.3). Recent advances in computer and information technologies have allowed the integration of both numeric and non-numeric data, i.e. of

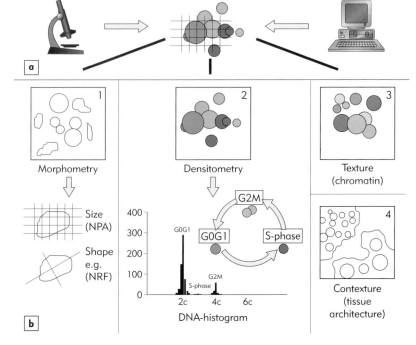

Fig. 13.1 (a) Image processing; **(b)** analysis. 1, morphometry; 2, densitometry (static cytophotometry); 3, texture; 4, contexture analysis. NRF, nuclear roundness factor; NPA, nuclear profile area. (Adapted from van der Poel et al. Quantitative light microscopy in urological oncology. J Urol 1992; 148:1–3.[41])

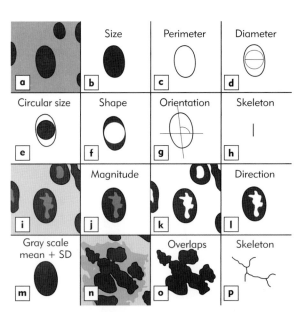

Fig. 13.2 Illustration of some simple object features. **(a)** A single nucleus (object) in a gray scale image; **(b)** the size of the object is calculated from the binary image; **(c)** the perimeter of the object; **(d)** the diameter (width) of the object is defined as the maximum (darkest) gray scale inside the object, measured from the distance image; **(e)** the circular size is defined as $\pi \times$ diameter/4; **(f)** the shape is defined as size/circular size; **(g)** the orientation of the principal axis of the object; **(h)** the skeleton of the object; **(i)** the gradient magnitude image in (a); **(j)** the gradient magnitudes of the object alone; **(k)** with gray scale, no significant edge; black/gray scale, 135° edge; lightest gray scale, 45° edge; **(m)** the image in (a) masked by the binary image (the resulting image is used to calculate the mean and standard deviation of the gray scale of the object); **(n)** touching nuclei in the gray scale image from a bladder cancer; **(o)** the binary image of the irregularly shaped object; **(p)** the skeleton of the irregularly shaped object. (Adapted from Jarkrans et al.[12])

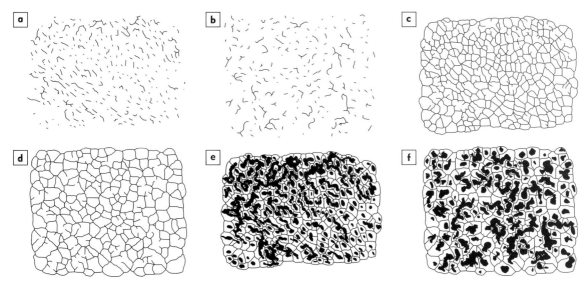

Fig. 13.3 The skeleton image for: **(a)** the grade 1 image; **(b)** the grade 3 image; **(c, d)** the ZOI images for (a) and (b); **(e, f)** the ZOI and the binary images merged. These images illustrate various ways to express the architectural differences of images from two extreme grade examples. (Adapted from Jarkrans et al.[12])

descriptive, linguistic terms. This has had a significant impact on our capabilities to derive diagnostic information from histopathologic materials.

There is an evolution of digital knowledge (i.e. of diagnostic information accessible only by digital processing) where computation is truly used to expand our ability to perceive. However, there is also a growing appreciation among researchers involved in the application of objective procedures to histopathologic diagnosis of the very high information content of traditional histopathologic diagnostic terminology and concepts.[9–15] The challenge is not only to take full advantage of numeric analytical procedures in support of visual expert diagnostic assessment, but also to have the objective methodology fully embody the traditional diagnostic concepts and terms and to enable a numeric/objective representation of that vast body of professional knowledge, insight and experience. This leads at one end of the spectrum of technology development to automated image analysis, and at the other to diagnostic decision support. In between, methods are evolving that use an interactive technique, aiming at analysis in representative areas of the specimens.[14]

EVALUATIONS WITH DATA EXPRESSED IN A NUMERIC FORM

There have been at least two practical reasons for applying analytical and quantitative methods in the evaluation of bladder neoplasms: low reproducibility and poor accuracy in the identification of the morphologic changes in histologic sections as well as in cytologic preparations obtained from voided urine or bladder wash.

The grading systems of papillary transitional cell carcinoma are based on multiple features such as number of cell layers, cell density, nuclear polarity, hyperchromasia, pleomorphism and mitoses.[16–26] As with all subjective systems, there is potential for marked inter- and intraobserver variation.[27] The considerable degree to which this occurs has been demonstrated in a study of 57 transurethrally resected bladder papillary carcinomas. These were graded based on the World Health Organization (WHO) system. The majority of pathologists assigned a different grade to the same lesion when it was reassessed in approximately 50% of cases. The level of interindividual (correlation coefficient 0.51–0.67) and intraindividual (correlation coefficient 0.46) inconsistency was disturbing. The recent WHO/International Society of Urologic Pathologists (ISUP) (1998) and WHO (1999) systems[24,25] use a far better set of linguistic criteria and are using pattern recognition parameters of variation and order–disorder, which are expected to improve reproducibility.

Such inconsistencies arise from at least two causes, the first related to the inherent vagueness of linguistic or descriptive terms, words and concepts used in the morphologic evaluation of bladder pathology. This means that almost all our knowledge in this field as well as in others is not expressed in numerical form. The second cause – inconsistency – is linked to the variability of biologic events: a diagnostic category is not precisely separated from another similar condition by a sharply delineated boundary. Extreme grades or categories in the urothelial papillary neoplasms, such as urothelial papilloma and papillary carcinoma grade 3, can be considered definitive sets because the cases in each set are unequivocally members of that set and cannot possibly be considered to belong to the other set as well. However, urothelial papilloma and papillary carcinoma grade 3 belong to a spectrum of morphologic changes and the boundaries of contiguous grades are drawn by histopathologists. Unequivocal membership for all cases is not possible and for cases falling close to the border or at the intersection between contiguous grades and categories (i.e. the area of overlap of diagnostic criteria), it is not 100% true or sure that they belong to a given group.[14]

Several papers have shown that such drawbacks in the morphologic evaluation of bladder lesions by pathologists can be overcome when analytical and quantitative methods are used.[28–32]

Concerning the bladder neoplasms examined in tissue sections, Ooms et al.[33] were among the first to show such a benefit. They found that the results of the histomorphometric grading are markedly better than those of the histologic grading. The percentage of tumors given the same grade is much higher using morphometry than for routine histologic assessment. Moreover, the differences in morphometric grading were never more than one grade, which is in striking contrast to the histologic grading where there is a difference of two grades in many cases.

Concerning the bladder neoplasms examined in cytologic preparations, Sherman et al.[27] evaluated the diagnostic performance of six observers with various degrees of experience in comparison with classification by computer. The study indicated considerable inter- and intraobserver differences, which appeared to be more closely related to the individual's perception of the visual targets than to the degree of experience. The performance of the programmed computer was well within the midrange of the human diagnostic performance. A recent study by van der Poel et al.[32] compared conventional bladder wash cytology performed by experts with quantitative image analysis. It was found that both the image analysis system and the cytologic examination detected all high-grade lesions. Image analysis was superior to cytologic analysis in the identification of tumor recurrence after normal cystoscopic findings.

Analytical and quantitative methods have yet to be implemented in the evaluation of bladder neoplasms in the daily routine. This is due in part to the fact that there is little interest among histopathologists in morphometry. Another reason is linked to the lack of standardization in the use of analytical and quantitative techniques. The DNA Cytometry Consensus Conference did not examine the clinical applications and technical aspects of image analysis in patients with bladder cancer, due to the paucity of reports on this modality.[34] However, a certain number of publications have shown that image analysis of DNA content in bladder irrigation specimens adds information of clinical value above and beyond that obtained by flow cytometry.[35,36]

IMAGE ANALYSIS IN BLADDER CANCER

Image cytometry has been used in bladder neoplasia to analyze cell features related to the size and shape of the epithelial nuclei and their DNA content or ploidy as well as their chromatin texture characterization.[9,37–46] Even though hematoxylin and eosin-, Papanicolaou- or Giemsa-stained material has been used in some studies, Feulgen-stained slide preparations are usually used for this assay, the Feulgen reaction producing a specific blue stain of the nuclear DNA. A wide range of factors – including sampling, fixation, staining procedure, preparation and analysis – affect nuclear size, staining intensity and chromatin texture and hence the results of image analysis.[47] Nevertheless, using several different fixatives, including formaldehyde, acceptable results are obtained. The types of slide preparation that have been used for image analysis include bladder washings or single nuclear suspensions of fresh or fixed embedded tissue, and sections of fixed embedded tissue.

Although tissue sections are not ideal when nuclear DNA content has to be determined, this type of slide preparation has been very useful for the evaluation of the architecture of the urothelium in normal and neoplastic conditions.[29,48] In particular, the determination of the so-called 'inclination angle of the non-round nuclei' has been found to be important for the accurate identification of the position of individual cases along the continuous spectrum of changes of bladder papillary neoplasia.[49] This quantitative feature evaluates the variations in nuclear polarity, i.e. a feature now recognized to be important in the morphologic evaluation of such lesions in tissue sections. For details regarding some morphometric principles and features, see Figures 13.1–13.3.

Quantitative immunohistochemistry

Quantitation of immunohistochemical stainings for various markers of bladder tumor behavior is slowly coming of age.[50–52] A study by Ranefall et al.[50,51] describes two methods for color quantification in immunohistochemistry, one supervised ('manual') and one unsupervised (automatic) (Figs 13.4, 13.5).

In some studies, analytical and quantitative methods, including image cytometry, have been adopted to analyze nuclear proliferation-related markers, such as

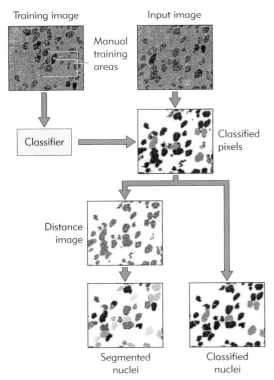

Fig. 13.4 A supervised algorithm for creating a color-based pixel classifier is applied to an image that is typical for the sample. The resulting classifier can be applied to all images. This method is suitable when a large number of images from the same staining session are to be classified, and when conditions such as illumination are considered to be constant. To be able to count the number of nuclei, all pixels are grouped into individual nuclei and touching nuclei are separated by using a watershed separation algorithm. Each nucleus is then classified into the class that has most pixels within the nucleus. (Adapted from Ranefall et al.[50])

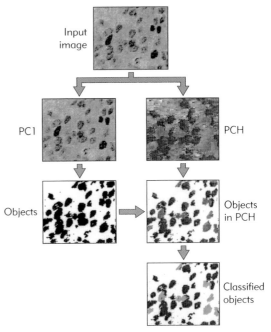

Fig. 13.5 Step one in unsupervised classification is to separate the nuclei from the rest of the tissue. This is done by automatically finding the optimal threshold value for the current image based on a transformation of the pixels into the first principal component (PC1). In step two the pixels within the nuclei are automatically classified as either positive or negative according to a transformation into principal component hue (PCH). ('PC1' and 'PCH' are transformations that in practice will work as normalized versions of 'lightness' and 'hue'.) This method is very robust with respect to changes in focus and illumination. Afterwards it is possible to separate the nuclei as above to be able to count the number of nuclei. (Adapted from Ranefall et al.[51])

MIB-1,[53] mitosis,[54–60] AgNORs[61] and p53.[62–65] In particular, investigation of the frequency and location of the mitotic figures has allowed determination of changes in the relationship between the proliferation and differentiation/differentiated compartments and the increasing grades of lesions. The determination of the frequency of mitoses together with their location is now recognized as having an important role in the diagnosis, grading and prognosis of bladder lesions (Figs 13.6–13.8).

Image cytometry has also been used to analyze the cytoplasmic immunostaining of endothelial cells (angiogenesis). Microvessels are immunostained for factor VIII-related antigen, CD34 or CD31, which decorate endothelial cytoplasm. Microvessel density (MVD) is

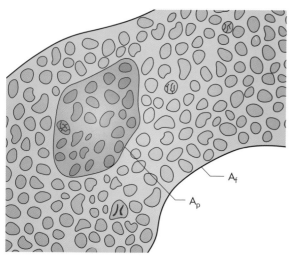

Fig. 13.6 Schematic picture of the computer screen visualizing one field of the tumor tissue. The tumor epithelium (A_f) and a representative part of it (A_p) are marked. The number of mitoses in A_f is 4 ($^nMA_f = 4$) (Adapted from Vasko et al.[60])

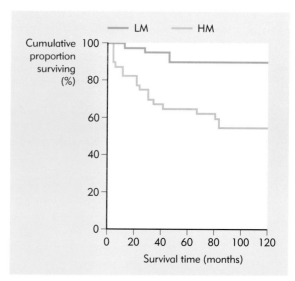

Fig. 13.8 Corrected survival rates of patients with grade 2 tumors related to MF. 54 low mitotic frequency (LM) and 43 high mitotic frequency (HM) cases ($p < 0.0003$). (Adapted from Vasko et al.[60])

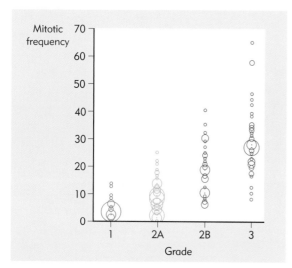

Fig. 13.7 Scatter diagram of mitotic frequencies in different grades. LM, low mitotic frequency, MF < 13; HM, high mitotic frequency, MF > 13. Grades 1, 2A, and 2B–3 are equivalent to PUNLMP, grades I, II and III, respectively, according to the WHO 1999 Classification of Bladder Tumours.[25]

semi-quantitated by light microscopy at a 200× or 400× magnification in the so-called neovascular 'hot spots', i.e. areas of greatest microvessel density. The integrated optical density (IOD) of immunostained endothelial cells is also used to measure microvessel density.[66–68] An automatic method for quantification of microvessel density in urinary bladder carcinoma was described by Wester et al.[67,68] (Fig. 13.9). Published results relating MVD to prognosis are not always concordant. This is due to several factors which include:

- the 'hot spot' sampled is subjectively chosen
- the number of fields semi-quantitated varies from one to four
- different antisera are used
- there are different interpretations of what are microvessels
- two different techniques are used (image analysis with the inherent problems and visual semi-quantitation with its tedium).

The cytoplasmic expression of various oncogenes has also been measured by image analysis of immuno-stained sections of bladder tumors.[30,31]

It will be crucial in the future to agree on principles for standardization of immunohistochemical methods as a baseline for standardization of quantitation. Based on principles described by Riera et al.,[69] immuno-histochemistry uses cultured cells in agarose gel as a multifunctional control. In short, the control cells are suspended in agarose tubing and stored at 4°C. Pieces of the tubing are cut and follow the actual biopsies through the preparation steps and staining.[70,71] Wester et al.[71] have suggested a technique for markers such as MIB-1 and p53 (Figs 13.10–13.12). In a study of the effects of time, temperature, fixation and different

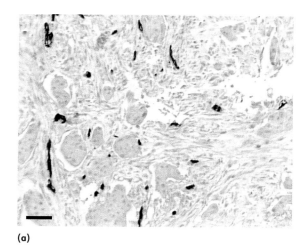

(a)

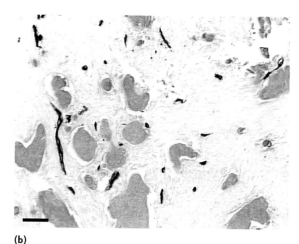

(b)

Fig. 13.9 Microvessels highlighted by: **(a)** single immunostaining outcome (IHC) protocol; **(b)** simultaneous IHC staining of epithelial cells, multiple IHC protocol. Scale bars 50 μm. (From Wester et al.[68])

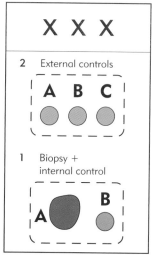

Fig. 13.10 Schematic drawing illustrating the placement of biopsy and controls on the objective slide. **1.** (A) Biopsy and (B) internal control, fixed, histoprocessed and paraffin-embedded controls. **2.** (A) 3-h fixation; (B) 6-h fixation; (C) 50-h fixation. This example represents a set-up for the control of the influence of a given fixation time on the immunodetection of any marker. (Adapted from Wester et al.[70] Cultured human fibroblasts in agarose gel as a multi-functional control for immunohistochemistry. Standardization of Ki67 (MIB1) assessment in routinely processed urinary bladder carcinoma tissue. J Pathol 2000; 190:503–511. © Pathological Society of Great Britain and Ireland. Reproduced with permission. Permission is granted by John Wiley & Sons of behalf of PathSoc.)

retrieval protocols of paraffin section storage and immunohistochemistry using bladder cancer specimens as well as bladder cancer cell lines with known p53 mutations and proliferation status, it was defined how standardization may be achieved for routine assessment of these markers.[71]

Morphometry and image analysis-based grading

While histopathologic grading of primary bladder cancer has proved to be of considerable value in predicting clinical outcome, its subjective nature and the rather poor descriptions of the grades in earlier classifications have precluded good reproducibility. For this reason there has been an increasing interest in quantitative methods.[72–75]

The longstanding WHO classification from 1973 had rather specific criteria for the lowest (grade I) and highest (grade III) grades.[23] As low-grade tumors are generally treated conservatively with either trans-urethral resection or intravesical chemotherapy (and conversely, high-grade tumors are treated more aggressively), a consistent and reproducible method of grading bladder tumors is essential. Identification of extreme examples of low- and high-grade tumors is generally not problematic. However, there are clear difficulties in tumors diagnosed as intermediate-grade regardless of the system used: it appears that some behave in a fairly indolent fashion while others are much more aggressive.

Using a variety of morphometric techniques it has been convincingly shown that the WHO (1973) grade II and a fraction of grade I tumors behave differently and show different characteristics regarding the properties

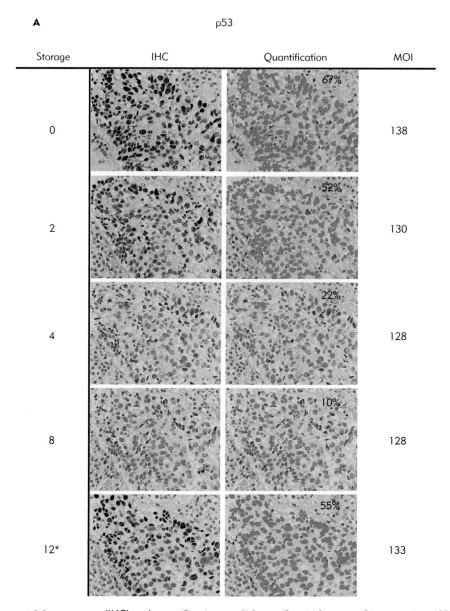

A   p53

Storage	IHC	Quantification	MOI
0		67%	138
2		52%	130
4		22%	128
8		10%	128
12*		55%	133

Fig. 13.11 Immunostaining outcome (IHC) and quantification result (quantification) assessed in two urinary bladder carcinoma biopsies in freshly cut sections (0) and sections stored for 2, 4, 8, and 12 weeks, respectively, at 20°C. Example of p53 immunostaining. MOI, mean object intensity. (From Wester et al: Paraffin Section Storage and Immunohistochemistry. Applied Immunohist & Molecular Morphology 2000; 8: 61–70.[71])

of – above all – the nuclei. This method involves analysis of the mean and standard deviation of nuclear size in histologic sections.[76] Thus early work[1–3,9] indicated that the mean area of the largest cells of each grade differed. Bjelkenkrantz et al.[2] concluded that a stepwise grading system such as the WHO system can never exactly reflect a continuously increasing nuclear atypia. They found that with increasing WHO grade there is a gradual increase in nuclear size and variability as well

as stainability. Helander et al.[4,6] reached similar conclusions with the addition that nuclear volume densities were higher in grade II than in grade I and they later showed that grade II could be split both by DNA ploidy measurements and by nuclear profile area. Similarly, Nielsen's groups[77–80] found that an increased mean nuclear volume indicated recurrence and invasion potential in primary non-invasive bladder tumors (Ta). A much larger study by Schapers and associates[81]

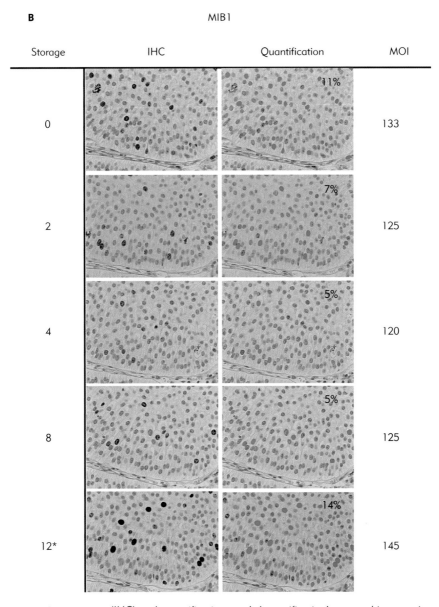

Fig. 13.12 Immunostaining outcome (IHC) and quantification result (quantification) assessed in two urinary bladder carcinoma biopsies in freshly cut sections (0) and sections stored for 2, 4, 8, and 12 weeks, respectively, at 20°C. Example of Ki-67 (MIB-1) immunostaining. MOI, mean object intensity. (From Wester et al: Paraffin Section Storage and Immunohistochemistry. Applied Immunohist & Molecular Morphology 2000; 8: 61–70.[71])

involving 294 patients with primary bladder cancer showed that morphometric grade as a single factor was correlated with tumor progression and a poorer overall survival. They used mean nuclear area to subdivide their cases into two groups where low-grade tumors had a mean nuclear area < 95 mm^2 and high-grade tumors > 95 mm^2.

Sowter et al. defined a novel variable, which carried the issue further. They used measurements of nuclear size, the mean area and the size distribution curve of nuclear area.[82,83] They found that separation between two groups was best achieved using a weighted distribution of nuclear size. De Meester et al.[84] provided an early step towards a more complex assessment of nuclear object features by measuring size, shape, optical density and texture features and found that there is a significant quantitative difference between grade I and grade III tumors. Grade II did not appear to represent a statistically distinct population. They also highlighted the problem of reproducibility depending on the field-of-view chosen for analysis.

The grading system of Malmstrom et al.[85] (developed as a modification of the Bergkvist classification[20]) was tested using image analysis in an attempt to achieve more objective texture- and object-based methods. The modification was based on the realization that the grades could be described using pattern recognition features. These included decisions regarding the predominance of order or disorder in the pattern and the existence of easily recognized variation or, in the case of predominant disorder, recognizable areas of order.

In fact, the architectural organization of bladder cancer epithelium as presented in two-dimensional images of stained sections is a visually interpreted sum of all morphologic features provided by the objects, the cells, their nuclei and cytoplasm as individual objects and their interrelationships. So, by combining object-based and texture-based (i.e. contexture-based) features, image analysis techniques have been developed.

In a study by Jarkrans et al.[12] an object-based method was used in which features were extracted from gray-scale images, from binary images obtained by thresholding the nuclei and from several other images through image processing operations. In a study by Choi et al.[11,13] graph-based features were extracted from minimal spanning trees connecting all nuclei (Fig. 13.13). A large number of extracted features were evaluated by making a comparison with the results of subjective grading and other factors related to prognosis using multivariate statistical methods. All the methods were originally developed and tested on one set of patient material and then tested for reproducibility on

an entirely different set of material. The results indicated that it is possible to describe in quantitative terms the features of the subjectively derived classes with reasonable reproducibility. Various levels of structural organization are analyzed by this system: individual objects, and features relating to individual objects, as well as the entire image ('contexture'). Interestingly, features describing variation of size, texture and internuclear distances proved to carry the highest weight in the selected set (Figs 13.14–13.16).

Work done using image texture analysis has shown that it is possible to select a set of factors on the basis of correlation to subjective grading and to surrogate end-points for prognosis, using multivariate statistical methods and so-called neural network analysis.[13] Van Velthoven et al.[29] used digital image analysis of chromatin texture in Feulgen-stained nuclei to predict recurrence of low-grade superficial transitional cell carcinoma of the bladder and concluded that quantitative description of chromatin patterns provided helpful information in predicting recurrence of these tumors. Apart from nuclear area, the following were all significant parameters in their study:

- the skewness index (i.e. the asymmetry in the distribution of densitometric values in the nuclei)
- the kurtosis index (i.e. the half-height width of the optical density value distribution histogram in the nucleus, measuring the homogeneity level of the optical density value distribution in the nucleus)
- the variance of the optical density (also describing the heterogeneity level)
- the frequency of small dense chromatin clumps
- the contrast measuring the number of boundaries between the nuclear regions of different extinction values.

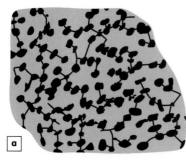 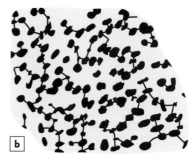

Fig. 13.13 **(a)** Minimum spanning tree of a tissue section with 153 vertices superimposed on the gray scale image; **(b)** Euclidean distance between vertices has been thresholded at 16 μm to create the 31 clusters. Thus, a minimum spanning tree connecting the centroids of all nuclei in a tissue section can be used as a basis for extracting features describing the tissue architecture. (Adapted from Choi et al.[13])

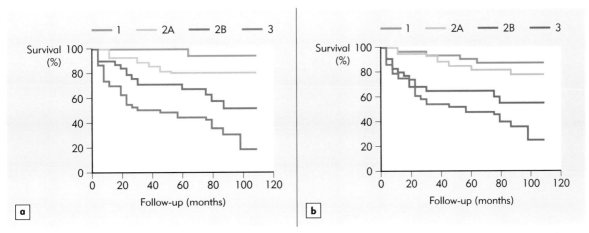

Fig. 13.14 Survival in bladder cancer graded (**a**) subjectively, and (**b**) using computer-assisted texture analysis based grade. Grades 1, 2A, and 2B–3 are equivalent to PUNLMP, grades I, II and III, respectively, according to the WHO 1999 Classification of Bladder Tumours.[25] (Adapted from Choi et al.[13])

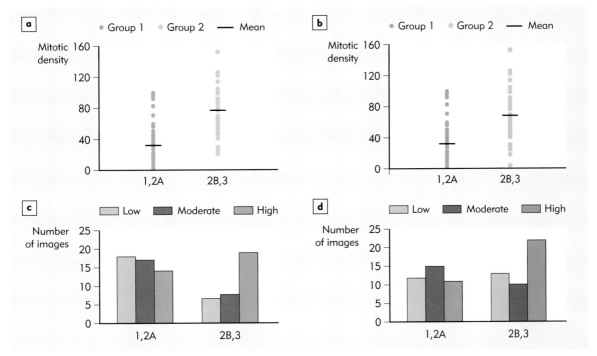

Fig. 13.15 Correlation between subjective and image analysis-based grading and mitotic density and p53 protein expression. Scatter diagrams for two groups: (**a**) mitotic density related to subjective grading; (**b**) mitotic density related to computer grading; (**c**) p53 expression related to subjective grading; (**d**) p53 expression related to computer grading. In this example the tumors have been subdivided into 'low grade' (1, 2A) and 'high grade' (2B, 3). Grades 1, 2A, and 2B–3 are equivalent to PUNLMP, grades I, II and III, respectively, according to the WHO 1999 Classification of Bladder Tumours.[25] Note the excellent correlation between subjective and computer grading and the chosen end-points. (Adapted from Choi et al.[13])

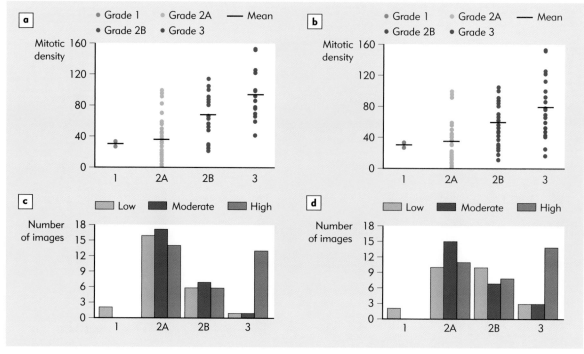

Fig. 13.16 Correlation between subjective and image analysis-based grading and mitotic density and p53 protein expression. Scatter diagrams for two groups: **(a)** mitotic density related to subjective grading; **(b)** mitotic density related to computer grading; **(c)** p53 expression related to subjective grading; **(d)** p53 expression related to computer grading. Grades 1, 2A, and 2B–3 are equivalent to PUNLMP, grades I, II and III, respectively, according to the WHO 1999 Classification of Bladder Tumours.[25] Note the excellent correlation between subjective and computer grading and the chosen end-points. (Adapted from Choi et al.[13])

By using image cytometry and the decision tree technique, Decaestecker et al.[86] characterized aggressiveness in WHO (1973) grade II superficial transitional cell carcinomas of the bladder. The latter technique belongs to the supervised learning algorithm and enables an objective assessment to be made of the diagnostic value associated with a given parameter. The image analysis technique in this study involved a determination of DNA histogram types based on a subclassification according to DNA index values; this yielded six classes named diploid, triploid, tetraploid, hyperdiploid, hypertriploid and polymorphic. The combined use of these two techniques enabled the authors to identify one subgroup of grade II tumors which behave clinically like grade I tumors and a second subgroup behaving like grade III tumors. Of the ploidy-related parameters it was the percentage of hyperdiploid and hypertetraploid cell nuclei which enabled identification.

In summary, many studies with different morphometric approaches have demonstrated that image analysis-based techniques can be used to reproduce quantitate parameters and combined sets of parameters, which serve to stratify bladder cancer into prognostically relevant classes. The addition of decision tree techniques and quantification of markers will undoubtedly lead to more objective diagnosis and grading of tumors in the future.

Investigations in bladder irrigation/washing and voided urine

Quantitation analysis, in particular DNA cytometry, should not be used to screen for bladder cancer or to investigate microscopic hematuria. Although the sensitivity of this technique on irrigation specimens is higher than cytology in detecting malignancy, the specificity is too low to screen low-risk patients. Irrigation specimens require invasive procedures for collection, thus precluding mass screening.[87]

Cytometry is recommended for use only in patients with bladder cancer, a history of cancer or where there is a strong suspicion of cancer. For instance, Ooms et al.[37] found that there are morphometric differences between urothelial cells in voided urine of patients with grade I and grade II bladder tumors. Subsequently, the same group developed a cytomorphometry-based classification rule to discriminate low-grade (grades I and II) from high-grade (grade III) bladder tumors, whereas Sherman et al.[38] used hierarchic analysis to formulate bladder cancer diagnosis of cells in voided urine using a small computer. Others have shown that DNA ploidy status of irrigation and tumor specimens correlates with grade and stage. Diploidy and tetraploidy must always be interpreted in conjunction with the patient's history. Cytometry has its main applications in the management of bladder cancer patients at the time of superficial tumor diagnosis and at follow-up evaluations.[88]

Detection of recurrent tumor

Patients with superficial bladder cancer (Ta, T1 and Tis) are treated conservatively. Cytologic examination of urothelial cells from voided urine, urinary bladder washing and upper urinary tract brushing specimens in combination with cystoscopic examination has been considered the gold standard for the detection of recurrent urothelial neoplasia. The sensitivity for the detection of recurrent urothelial neoplasms has shown a wide variation in the published literature. Despite the high sensitivity and specificity for the detection of both low- and high-grade urothelial neoplasms achievable in those laboratories directed by expert cytopathologists, the general consensus is that cytologic techniques are not capable of identifying all cases of recurrent disease. The development of ancillary techniques, such as image analysis, to complement the relatively inexpensive and convenient cytologic methods has appeared relevant to both clinical patient outcome and financial outcome in an era of health care cost containment.[89]

In the early 1980s flow cytometry was introduced to detect abnormal total DNA content in urothelial cells obtained from urothelial cytologic specimens. Early hope that DNA aneuploidy would be a major adjunct to the cytologic detection of recurrent urothelial carcinoma ultimately gave way to the reality that the technique could improve on the sensitivity and specificity of cytology only to a marginal degree.[36] Improvements in flow cytometric techniques, including dual parameter immunoflow cytometry, have achieved an increased sensitivity for the detection of WHO system grade I urothelial papillary carcinomas (i.e. papillary urothelial neoplasms of low malignant potential) to 86%.

The introduction of DNA content measurements by digital static image analysis in the late 1980s also

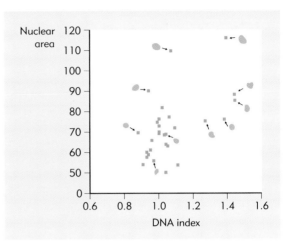

Fig. 13.17 Scattergram of nuclear area versus DNA index. Each square in the graph represents a nucleus. Two populations are detected, one with a DNA index in the diploid range and the other in the triploid range. The digitized images of some examples from the two nuclear populations are included. The cytologist reported the cytologic preparation as 'urine with normal urothelial cells'. Cytometry was done in the bladder washing of a patient with recurrent papillary carcinoma, grade 3.

reported an increase in the sensitivity and specificity for the detection of recurrent urothelial malignancies (Fig. 13.17). Subsequently, it was reported that for patients with urothelial neoplasms, approximately 33% of cases with diploid urothelial cytology samples are ultimately associated with progression to muscle-invasive disease. In addition, although the combination of conventional cytology with DNA ploidy measurement by image analysis has been reported to be capable of detecting up to 85% of cases of recurrent urothelial neoplasms, it has not appeared to be able to identify all patients with disease recurrence.

The Quanticyt™ karyometric analysis was developed as an automated system for urothelial cell grading using Feulgen-stained cytospin preparations and a digital analysis system.[39,89] The system combines DNA content analysis with nuclear shape calculations to calculate a low-, an intermediate- and a high-risk factor for bladder cancer.[39] According to the developers, this system provides significant additional prognostic information that could be used to reduce the number of cystoscopies needed to care for patients with superficial bladder cancer.

Monitoring intravesical therapy

A major application of DNA ploidy analysis in urothelial cytology samples has been to differentiate recurrent urothelial malignancy (diploid or aneuploid) from cytologic atypia associated with intravesical instillation of chemotherapy and immunotherapy (uniformly diploid). Using aneuploidy and tetraploidy (> 10% of cell population) as positive markers for malignancy, sensitivity and specificity are markedly reduced after local chemotherapy as compared with surgery.[90] This may be explained by an increase in certain cases of tetraploid cells in a proliferative state due to regenerative and inflammatory phenomena. An increased false positivity was also reported after intravesical bacillus Calmette-Guérin treatment. At 6 months or more after intravesical treatment of superficial tumors (Ta, T1 and Tis), a DNA aneuploid histogram is a good predictor of progression and treatment failure. A negative DNA analysis (a DNA diploid histogram) following an initial aneuploid histogram is a strong indicator of response and a good prognostic sign. The value of an elevated hyperdiploid fraction alone is not proven and interpretation must consider the clinical setting.[34]

Bladder-sparing treatment of invasive (T2–T4) cancer

After radiation therapy, an increased tetraploid population is to be expected for up to 2 years. Only 'non-tetraploid' aneuploid populations are indicative of cancer during this period. The significance of a DNA 'non-tetraploid' aneuploid population is not altered by a history of chemotherapy and/or radiotherapy and indicates treatment failure. Because of the nature of invasive cancer, however, a negative DNA analysis should not be relied on to rule out persistent or recurrent disease, as the tumor may not be adequately sampled.[34]

Combination of image analysis with ancillary methods

The technique of fluorescent in situ hybridization (FISH) has been applied to urothelial cytology specimens to detect chromosomal aneusomy.[91–93] The success of this technique is dependent on the number of chromosomal centromeric probes used to detect gains or losses and will have relatively low sensitivity if insufficient numbers of probes are utilized. In one study, routine ploidy analysis was combined with FISH-based assessment for chromosome 9 and resulted in an increased sensitivity compared with that of either technique alone. Chromosome 9 has also been evaluated by single strand conformational polymorphism (SSCP) analysis, with loss of heterozygosity found to be a marker of recurrent urothelial cancer that was more

sensitive than routine cytology. However, urothelial carcinomas are a heterogeneous group of neoplasms and multiple probes must be used to detect recurrent disease. The FISH and SSCP methods are too complex, time-consuming and expensive for general use in most laboratories.[90]

Image analysis versus ancillary methods

A variety of wet laboratory immunoassays, on-slide immunoassays, in situ hybridization procedures and postnucleic acid extraction molecular techniques have been designed to complement cytology and improve the overall sensitivity and specificity for the detection of recurrent urothelial neoplasia. This was demonstrated in a recent study published by Wiener et al.[87,89] These authors compared the diagnostic value of NMP22™ (nuclear matrix protein) and Bard's BTA™ (bladder tumor antigen) stat testing and Quanticyt computer-assisted dual parameter image analysis to cytology and cystoscopy in patients who had symptoms suggestive of transitional cell cancer or who were being followed up after treatment for that disease. They found that BTA stat and NMP22 tests, and Quanticyt computer-assisted analysis, improve the detection of urothelial carcinoma, particularly grade I tumors, compared to cytologic evaluation. Additionally, van der Poel et al.[94] found that the BTA test is useful in patients with recurrent low-grade papillary lesions. The value of the immunologic markers is limited by low sensitivity in grade III transitional cell carcinoma as well as low specificity. None of the urine-bound diagnostic tools that were investigated replaced cystoscopy.

Although the current consensus maintains that no new individual marker can eliminate the need for follow-up cystoscopy, there is significant agreement that, with the use of the ancillary tests, the sensitivity and specificity of cytologic diagnosis can be increased and the intervals between surveillance cystoscopies for the management of urothelial neoplasia can be lengthened.

EVALUATIONS WITH DATA NOT EXPRESSED IN A NUMERIC FORM

Objective numeric features can establish the grade of bladder cancer or classify the case into a diagnostic or prognostic category. Multivariate statistics provide precisely defined algorithmic procedures for the analyses of numeric data. However, most knowledge in histopathology exists in mental imagery and is communicated by linguistic, descriptive terms, not in numeric form. Data of the descriptive, linguistic form have not generally been processed in a systematic manner.[14] Descriptive diagnostic terms are not burdened in the way numerical data are and yet, from an information carrying point of view, are generally much more encompassing and informative than numeric features. Descriptive linguistic data not only carry a very large amount of information in the terms themselves, but, through the associations which they evoke, they also carry interpretive and diagnostic meaning. They are highly specific and greatly invariant to many sources of variation that would affect numeric analysis. Moreover, there are ways in which linguistic data can be numerically evaluated.

Diagnostic distance measures

The pathologist compares features in a sample (e.g. a urothelial papillary lesion) with some standard or baseline in memory (e.g. normal urothelium). Given a suitable baseline, determination is then made as to how far removed the features are from that point and thus the degree of abnormality to make a diagnostic decision. The case is then positioned either along a univariate axis or in multidimensional feature space, and it is convenient to express cases by their distance from baseline. This is achieved with diagnostic distance measures. The spectrum of the potential morphologic changes, such as papillary neoplasia or the preneoplastic non-papillary (or flat) lesions of the urothelium, can be represented – and objective thresholds set – at what are considered to be clinically relevant points along the distance scale. Thus, quantitative data are derived from morphologic observations. The practical value of the diagnostic distance measure has already been shown for diseases of other organs, such as those of the prostate. Little as been done in this respect in the bladder.[14,15]

Inference networks

The processing of linguistic data in the histopathologic grading as well as morphologic diagnosis of preneoplastic and neoplastic lesions of the bladder results in the central problem of uncertainty management. The systematic combining of diagnostic clues in an algorithmic fashion which utilizes traditional diagnostic concepts is enabled by inference networks.

An inference network consists of a decision node in which diagnostic alternatives are evaluated as a set of clues at evidence nodes in the network. Each clue is

observed, rated and assigned to a function with a given probability. This models the vagueness or uncertainty of the diagnostic clue. In an inference network, the evidence is then forwarded to the decision node via a conditional probability link matrix. This models the uncertainty with which a given clue predicts a specific diagnostic outcome. For instance, the conditional probability may be 0.70, meaning 'given the presence of prominent nucleoli, there is a 70% probability that papillary carcinoma grade III exists'. At the decision node, the belief in each diagnostic alternative is accumulated. Recent studies have shown that an inference or Bayesian belief network (BBN) offers a descriptive classifier useful for accurate and reproducible analysis of the urothelial papillary and flat lesions[15] (Figs 13.18, 13.19).

TELEPATHOLOGY

The first telepathology-based Virtual Reference and Certification Centre for DNA image cytometry has been established in Dresden by Haroske et al.[95,96] The authors conclude that quantitation methods in clinical pathology have to be normalized and standardized on their instrumental and methodologic basis so as to guarantee a defined level of precision and accuracy independent of the site they are applied. The group has established a system for a remote DNA ploidy analysis, based on client server technology and accessible via Internet or ISDN connections (Quantitation Server EUROQUANT). This system enables the cytometric measurement of the DNA content of cells for diagnostic purposes, provides the user with comprehensive quality control of such measurements and helps in trouble-shooting as well as giving assistance in diagnostic interpretation. To date, more than 40 laboratories from Europe, USA and Asia are involved. The Quantitation Server of the EUROQUANT can be reached at: http://euroquant.med.tu-dresden.de.

FUTURE DIRECTIONS

The future directions in the diagnosis and prognosis of bladder neoplasms by analytical and quantitative techniques include the development of advanced image analysis techniques that allow the automated simultaneous evaluation of morphologic, immunohisto-chemical and molecular markers as well as the development of classification/identification techniques more suited to individual patients. Artificial neural

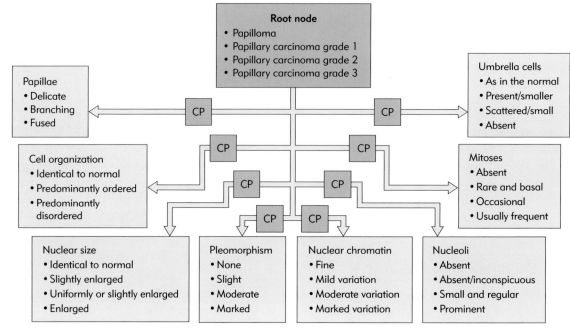

Fig. 13.18 Shallow network with an open-tree hierarchic topology with a diagnostic decision node and eight first-level descendant nodes.

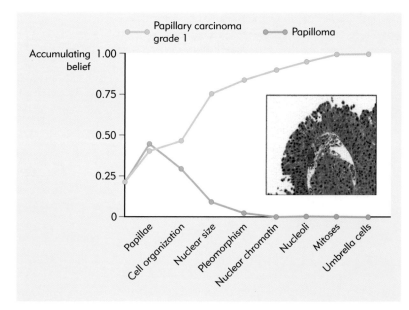

Fig. 13.19 When evidence for all the eight features is entered, the accumulation of belief for papillary carcinoma grade 1 is progressive and monotonic towards 1.0 whereas the belief for papilloma and papillary carcinoma grades 2 and 3 decreases to 0.0 (the belief curves for the latter two are not shown). This figure also shows the histologic image of the urothelial papillary lesion used to derive the evidence for the features.

networks and case-based reasoning are examples of the latter.

Artificial neural networks

Artificial neural networks (ANNs) are powerful, non-linear statistical classifiers which can be trained to generate highly convoluted decision boundaries between data sets. ANN classifiers offer several practical advantages. ANNs learn by example and there is no need to develop specific computer codes for a classification procedure, feature selection, feature weighting and feature combination. They can be particularly robust, and can tolerate missing data. They naturally incorporate redundancies in data representation so that bad data associated with one feature of a case might be compensated for by correct information from another feature. True parallelism in ANN processing suggests time saving from execution of complex classification tasks.[14]

Case-based reasoning

Case-based reasoning establishes a prognosis for a particular patient, and thus differs significantly from statistical classification in which the patient is assigned to a group, all of whose members were given the same diagnosis. Statistical classification allows a prognosis on the basis of what is known for the group (e.g. a probability to progress or survive for a certain period of time). However, statistical procedures are neither usually intended nor designed to characterize individuals. For example, for a given patient it is not possible to say whether the prognostic outlook is poorer or better within the bounds given for the group. Case-based reasoning, on the other hand, is designed to provide individual patient prognosis. Case-based reasoning compares the new case with cases from a large database of cases for which the clinical outcome is known. From such a database, only the most similar cases are retrieved and used to predict the outcome. The data may include qualitative and quantitative histopathologic feature values, patient anamnestic data, treatment and observed response to treatment, thus providing a very detailed characterization of the patient's situation.[14]

CONCLUSION

Measurement of histologic and cell features has provided objective data that significantly improve the ability to make diagnostic decisions in bladder tumor interpretation. Histometric and karyometric measurements can be made that objectively reflect tissue characteristics that are visually apparent and are assessed routinely, in a subjective fashion, for the diagnosis and prognosis of the diseases. In addition, measurements can reveal subtle changes in tissues or cells not visually apparent to the eye. In both instances, measurement can be an invaluable tool for objective interpretation of morphologic abnormalities and quantitative assessment of bladder neoplasms.

REFERENCES

1. Herder A, Bjelkenkrantz K, Gröntoft O. Histopathological subgrouping of WHO II urothelial neoplasms by cytophotometric measurements of nuclear atypia. Acta Pathol Microbiol Scand 1982;90:405–408.
2. Bjelkenkrantz K, Herder A, Gröntoft O, Stål O. Cytophometric characterization of the WHO grades of transitional cell neoplasms. Pathol Res Pract 1982;174:68–77.
3. Ooms ECM, Kurver PHJ, Veldhuizen RW, Alons CL, Boon ME. Morphometric grading of bladder tumours in comparison with histologic grading by pathologists. Hum Pathol 1983;14:144–150.
4. Helander K, Hofer P-Å, Holmberg G. Karyometric investigations on urinary bladder carcinoma, correlated to histopathological grading. Virchows Arch [Pathol Anat] 1984;403:117–125.
5. Kieler J, Ostrowski K, Strojny P, et al. Fourier analyses of the shape of normal and transformed epithelial cells derived from human transitional epithelium. Histochemistry 1984;81:119–128.
6. Helander K, Kirkhus B, Iversen OH, et al. Studies on urinary bladder carcinoma by morphometry flow cytometry, and light microscopic malignancy grading with special reference to grade II tumours. Virchows Arch [Pathol Anat] 1985;408:117–126.
7. Montironi R, Scarpelli M, Sisti S, et al. Quantitative analysis and malignancy progression of the papillary neoplasia of urinary bladder. Pathol Res Pract 1987;182:528–529.
8. Montironi R, Scarpelli M, De Nictolis M, et al. Comparison of computerized analysis of nuclear DNA changes in uterine cervix dysplasia and in urothelial non-invasive papillary carcinoma. Pathol Res Pract 1988;183:489–496.
9. Boon ME, Kurver PHJ, Baak JPA, Ooms ECM. Morphometric differences between urothelial cells in voided urine of patients with grade I and grade II bladder tumours. J Clin Pathol 1981;34:612–615.
10. Henstreet GP, West SS, Weems WL, et al. Quantitative fluorescence measurements of OA-stained normal and malignant bladder cells. Int J Cancer 1983;31:577–585.
11. Choi HK, Vasko J, Bengtsson E, et al. Grading of transitional cell bladder carcinoma by texture analysis of histological sections. Anal Cell Pathol 1994;6:327–343.
12. Jarkrans T, Vasko J, Bengtsson E, et al. Grading of transitional cell bladder carcinoma by image analysis of histological sections. Anal Cell Pathol 1995;8:135–158.
13. Choi HK, Jarkrans T, Bengtsson E, et al. Image analysis based grading of bladder carcinoma.Comparison of object, textures and graph based methods and their reproducibility. Anal Cell Pathol 1997;15:1–18.
14. Montironi R, Mazzucchelli R, Bostwick DG, et al. Recent advances in the quantitative morphological evaluation of prostate neoplasia. J Urol Pathol 2000;12:133–168.
15. Mazzucchelli R, Santinelli A, Colanzi P, et al. Urothelial papillary lesions. Development of a Bayesian belief network for diagnosis and grading. Anticancer Res 2001;21:1157–1162.

16. Broders AC. Epithelioma of the genitourinary organs. Ann Surg 1922;75:574–604.

17. Broders AC. Grading of cancer: its relationship to metastasis and prognosis. Texas State J Med 1933;29:520–525.

18. Ash JE. Epithelial tumors of the bladder. J Urol 1940;44:135–145.

19. Franksson C. Tumors of the urinary bladder. Acta Chir Scand (Suppl) 1950;151:1–203.

20. Bergkvist A, Ljungquist A, Moberger G. Classification of bladder tumours based on the cellular pattern. Acta Chir Scand 1965;130:371–378.

21. Esposti PL, Moberger G, Zajicek J. The cytologic diagnosis of transitional cell tumors of the urinary bladder and its histologic basis. A study of 567 cases of urinary-tract disorder including 170 untreated and 182 irradiated bladder tumors. Acta Cytol 1970;14:145–155.

22. Esposti PL, Zajicek J. Grading of transitional cell neoplasms of the urinary bladder from smears of bladder washings. Acta Cytol 1972;16:529–537.

23. World Health Organization. Histological typing of urinary bladder tumours. International Histological Classification of Tumours. No 10. Geneva: WHO, 1973.

24. Epstein JI, Amin MB, Reuter VR, Mostofi FK and the Bladder Consensus Conference Committee. The World Health Organization/International Society of Urological Pathology consensus classification of urothelial (transitional cell) neoplasms of the urinary bladder. Am J Surg Pathol 1998;22:1435–1448.

25. World Health Organization. Histological Typing of Urinary Bladder Tumours. International Classification of Tumours. No 10, 2nd edn. Geneva: WHO, 1999.

26. Holmang S, Hedelin H, Anderstrom C, et al. Recurrence and progression in low grade papillary urothelial tumors. J Urol 1999;162:702–707.

27. Sherman AB, Koss LG, Adams SE. Interobserver and intraobserver differences in the diagnosis of urothelial cells. Anal Quant Cytol Histol 1984;6:112–120.

28. Montironi R, Scarpelli M, Pisani E, et al. Non-invasive papillary transitional-cell tumors: karyometric and DNA content analysis. Anal Quant Cytol Histol 1985;7:337–342.

29. van Velthoven R, Petein M, Oosterlinck WJ, et al. The use of digital image analysis of chromatin texture in Feulgen-stained nuclei to predict recurrence of low grade superficial transitional cell carcinoma of the bladder. Cancer 1995;75:560–568.

30. True LD. Morphometric applications in anatomic pathology. Hum Pathol 1996;27:450–467.

31. Cohen C. Image cytometric analysis in pathology. Hum Pathol 1996;27:482–493.

32. van der Poel HG, Boon ME, van Stratum P, et al. Conventional bladder wash cytology performed by four experts versus quantitative image analysis. Mod Pathol 1997;10:976–982.

33. Ooms ECM, Anderson WAD, Alons CL, Boon ME, Veldhuizen RM. Analysis of the performance of pathologists in the grading of bladder tumors. Hum Pathol 1983;14:140–143.

34. Wheeless LL, Badalament RA, deVere RW, Fradet Y, Tribukait B. Consensus review of the clinical utility of DNA cytometry in bladder cancer. Cytometry 1993;14:478–481.

35. Koss LG, Wersto RP, Simmsons DA, Deitch DS, Herz F, Freed SZ. Predictive value of DNA measurements in bladder washings. Cancer 1989;64:916–924.

36. Chabanas A, Rambeaud JJ, Seigneurin D, et al. Flow and image cytometry for DNA analysis in bladder washings: improved concordance by using internal reference for flow. Cytometry 1993;14:943–950.

37. Ooms ECM, Kurver PJH, Boon ME. Morphometrical analysis of urothelial cells in voided urine of patients with low and high grade bladder tumours. J Clin Pathol 1982;35:1063–1065.

38. Sherman A, Koss LG, Adams S, et al. Bladder cancer diagnosis by cell image analysis of cells in voided urine using a small computer. Anal Quant Cytol Histol 1981;3:239–249.

39. van der Poel HG, Witjes, JA, van Stratum P, et al. Quanticyt: karyometric analysis of bladder washing for patients with superficial bladder cancer. Urology 1996;48:357–364.

40. van der Poel HG, Witjes JA, Schalken JA, Deruyne FMJ. Automated image analysis for bladder cancer. Urol Res 1998;26:1–5.

41. van der Poel HG, Schaafsma E, Vooijs P, Debruyne FMJ, Schalken JA. Quantitative light microscopy in urological oncology. J Urol 1992;148:1–13.

42. Fosså SD, Kaalhus O, Scott-Knudsen O. The clinical and histopathological significance of Feulgen DNA values in transitional cell carcinoma of the human urinary bladder. Eur J Cancer 1977;13:1155–1162.

43. Tribukait BT, Gustafson H, Esposti P. Ploidy and proliferation in human bladder tumours as measured by flow cytometric DNA analysis and its relations to histopathology and cytology. Cancer 1979;43:1742–1751.

44. Loerum OD, Farsund T. Clinical application of flow cytometry; a review. Cytometry 1981;2:1–13.

45. Farsund T, Hoestmark JG, Loerum OD. Relation between flow cytometric DNA distribution and pathology in human bladder cancer: a report on 69 cases. Cancer 1984;54:1771–1777.

46. Kirkhus B, Clausen OPF, Fjordvang H, et al. Characterization of bladder tumours by multiparameter flow cytometry with special reference to grade II tumours. APMIS 1988;96:783–792.

47. van Velthoven R, Petein M, Zlotta A, et al. Computer-assisted chromatin texture characterization of Feulgen-stained nuclei in a series of 331 transitional bladder cell carcinomas. J Pathol 1994;173:235–242.

48. Montironi R, Scarpelli M, Pisani E, et al. Multivariate classifications of transitional tumors of the bladder: nuclear abnormality index and pattern recognition analysis. Appl Pathol 1986;4:48–54.

49. Montironi R, Scarpelli M, Sisti S, et al. Prognostic value of computerized DNA analysis in non-invasive papillary carcinomas of the urinary bladder. Tumori 1987;73:567–574.

50. Ranefall P, Egevad L, Nordin B, Bengtsson E. A new method for segmentation of colour images applied to immunohistochemically stained cell nuclei, Anal Cell Pathol 1997;15:145–156.

51. Ranefall P, Wester K, Busch C, Malmström P-U, Bengtsson E. Automatic quantification of immunohistochemically stained cell nuclei using unsupervised image analysis. Anal Cell Pathol 1998;16:29–43.

52. Ranefall P, Wester K, Andersson AC, Busch C, Bengtsson E. Automatic quantification of immunohistochemically stained cell nuclei based on standard reference cells. Anal Cell Pathol 1998;17:111–123.

53. Helpap B, Kollermann J. Assessment of basal cell status and proliferative patterns in flat and papillary urothelial lesions: a contribution to the new WHO classification of urothelial tumors of the urinary bladder. Hum Pathol 2000;31:745–750.

54. Montironi R, Scarpelli M, Sisti S, et al. Quantitation of malignancy progression in the urothelial non-invasive papillary carcinoma. In: Castagnetta L, Nenci I. (eds) Biology and Biochemistry of Normal and Cancer Cell Growth. New York: Harwood Academic, 1988, pp 85–89.

55. Busch C, Vasko J. Differential staining of mitoses in tissue sections and cultured cells by a modified methanamine-silver method. Lab Invest 1988;59:876–878.

56. Lipponen PK, Kosma VM, Collan Y, et al. Potential of nuclear morphometry and volume-corrected mitotic index in grading transitional cell carcinoma of the urinary bladder. Eur Urol 1990;17:333–337.

57. Lipponen PK, Collan Y, Eskelinen MJ, Pesonen E, Sotarauta M. Volume corrected mitotic index (M/V index) in human bladder cancer; relation to histological grade (WHO), clinical stage (UICC) and prognosis. Scand J Urol Nephrol 1990;24:39–45.

58. Lipponen PK, Eskeline MJ, Kiviranta J, Nordling S. Classic prognostic factors, flow cytometric data, nuclear morphometric and mitotic indexes as predictors in transitional cell bladder cancer. Anticancer Res 1991;11:911–916.

59. Hapsalo H. Grading of superficial bladder cancer by quantitative mitotic frequency analysis. J Urol 1993;149:36–41.

60. Vasko J, Malmström P-U, Taube A, Wester K, Busch C. Toward an objective method of mitotic figure counting and its prognostic significance in bladder cancer. J Urol Pathol 1995;3:315–326.

61. Cairns P, Suarez V, Newman J, Crocker J. Nucleolar organizer regions in transitional cell tumors of the bladder. Arch Pathol Lab Med 1989;113:1250–1252.

62. Fujimoto K, Yamada Y, Okajima E, et al. Frequent association of p53 gene mutation in invasive bladder cancer. Cancer Res 1992;52:1393–1398.

63. Spruck CH, Ohneseit PF, Gonzalez-Zulueta M, et al. Two molecular pathways to transitional cell carcinoma of the bladder. Cancer Res 1994;54:784–788.

64. Uchida T, Wada C, Ishida H, et al. p53 mutations and prognosis in bladder tumors. J Urol 1995;153:1097–1104.

65. Cote RJ, Esrig D, Groshen S, Jones PA, Skinner DG. p53 and treatment of bladder cancer. Nature 1997;385:123–124.

66. Bochner BH, Cote RJ, Weidner N, et al. Angiogenesis in bladder cancer: relationship between microvessel density and tumor prognosis. J Natl Cancer Inst 1995;87:1603–1612.

67. Ranefall P, Wester K, Busch C, Malmstrom PU, Bengtsson E. Automatic quantification of microvessels using unsupervised image analysis. Anal Cell Pathol 1998;17:83–92.

68. Wester K, Ranefall P, Bengtsson E, Busch C, Malmstrom PU. Automatic quantification of microvessel density in urinary bladder carcinoma. Br J Cancer 1999;81:1363–1370.

69. Riera J, Simpson JF, Tamayo R, Battifora H. Use of cultured cells as a control for quantitative immunocytochemical analysis of estrogen receptor in breast cancer. The Quickgel method. Am J Clin Pathol 1999;11:329–335.

70. Wester K, Andersson AC, Ranefall P, et al. Cultured human fibroblasts in agarose gel as a multi-functional control for immunohistochemistry. Standardization of Ki67 (MIB1) assessment in routinely processed urinary bladder carcinoma tissue. J Pathol 2000;190:503–511.

71. Wester K, Wahlund E, Sundström C, et al. Paraffin section storage and immunohistochemistry. Appl Immunohistochem Mol Morphol 2000;8:61–70.

72. Oooms ECM, Blok APR, Veldhuizen RW. The reproducibility of a quantitative grading system of bladder tumours. Histopathology 1985;9:501–509.

73. Pauwels RPE, Schapers FM, Smeets WGB, Debruyne FMJ, Geraedts JPM. Grading in superficial bladder cancer. (1) Morphological criteria. Br J Urol 1988;61:129–134.

74. Abel PD, Henderson D, Bennet MK, Hall RR, Williams G. Differing interpretations by pathologists of the pT category and grade of transitional cell cancer of the bladder. Br J Urol 1988;62:339–342.

75. van der Poel HG, Boon ME, Kok LP, et al. Can cytomorphometry replace histomorphometry for grading of bladder tumours? Virchows Arch [Pathol Anat] 1988;413:249–255.

76. De Prez C, de Launoit Y, Kiss R, et al. Computerized morphonuclear cell image analyses of malignant disease in bladder tissues. J Urol 1990;143:694–699.

77. Nielsen K, Colstrup H, Nilsson T, Gundersen HJ. Stereological estimates of nuclear volume correlated with histopathological grading and prognosis of bladder tumours. Virchows Arch [Cell Pathol] 1986;52:41–54.

78. Nielsen K. Stereological estimates of nuclear volume in normal mucosa and carcinoma in situ of the human urinary bladder. Virchows Arch [Cell Pathol] 1988;55:233–236.

79. Nielsen K, Petersen SE, Örntoft T. A comparison between stereological estimates of mean nuclear volume and DNA flow cytometry in bladder tumours. APMIS 1989;97:949–956.

80. Nielsen K, Örntoft T, Wolf H. Stereological estimates of nuclear volume in non-invasive bladder tumours (Ta) correlated with the recurrence pattern. Cancer 1989;64:2269–2274.

81. Schapers FM, Pauwels RPE, Wijnen JTM, Smeets WGB, Bosman FT. Morphometric grading of transitional cell carcinoma of the urinary bladder. J Urol Pathol 1995;3:107–118.

82. Sowter C, Slavin G, Rosen D. Morphometry of bladder carcinoma: I. The automatic delineation of urothelial nuclei in tissue sections using an IBAS II image array processor. J Pathol 1987;153:289–297.

83. Sowter C, Sowter G, Slavin G, Rosen D. Morphometry of bladder carcinoma: definition of a new variable. Anal Cell Pathol 1990;2:205–213.

84. De Meester U, Young IT, Lindeman J, van der Linden HC. Towards a quantitative grading of bladder tumors. Cytometry 1991;12:602–613.

85. Malmstrom P-U, Busch C, Norlen BJ. Recurrence, progression and survival in bladder cancer. Scand J Urol Nephrol 1987;21:185–195.

86. Decaestecker C, van Velthoven R, Petein M, et al. The use of the decision tree technique and image cytometry to characterize aggressiveness in World Health Organization (WHO) grade II superficial transitional cell carcinomas of the bladder. J Pathol 1996;178:274–283.

87. Wiener HG, Mian CH, Haitel A, et al. Can urine bound diagnostic tests replace cystoscopy in the management of bladder cancer? J Urol 1996;159:1876–1880.

88. Ross JS, Cohen MB. Ancillary methods for the detection of recurrent urothelial neoplasia. Cancer 2000;90:75–86.

89. Wiener HG, Remkes GW, Schtzl G, Breitencker G. Quick-staining urinary cytology and bladder wash image analysis with an integrated risk classification. Cancer 1999;87:263–269.

90. Tetû B, Katz R, Kalter SP, von Eschenbach AC, Barlogie B. Flow cytometry of transitional cell carcinoma of the urinary bladder: influence of prior local therapy. Semin Diagn Pathol 1987;4:243–250.

91. Sauter G, Gasser TC, Moch H, et al. DNA aberrations in urinary bladder cancer detected by flow cytometry and FISH. Urol Res 1997;1(Suppl 1):37–43.

92. Zhang FF, Arber DA, Wilson TG, Kawachi MH, Slovak ML. Toward the validation of aneusomy detection by fluorescence in situ hybridization in bladder cancer: comparative analysis with cytology, cytogenetics, and clinical features predicts recurrence and defines clinical testing limitations. Clin Cancer Res 1997;3:2317–2328.

93. Junker K, Werner W, Mueller C, et al. Interphase cytogenetic diagnosis of bladder cancer on cells from urine and bladder washing. Int J Oncol 1999;14:309–313.

94. van der Poel HG, van Balken MR, Schmhart DHJ, et al. Bladder wash cytology, quantitative cytology, and the qualitative BTA test in patients with superficial bladder cancer. Urology 1998;51:44–50.

95. Haroske G, Meyer W, Oberholzer M, Böcking A, Kunze KD. Competence on demand in DNA image cytometry. Pathol Res Pract 2000;196:285–291.

96. Haroske G, Giroud F, Kunze KD, Meyer W. A telepathology based Virtual Reference and Certification Centre for DNA image cytometry. Anal Cell Pathol 2000;21:149–159.

14

CONVENTIONAL MORPHOLOGIC, PROGNOSTIC AND PREDICTIVE FACTORS FOR BLADDER CANCER

Sanjay Logani and Mahul B. Amin

INTRODUCTION

There are well-known histopathologic features of urothelial carcinoma of the bladder that have prognostic significance and are crucial for patient management. These vary according to the type of bladder cancer presentation in the patient: non-invasive papillary tumors, primary urothelial carcinoma in situ or invasive urothelial carcinoma. The prognostic factors are discussed separately for each category and are summarized in Table 14.1. There are several molecular/chromosomal markers (e.g. loss of chromosome 9, loss of material on chromosome 17, p53, retinoblastoma tumor suppressor gene status) that are likely to complement traditional morphologic markers in the future; these are discussed in detail in Chapter 22. Additionally, clinical parameters (co-morbid disease etc.) as well as clinical presentation (frequency of recurrence and interval between recurrences) influence progression and disease outcome.

NON-INVASIVE PAPILLARY TUMORS

Histologic grade

Histologic grade is a powerful prognostic factor for recurrence and progression in non-invasive tumors. Using the restrictive criteria outlined by the World Health Organization/International Society of Urological Pathology (WHO/ISUP) classification[1] for the histologic diagnosis of papilloma, these lesions have the lowest risk for either recurrence or progression and the majority of papillomas, particularly the lesions that occur de novo, once resected will not recur.[2] Papillary urothelial

Table 14.1 Morphologic prognostic and predictive factors of bladder cancer

- Non-invasive papillary tumors
  - histologic grade
  - size of tumor
  - multifocality
  - status of non-papillary urothelium: carcinoma in situ
- Urothelial carcinoma in situ
  - mode of presentation: primary (de novo) or secondary
  - multifocality
  - failure to respond to typical therapy
- Invasive urothelial carcinoma
  - depth of invasion in bladder wall (pT stage)
  - lymph node involvement (pN stage)
  - involvement of prostate gland and seminal vesicles
  - histologic type
  - histologic grade (controversial)
  - vascular–lymphatic invasion (controversial)
  - surgical margin status for invasive carcinoma
  - multifocality and carcinoma in situ of urethra or ureters

neoplasm of low malignant potential (PUNLMP), a newly introduced term in the WHO/ISUP classification, has now been shown in numerous studies to have a recurrence rate between that observed for papilloma and low-grade carcinoma. Progression in grade or stage in these lesions is unusual. In one study, up to 33% of PUNLMP recurred; however, none progressed to invasive disease.[3] Patients with papilloma and PUNLMP have essentially a normal age-related life expectancy. It is important to clarify at this point that PUNLMP is not synonymous with the 1973 WHO grade I transitional cell carcinoma, although many lesions classified as such would have been graded as WHO grade I using the previous system. The criteria for grading these urothelial tumors are outlined in detail in Chapter 13.

Progression risk in grade, stage and mortality increases across the spectrum of grades of bladder neoplasia. In 2000, Desai et al. (using the WHO/ISUP classification of bladder tumors) found that cases of papilloma in their series did not progress or recur, PUNLMP tumors frequently recurred but rarely progressed and patients with low- and high-grade carcinomas experienced progression and death though at very

different rates.[3] Similar results were obtained by other studies using the same grading system[3–9] (Table 14.2).

As experience with this classification system accumulates, it is becoming increasingly clear that the designation of a tumor as PUNLMP identifies patients with negligible risk for disease progression and avoids labeling the patient with a diagnosis of carcinoma and its associated psychosocial and financial (insurance) implications. On the other hand, high-grade carcinoma shows a significant rate of recurrence and progression.

Size of tumor

Large tumors (often greater than 3 cm) are at an increased risk for recurrence and progression.[10] Heney et al.[11] found a direct correlation between tumor size and invasiveness. In their study, 35% of tumors that were larger than 5 cm progressed to muscle-invasive disease whereas only 9% of tumors smaller than 5 cm progressed.

Multifocality

Patients with multifocal tumors in the bladder and involving other regions of the urothelial tract (ureters, pelvicalyceal system and urethra) are at increased risk for recurrence, progression or death due to disease. Lutzeyer et al.[12] reported that solitary stage Ta and T1 tumors had recurrence rates of 18% and 33%, respectively, whereas multiple stage Ta and T1 lesions had recurrence rates approaching 46%. More recently, Millan-Rodriguez et al.[13] evaluated prognostic factors in 'superficial' bladder carcinoma. In this study, multiple tumors had a statistically significant correlation with both rate of recurrence as well as progression.

Urothelial carcinoma in situ in non-papillary mucosa

Although the impact of the presence of dysplasia in the non-papillary urothelium is controversial as a prognostic factor and at best may represent a marker of urothelial instability, the presence of urothelial carcinoma in situ (CIS) is a known adverse prognostic factor in terms of recurrence and progression. The occurrence of CIS in the absence of an associated urothelial tumor is rare and when extensive has a 60–80% risk of progression at 5 years.[14] More commonly, CIS is present synchronously with urothelial tumors and is more frequent with increasing grade and stage of the associated tumor.[15]

Table 14.2 Relation of WHO/ISUP grades to recurrence and progression in pTa and pT1 papillary urothelial neoplasia

Reference	Papilloma	PUNLMP	Low grade	High grade
Cheng et al.[8]	n = 0	n = 112	n = 0	n = 0
Recurrence	–	25.9%	–	–
Progression	–	3.5%	–	–
Desai et al.[3]	n = 8	n = 8	n = 42	n = 62
Recurrence	0%	33.3%	64%	56.4%
Progression	0%	0%	10.5%	27.1%
Holmang et al.[5]	n = 0	n = 95	n = 160	n = 103
Recurrence	–	35%	71%	73%
Progression	–	0%	4%	23%
Alsheikh et al.[4]	n = 0	n = 20	n = 29	n = 0
Recurrence	–	25%	48.2%	–
Progression	–	0%	6.8%	–
Pich et al.[6]	n = 0	n = 19	n = 43	n = 0
Recurrence	–	47.4%	76.7%	–
Progression	–	0%	11.6%	–
Oosterhuis et al.[7]	n = 18	n = 116	n = 141	n = 45
Recurrence	16.6%	25.8%	30.4%	40%
Progression	0%	2.5%	3.5%	4.4%
Samaratunga et al.[9]	n = 3	n = 29	n = 73	n = 29
Progression	0%	8%	13%	51%

PUNLMP, papillary urothelial neoplasm of low malignant potential.

UROTHELIAL CARCINOMA IN SITU

Urothelial carcinoma in situ (TCIS) is defined as a flat urothelial neoplasm of high cytologic grade without stromal invasion. It usually presents as an associated finding with prior or synchronous urothelial tumors; however, in rare cases it may be the sole form of urothelial cancer present in the patient (de novo or primary CIS).

The natural history of TCIS is one of progression, with most cases of untreated CIS having the ability to develop invasive carcinoma. In a study by Zincke et al., 34% of patients undergoing cystectomy for CIS showed evidence of microinvasion.[16] In a multivariate analysis of prognostic factors for Ta and T1 bladder carcinoma, Millan-Rodriguez et al.[13] found that the presence of TCIS was a predictor for both recurrence and progression of the disease. In a study of 192 radical cystectomy specimens by Nixon et al., CIS was present in 31% of cases with concomitant prostatic urethral involvement whereas only 4.5% of cases without CIS showed prostatic urethral involvement.[17] Patients with primary (de novo) CIS are more likely to have no evidence of disease

(62% versus 45%), and are less likely to progress (28% versus 59%) or die of disease (7% versus 45%) when compared to CIS occurring in patients with papillary bladder carcinoma. Patients with multifocal disease and those who fail to respond to intravesical therapy have a worse outcome.

INVASIVE UROTHELIAL CARCINOMA

Depth of invasion in bladder wall

Invasion in urothelial carcinoma may arise at the base of the papillary neoplasm or within it. It may also be seen in association with a flat lesion (CIS with microinvasion). Invasion into the muscularis mucosae (thin, often discontinuous muscle fibers) and muscularis propria (compact smooth muscle bundles) is the basis for distinguishing invasive disease into T1 and T2 stages, the distinction between the two being one of immense therapeutic importance. Most patients with T1 disease are managed conservatively. The American Joint Commission on Cancer/International Union Against

Table 14.3 AJCC/UICC staging system for bladder cancer[18]

Primary tumor (T)*

TX Primary tumor cannot be assessed
T0 No evidence of primary tumor
Ta Non-invasive papillary carcinoma
Tis Carcinoma in situ: 'flat tumor'
T1 Tumor invades subepithelial connective tissue
T2 Tumor invades muscle:
    T2a Tumor invades superficial muscle (inner half)
    T2b Tumor invades deep muscle (outer half)
T3 Tumor invades perivesical tissue:
    T3a Microscopically
    T3b Macroscopically (extravesicular mass)
T4 Tumor invades any of the following: prostate, uterus, vagina, pelvic wall, and abdominal wall
    T4a Tumor invades prostate or uterus or vagina
    T4b Tumor invades pelvic wall or abdominal wall

Regional lymph nodes (N)

Regional lymph nodes are those within the true pelvis; all others are distant nodes.

NX Regional lymph nodes cannot be assessed
N0 No regional lymph node metastasis
N1 Metastasis in a single lymph node, 2 cm or less in greatest dimension
N2 Metastasis in a single lymph node, more than 2 cm but not more than 5 cm in greatest dimension, or multiple lymph nodes, none more than 5 cm in greatest dimension
N3 Metastasis in a lymph node more than 5 cm in greatest dimension

Distant metastasis (M)

MX Distant metastasis cannot be assessed
M0 No distant metastasis
M1 Distant metastasis

TNM stage grouping: bladder

Stage 0a	Ta	N0	M0
Stage 0is	Tis	N0	M0
Stage I	T1	N0	M0
Stage II	T2a	N0	M0
	T2b	N0	M0
Stage III	T3a	N0	M0
	T3b	N0	M0
Stage IV	T4a	N0	M0
	T4b	N0	M0
	Any T	N1,2,3	M0
	Any T	Any N	M1

*The suffix 'm' should be added to the appropriate T category to indicate multiple tumors. The suffix 'is' may be added to any T to indicate the presence of associated carcinoma in situ.

Cancer (AJCC/UICC) pathologic staging[18] of urothelial carcinoma is outlined in Table 14.3. Although several studies have documented that T1 tumors have a less favorable outcome compared to Ta (non-invasive) tumors, for treatment purposes Ta and T1 tumors are usually lumped together by the urologist under the designation of 'superficial' tumors. The use of this term is inappropriate in a pathology report of bladder cancer. The pT system of staging has excellent correlation with prognosis and distinguishes distinct prognostic groups: patients with tumors invasive into the lamina propria (pT1) have a better survival than those with tumors invasive into the muscularis propria (pT2), with poor survival for patients with tumors with extravesicular extension (pT3, pT4). Moreover, as alluded to before, the distinction between pT1 and pT2 tumors is vitally important in stratifying patients for further therapy as patients with pT1 tumors are often managed conserva-

tively (bladder-sparing treatment) compared to patients with pT2 tumors who are usually candidates for more aggressive approaches including cystectomy or radiotherapy.

Although substaging of urothelial tumors (pT1a, tumors invasive up to muscularis mucosae; pT1b, tumors invasive into or beyond muscularis mucosae) has shown prognostic value,[19] this is currently not recommended as it may not always be possible to substage pT1 tumors due to absence of muscularis mucosae in some bladders or because of a lack of orientation in transurethral resection specimens.[1] The cumulative data suggest that pT1b tumors tend to behave more like pT2 tumors whereas pT1a tumors have an outcome between that of pTa and pT2 tumors. The 5-year survival in patients with pT1 disease is approximately 75% and this decreases to about 40% for pT2 and to 20% for pT3 or pT4 disease.[20]

Lymph node involvement

Lymph node metastases have been reported in approximately 15% of patients undergoing cystectomy for muscle-invasive disease.[21] Patients with regional spread of tumor (node-positive) have a poor prognosis although a small percentage of patients with lymph node involvement may be cured.[22,23] Jimenez et al. found a median survival of 23 months for patients with lymph node involvement as compared to 63 months for patients with negative lymph nodes at the time of cystectomy.[24] Immunohistochemical detection of micrometastasis has no established prognostic value.[25]

Involvement of prostate gland and seminal vesicles

Involvement of the prostate gland may be by urothelial carcinoma extending along the luminal aspect (mucosal spread of CIS) of prostatic ducts and acini (CIS of prostatic ducts and acini/urothelial carcinoma involving prostatic ducts and acini). This pattern of disease predicts a high recurrence[26] on a stage-adjusted basis, but is not equivalent to pT4 disease. Invasion of the prostatic or seminal vesicle stroma secondary to CIS involving prostatic ducts and acini or seminal vesicle epithelium is usually a microscopic disease but when present portends a very poor prognosis. Wishnow et al.[27] reported the development of metastatic cancer in all five of their patients with prostatic stromal involvement. In contrast, only 2 of 11 patients developed metastases when the prostatic involvement was confined to prostatic ducts and acini.

The precise stage designation for this form of invasion is not recognized in the current TNM classification. Rarely, invasive urothelial carcinoma may involve the prostatic gland without any documentable bladder disease and such cases represent a prostatic urothelial primary, an occurrence seen in less than 1% of primary prostatic tumors.

Histologic type

Aberrant differentiation (squamous or glandular) in urothelial carcinoma has no known prognostic significance except that the frequency and extent are directly proportional to the grade of urothelial carcinoma. Pure squamous carcinomas and adenocarcinomas tend to present at higher stage but when corrected for stage have an outcome similar to that of urothelial carcinoma

of comparable stage. The nested variant of urothelial carcinoma, micropapillary urothelial carcinoma, sarcomatoid carcinoma (carcinosarcoma) and small cell carcinoma are histologic patterns associated with poor outcome, usually due to the high stage at presentation.[28–30] The diagnoses of urachal adenocarcinoma, lymphoepithelioma-like carcinoma and small cell carcinoma have additional therapeutic relevance; for example, urachal carcinomas are often treated with partial cystectomy, excision of urachal tract and umbilectomy, in contrast to primary mucosal bladder muscle-invasive adenocarcinomas, which are usually treated with radical cystectomy. Chemotherapy may be an important component of therapy in patients with lymphoepithelioma-like[28] or small cell carcinoma (particularly pure tumors).

Histologic grade

Once invasive into muscularis propria, the importance of histologic grade is controversial and not shown to be of additional prognostic value,[24] although it should not be assumed that all invasive tumors are likely to be high-grade. Angulo et al.[31] reported 41% of their pT1 tumors and 18% of their pT1b tumors to be grade I (using the 1973 WHO classification). There is, in fact, often an outcome paradox: for example, nested variants, which histologically may be low-grade, have a poor outcome.[32–34]

Vascular–lymphatic invasion

The importance of this feature is controversial as retraction artifact around tumor is often overdiagnosed as such. Unequivocal invasion into endothelial-lined spaces has been shown to be significant in univariate analysis. Bell et al.[35] reported 5-year survival rates of 29% and 51% for patients with and without vascular invasion, respectively. Lopez et al.[36] have reported a 5-year survival rate of 81% for patients with T1 tumors without vascular invasion versus a 44% 5-year survival rate for those patients with T1 tumors that had vascular invasion. Since the presence of vascular invasion may influence therapeutic choices, strict morphologic criteria should be utilized for the accurate reporting of vascular invasion. Criteria for its recognition have been well defined.[19]

The study by Larsen et al.[37] underscores the importance of accurate diagnosis of vascular invasion, where only 14% of cases were determined to be true vascular invasion after immunohistochemical confirmation. A similar study by Ramani et al.[38] confirmed lympho-vascular invasion in only 40% of cases using multiple endothelial markers. Furthermore, this study showed that the presence of lymphovascular invasion did not confer an adverse prognosis in stage T1 tumors although the number of patients evaluated was small. More recently, Leissner et al. reaffirmed the prognostic significance of vascular invasion in their study of 283 radical cystectomy specimens. Blood vessel invasion was identified as an adverse prognostic variable on both univariate and multivariate analysis.[39]

Surgical margin status

Presence of invasive carcinoma at the resection margin is an adverse prognostic parameter, primarily for local recurrence.[40]

Multifocality and CIS of urethra or ureters

Patients with multifocal high-grade papillary or inva-sive tumors and/or multifocal CIS are at an increased risk for recurrence.[41] Presence of CIS at the urethral margin at cystoprostatectomy may be an indication for urethrectomy.

REPORTING OF BLADDER CANCER

The elements that should be included in the surgical pathology report must have prognostic significance and should very likely be important for patient man-agement. Checklists for reporting bladder cancer have been developed by the Association of Directors of Anatomic and Surgical Pathology[42] and the College of American Pathologists.[43] While evaluating bladder tumor specimens, the most important role of the pathologist is to grade non-invasive tumors accurately, to ascertain the invasion status diligently and, if inva-sive, to assign a tumor stage accurately.[18] Table 14.4 summarizes the essential elements to be reported in biopsy/transurethral resection and radical cystectomy/cystoprostatectomy specimens. This is discussed in greater detail in Chapter 19.

Table 14.4 Elements to be included in bladder cancer surgical pathology reports

Biopsy/transurethral resection
- Essential
  - histologic type (urothelial, squamous cell, etc.)
  - histologic grade (WHO/ISUP for urothelial carcinoma)
  - pathologic stage (pT) (only pTa, pT1 or pT2)
  - presence or absence of muscularis propria in specimen
  - presence or absence of urothelial carcinoma in situ
- Optional
  - configuration of tumor: papillary, flat, ulcerative, solid, etc.
  - unequivocal vascular–lymphatic invasion
  - urothelial dysplasia
  - other benign/proliferative, inflammatory or therapy-related changes

Cystectomy/cystoprostatectomy/anterior exenteration
- Essential
  - histologic type (urothelial, squamous cell, etc.)
  - histologic grade (WHO/ISUP for urothelial carcinoma)
  - pathologic stage (pT and pN status)
  - presence or absence of urothelial carcinoma in situ
  - involvement of prostate:
    - direct extension
    - involvement of prostatic ducts and acini without stromal invasion
    - involvement of prostatic ducts and acini with stromal invasion
  - direct involvement of adjacent viscera (exenteration specimen)
  - margins of excision for carcinoma in situ (mention all negative and positive margins)
  - margins of excision for invasive carcinoma (mention all negative and positive margins)
- Optional
  - configuration of tumor: papillary, flat, ulcerative, solid, etc.
  - unequivocal vascular–lymphatic invasion
  - multifocal tumors
  - urothelial dysplasia
  - other benign/proliferative, inflammatory or therapy-related change

REFERENCES

1. Epstein JI, Amin MB, Reuter VR, Mostofi FK. The World Health Organization/International Society of Urological Pathology consensus classification of urothelial (transitional cell) neoplasms of the urinary bladder. Bladder Consensus Conference Committee. Am J Surg Pathol 1998;22:1435–1448.

2. McKenney JK, Amin MB, Young RH. Urothelial (transitional cell) papilloma of the urinary bladder: a clinicopathologic study of 26 cases. Mod Pathol 2003;16:623–629.

3. Desai S, Lim SD, Jimenez RE, et al. Relationship of cytokeratin 20 and CD44 protein expression with WHO/ISUP grade in pTa and pT1 papillary urothelial neoplasia. Mod Pathol 2000;13:1315–1323.

4. Alsheikh A, Mohamedali Z, Jones E, Masterson J, Gilks CB. Comparison of the WHO/ISUP classification and cytokeratin 20 expression in predicting the behavior of low-grade papillary urothelial tumors. World Health Organization/International Society of Urologic Pathology. Mod Pathol 2001;14:267–272.

5. Holmang S, Andius P, Hedelin H, et al. Stage progression in Ta papillary urothelial tumors: relationship to grade, immunohistochemical expression of tumor markers, mitotic frequency and DNA ploidy. J Urol 2001;165:1124–1128, discussion 1128–1130.

6. Pich A, Chiusa L, Formiconi A, et al. Biologic differences between noninvasive papillary urothelial neoplasms of low malignant potential and low-grade (grade 1) papillary carcinomas of the bladder. Am J Surg Pathol 2001;25:1528–1533.

7. Oosterhuis JW, Schapers RF, Janssen-Heijnen ML, et al. Histological grading of papillary urothelial carcinoma of the bladder: prognostic value of the 1998 WHO/ISUP classification system and comparison with conventional grading systems. J Clin Pathol 2002;55:900–905.

8. Cheng L, Neumann RM, Bostwick DG. Papillary urothelial neoplasms of low malignant potential. Clinical and biologic implications. Cancer 1999;86:2102–2108.

9. Samaratunga H, Makarov DV, Epstein JI. Comparison of WHO/ISUP and WHO classification of noninvasive papillary urothelial neoplasms for risk of progression. Urology 2002;60:315–319.

10. Rodriguez Alonso A, Pita Fernandez S, Gonzalez-Carrero J, Nogueira March JL. Multivariate analysis of recurrence and progression in stage T1 transitional-cell carcinoma of the bladder. Prognostic value of p53 and Ki67. Actas Urol Esp 2003;27:132–141.

11. Heney NM, Ahmed S, Flanagan MJ, et al. Superficial bladder cancer: progression and recurrence. J Urol 1983;130:1083–1086.

12. Lutzeyer W, Rubben H, Dahm H. Prognostic parameters in superficial bladder cancer: an analysis of 315 cases. J Urol 1982;127:250–252.

13. Millan-Rodriguez F, Chechile-Toniolo G, Salvador-Bayarri J, Palou J, Vicente-Rodriguez J. Multivariate analysis of the prognostic factors of primary superficial bladder cancer. J Urol 2000;163:73–78.

14. Birch BR, Harland SJ. The pT1 G3 bladder tumour. Br J Urol 1989;64:109–116.

15. Wolf H, Olsen PR, Fischer A, Hojgaard K. Urothelial atypia concomitant with primary bladder tumour. Incidence in a consecutive series of 500 unselected patients. Scand J Urol Nephrol 1987;21:33–38.

16. Zincke H, Utz DC, Farrow GM. Review of Mayo Clinic experience with carcinoma in situ. Urology 1985;26:39–46.

17. Nixon RG, Chang SS, Lafleur BJ, Smith JJ, Cookson MS. Carcinoma in situ and tumor multifocality predict the risk of prostatic urethral involvement at radical cystectomy in men with transitional cell carcinoma of the bladder. J Urol 2002;167:502–505.

18. American Joint Commission on Cancer. AJCC Cancer Staging Manual, 6th edn. Philadelphia: Lippincott-Raven, 2002.

19. Jimenez RE, Keane TE, Hardy HT, Amin MB. pT1 urothelial carcinoma of the bladder: criteria for diagnosis, pitfalls, and clinical implications. Adv Anat Pathol 2000;7:13–25.

20. Skinner DG. Current state of classification and staging of bladder cancer. Cancer Res 1977;37:2838–2842.

21. Skinner DG. Management of invasive bladder cancer: a meticulous pelvic node dissection can make a difference. J Urol 1982;128:34–36.

22. Laplante M, Brice M, 2nd. The upper limits of hopeful application of radical cystectomy for vesical carcinoma: does nodal metastasis always indicate incurability? J Urol 1973;109:261–264.

23. Vieweg J, Gschwend JE, Herr HW, Fair WR. Pelvic lymph node dissection can be curative in patients with node positive bladder cancer. J Urol 1999;161:449–454.

24. Jimenez RE, Gheiler E, Oskanian P, et al. Grading the invasive component of urothelial carcinoma of the bladder and its relationship with progression-free survival. Am J Surg Pathol 2000;24:980–987.

25. Yang XJ, Lecksell K, Epstein JI. Can immunohistochemistry enhance the detection of micrometastases in pelvic lymph nodes from patients with high-grade urothelial carcinoma of the bladder? Am J Clin Pathol 1999;112:649–653.

26. Richie JP, Skinner DG. Carcinoma in situ of the urethra associated with bladder carcinoma: the role of urethrectomy. J Urol 1978;119:80–81.

27. Wishnow KI, Ro JY. Importance of early treatment of transitional cell carcinoma of prostatic ducts. Urology 1988;32:11–12.

28. Amin MB, Ro JY, Lee KM, et al. Lymphoepithelioma-like carcinoma of the urinary bladder. Am J Surg Pathol 1994;18:466–473.

29. Maranchie JK, Bouyounes BT, Zhang PL, et al. Clinical and pathological characteristics of micropapillary transitional cell carcinoma: a highly aggressive variant. J Urol 2000;163:748–751.

30. Amin MB, Ro JY, el-Sharkawy T, et al. Micropapillary variant of transitional cell carcinoma of the urinary bladder. Histologic pattern resembling ovarian papillary serous carcinoma. Am J Surg Pathol 1994;18:1224–1232.

31. Angulo JC, Lopez JI, Grignon DJ, Sanchez-Chapado M. Muscularis mucosa differentiates two populations with different prognosis in stage T1 bladder cancer. Urology 1995;45:47–53.

32. Holmang S, Johansson SL. The nested variant of transitional cell carcinoma – a rare neoplasm with poor prognosis. Scand J Urol Nephrol 2001;35:102–105.

33. Ozdemir BH, Ozdemir G, Sertcelik A. The nested variant of the transitional cell bladder carcinoma: a case report and review of the literature. Int Urol Nephrol 2000;32:257–258.

34. Drew PA, Furman J, Civantos F, Murphy WM. The nested variant of transitional cell carcinoma: an aggressive neoplasm with innocuous histology. Mod Pathol 1996;9:989–994.

35. Bell JT, Burney SW, Friedell GH. Blood vessel invasion in human bladder cancer. J Urol 1971;105:675–678.

36. Lopez JI, Angulo JC. The prognostic significance of vascular invasion in stage T1 bladder cancer. Histopathology 1995;27:27–33.

37. Larsen MP, Steinberg GD, Brendler CB, Epstein JI. Use of *Ulex europaeus* agglutinin I (UEAI) to distinguish vascular and 'pseudovascular' invasion in transitional cell carcinoma of bladder with lamina propria invasion. Mod Pathol 1990;3:83–88.

38. Ramani P, Birch BR, Harland SJ, Parkinson MC. Evaluation of endothelial markers in detecting blood and lymphatic channel invasion in pT1 transitional carcinoma of bladder. Histopathology 1991;19:551–554.

39. Leissner J, Koeppen C, Wolf HK. Prognostic significance of vascular and perineural invasion in urothelial bladder cancer treated with radical cystectomy. J Urol 2003;169:955–960.

40. Herr HW. Extent of surgery and pathology evaluation has an impact on bladder cancer outcomes after radical cystectomy. Urology 2003;61:105–108.

41. Solsona E, Iborra I, Ricos JV, et al. Clinical panurothelial disease in patients with superficial bladder tumors: therapeutic implications. J Urol 2002;167:2007–2011.

42. Recommendations for the reporting of urinary bladder specimens containing bladder neoplasms. Association of Directors of Anatomic and Surgical Pathology. Hum Pathol 1996;27:751–753.

43. Amin MB, Srigley JR, Grignon DJ, et al. Updated protocol for the examination of specimens from patients with carcinoma of the urinary bladder, ureter and renal pelvis. Arch Pathol Lab Med 2003;127:1263–1279.

15

EXAMINATION OF URINARY BLADDER SPECIMENS

John N. Eble

INTRODUCTION

A variety of specimens from the urinary bladder are submitted for surgical pathologic examination. The origin of these specimens may be cystoscopic biopsy, transurethral resection, partial cystectomy, total cystectomy or radical cystoprostatectomy. In the gross room, each must be examined with a different protocol. Likewise, the microscopic examination and reporting of each type of specimen are different. This chapter recommends a practical approach to the examination of each type of specimen.

CYSTOSCOPIC BIOPSIES

The invention of the cystoscope by Nitze in 1878 made the mucosa of the urinary bladder accessible to examination and biopsy. Cystoscopic biopsy specimens are usually small (in the range 1–3 mm), irregularly shaped fragments of soft grayish tissue. They may be directed to the diagnosis of a visible lesion or randomly selected in a search for urothelial carcinoma in situ which is invisible macroscopically via the cystoscope. These specimens are generally impossible to orient and gross examination mainly confirms the number and size of the fragments. However, these data are essential to ensure that the histologic section presents all fragments adequately.

The location from which each biopsy was obtained must be recorded and a separate diagnosis rendered for each site to guide the urologist in later cystoscopic examinations and in planning treatment. In some centers, urologists employ a cumulative 'bladder map' upon which to record the location of biopsies taken at each examination (Fig. 15.1). Such a record is of

Royal Liverpool
......
....
....

PATIENT IDENTIFYING DETAILS (ADDRESSOGRAM)

AGE	NAME GROUP	RADIOTHERAPY No.

FAMILY HISTORY

DIAGNOSIS	YEAR

OCCUPATION

HISTORY

DURATION (in weeks)

PYELOGRAM (At least every two years)

Date	Report

RADIOTHERAPY

Date	Dose	Duration

ORIGINAL TUMOUR

DATE

MED/C 335.61   1.76

E.U.A

a

DESCRIPTION		FIRST TREATMENT	
SINGLE		SURGICAL	Fulguration	
MULTIPLE			T.U.R	
SIZE (CMS)	<3		Suprapubic Excision	
	3-5		Partial Cystectomy	
	>5		Total Cystectomy	
MUCOSAL			Other	
MUCOSAL–SUPERFICIAL		Radio-therapy	Interstitial	
MUSCLE–DEEP			H.E.R.	
EXTRAVESICAL		Chemo-therapy	Local	
FIXED			General	
METASTASIS		OTHER		
HISTOLOGY		DIAGNOSIS ONLY		
		INOPERABLE		
PAPILLARY		PALLIATIVE ONLY		
MIXED		COMPLICATIONS		
SOLID				
WELL DIFFERENTIA'D				
POORLY DIFFERENTIA'D				
ANAPLASTIC				
NO INVASION				
INVASION				
METAPLASIA				
SARCOMA AND OTHER				

Illustration continued on following page

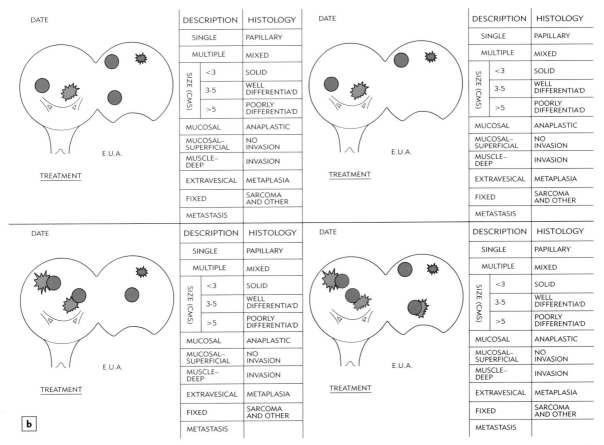

Fig. 15.1 (a) Outline 'bladder map' used routinely for patients with urinary bladder tumors referred to the Royal Liverpool University Hospital, UK. The map contains all of the initial information concerning the primary tumor, including the location of the sites from which biopsies have been taken. In this diagram, probable confirmed tumors are indicated in red. Biopsy sites are identified as blue circles. **(b)** During the patient's clinical progress, whenever cystoscopies are performed and biopsies taken, these data are recorded systematically together with other salient findings. Separately, a database of longitudinal phenotypic and genotypic information derived from these specimens (see Chapter 20) correlates these data and allows rapid assessment of each patient's progress, in a comprehensive manner, as their tumor status is reviewed. In this diagram, sites of previous tumors (or residual scar tissues) are indicated in green.

particular value to the urologic pathologist who is then able to assemble, in a temporally sequential manner, the distribution and spread of malignant, neoplastic and dysplastic lesions. With increasingly sophisticated analytical techniques, particularly that of molecular biology (see Chapter 1), this approach is becoming increasingly relevant to the proactive clinical management of individual patients with bladder neoplasia.

TRANSURETHRAL RESECTION SPECIMENS

When a papillary lesion is seen, a urologist usually resects the entire visible tumor cystoscopically. If the tumor is small, there are only a few fragments which could be confused with biopsy specimens. When a papillary tumor is identified microscopically, and no information to the contrary is provided by the urologist (e.g. a note saying that the specimen is a biopsy of a larger tumor), it is safe to assume that the urologist intended a transurethral resection and the report should reflect this. Transurethral resection specimens range in volume from less than 1 cm^3 up to more than 100 cm^3 such that each specimen consists of irregular fragments of soft gray tissue ranging in size from a few millimeters up to a centimeter or more. Even larger fragments are often impossible to orient.

When an entire specimen is processed for histology, the gross examination contributes mainly the aggregate volume of the fragments and the number of blocks prepared, both of which must be included in the report. While the great majority of transurethral resection specimens should be processed in their entirety for histologic examination, occasionally a specimen is so large that this is impractical. Whenever less than the entire specimen is processed for histology, the fragments must be spread out in a single layer on the cutting board and closely examined in an attempt to identify fragments containing muscle. Usually, these are firmer and slightly different in color from urothelial carcinoma. All fragments considered to contain muscle must be processed for histology since the identification of invasive malignancy in the muscularis propria materially affects the pathologic staging of each carcinoma.

The examination of a transurethral resection specimen is aimed at providing diagnostic, grading and staging information. The diagnosis should follow the generally accepted classification scheme of the 1998 World Health Organization and International Society of Urologic Pathology classification (WHO/ISUP)[1] or the 2003 WHO classification (see Chapter 9 for a detailed appraisal of this system). Similarly, the tumor should be graded according to the WHO/ISUP system or the 2003 WHO grading system. Invasion must be assessed and its extent reported: 'no invasion', 'invasion of lamina propria' or 'invasion of muscularis propria'. Assessment of invasion in transurethral resection specimens can be challenging.[2] Particular attention must be paid to distinguishing muscularis mucosae from muscularis propria.[3] Invasion of the lamina propria to or beyond the level of the muscularis mucosae is not presently part of the internationally accepted criteria for staging but there is evidence that it has prognostic significance and should be reported.[4,5] Invasion of muscularis propria is of great importance in staging, distinguishing pathologic stage T2 from T1.[6] While the staging system divides stage T2 into two parts (T2a and T2b) according to the depth of invasion of the muscularis propria, it is not possible to make this distinction in transurethral resection specimens. The presence of adipose tissue does not per se indicate that the fragment is derived from the outer half of the muscularis propria or from perivesical soft tissue,[7] since appreciable amounts of adipose connective tissue may naturally occur at any level within the muscularis propria. Sometimes the urologist specifically samples the bladder wall deep to the tumor. These specimens should be analyzed and reported separately.

TOTAL CYSTECTOMY AND CYSTOPROSTATECTOMY SPECIMENS

Total cystectomy specimens

Orientation of a total cystectomy specimen can be accomplished by recognizing that the peritoneum extends low on the posterior wall of the bladder but terminates high on the anterior wall. Once the specimen is oriented, the stumps of the ureters should be identified within the fatty tissues at each side of the bladder. This is more easily done when the specimen is not fixed. Once found, these structures should be marked with pins or sutures for later retrieval. Clips or ligatures attached by the urologist to the ends of the ureters may facilitate their identification. Some pathologists record the weight and dimensions of cystectomy specimens,[8] although the value of these observations is dubious. Measurement of the length of the urethral segment should be recorded to determine whether a urethrectomy has been performed.

Overnight fixation makes the preparation of blocks with intact mucosa overlying bladder wall structures much easier, although exposure of the mucosa to fixative must be ensured. This can be done by filling the bladder with fixative, either instilled through a catheter or injected with a hypodermic needle. A better method is to open the bladder from urethra to dome with an incision in the midline of the anterior wall (Fig. 15.2). (The precise location and extent of the sampling will depend upon the individual specimen. However, it is advised that adequate samples of the tumor be taken in order to assess the amount and the extent of malignant tissue, both laterally and in depth. Tissues taken routinely should include both ureteric resection margins and the urethral resection margin. If indicated, intramural portions of each ureter should be sampled. Specimens sampled routinely should also include both seminal vesicles and at least two blocks from the prostate. A series of random samples from macroscopically uninvolved bladder, including the trigone and periureteric tissues, is recommended in order to complete a comprehensive assessment of the specimen.) The specimen can then be pinned to a dissecting board or propped open with wooden or plastic supports. This method allows the pathologist to examine the fresh mucosa and to collect samples for special studies before fixation. Some recommend covering the surface of the specimen with ink before these procedures. This can be messy and is often unnecessary.

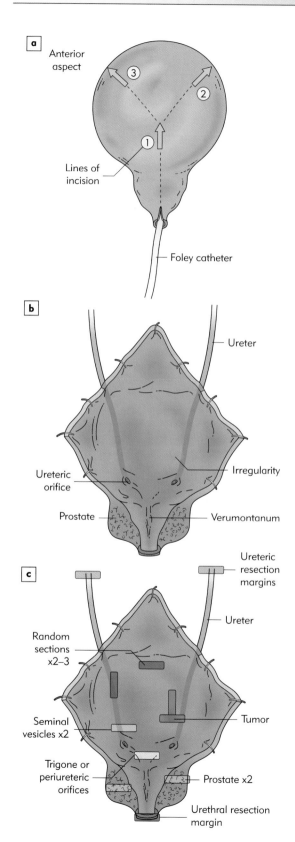

a

Anterior
aspect

③
②
①

Lines of
incision

Foley catheter

b

Ureter

Ureteric
orifice

Irregularity

Prostate

Verumontanum

c

Ureteric
resection
margins

Ureter

Random
sections
x2–3

Seminal
vesicles x2

Tumor

Trigone or
periureteric
orifices

Prostate x2

Urethral resection
margin

Fig. 15.2 **(a)** Schematic representation of a cystoprostatectomy specimen, including Foley catheter, indicating the preferred manner in which the specimen is opened using sharp scissors. **(b)** The open specimen is pinned out on a corkboard, but is separated from the latter by several sheets of absorbent paper, to allow penetration by fixative. In laboratories where specimens are analyzed for genotypic and phenotypic information, these specimens are taken prior to fixation. The sites and location of each of these specimens should be recorded, preferably on a schematic diagram of the type shown in **(a)**. Each diagram is then returned with the particular laboratory records. **(c)** For routine histopathologic examination, cystectomy specimens require adequate fixation of at least 24 hours to stabilize the specimen and to prevent disintegration of small pieces during subsequent manual handling. Total immersion of the pinned-out specimen is performed routinely. Following fixation, a series of routine blocks is taken, using a sharp-pointed scalpel, for histologic examination.

When a tumor is seen in the opened bladder, it is easy and effective to ink only the relevant external surface over the tumor. Following fixation, the urethral margin should be collected as a circumferential shave margin. When the urethra is resected at the same time as the bladder, the urethra should be completely processed for histology.[9] The ureteral ends should also be collected as complete cross-sections. Often, these are not surgical margins since the true ureteral margins may have been examined with frozen sections performed to exclude tumor in these locations. Whether or not carcinoma in situ at the ureteral margin is important is not completely clear.[10] Next, the mucosa of the bladder should be examined and each of the lesions described: size; shape (flat, papillary, ulcerated); location (trigone or bladder base; dome; left, right, anterior and posterior walls). Identified tumors should be deeply incised with a clean vertical incision to the perivesical tissue to permit assessment of the depth of invasion of the tumor. Sections from the deepest point of invasion to the surgical resection margin of the specimen should be processed for histology, as well as sections showing the relationship of the tumor to surrounding tissue.

Not infrequently, any previous transurethral resection will have left no visible tumor. The precise appearance of the mucosa will depend, in part, on the interval from the previous resection and the extent of the surgery performed at that time. When this is the case, the site of the transurethral resection should be extensively sampled to search for microscopic residual carcinoma. Urothelial neoplasia is often multifocal. The mucosa should be scrutinized for subtle areas of congestion or slight surface irregularity which may be clues to the presence of urothelial carcinoma in situ. Even if none is found, samples from all six surfaces of the bladder mucosa should be processed for histology. It is recommended that the specimen is sampled in a manner to leave it as intact as possible – rather than fragmenting the specimen into multiple pieces. It is not infrequent that, following identification of a part of a residual tumor, additional blocks of tissue will be required for further examination. Thus, it is imperative that the pathologist can return, with as little difficulty as possible, to the exact site of the particular block from which tissue containing tumor was taken.

Perivesical soft tissues should be examined for extension of the tumor and for any lymph nodes, which are occasionally present. However, often there are no lymph nodes in the perivesical soft tissue. The essential samples for histologic examination are listed in Table 15.1.

Table 15.1 Essential samples for histology of total cystectomy specimens

1. Urethral margin (1 block)
2. Remainder of urethra
3. Ends of right and left ureteral segments (2 blocks)
4. Tumor with full thickness of bladder wall (3 blocks unless tumor is very small)
5. Mucosa of bladder:
   — dome (2 blocks)
   — trigone (2 blocks)
   — left wall (2 blocks)
   — right wall (2 blocks)
   — anterior wall (2 blocks)
   — posterior wall (2 blocks)
6. Perivesical lymph nodes, if present (blocks as needed)

Cystoprostatectomy specimens

The bladder component of cystoprostatectomy specimens is examined with the same procedures as total cystectomy specimens. Clinically undetected prostatic adenocarcinoma is present in approximately one-third to one-half of cystoprostatectomy specimens.[11–13] Therefore, it is prudent to examine the prostate in these specimens as if they were prostatectomy specimens received from patients known to have prostatic adenocarcinoma, i.e. by marking the margins with ink and selecting blocks which support accurate staging and assessment of margins. This includes the use of different colored paints or inks to distinguish left and right lobes, and anterior and posterior aspects.[14] Since urothelial carcinoma may extend into the prostatic urethra, prostatic ducts or prostatic stroma, the prostatic urethra should be sampled generously.[15,16]

PARTIAL CYSTECTOMY SPECIMENS

Occasionally, in an attempt to retain bladder function, a partial cystectomy is performed. This usually removes part of the superior portion of the bladder. In these specimens, visible lesions should be sampled with full-thickness sections, from lumen to anatomic or resection margin, as in a total cystectomy specimen. Additionally, the mucosal margins must be generously sampled for histologic examination. Tumors of the urachus are sometimes treated with a partial cystectomy by removing the dome of the bladder along with the contents of the space of Retzius (including the urachus) superiorly to include the umbilicus. The bladder component should be examined as a partial cystectomy specimen. The surfaces of the supravesical tissues should be marked with ink and then sectioned at right angles to the long axis. If tumor is visible in this tissue, blocks including the soft tissue margin adjacent to the tumor should be processed for histology. Otherwise, four or five blocks from different levels should be processed for histology. If tumor is visible in the umbilicus, the cutaneous margins of the umbilicus should be marked with ink and processed for histology.

CONCLUSION

The vast majority of urinary bladder specimens are removed to exclude malignancy. This factor must receive utmost consideration when embedding small specimens for histologic examination and when taking tissue blocks from large specimens so that the distribution of any malignancy within the tissues might be accurately determined. Aides-mémoire and written protocols on paper (Table 15.2) or on VDU screens are invaluable in busy laboratories to ensure that all of the essential information is gathered at one time without recourse to taking additional specimens. Printed diagrams on which details of any irregularity noted and blocks taken are also extremely valuable practice in addition to being valuable assets when formulating reports of both the macroscopic (gross) and microscopic appearance.

Table 15.2 Checklist for cystectomy reports

1. What structures and organs are present and what surgical procedure was done?
2. Is there a visible tumor?
3. Is there more than one tumor or urothelial carcinoma in situ remote from the tumor?
4. What is the location of the tumor?
5. What is the size of the tumor?
6. What is the appearance of the tumor: flat, papillary, ulcerated?
7. What are the histologic type and grade of the tumor?
8. Is the tumor invasive and if so, how deeply does it extend: lamina propria, inner half of muscularis propria, outer half of muscularis propria, perivesical soft tissue?
9. Is tumor present at any of the margins?
10. Were there any lymph nodes in the specimen and did they contain metastases?

REFERENCES

1. Epstein JI, Amin MB, Reuter VE, et al. The World Health Organization/International Society of Urological Pathology consensus classification of urothelial (transitional cell) neoplasms of the urinary bladder. Am J Surg Pathol 1998;22:1435–1438.
2. Jimenez RE, Keane TE, Hardy HT, Amin MB. PT1 Urothelial carcinoma of the bladder: criteria for diagnosis, pitfalls, and clinical implications. Adv Anat Pathol 2000;7:13–25.
3. Ro JY, Ayala AG, El-Naggar A. Muscularis mucosa of urinary bladder: importance for staging and treatment. Am J Surg Pathol 1987;11:668–673.
4. Younes M, Sussman J, True LD. The usefulness of the level of the muscularis mucosae in the staging of invasive transitional cell carcinoma of the urinary bladder. Cancer 1990;66:543–548.
5. Bernardini S, Billerey C, Martin M, et al. The predictive value of muscularis mucosae invasion and p53 overexpression on progression of stage T1 bladder carcinoma. J Urol 2001;165:42–46.
6. Greene FL, Page DL, Fleming ID, et al. (eds) American Joint Committee on Cancer, AJCC Cancer Staging Handbook, 6th edn. New York: Springer-Verlag, 2002.
7. Association of Directors of Anatomic and Surgical Pathology. Recommendations for the reporting of urinary bladder specimens containing bladder neoplasms. Hum Pathol 1996;27:751–753.
8. Murphy WM. ASCP survey on anatomic pathology examination of the urinary bladder. Am J Clin Pathol 1994;102:715–723.
9. De Paepe ME, André R, Mahadevia P. Urethral involvement in female patients with bladder cancer, A study of 22 cystectomy specimens. Cancer 1990;65:1237–1241.
10. Silver DA, Stroumbakis N, Russo P, et al. Ureteral carcinoma in situ at radical cystectomy: does the margin matter? J Urol 1997;158:768–771.
11. Pritchett TR, Moreno J, Warner NE, et al. Unsuspected prostatic adenocarcinoma in patients who have undergone radical cystoprostatectomy for transitional cell carcinoma of the bladder. J Urol 1988;139:1214–1216.
12. Montie JE, Wood DP Jr, Pontes JE, et al. Adenocarcinoma of the prostate in cystoprostatectomy specimens removed for bladder cancer. Cancer 1989;63:381–385.
13. Abbas F, Hochberg D, Civantos F, Soloway M. Incidental prostatic adenocarcinoma in patients undergoing radical cystoprostatectomy for bladder cancer. Eur Urol 1996;30:322–326.
14. Bostwick DG, Foster CS. Examination of radical prostatectomy specimens: therapeutic and prognostic significance. In: Foster CS, Bostwick DG (eds) Pathology of the Prostate. Philadelphia: W.B. Saunders, 1998, Vol. 34, pp 172–189.
15. Esrig D, Freeman JA, Elmajian DA, et al. Transitional cell carcinoma involving the prostate with a proposed staging classification for stromal invasion. J Urol 1996;156:1071–1076.
16. Reese JH, Freiha FS, Gelb AB, et al. Transitional cell carcinoma of the prostate in patients undergoing radical cystoprostatectomy. J Urol 1992;147:92–95.

16

URO-ONCOLOGICAL MANAGEMENT OF BLADDER TRANSITIONAL CELL CARCINOMA: CLINICAL ASPECTS

Philip Cornford and Keith Parsons

INTRODUCTION

Bladder cancer is one of the most common diseases treated by urologists. In the UK more than 90% of these tumors are transitional cell carcinomas. They show a wide range of biological behavior but can be broadly divided into three groups: low-grade superficial tumors, high-grade superficial tumors and high-grade invasive tumors; a variety of phenotypic and genotypic attributes are considered in Chapters 9 and 20.

While the presumptive diagnosis of the majority of papillary carcinomas may be made macroscopically at cystoscopy, other primary tumors, including all of the flat lesions, require detailed pathologic assessment. Thereafter, the follow-up of all patients subsequent to the diagnosis of bladder cancer must include a detailed and accurate assessment of cystoscopic biopsy specimens to ensure that the apparent clinical stage of earlier cancer is supported by the pathologic evaluation of grade and stage. Such a dialogue between clinician and pathologist is fundamental to understanding the tumor biology of each neoplasm and to managing individual patients with urinary bladder cancer. This relationship is already evident where the pathologist performs a range of immunohistochemical assessments (e.g. Ki-67 for proliferation, p53 or Rb-1 mutation analysis) and then interprets the findings with respect to predictive likely tumor behavior, including response to therapy. The open dialogue between clinician and pathologist will be of even greater importance when molecular genetic analyses of multiple genes expressed by different cancers are performed routinely. Hence, it is opportune to identify, as precisely as possible, the information required by clinicians to treat an individual patient. Conversely, it is equally important for the pathologist to receive appropriate and adequate information with which to support the analysis of individual specimens.

INCIDENCE AND PREVALENCE

Since the 1950s, the incidence of bladder cancer has risen by approximately 50%. This does not appear to relate to alteration in medical practice, and as bladder cancers are rarely reported as an incidental at post-mortem examination,[1,2] this would appear to represent a clinically significant change. In part this can be explained by our aging population. The incidence of bladder cancer increases directly with age – from roughly 142 per 100,000 men and 33 per 100,000 women aged 65–69 years to 296 per 100,000 men and 74 per 100,000 women aged 85 years or older.[3] Consequently, it is to be anticipated with the aging of the United Kingdom population that this trend will continue.

Bladder cancer is 2.5 times more common in men than in women.[4] In men it is the fourth most common cancer after prostate, lung and colorectal cancer, accounting for 6.2% of all cancer cases.[4] In women, it is the eighth most common cancer, accounting for 2.5% of all cancers. Interestingly, the incidence of bladder cancer appears to be increasing[4,5] and this is occurring more rapidly in men than in women.[5,6] This is particularly surprising because since the 1960s women have worked outside the home and have changed habits, exposing them to both industrial and environmental carcinogens (e.g. cigarette smoking) from which they had previously been excluded. One would expect that these changes would result in a disproportionate increase in women having bladder cancer, as has been seen in lung cancer during this interval.[4] It is possible that genetic,[7] hormonal,[8] anatomic (e.g. relative urinary retention in older men because of prostatic enlargement) and/or other factors may explain this puzzling trend. However, outcome in women diagnosed with the disease is worse, with an approximate 50% higher lifetime risk of dying from the disease in women who contract it when compared to men.[4,9] This may be due to differences in the stage at diagnosis, disease characteristics or treatment between the sexes.

Because so many patients with bladder cancer experience recurrences but do not succumb to the disease, and while bladder cancer is only the fourth most common cancer in terms of incidence in men, it is the second most prevalent malignancy in middle-aged and elderly men (after prostate cancer).

NATURAL HISTORY

At diagnosis approximately 60% of bladder transitional cell carcinomas are superficial and either well or moderately differentiated.[10] The majority of these patients develop recurrences, of which 16–25% are of a higher grade.[11] Eventually up to 10% of these patients will develop invasive or metastatic cancer.[11,12] At presentation, 20–25% of tumors are poorly differentiated and yet still apparently superficial.[10] In addition, 15–20% are muscle-invasive.[12]

High-grade superficial tumors have a much higher chance of progressing to muscle-invasive or metastatic disease.[13,14] Almost 50% of patients with muscle-invasive bladder cancer already have occult distant metastases. This limits the efficacy of local or regional forms of therapy for invasive tumors. Most patients with occult metastases develop overt clinical evidence of distant metastases within 1 year.[15] Consequently, histopathologic examination plays a crucial role in planning appropriate treatment regimes.

The most useful prognostic parameters for tumor recurrence and subsequent cancer progression in a patient with a superficial tumor are tumor grade, depth of tumor penetration (stage), lymphatic invasion, tumor size, urothelial dysplasia or carcinoma in situ (CIS) in neighboring or distant urothelial areas, papillary or solid tumor architecture, multifocality, and frequency of prior tumor recurrences. Of these, the most important are grade, stage and presence of CIS.[16,17] In patients with lamina propria-invading, grade 3 transitional cell carcinomas, at least one-third exhibit stage progression to muscle invasion,[16] even with complete endoscopic resection and intravesical therapy with bacille Calmette–Guérin (BCG).[14]

DIAGNOSIS

Signs and symptoms

Transitional cell carcinoma of the bladder presents most commonly (> 85% of cases) with painless frank hematuria[18] and in reality almost all cystoscopically detectable tumors have at least microscopic hematuria.[19] The symptom complex of bladder irritability and urinary frequency, urgency and dysuria is the second most common presentation and is usually associated with diffuse CIS or invasive bladder cancer. However, these symptoms almost never occur without (at least) microscopic hematuria. Other signs and symptoms of bladder cancer include flank pain from ureteral obstruction, lower-extremity edema and pelvic mass. Very rarely, patients present with symptoms of advanced disease, such as weight loss and abdominal or bone pain.

Investigations

Mid-stream specimen of urine

Hematuria is frequently intermittent and consequently a clear second sample is insufficient reason not to investigate hematuria. However, a mid-stream specimen of urine may allow diagnosis of a urinary tract infection that may affect management decisions.

Urine cytology

The specificity and positive predictive value of cytology are generally high, provided that only unequivocally malignant or highly suspicious samples are considered as positive.[20] However, the limitations of microscopic cytology are the cytologically normal appearance of cells from well-differentiated tumors. Since well-differentiated cancer cells are more cohesive, they are not readily shed into the urine. Therefore, microscopic cytology is more sensitive in patients with high-grade tumors or CIS. Even in patients with high-grade tumors, however, urinary cytology may be falsely negative in 20%. In addition false-positive cytology may occur in 1–12% of patients and is usually due to urothelial atypia, inflammation, or changes caused by radiation therapy or chemotherapy.[21]

Intravenous urogram

An intravenous urogram (IVU) is indicated in all patients with signs and symptoms suggestive of bladder cancer. Urography is not a sensitive means of detecting bladder tumors, particularly small ones. However, it is useful in examining the upper urinary tracts for associated urothelial tumors. Large tumors may appear as filling defects in the bladder on the cystogram phase of the urogram. Ureteral obstruction caused by a bladder tumor is usually a sign of muscle-invasive cancer. Additionally, of course, urography can assess other upper tract abnormalities that may affect management decisions.

Renal tract ultrasound scan

A renal tract ultrasound scan is an excellent modality for investigating hematuria. Small bladder tumors may be detected but it is most useful in detecting lesions of the renal cortex, which might be missed on an IVU.

Cystoscopy

All patients suspected of having bladder cancer should have careful cystoscopy. Abnormal areas should be biopsied. Random or selected-site mucosal biopsy specimens may also be obtained. Retrograde pyelography should be performed if the upper tracts are not adequately visualized on the IVU.

RESECTION OF BLADDER TUMORS

Ideally the bulk of a tumor should first be resected. Then the base of each tumor should be resected separately, together with some underlying muscle. Each specimen is then sent separately for histologic analysis. In addition, mucosal biopsies are taken from the opposite bladder wall, bladder dome and trigone. These biopsies provide important prognostic information about the likelihood of tumor recurrence, with approximately 20–25% of patients found to have dysplasia or CIS on such biopsies.[11]

Clearly, selected mucosal biopsies run the risk of missing premalignant or malignant areas because of sampling issues. Consequently, it has been suggested that taking advantage of the propensity of tumors to retain fluorescing porphyrin derivatives, such as protoporphyrin IX (PPIX), may reduce this problem. The PPIX precursor, 5-aminolevulinic acid (ALA), when administered intravesically in conjunction with fluorescent cystoscopy using blue light at 375–440 nm, enables detection of lesions invisible with white light cystoscopy.[22] This has been claimed to increase sensitivity in detecting small tumors and CIS from 77% with white light to nearly 98% with fluorescent cystoscopy; however, the number of tumors missed is uncertain.[22] Moreover, more than half the regions biopsied because of fluorescence were histologically normal or inflamed without neoplasia. Although it is likely that some 'false-positive' regions contained patches of genetically altered cells destined to become tumors, this technique might decrease the likelihood of tumor recurrence. However, compelling data in support of either of these contentions are limited.

TUMOR EVALUATION

Accurate pathologic staging of the tumor, confirming the clinical evaluation, is important because this will determine the treatment offered. However, current staging methods remain imprecise. Understaging occurs most frequently in patients with high-grade and intermediate-stage tumors, of whom approximately one-third are understaged and 10% are overstaged.[23]

Treatment decision 1

The first treatment decision, based on tumor stage, is whether the patient has a superficial or a muscle-invasive tumor. If the tumor is superficial, more elaborate staging techniques such as bone scan and computed tomography (CT) are not usually indicated, since metastatic spread is extremely rare with superficial disease.

Primary transurethral resection (TUR) of a tumor is the most important test by which to judge its depth of penetration. However, variation in the interpretation of histology sections occurs between different pathologists assessing tumor grade and depth of infiltration. Part of the reason for these discrepancies is related to the smooth muscle fibers of the muscularis mucosa in the lamina propria of the bladder wall (see Fig. 1.7b), which may be confused with detrusor muscle.[24] The presence of deep lamina propria involvement (pT1b) probably confers a worse outlook than superficial lamina propria invasion in terms of disease progression and survival, especially for high-grade cancer, when it is treated with local resection alone.[16] In those patients in whom muscularis mucosa is not consistently identified on transurethral biopsies (current estimates range from 11 to 46%),[25] defining the extent of invasion below the urothelial surface (above or below 1.5 mm) has correlated well with progression-free 5-year survival (67% for more than 1.5 mm versus 93% for 1.5 mm or less) in a retrospective series of 83 patients.[26] Bimanual physical examination provides little information about whether or not there is infiltration of the bladder wall. In this regard, if the tumor is palpable on bimanual examination before resection, it is usually infiltrating into detrusor or perivesical tissues.

Should invasion of the detrusor muscle be identified (pathologic stage pT2), the next important determinant is: Has the tumor invaded through the bladder wall? Obviously this is not possible to assess histologically. However, an interesting report has suggested that transurethral ultrasonography may be effective. Koraitim et al.[27] reported 100% sensitivity and more than 98% specificity in distinguishing muscle-invasive from superficial bladder cancers, more than 90% accuracy in distinguishing superficial muscularis invasion from deeper muscle invasion, and 70% positive pre-

dictive value in distinguishing vesical-confined from extravesical disease. This study is awaiting independent confirmatory evidence.

Treatment decision 2

The second treatment decision made on the basis of staging is identifying patients with invasive tumors who may benefit from aggressive, potentially curative therapy. For this purpose, CT scanning, ultrasonography and magnetic resonance imaging (MRI) have been used to evaluate the local extent of bladder tumors. These staging studies may provide valuable information, but appear to be inaccurate in determining the presence or absence of microscopic muscle infiltration and minimal extravesical tumor spread. Moreover, postoperative changes produced by TUR of the primary tumor, as well as postradiation therapy or postchemotherapy fibrosis, may also cause difficulties in interpreting CT, MRI and ultrasound scans.

Computed tomography scan

In addition to assessing the extent of the primary tumor, CT scanning also provides information about the presence of pelvic and para-aortic lymphadenopathy and visceral metastases.[28] To assess the depth of penetration accurately, CT scanning should be performed before TUR[29], but this is rarely practical. Contrast-enhanced CT scanning improves accuracy of staging.[30] Studies with spiral CT imaging have not yet been fully assessed to determine if they can improve staging further, but preliminary information indicates little additional benefit.[31]

CT scanning is limited in accuracy because it can detect only gross extravesical tumor extension, lymph nodes that are significantly enlarged, and liver metastases larger than 2 cm in diameter.[32] CT scans fail to detect nodal metastases in up to 40–70% of patients in which these are present.[28,31] Although some authors have questioned the practical utility of using CT scans for local staging of bladder cancer,[31,33] the scans are undoubtedly more sensitive than physical examination in evaluating both regional and metastatic disease. Also, because of the magnitude of the treatments considered for invasive bladder cancer, it would seem prudent to perform CT scans before embarking on such therapy.

Magnetic resonance imaging scan

MRI scanning is not much more helpful than CT scanning. With few exceptions,[34] resolution of the pelvic and abdominal anatomy with traditional MRI has not been reported to be as good as CT scanning.[29,35] A double-surface coil may permit more accurate MRI staging of bladder cancer than with conventional coil MRI.[36] However, the possibility of multiplane MRI imaging should theoretically provide better visualization of the anatomy.

Soft tissue contrast may be enhanced by use of paramagnetic contrast agents, such as gadolinium-diethylenetriamine-penta-acetic acid complex (Gd-DTPA) and iron-containing materials.[37,38] Indeed, using these agents, Barentsz[38] reported a small series in which three-dimensional MRI had a 75% sensitivity and a 96% specificity in detecting nodal metastases in patients with muscle-invasive bladder cancer who eventually underwent surgical staging. Successful percutaneous biopsy of nodes deemed suspicious by this mode of imaging has also been done.

MRI spectroscopy in the future may also have the capacity to provide information about the states of different tissues, but this possibility has not yet been realized for bladder cancer. As might be expected, both CT and MRI scanning are more accurate in very advanced tumors.[39] MRI has become particularly useful in clinical management in that it appears to be more sensitive than CT scans or, for that matter, radionuclide bone scans for determining the presence of bone metastases. Thus, if clinical symptoms, pelvic extension on CT scan, bimanual examination or nuclear bone scan indicate suspicious sites of osseous metastases, MRI may be appropriate in such cases.

Chest x-ray

Metastatic evaluation to exclude distant metastases should be performed before proceeding to radical surgery. The most sensitive means of detecting pulmonary metastasis is chest CT scan. However, CT scans frequently detect small, non-calcified pulmonary lesions, most of which are granulomas. There is a direct correlation between the size of a pulmonary lesion and the likelihood of its being a metastasis. Most non-calcified lesions that are 1 cm or larger are metastases (or primary pulmonary neoplasms). Because standard films do not have sufficient resolution to demonstrate small granulomas but rather only detect lesions larger than 1 cm in diameter, routine chest radiographs, rather than CTs, are usually relied on to rule out pulmonary metastases in bladder cancer patients.

Bone scans

Bone scans seldom reveal metastatic disease in patients with normal liver function tests, especially if the alkaline phosphatase level is normal.[40] However, a bone scan may be useful as a baseline for future reference. Thus, the recommended metastatic evaluation for patients with invasive bladder cancer includes chest radiograph, excretory urogram, abdominal–pelvic CT scan, bone scan and liver function tests.

Grade

For a comprehensive review of urothelial cancer grading according to World Health Organization (WHO) guidelines, see Chapter 9. Bladder cancers are classified into three grades: G1 (well differentiated), G2 (intermediate differentiation) and G3 (undifferentiated).[41]

Staging

This is based upon TNM classification of malignant tumors,[41] developed jointly by the International Union Against Cancer (UICC) and the American Joint Commission on Cancer (AJCC) (see Table 17.3).

TREATMENT

For the purpose of documenting the current situation, several different grading systems are employed by pathologists in different laboratories and in different countries. No single consensually agreed system is employed universally. Such lack of consensus emphasizes the paucity of knowledge with respect to the tumor biology of urinary bladder cancer. It also allows political rivalry to flourish between competitive groups. Such competition will only be alleviated when the true tumor biology of individual lesions can be precisely defined.

In the meantime, since Broders first described the prognostic significance of this system regarding bladder lesions,[42] several others have been devised, including those of Franksson[43] and Bergkvist et al.[44] Currently, in most common usage are the UICC system[45] and the new WHO classification.[46] Differences between these systems are subtle but important, especially clarifying their precise usage when communicating between clinicians and pathologists.

Superficial bladder tumors

Low-grade superficial transitional cell carcinomas are managed by endoscopic resection. This is commonly followed by a single shot of intravesical chemotherapy with a drug such as mitomycin C. Such treatment has been shown to decrease the number of local recurrences,[47] although it is not thought to decrease the risk of disease progression. The overall survival rates are excellent,[48] with less than 10%[49] of patients ultimately requiring more aggressive therapy. It is usual to follow up the majority of such tumors with flexible check cystoscopy at regular and lengthening intervals. Any recurrent tumors are biopsied and resected or coagulated with diathermy as long as they are few and solitary. When tumors recur often and in large numbers, then adjuvant intravesical chemotherapy with eight once-weekly instillations is indicated.[50] Table 16.1 summarizes the response rate to various treatments.

All G3 tumors, along with CIS, are considered to be high-risk superficial tumors. Such tumors have a much higher risk of subsequently becoming muscle-invasive[14] and require close surveillance. It is particularly important to ensure that at presentation complete resection, and therefore accurate staging, is achieved. Subsequently, it is proposed that a separate biopsy of the base of the resection area is sent. Unfortunately, even when the surgeon believes complete resection has been accomplished, re-resection at 6 weeks may show residual tumor in more than 40% of patients,[51] and in 25% there may be a worsening of the stage.[52] As a consequence, early re-resection is recommended for all G3pT1 bladder tumors.

High-risk superficial tumors, especially G3pT1 lesions, have a significant chance of recurrence (80%) and progression (50% by 3 years),[53] and adjuvant treatment should therefore be considered. BCG is the standard treatment of choice for G3pT1 tumors and CIS. It is routinely given in six once-weekly instillations, commencing 2 weeks after TUR. Studies comparing TUR plus BCG versus BCG alone suggest a 30% decrease in recurrence rates.[54] It has been suggested that BCG may also decrease disease progression.[55] In addition, Herr et al.[56] reported an improved survival rate of 75% for patients given BCG, versus 55% for those with TUR alone, at 10-year follow-up. Approximately 25% of

patients whose disease fails to respond to an initial 6-week course may still respond to a second course.[57] In healthy patients with persistent or recurrent high-risk superficial disease who have failed intravesical therapy, it is appropriate to perform cystectomy as repeated attempts at intravesical therapy carry a significant potential for disease progression. Early (3-month) failure after BCG is associated with an 82% progression rate, compared with a 25% progression rate in patients who do not fail at 3 months.[58] Ten-year survival after cystectomy for superficial disease can range from 67 to 92%.[13,59]

Since those patients who respond initially may later relapse, the concept of maintenance treatment has been investigated. The Southwest Oncology Group[60] showed significant differences between those who received only standard (protocol) maintenance (the non-maintenance arm) and those who also received maintenance BCG. Median recurrence-free survival was 76.8 months in the maintenance arm and 35.7 months in the non-maintenance arm ($p < 0.0001$). Time until failure-free survival was 111.5 months in the non-maintenance arm and not estimable in the maintenance arm ($p = 0.04$). Overall 5-year survival was 78% in the non-maintenance arm compared with 83% in the maintenance arm. However, only 16% of patients could tolerate the full dose-schedule regimen and required reduction of the three booster treatments.

Muscle-invasive cancer

TUR of a bladder lesion provides essential information used to identify invasive carcinoma. At this time, bimanual palpation of the bladder before and after tumor resection is performed. Wijkstrom and colleagues[61] suggested that the presence of a palpable mass after TUR correlates with stage T3 cancer and prognosis after treatment. Once a histologic diagnosis of invasion is made, non-invasive imaging may provide valuable insight into the extent of the tumor diathesis. However, for those patients in whom an invasive lesion is suspected before TUR, axial staging should be performed before resection because of the confounding artifact produced by endoscopic surgery, as shown in postoperative studies.

Radical cystoprostatectomy in the male patient and anterior exenteration in the female patient, coupled with en bloc pelvic lymphadenectomy, remain the standard surgical approaches to muscle-invasive bladder carcinoma in the absence of metastatic disease. Patients with significant medical co-morbidity or evidence of

Table 16.1 Response rate to various treatments for superficial bladder tumors

	Decrease in recurrence (%)	Decrease in progression (%)
Doxorubicin	15	Ns
Epirubicin	12–15	Ns
Mitomycin C	19–42	Ns
Valrubicin	21	Ns
BCG	40	25

Ns, Not stated

metastatic disease are better served by alternative management approaches. Male patients undergoing cutaneous diversion should be encouraged to undergo simultaneous or delayed urethrectomy if CIS or gross tumor involves the prostatic urethra. Female patients with overt cancer at the bladder neck and urethra, diffuse CIS, or a positive margin at surgery are poor candidates for orthotopic reconstruction and should be treated by immediate en bloc urethrectomy as part of the radical cystectomy. Patients considered candidates for orthotopic reconstruction should be cautioned that the final commitment to using the residual urethra cannot be made until frozen-section analysis demonstrates a tumor-free distal urethral margin.[62] Numerous series have demonstrated that, with improvements in pre- and postoperative care, refinements in surgical technique, and better appreciation of the long-term metabolic consequences of urinary tract reconstruction, patients with organ-confined disease can anticipate long-term disease-specific survival. Data from international series reveal similar outcomes for surgically treated patients (Table 16.2).

After radical surgery and reconstruction, patients require long-term surveillance for two specific problems: tumor recurrence, and complications related to the interposition of bowel in the urinary tract.

Pelvic lymphadenectomy remains an important part of the management of patients with muscle-invasive bladder cancer since it provides an assessment of the local extent of disease. In addition, some patients with limited nodal tumor burden can experience unexpectedly high rates of long-term survival in the absence of additional intervention.[63,64] The risk of pelvic lymph node metastases increases with tumor stage, such that patients with stage pT2 disease have a 10–30% risk of positive lymph nodes at the time of surgery, whereas patients with disease higher than stage pT3 have a 30–65% risk.

Table 16.2 Percentage disease-specific survival by pathologic stage after radical cystectomy with and without pelvic lymph node metastasis

		P2	P3	P4a	N+
Bassi	369	63	33	28	15
Schoenberg	101	84	56	NA	48
Skinner	197	64	44	36	44
Waehre	227	79	36	29	22

Adjuvant chemotherapy

Approximately 40% of patients with muscle-invasive disease will be metastatic at presentation. Therefore, in an attempt to improve long-term survival in those patients whose disease is not confined to the bladder at cystectomy, adjuvant chemotherapy has been explored. Reports suggest that for patients with locoregional disease and pelvic lymph node involvement, cisplatin-based adjuvant therapy may provide a survival advantage worth discussing with appropriately selected patients.[65] There is no evidence to suggest that the administration of adjuvant chemotherapy to patients with organ-confined bladder cancer (stage T1–T2) provides either a survival advantage or an improvement in local control after cystectomy.

Bladder preservation protocols

Combined modality bladder preservation protocols have been proposed as an alternative to radical cystectomy, motivated by a rationale with two components:

- Many patients with invasive bladder cancer already have micrometastatic disease at the time of presentation. Lymphovascular space involvement is a common finding on histopathologic examination of urinary bladder mucosal biopsies containing tumor. However, the significance of micrometastatic tumor within the circulatory space is not fully appreciated and the finding does not form part of any current staging system. Patients with micrometastatic disease, when asymptomatic, may not derive significant benefit from local intervention without concomitant systemic therapy.
- Removal of the bladder and the associated consequences in terms of continence, sexual function and body image affects the quality of life even when the bladder cancer is eradicated.

Well-defined, small, superficially invasive bladder cancers have been managed by TUR for many years. The results of these experiences suggest that in highly selected patients with small, low-stage (T2) lesions, conservative surgical monotherapy can provide excellent local and distant control.[66] Conventional radiotherapy controls muscle-invasive bladder cancer in 30–50% of cases[67] and although some increase in frequency may been seen, this is rarely clinically significant. Even with more advanced disease, long-term disease control is possible with combination therapy in carefully selected patients. Kaufman et al.[68] treated 106 patients with stage T2–T4NXM0 bladder cancer by TUR, neoadjuvant chemotherapy (MCV) and subsequent radiation therapy. Patients not responding were treated by radical cystectomy. These authors reported a 52% overall survival. Of the patients completing the full course of therapy, 75% retained bladders free of disease with a median follow-up of 64 months. These authors observed that smaller tumors, those not associated with hydronephrosis, and those amenable to complete TUR were the most likely to achieve a favorable outcome using this strategy. Structural and histologic features that argue against the use of bladder preservation include the presence of hydronephrosis, CIS (which responds poorly to multimodality therapy), and a tumor that cannot be completely resected transurethrally.

Metastatic disease

Patients with metastatic bladder cancer are routinely treated with systemic chemotherapy, particularly in the setting of unresectable, diffusely metastatic, measurable disease. The most commonly employed agents are methotrexate, vinblastine, doxorubicin and cisplatin (MVAC).[69] Regimens containing these drugs produce a complete response (CR) in approximately 20% of patients, although long-term disease-free survival is rare. MVAC, although superior to single-agent therapy, is associated with significant toxicity (more than 20% experience neutropenic fever). Death from sepsis has been reported in 3–4% of patients receiving MVAC.

Of the newer drugs available, gemcitabine and the taxoids look most promising. Gemcitabine, a new anti-metabolite chemotherapeutic agent, has been used as a single agent (higher than 25% CR) and in combination with cisplatin (40% partial response (PR) and CR) with encouraging initial results in patients with metastatic disease.[70] Taxoids are microtubule disassembly inhibitors. Paclitaxel (Taxol) and docetaxel (Taxotere), the latter a semi-synthetic taxane, have been used in clinical trials of patients with advanced bladder cancer, with response rates ranging from 25 to 83% in combination regimens.[71]

CONCLUSION

Management options for urothelial malignancy are varied and range from conservative bladder preservation techniques (utilizing a combination of endoscopic surgical procedures with intravesical chemo- or immunotherapy) to excisional surgery with complex

urinary reconstruction. The importance of accurate histologic diagnosis and staging of the disease thus cannot be overstated. The role of the histopathologist is especially important in the following areas:

- *Initial diagnosis:* The prognosis of disease in each individual patient is best predicted by the stage and grade at presentation. Consequently it is vital that this is as accurate as possible and that the urologist understands the level of uncertainty in any given report. In practical terms, this means that histopathologic reports must contain all relevant information written in a clear and logical format, without ambiguity, while remaining succinct and concise. Since biopsy specimens are individual, the reports should be written individually without resorting to the shorthand of 'canned text' or 'macros'. Conversely, there is value in employing a protocol as an aide-mémoire such that reports are written with a similar format, either containing all the information, or at least addressing the individual items that the urologist expects. There is great value in placing the salient information (e.g. the presence and type of malignancy) at the beginning of a report rather than embedded somewhere in the body of the text. Short summaries of pathologic stage and grade placed at the end of a report are also of value in assisting communication.

- *Progression of disease:* Changes in the phenotype or behavior of tumors over time (if noticed) will allow more aggressive early intervention to be considered. Although not yet common to all routine diagnostic laboratories, immunophenotyping to detect gene expression or mutation (e.g. phosphatase and tensin homolog (PTEN), p53 or pRb-1), together with markers of proliferation (e.g. Ki-67), are becoming more frequent. Analysis of these tumors by DNA array is being introduced and is likely to become common within the foreseeable future. Assessment, interpretation and reporting of such data will be required as a routine component of the pathology report.

- *Prognostic indicators:* Currently under evaluation are individual immunohistochemical markers or groups of markers that may allow us to predict which tumors will progress and which are safe to treat with conservative surgery, or which will be in the 50% that respond to radiotherapy versus those that need to proceed direct to cystectomy.

- *During radical surgery:* Tissue is commonly sent to ensure the ureteric margin is free of tumor prior to anastomosis or that the urethral margin is tumor-free prior to orthotopic bladder reconstruction.

Open intelligible communication between clinicians and pathologists is fundamental to the diagnosis and management of patients with urothelial cancer. There must be a clear, bidirectional transfer of accurate information without impediment or interference so that the pathologist is able to analyze submitted tissues comprehensively and also that the clinician receives the appropriate and necessary information with which to manage individual patients in an ongoing manner, possibly over many years. From the clinician, information must be clearly documented on the initial request form accompanying each specimen. Conversely, the pathologist should return the analysis of the tissue in a timely, succinct and coherent manner. Whenever such communication occurs, then there is not only the foundation for the clinically appropriate treatment of individual patients with bladder cancer, but also for further investigating this disease and of managing its tumor biology.

REFERENCES

1. Resseguie LJ, Norbrega FT, Farrow GM, et al. Epidemiology of renal and ureteral cancer in Rochester, Minnesota, 1950–1974, with special reference to clinical and pathologic features. Mayo Clin Proc 1978;53(8):503–510.

2. Kishi K, Hirota T, Matsumoto K, et al. Carcinoma of the bladder: a clinical and pathological analysis of 87 autopsy cases. J Urol 1981;125:36–39.

3. Lynch CF, Cohen MB. Urinary system. Cancer 1995;75(Suppl.):316.

4. Greenlee RT, Murray T, Bolden S, Wings PA. Cancer statistics, 2000. CA Cancer J Clin 2000;50:7–33.

5. Silverberg E. Cancer statistics 1985. CA Cancer J Clin 1985;35:19–35.

6. Boring CC, Squires TS, Tong T. Cancer statistics 1993. CA Cancer J Clin 1993;43:7–26.

7. Risch A, Wallace DM, Bathers S, Sim E. Slow N-acetylation genotype is a susceptibility factor in occupational and smoking related bladder cancer. Hum Mol Genet 1995;4:231–236.

8. Horn EP, Tucker MA, Lambert G, et al. A study of gender-based cytochrome P4501A2 variability: a possible mechanism for the male excess of bladder cancer. Cancer Epidemiol Biomarkers Prev 1995;4:529–533.

9. Mungan NA, Kiemeney L, van Dijck J, et al. Gender differences in stage distribution of bladder cancer. Urology 2000;55:368–371.

10. Messing EM, Young TB, Hunt VB, et al. Comparison of bladder cancer outcome in men undergoing hematuria home screening versus those with standard clinical presentations. Urology 1995;45:387–396.

11. Althausen AF, Prout GR Jr, Daly JJ. Non-invasive papillary carcinoma of the bladder associated with carcinoma in situ. J Urol 1976;116:575–580.

12. Cheng L, Neumann RM, Bostwick DG. Papillary urothelial neoplasm of low malignant potential. Clinical and biologic implications. Cancer 1999;86:2102–2108.

13. Freeman JA, Esrig DE, Stein JP, et al. Radical cystectomy for high risk patients with superficial bladder cancer in the era of orthotopic urinary reconstruction. Cancer 1995;76:833–839.

14. Cookson MS, Sarosdy MF. Management of stage T1 superficial bladder cancer with intravesical bacillus Calmette-Guérin therapy. J Urol 1992;148:797–801.

15. Babaian RJ, Johnson DE, Llamas L, Ayala AG. Metastases from transitional cell carcinoma of the urinary bladder. Urology 1980;16:142–144.

16. Holmang S, Hedelin H, Anderstrom C, et al. The importance of the depth of invasion in stage T1 bladder carcinoma: a prospective cohort study. J Urol 1997;157:800–803.

17. Millan-Rodriquez F, Chechile-Tomiolo G, Salvador-Bayarri J, et al. Multivariate analysis of the prognostic factors of primary superficial bladder cancer. J Urol 2000;163:73–78.

18. Varkarakis MJ, Gaeta J, Moore RH, Murphy GP. Superficial bladder tumor. Aspects of clinical progression. Urology 1974;4:414–420.

19. Messing EM, Vaillancourt A. Hematuria screening for bladder cancer. J Occup Med 1990;32:838–845.

20. Schwalb DM, Herr HW, Fair WR. The management of clinically unconfirmed positive urinary cytology. J Urol 1993;150:1751–1756.

21. Koshikawa T, Leyh H, Schenck U. Difficulties in evaluating urinary specimens after local mitomycin therapy of bladder cancer. Diagn Cytopathol 1989;5:117–121.

22. Filbeck T, Roessler W, Kneichel R, et al. Improved bladder cancer detection and resection using 5-aminolevulinic acid and induced fluorescence diagnosis: a prospective trial on 310 patients. J Urol 2000;163(Suppl.):589A.

23. Wijkstrom H, Edsmyr F, Lundh B. The value of preoperative classification according to the TNM system. A critical examination of Category T2 in 96 patients with grade 3 transitional cell bladder carcinoma subjected to preparative irradiation and cystectomy. Eur Urol 1984;10:101–106.

24. Younes M, Sussman J, True LD. The usefulness of the level of the muscularis mucosae in the staging of invasive transitional cell carcinoma of the urinary bladder. Cancer 1990;66:543–548.

25. Engel P, Anagnostaki L, Braendstrap O. The muscularis mucosae of the human urinary bladder. Implications for tumor staging on biopsies. Scand J Urol Nephrol 1992;26:249–252.

26. Cheng L, Weaver AL, Bostwick DG. Predicting extravesical extension of bladder carcinoma: a novel method based on micrometer measurement of the depth of invasion in transurethral resection specimens. Urology 2000;55:668–672.

27. Koraitim M, Kamal B, Metwalli, N, Zaky Y. Transurethral ultrasonic assessment of bladder carcinoma: its value and limitation. J Urol 1995;154:375–378.

28. Lantz EJ, Hattery RR. Diagnostic imaging of urothelial cancer. Urol Clin North Am 1984;11:576–583.

29. Husband JE, Olliff JF, Williams, MP, et al. Bladder cancer: staging with CT and MR imaging. Radiology 1989;173:435–440.

30. Sager EM, Talle K, Fossa SD, et al. Contrast-enhanced computed tomography to show perivesical extension in bladder carcinoma. Acta Radiol 1987;28:307–311.

31. Paik ML, Scolieri MJ, Brown SL, et al. Limitations of computerized tomography in staging invasive bladder cancer before radical cystectomy. J Urol 2000;163:1693–1696.

32. Voges GE, Tauschke E, Stockle M, et al. Computerized tomography: an unreliable method for accurate staging of bladder tumors in patients who are candidates for radical cystectomy. J Urol 1989;142:972–974.

33. Nishimura K, Hida S, Nishio Y. The validity of magnetic resonance imaging (MRI) in the staging of bladder cancer: comparison with computed tomography (CT) and transurethral ultrasonography (US). Jpn J Clin Oncol 1988;18:217–226.

34. Johnson RJ, Carrington BM, Jenkins JP, et al. Accuracy in staging carcinoma of the bladder by magnetic resonance imaging. Clin Radiol 1990;41:258–263.

35. Tavares NJ, Demas BE, Hricak H. MR imaging of bladder neoplasms: correlation with pathologic staging. Urol Radiol 1990;12:27–33.

36. Barentsz JO, Lemmens JA, Ruijs SH, et al. Carcinoma of the urinary bladder: MR imaging with a double surface coil. AJR Am J Roentgenol 1988;151:107–112.

37. Sohn M, Neuerburg J, Teufl F, Bohndorf K. Gadolinium-enhanced magnetic resonance imaging in the staging of urinary bladder neoplasms. Urol Int 1990;45:142–147.

38. Barentsz JO. Imaging: old and new issues. Presented at 3rd International Symposium on Bladder Cancer. Invasive Bladder Cancer: the State of the Art. Padova, Italy, September 24, 1999.

39. Vock P, Haertel M, Fuchs WA, et al. Computed tomography in staging of carcinoma of the urinary bladder. Br J Urol 1982;54:158–163.

40. Brismar J, Gustafson T. Bone scintigraphy in staging of bladder carcinoma. Acta Radiol 1988;29:251–252.

41. Sobin LH, Wittekind C (Eds.). Urinary bladder. In: TNM Classification of Malignant Tumours. New York: Wiley-Liss, 1997, pp 187–190.

42. Broders AC. Epithelioma of the genitourinary organs. Ann Surg 1922;75:574–604.

43. Franksson C. Tumors of the urinary bladder. A pathological and clinical study of 434 cases. Acta Chir Scand Suppl 1950;100(6);Suppl 151,664–667.

44. Bergkvist A, Ljungquist A, Morberger G. Classification of bladder tumours based on the cellular pattern. Acta Chir Scand 1965;130:371–378.

45. Sobin LH, Wittekind C. TNM Classification of Malignant Tumours, 6th edn. New York: Wiley-Liss, 2002.

46. Epstein JI, Amin MB, Reuter VR, Mostofi FK. The World Health Organization/International Society of Urological Pathology consensus classification of urothelial (transitional cell) neoplasms of the urinary bladder.

Bladder Consensus Conference Committee. Am J Surg Pathol 1998;22(12):1435–1448.

47. Tolley DA, Hargreave TB, Smith PH, et al. Effect of intravesical mitomycin C on recurrence of newly diagnosed superficial bladder cancer: interim report from the Medical Research Council Subgroup on Superficial Bladder Cancer (Urological Cancer Working Party). Br Med J 1988;296:1759–1761.

48. Prout GR, Barton BA, Griffin PP, Friedell GH. Treated history of noninvasive grade 1 transitional cell carcinoma. J Urol 1992;148:1413–1419.

49. Lamm DL, Riggs DR, Traynelis CL, Nseyo UO. Apparent failure of current intravesical chemotherapy prophylaxis to influence the long-term course of superficial transitional cell carcinoma of the bladder. J Urol 1995;153:1444–1450.

50. Soloway MS. Treatment of superficial bladder cancer with intravesical mitomycin C. Analysis of immediate and long-term response in 70 patients. J Urol 1985;134:1107–1109.

51. Klan R, Loy V, Huland H. Residual tumour discovered in routine second transurethral resection in patients with stage T1 transitional cell carcinoma of the bladder. J Urol 1991;146:316–318.

52. Schwaibold HE, Treiber U, Kuebler H, et al. Second transurethral resection detects histopathological changes worsening the prognosis in 25% of patients with T1 bladder cancer. J Urol 2000;163:153.

53. Evans CP, Busby JE. The management of stage T1 grade 3 transitional cell carcinoma of the bladder. BJU Int 2003;92:345–348.

54. Morales A, Nickel JC, Wilson JWL. Dose response of bacillus Calmette-Guérin in the treatment of superficial bladder cancer. J Urol 1992;157:1256–1258.

55. Lamm DL, Blumenstein BA, Crawford ED, et al. A randomized trial of intravesical doxorubicin and immunotherapy with bacille Calmette-Guérin for transitional cell carcinoma of the bladder. N Engl J Med 1991;325:1205–1209.

56. Herr HW, Schwalb DM, Zhang ZF, et al. Intravesical bacillus Calmette-Guérin therapy prevents tumour progression and death from superficial bladder cancer: ten-year follow-up of a prospective randomised trial. J Clin Oncol 1995;13:1404–1408.

57. Bretton PR, Herr HW, Kimmel M, et al. The response of patients with superficial bladder cancer to a second course of intravesical bacillus Calmette-Guérin. J Urol 1990;143:710–712.

58. Herr HW. Timing of a cystectomy for superficial bladder tumors. Urol Oncol 2000;5:162–165.

59. Amling C, Thrasher J, Frazier HA, et al. Radical cystectomy for stages Ta, Tis and T1 transitional cell carcinoma of the bladder. J Urol 1994;151:31–35, discussion 35–36.

60. Lamm DL, Blumenstein BA, Crissman JD et al. Maintenance bacillius Calmette-Guérin immunotherapy for recurrent Ta, T1 and carcinoma in situ transitional cell carcinoma of the bladder: a randomised Southwest Oncology Group Study. J Urol 2000;163:1124–1129.

61. Wijkstrom H, Lagerkvist M, Nilsson B, et al. Evaluation of clinical staging before cystectomy in transitional cell bladder carcinoma: a long-term follow-up of 276 consecutive patients. Br J Urol 1998;81:686–691.

62. Lebret T, Herve JM, Barre P, et al. Urethral recurrence of transitional cell carcinoma of the bladder. Predictive value of preoperative latero-montanal biopsies and urethral frozen sections during prostatocystectomy. Eur Urol 1998;33(2):170–174.

63. Schoenberg MP, Walsh PC, Breazeale DR, et al. Local recurrence and survival following nerve sparing radical cystoprostatectomy for bladder cancer: 10-year followup. J Urol 1996;155(2):490–494.

64. Vieweg J, Whitmore WF Jr, Herr HW, et al. The role of pelvic lymphadenectomy and radical cystectomy for lymph node positive bladder cancer. The Memorial Sloan-Kettering Cancer Center experience. Cancer 1994;73(12);3020–3028.

65. Dimopoulos MA. Role of adjuvant chemotherapy in the treatment of invasive carcinoma of the urinary bladder. J Clin Oncol 1998;16:1601–1612.

66. Solsona E, Iborra I, Ricos JV, et al. Feasibility of transurethral resection for muscle infiltrating carcinoma of the bladder: long-term follow up of a prospective study. J Urol 1998;159:95–98.

67. Hayter CR, Groome PA, Schulze K, et al. A population-based study of the use and outcome of radical radiotherapy for invasive bladder cancer. Int J Radiat Oncol Biol Phys 1999;45:1239–1245.

68. Kaufman DS, Shipley W, Griffen PP, et al. Selective bladder preservation by combination treatment of invasive bladder cancer. N Engl J Med 1993;329:1377–1382.

69. Sternberg CN, Scher HI, Watson RC, et al. Methotrexate, vinblastine, doxorubicin, and cisplatin for advanced transitional cell carcinoma of the urothelium. Efficacy and patterns of response and relapse. Cancer 1989;64:2448–2458.

70. Moore MJ, Murray N, Tannock IF, et al. Gemcitabine plus cisplatin, an active regimen in advanced urothelial cancer: a phase II trial of the National Cancer Institute of Canada Clinical Trials Group. J Clin Oncol 1999;17:2876–2881.

71. Pycha A, Posch B, Schnack B, et al. Paclitaxel and carboplatin in patients with metastatic transitional cell cancer of the urinary tract. Urology 1999;53:510–515.

17

SCHISTOSOMIASIS
Manal Ismail Abd-Elghany

INTRODUCTION

Schistosomiasis is a parasitic waterborne trematode infection. It is one of the major public health issues and the second most prevalent tropical disease after malaria in the developing countries. It is often suggested that urinary schistosomiasis originated in the Nile Valley. Interestingly, hematuria was described in the 'Gynecological' Papyrus of Kahun written about 1900 BC and several remedies for hematuria are recorded in other papyri. The long existence of this human infection was confirmed in 1910 by Ruffer, who found large numbers of calcified eggs in the kidneys of Egyptian mummies of the Twentieth Dynasty (1250–1000 BC).[1] Discovery of schistosome worms had not been identified until the middle of the 19th century. In 1851 in Cairo's Kasr El-Aini Hospital, a German pathologist, Theodor Bilharz, discovered *Schistosoma haematobium* worms in the mesenteric veins while performing an autopsy. The genus was originally named *Distomum haematobium*, but in 1858 it was found that only one of the suckers had an oral cavity and Weinland renamed it *Schistosoma*, referring to the cleft (schistose) and the body (soma) of the male worm. The name bilharzia was suggested for the worm but rules of nomenclature gave priority to *Schistosoma* to refer to the genus and schistosomiasis when referring to the disease.[2] However, the infection is sometimes known as bilharziasis, especially in endemic areas. It is also known by many local names such as red-water fever, snail fever, big-belly and Katayama disease.

In 1915, Leiper worked out the life cycle of *S. haematobium* and *S. mansoni* and identified the snail intermediate hosts for the trematode infection. To this day, his report remains a classic and the preventive measures he suggested are similar to those currently recommended.[2,3]

BURDENS AND TRENDS

The global distribution of schistosomiasis has changed significantly over the past 50 years due to successful control in some countries. This success has been consistently linked to the implementation of a concerted control strategy.[4] A number of endemic countries such as Brazil, China, the Philippines and Egypt have been unable to sustain national control programs for a prolonged period. On the other hand, countries such as Puerto Rico, Venezuela, Saudi Arabia and Morocco are approaching eradication, while some have already achieved this goal (Japan, Lebanon, Monteserrat, Tunisia). However, an estimated 200 million people are still infected, of which 120 millions have symptoms and 20 million are thought to suffer severe consequences of the infection, particularly in sub-Saharan Africa.[5] Schistosomiasis therefore ranks high among other human endemic infections.[6]

Urinary schistosomiasis affects 53 countries in Africa and the eastern Mediterranean. It has been estimated that 39 million people have urinary schistosomiasis in Africa,[7] of whom nearly 50% may have apparently severe pathologic changes in the urinary tract that are readily demonstrated on radiography.[8]

People are infected by contact with infested water used in normal daily activities for personal or domestic hygiene and when swimming, or through occupational activities such as fishing, rice cultivation, irrigation, etc. A higher proportion of children of school age are affected by the disease. It also affects adult workers in rural areas employed in either agriculture or fresh water fishing. In some villages in Ghana around Lake Volta, the world's largest artificial lake, over 90% of children suffer from subtle morbidity such as anemia, impaired growth, development and cognition, and poor school performance. Poverty with deplorable unsanitary conditions, the lack of public health measures and facilities, and the unawareness of the risks are all factors contributing to the risk of infection. While direct mortality is relatively low, the disease burden is high in terms of chronic pathology and disability. Around 20,000 deaths annually are estimated to be associated with schistosomiasis. In urinary schistosomiasis, this is mostly due to associated bladder cancer or renal failure.[7]

PATHOGENESIS

The main forms of human schistosomiasis are caused by five species of flatworms, or blood flukes, known as schistosomes. Urinary schistosomiasis, caused by *S. haematobium*, affects mainly the urinary bladder, ureters and genitalia. Man is the only natural host.

Infected individuals contaminate fresh water with their excreta containing *Schistosoma* eggs. On contact with water, the eggs hatch and release the ciliated miracidia (larvae). *S. haematobium* is transmitted by species of fresh water pulmonate snails belonging to the various species complexes of the genus *Bulinus*.[9] If fresh water snails (intermediate host) are present, the miracidium multiplies, producing large numbers of fork-tailed cercariae. Cercariae are liberated into the water where they swim freely and may survive for 2–3 days until they encounter the definitive host (man). On contact with skin, cercariae attach themselves firmly with their oral sucker and mucinous secretions, which can be seen within the epidermis as periodic acid–Schiff (PAS)-positive masses.[10] They then penetrate the papillary dermis of the skin (which may be facilitated by their secretion of collagenases) where they continue their biological cycle.[11] In the dermis, cercariae enter the venules and are carried by the blood stream to the lungs, where many of them are destroyed; however, some survive and manage to find their way to the systemic circulation, lodging in mesenteric veins. Subsequently, they migrate via the inferior hemorrhoidal and pudendal veins to the vesical and pelvic plexuses.[10]

Over a period of 4–6 weeks the worms grow inside the blood vessels where they mature and females produce small clusters of eggs in venules of lamina propria.[12] The eggs are ovoid in shape, yellowish in color and translucent with a terminal spine. They are partly mature when laid, and measure about 50×100 microns.[13] One female may produce between 20 and 290 eggs per day.[1] Nearly 50% of the eggs are excreted in the urine, while the remainder are trapped in the body tissues, where they excite an intense inflammatory reaction.

Migration of either adult worms or ova may rarely occur resulting in dissemination of eggs in ectopic locations such as the central nervous system (CNS). However, the factors influencing ectopic migration are not clear. In fact, it is not the worm but the eggs which produce severe damage and chronic illness to the bladder and other vital organs. Adult schistosomes do not usually provoke any sort of inflammation while alive in the venules. On the other hand, dead worms killed by drugs may become entangled as verminous emboli and be swept to the lungs, where they provoke a severe reaction.[14] However, as the adult worms can live for nearly 20 years, progressive lesions may develop if treatment is not given.

PATHOLOGY

Schistosoma eggs are responsible for most of the lesions. Miracidia of retained ova in the wall of the bladder produce egg antigens, through the porous eggshells, resulting in sensitization of T lymphocytes (delayed hypersensitivity reaction) which in turn release lymphokines. Eventually a granuloma is formed around the ova. The early inflammatory response includes neutrophils and eosinophils. Later, more inflammatory cells accumulate to form a granuloma which consists of epithelioid cells, lymphocytes and giant cells surrounded by a zone of plasma cells, eosinophils and fibroblasts; its diameter is approximately 500 microns.[13]

When the eggs are close to the mucosal surface, the miracidia secrete a cytolytic enzyme to facilitate discharging of the ova into the bladder. If, however, the ova are retained in the tissues, the miracidia die and the ova then either disintegrate or calcify. Vascular congestion, hemorrhage and cytolytic secretions from the miracidia may enhance the passage of the ova into the surrounding stroma.[11] Later, as the infection turns chronic, the granuloma becomes fibrocellular surrounded by more fibroblasts and granulation tissues. Each individual granuloma then undergoes healing with or without fibrosis. The healed (fibrous) granuloma is smaller. Extensive fibrosis may involve all layers of the bladder, leading to a reduced bladder capacity of 300 ml or less with an associated increase in intravesical pressure and frequency. Unless the adult worms are killed or rendered infertile, new crops of granulomas continue to form.

PATHOLOGIC CHANGES OF THE URINARY BLADDER

Because of retention of the ova, a variety of changes may occur. The severity of these varies, due to variations in the intensity of infection and the duration of the disease.[15] The earliest lesion seen using a cystoscope was in the bladder in the form of a small grayish pseudotubercle, surrounded by an area of congestion. Such tubercles can occur anywhere in the bladder but are predominantly found around the ureteric orifices and on the fundus. Several other changes have been observed such as nodules, ulcers, polyps, leukoplakia

patches, trabeculations or fasciculation.[1] The picture may vary in different parts of the bladder between the acute and the chronic stage. In light infections, ova are generally restricted to the submucosa and mucosa; however, in heavy infections, involvement of all bladder layers may be seen. Early bladder changes usually consist of hyperemia and petechial hemorrhages of the bladder mucosa, followed by the development of more specific lesions.

Sandy patches

Sandy patches are a typical finding in longstanding infection due to heavy deposition within the submucosa of the calcified ova, surrounded by chronic inflammatory cells encased in fibrous tissue. They are generally irregular, yellowish to gray in color, of variable size, and appear as granular rough mucosal patches. Sandy patches are surrounded by dense hyaline fibrous tissue with an atrophic mucosal covering, which may either be intact or show single or multiple ulcers. The most common sites are the trigone and the ureteric orifices.[16–18] The calcification of numerous eggs in the bladder submucosa gives rise to a 'calcified bladder', which may appear on x-ray as a thin opaque rim outlining the bladder. In such cases, it has been calculated that there are 100,000 ova per square centimeter,[19] or 20,000 eggs per gram (epg).[17]

Schistosomal ulcers

Schistosomal ulcers are common bladder lesions. They occur frequently in areas of thin atrophic mucosa covering the sandy patches. Ulcers are variable in size and shape and have sharp edges, a granular floor (due to deposition of ova) and a firm (fibrotic) base. Acute ulcers can be very small, irregular defects (mucosal shedding) at the site of penetration of extruded eggs, or larger ulcers resulting from avulsed polypoid lesions. Chronic ulcers are usually transverse fissures, irregular and deep, due to retraction produced by extensive fibrosis, and they sometimes reach the muscle layer.[20] Microscopically, ulcers show schistosomal granulomas, formed of multiple ova surrounded by chronic inflammatory cells and fibrosis (Fig. 17.1).

Schistosomal polyps

Schistosomal polyps are less common lesions, but are observed in all stages of the disease. Polyps are either single or multiple, and appear reddish with a granular

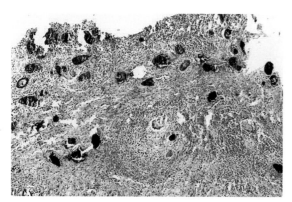

Fig. 17.1 Section of the urinary bladder showing typical granulomatous reaction (center) produced by *Schistosoma haematobium* eggs in the submucosa. The mucosa is ulcerated. Some eggs appear in nests, most of them showing calcification. Note the intense tissue reaction around the ova. H&E, ×100.

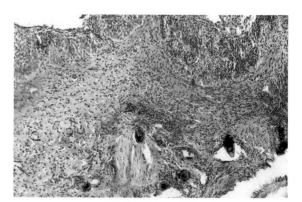

Fig. 17.2 Section in the urinary bladder showing deposition of *S. haematobium* ova in the lamina propria. The ova are surrounded with chronic inflammatory cells, fibrosis and areas of hemorrhage. The covering transitional epithelium is hyperplastic (top) with downgrowth of nest-like process into the submucosa (top right). H&E, ×100.

surface. Polyp size is variable, between 2 and 20 mm in diameter. In early active lesions, small polypoid projections may occur where hyperplastic urothelial cells cover large collections of inflammatory cells surrounding the ova. Larger polypoid lesions with fibrotic cores entangling a huge number of scattered fresh and calcified eggs are more common in longstanding cases.[21]

Associated changes in the urothelium

Associated changes in the urothelium, such as hyperplasia (Fig. 17.2), squamous metaplasia, leukoplakia (precancerous) and dysplasia, commonly arise in response to the persistent chronic irritation by ova. Dysplasia develops on top of transitional or metaplastic squamous epithelium and it may progress to carcinoma. Other urothelial changes include von Brunn's nests, cystitis cystica and cystitis glandularis.

von Brunn's nests

These are foci of solid buds projecting downward from the hyperplastic urothelium into the lamina propria (Fig. 17.3). According to von Brunn, cystitis cystica are derived from these nests with subsequent central degeneration in the center of these structures.[22] At cystoscopy, cystitis cystica appear as translucent to pearly white cysts about 1–5 mm in diameter. They are multiple, regular, rounded and – if present in excessive numbers – may give the mucosa a cobblestone appearance. Lesions are common around the trigone or ureteral orifices. The ureter and renal pelvis are less

frequently affected. However, involvement of the ureters may contribute to reflux or obstruction. Occasionally, cystitis cystica may occur in the posterior urethra leading to a variable degree of outlet obstruction.[10]

Cystitis glandularis

This type of cyst, first described by Morgagni in 1761, is lined by mucin-secreting columnar cells.[10] It may develop as a result of mucinous metaplasia in cells in the center of von Brunn's nests.[23] Cysts may dilate markedly and frank gland formation may occur. In the most mature glands prominent goblet cells can be seen and, rarely, Paneth cells.[24] Massive glandular proliferation (colonic metaplasia) may develop, and may grossly mimic adenocarcinoma, which can be excluded microscopically by the absence of cytologic atypia and muscle invasion.[25–27]

Schistosoma-associated carcinoma

In 1911, Ferguson was in no doubt that *S. haematobium* was the direct cause of the several squamous cancers that he saw at autopsy in Egypt. However, there was controversy as to whether such cancers are of bilharzial origin.[28] Bilharzial bladder cancer is one of the most common types of malignancy in both men and women in several developing countries, including Egypt. It has several unique clinical, epidemiologic and histologic characteristics, suggesting that it is an entity distinct from bladder cancer seen in Western countries.[29] *Schistosoma*-associated carcinoma (mostly squamous rather than the transitional cell type) is of common

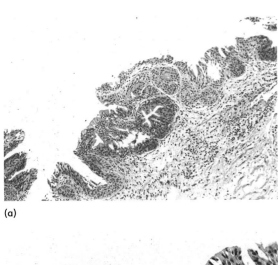

(a)

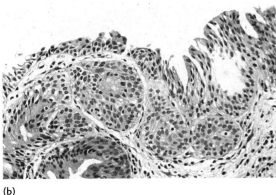

(b)

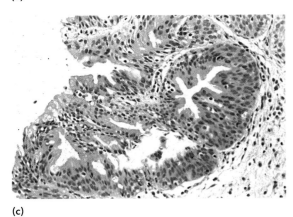

(c)

Fig. 17.3 Section of the urinary bladder showing some urothelial changes in the form of von Brunn's nests, cystitis cystica and cystitis glandularis. All figures are for the same area of the lesion with different magnifications, H&E stain: (a) ×100; (b) ×250; (c) ×150.

occurrence in some endemic areas. It occurs in relatively young people and is more prevalent in male hosts.[30] The common sites of *Schistosoma*-associated squamous cell carcinoma are the lateral and posterior walls of the bladder.

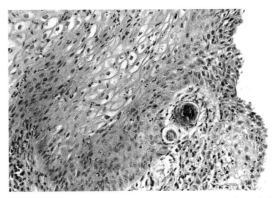

Fig. 17.4 Section in the bladder showing partially calcified eggs surrounded by chronic inflammatory cellular infiltrate, mainly plasma cells and lymphocytes. The mucosa shows squamous metaplasia. H&E, ×250.

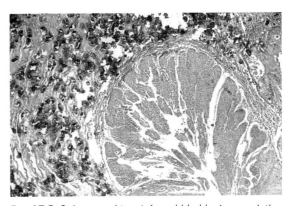

Fig. 17.5 *S. haematobium*-infected bladder in association with carcinoma. This lesion contains areas of both transitional cell carcinoma and squamous cell carcinoma. The stroma is heavily infiltrated by ova with variable degrees of degeneration and calcification which are surrounded by chronic inflammatory cells. H&E, ×100.

Grossly, bilharzial squamous cell carcinoma may occur in many patterns, such as invasive, fungating, infiltrative or ulcerative. True papillary patterns are very rare. The level of cytologic differentiation varies widely from the highly differentiated lesions to the undifferentiated, anaplastic giant cell tumors (Figs 17.4–17.6). The latter generally cover large areas of the bladder and are deeply invasive by the time of diagnosis.[13]

An interesting study was performed by Dimmette et al. on 90 cases of schistosomal carcinoma: 50 cases were squamous cell carcinoma, 33 transitional cell carcinoma, 6 adenocarcinoma and only 1 mixed transitional cell carcinoma/adenocarcinoma.[31]

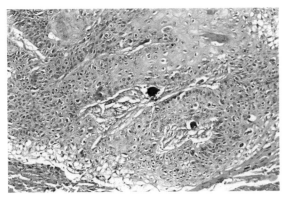

Fig. 17.6 Squamous cell carcinoma of bladder associated with *S. haematobium* infection. There are some ova within the sheets of a well-differentiated squamous cell carcinoma. H&E, ×250.

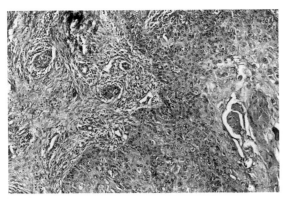

Fig. 17.7 *S. haematobium*-infected bladder in association with squamous cell carcinoma. Squamous cell carcinoma of bladder arises from transitional epithelium that has undergone metaplasia into squamous epithelium as a result of chronic irritation. Magnification ×250 shows a bladder lesion consisting of sheets of moderately differentiated squamous cell carcinoma cells with keratin formation (right). The stroma is fibrous and shows some calcified ova (left) surrounded by a heavy cellular infiltrate of chronic inflammatory cells.

The predisposing factors for schistosomal cancer are squamous metaplasia (Fig. 17.7), leukoplakia and dysplasia. As schistosomal cancers have a different distribution within the bladder from other non-schistosomal cancers, a local effect can be the cause. It is not fully understood whether the worms excrete a carcinogenic agent into the urine in increased amounts or cause local inflammation with subsequent development of urothelial changes and ultimately neoplastic transformation.[32] A potential role for p21WAF1/CIP1 alteration was suggested as contributing to schistosomal carcino-

genesis in the bladder.[33] In longstanding cases of schistosomiasis, secondary urinary tract infection is a common occurrence. Gram-negative bacteria such as *Escherichia coli* may change urinary nitrates and nitrites into carcinogenic nitrosamines. It has recently been reported that nitrates, nitrite and N-nitroso compounds in human bladder cancer are associated with schistosomiasis.[34] Recent studies have shown that schistosome-related cancers show different clinical and pathologic features compared with non-schistosome-related bladder cancers, i.e. they occur in younger patients and are predominantly of squamous cell type.

Genetic influences

Since bilharzia-associated bladder cancer (BAC) is a major health problem in countries where urinary schistosomiasis is endemic, characterization of the genetic alterations in this cancer might enhance our understanding of the pathogenetic mechanisms of that disease. In contrast to non-bilharzia bladder cancer, BAC has rarely been the subject of such scrutiny. A number of studies have been conducted in this area of research. For a better understanding of the underlying genetic influences on *Schistosoma*-associated carcinoma, DNA copy number changes were investigated in a number of *Schistosoma*-associated and non-*Schistosoma*-associated squamous cell carcinomas and transitional cell carcinomas of the bladder by comparative genomic hybridization (CGH).[35] Variations in the DNA copy number changes in all samples suggested that these tumors have different genetic pathways.

In another study, a molecular genetic model of schistosomal bladder cancer has been proposed. Interphase cytogenetics by fluorescence in situ hybridization (FISH) using a panel of centromere-associated DNA probes for chromosomes 1, 2, 5, 6, 12, 13, 14, 15, 18, 19, 20, and X and Y was performed on paraffin-embedded bladder specimens from 25 patients with schistosomal bladder cancer. No numerical aberrations were detected in all patients for all chromosomes except chromosome Y, where its loss was observed in 7 of the 17 male patients studied. However, no significant correlation was found between loss of chromosome Y and the clinicopathologic characteristics of those patients. The data suggest that loss of chromosome Y is the second frequent event that can occur in *Schistosoma*-associated bladder cancer.[36]

Muscheck et al. have addressed the difference between squamous and transitional tumor types in the presence of schistosome infection as a measure of the relationship between tumor genotype and phenotype.[37]

They used comparative genomic hybridization to analyze primary muscle-invasive schistosome-related bladder tumors in 54 patients. Of these tumors, 26 were squamous cell carcinomas and the remaining 28 were of transitional cell type. On average, transitional cell cancers showed 1.8 times the number of chromosomal aberrations as squamous cell tumors (14.4 versus 8.2, $p < 0.001$). For both groups combined, the most prevalent genetic alterations were losses of 8p and 18q, and gains of 8q. Transitional cell cancers also showed frequent losses involving 5q, 9p, 10q, 11p and 11q, and gains at 1q and 17q. Loss of 11p was significantly more frequent in transitional cell tumors than in squamous cell tumors (50 versus 4, $p = 0.01$). Squamous cell cancers showed more frequent losses of 17p and 18p than transitional cell tumors, which was clearly significant given the overall reduced frequency of changes in squamous cell cancers ($p = 0.001$ and $p = 0.03$, respectively). These data have shown that different histologic subgroups of bladder tumors were characterized by distinct patterns of chromosomal alterations. The genetic changes found in the transitional cell group were similar to those reported in non-schistosome-related transitional cell tumors, but differ from tumors exhibiting squamous differentiation.

A recent study has aimed to characterize chromosomal imbalances in benign and malignant post-bilharzial lesions, and to determine whether their unique etiology yields a distinct cytogenetic profile as compared to chemically induced bladder tumors.[38] DNA from 20 archival paraffin-embedded post-bilharzial bladder lesions (6 benign and 14 malignant) obtained from Sudanese patients (12 males and 8 females) with a history of urinary bilharziasis were investigated for chromosomal imbalances using CGH. Subsequent FISH analysis with pericentromeric probes was performed on paraffin sections of the same cases to confirm the CGH results. Seven of the 20 lesions (six carcinomas and one granuloma) showed chromosomal imbalances varying from one to six changes. The most common chromosomal imbalances detected were losses of 1p21–31, 8p21–pter and 9p, and gain of 19p material, seen in three cases each, including the benign lesion. Most of the detected imbalances have been repeatedly reported in non-bilharzial bladder carcinomas, suggesting that the cytogenetic profiles of chemical- and bilharzia-induced carcinomas are largely similar. However, loss of 9p seems to be more ubiquitous in BAC than in bladder cancer in industrialized countries.

Genetic alterations in bilharzial-related bladder cancer have been studied infrequently, especially in the advanced stages of disease, i.e. T3 and T4 classifications. One study tried to extend establishing the baseline cytogenetic profile of this type of malignancy to early T1 and T2 classifications.[29] This was performed by the application of FISH to interphase nuclei of frozen-stored samples with biotinylated repetitive DNA probes specific for all chromosomes to detect numerical chromosome changes in 35 patients presenting with relatively early-stage pT1 and pT2 disease. Of these 35 patients, 11 had squamous cell carcinoma and 24 had transitional cell carcinoma, with 6 of the 24 transitional cell carcinoma patients displaying diploid chromosome counts with all the probes. Numerical chromosome aberrations were detected in 18 cases (75%). In 12 cases, a loss of chromosome 9 was observed. In three cases, an additional loss of chromosome 17 was detected. One case demonstrated a loss of chromosome 10, whereas another two cases showed a gain of chromosome 7, next to a loss of chromosome 9. Loss of chromosome Y was observed in nine (33.3%) of the 27 male patients studied, in which only one case showed an abnormality whereas four cases were detected next to loss of chromosome 9, and one case showed gain of chromosome 7. Five cases showed loss of chromosome 19 whereas gain of chromosome 4 was detected in two cases. Two of 11 samples of squamous cell carcinoma had normal diploid chromosome counts with all the probes used. In four (36.4%) of 11 cases, under-representation of chromosome 9, compared with the other chromosomes, was detected. An additional loss of chromosome 17 and gain of chromosome 7, next to loss of chromosome 9, was detected in three cases. One case showed loss of chromosome 17 as the only numerical aberration. Loss of the Y chromosome was detected in three cases, of which one case had gain of chromosome 7 and one had loss of chromosome 19. No correlation was found between any of the clinicopathologic parameters examined in this study and the presence or absence of any numerical chromosomal aberrations except for the significant association between schistosomal history and loss of Y chromosome ($p = 0.007$).

Another study employing FISH, using repetitive alpha satellite probes to chromosomes 9 and 17, was performed on 27 paraffin-embedded bladder specimens from 18 Egyptian patients affected with bilharzial carcinoma.[39] The results of FISH in the carcinomas and benign mucosa of patients with schistosomiasis were compared with flow cytometric DNA ploidy and cell cycle assays. These results confirmed the feasibility of this technique for studies of the archival specimens, and suggested an early onset of chromosomal aberrations in histologically benign mucosa of schistosomal cystitis with progression during the development of bladder cancer. The study also suggested that monosomy 9 may be an early chromosomal change in urothelium of the bilharzia-infested bladder, and a predictor of incipient carcinoma in patients with bilharzial cystitis.

SCHISTOSOMIASIS OF THE UROGENITAL SYSTEM AND OTHER ORGANS

The ureters

Similar tissue reactions to those seen in the bladder may be seen in the ureter. Such changes are mostly secondary consequent on involvement of the bladder and less frequently due to primary involvement of the ureters by the disease. However, severe involvement of the ureters in the absence of bladder changes is unusual. The resulting pathologic changes are similar to those seen in the bladder, such as pseudotubercles, sandy patches, cysts, fibrosis and calcification. Dilatation (hydroureter), deformity, fibrosis, calcification or stenosis of the ureter is especially pronounced at its lower end, but occasionally may involve its whole length. There is usually a fusiform narrowing at the ureterovesical junction, with various degrees of dilatation above. These changes result in atony and dyskinesia, which appear radiographically.[40] With advanced cases, there may be obstructive uropathy (e.g. hydroureter and hydronephrosis). Such late complications are common findings in the hyperendemic areas to an extent that 10–17% of unselected patients may have already developed severe pathologic changes in the urinary tract, which appear radiographically.[41–43] As hydronephrosis develops, there is gradual compression of the kidneys leading eventually to renal failure, which is commonly complicated with secondary bacterial infection of the urinary tract and calculi formation (calcium phosphate stones).[44]

Male genital organs

Male genital organs are secondarily involved since *S. haematobium* infects the vesical plexus. The seminal vesicles are heavily infected with *S. haematobium* eggs, calculated to be 20,000 eggs per gram of seminal vesicle tissue. The seminal vesicle is therefore frequently enlarged with muscular hypertrophy and fibrosis. Such enlargement was suggested to correlate well with obstructive uropathy which can be assessed by manual examination of seminal vesicle size.[45] Disease of the seminal vesicles may result in hemospermia. The prostate is less commonly affected and eggs are more often found in the ejaculatory ducts where egg deposition may produce damage in the form of indurated lesions of granulomatous reaction which is later surrounded by marked fibrosis. Very rarely, testis, epididymis and penis are involved.[44] Rarely obstructive azoospermia and consequent sterility may develop as a complication.[46]

Female genital organs

Female genital organs can be involved by *S. haematobium* ova but this is not as common as in male genital organs. Sites of predilection are the vulva, vagina and cervix. Ovaries, Fallopian tubes and uterus are less commonly affected.[47] Schistosomal lesions can be polyps or ulcers in these sites and can be mistaken for carcinoma if they occur in the cervix. Schistosomal lesions may lead to sterility in some cases. Fistulae within the vagina or rectum may complicate schistosomal cystitis.

Other organs

Emboli of schistosomal ova can reach any organ. They may be carried to the lung, brain, spinal cord, lymph nodes, skin and elsewhere. Deposition of ova in the pulmonary arterioles may lead to pulmonary hypertension and cor pulmonale. These lung changes are especially frequent in combined infections with *S. haematobium* and *S. mansoni*. Most reported cases of acute cerebral schistosomiasis are caused by *S. japonicum* and most cases of schistosomal transverse myelitis by *S. mansoni*.[48,49]

CNS disease caused by *S. haematobium* is rare. Based on autopsy studies of patients with urinary schistosomiasis, *S. haematobium* ova may involve the brain in 30–50% of infected patients. However, CNS complications are uncommon.[50,51]

CLINICAL FEATURES

Invasive stage of dermatitis

The earliest symptoms are associated with invasion of skin by cercariae leading to swimmer's itch or cercarial dermatitis. This develops within a few minutes after exposure and appears as small red papules.[52] Cercarial dermatitis is usually mild but can occasionally be severe, especially in persons exposed for the first time to large numbers of cercariae.[53] It disappears within a few days and there are usually no other indications of the infection until the end of the pre-patent period when symptoms of toxemia may develop (approximately 8 weeks after initial infection).

Acute or toxemic stage

This stage was originally described by Walt in 1954,[1] where symptoms of toxemia were observed in relation to *S. japonicum* infection. Toxemic symptoms include pyrexia, anorexia, headache, malaise, mild abdominal pain, urticaria and cough. Commonly, in that early stage of infection, there may be few symptoms suggesting the true etiology of the parasitic infection, such as significant eosinophilia (as high as 80%).

Established infection stage

This is the stage of active egg deposition in the bladder wall, when the severity of *S. haematobium* infection varies greatly. The onset of egg appearance in the urine usually occurs 10–12 weeks after initial infection. Painless recurrent terminal hematuria is usually the first symptom. Chronic infection can lead to persistent cystitis, in the form of frequency of micturition and dysuria. Lower abdominal pain is common, localized either over the bladder region or in the suprapubic region, and may radiate to the groin. In endemic areas the majority of infected patients, usually children and young adults, are in this stage, suffering from hematuria. Although common, hematuria was not always considered abnormal; in some areas it was thought to be a normal process of puberty. It has been recorded that, during the Egyptian Campaign, many of Napoleon's troops suffered from its effects.[1] Hematuria is usually transient for a number of years in untreated cases, but microscopic blood cells can be seen between episodes in the majority of cases, accompanied by eggs, although the latter are excreted in decreased numbers over the years. Regrettably, many eggs are retained in the tissues of the host.

In advanced cases, hydronephrosis, pyelonephritis or pyonephrosis may develop and renal failure follows. Amyloid disease may arise in established cases. Schistosomal antigens (either by the worms or eggs) may lead to hyperplasia of lymphoid and reticuloendothelial cells. There is a high incidence of bladder carcinoma in patients with urinary schistosomiasis.

DIAGNOSIS

The simplest and easiest way to diagnosis schistosomiasis is by finding the characteristic schistosome eggs in the urine. In fact, schistosome granulomas process egg antigens and somatic components, in addition to generating a host of enzymes, lymphokines and other mediators.[54] As a result, a number of sensitive and specific serologic tests for diagnosing schistosomiasis have been developed;[55–57] those employing egg antigens are preferred.[58] However, abnormalities in the bladder and ureters are readily demonstrated by x-ray techniques, which may involve intravenous and retrograde pyelography and immediate, delayed and micturating cystograms to investigate ureteric reflux.

Clinically, the bladder shows variable filling defects, with eventual calcification and mural fibrosis. Cystometric measurements to determine bladder capacity may be required. Imaging techniques such as ultrasonography, computed tomography or magnetic resonance imaging scans may be helpful in indicating and defining the various organs and structures involved.[59]

TREATMENT

S. haematobium is treatable and the changes are only reversible in the early stages before the development of fibrosis.[60] Since there is no vaccine available,[61] chemotherapy is the current strategy for schistosomiasis control, with praziquantel being the drug of choice. Treatment with a single dose of praziquantel (40–60 mg per kg body weight) is safe and effective therapy against the adult worms of the three major species of schistosomes infecting humans (*S. haematobium*, *S. mansoni* and *S. japonicum*). Significant changes in the urogenital tract are reversed in as little as 6 months after treatment, particularly in children. Adult worms are more susceptible to praziquantel than 2–4-week-old immature schistosomes, and praziquantel does not kill immature eggs.[62] However, resistance to praziquantel has been reported in some endemic areas. Its resistance is species-specific and is stable, but is not field/laboratory consistent. There is no in vitro test for such resistance and there is less than a one-order magnitude in ED_{50} difference between resistant and susceptible worms. As yet, there is no evidence of resistance being genetically determined.[63]

Corticosteroids are often useful in neuroschistosomiasis to reduce edema and inflammation. Although

CNS schistosomiasis is rare, substantial morbidity from this condition is preventable by early diagnosis and rapid treatment.[64]

REFERENCES

1. Jordan P, Webbe G. Human Schistosomiasis. London: Heinemann Medical, 1969, pp 1–3.
2. Jordan P. Schistosomiasis – The St Lucia Project. Cambridge: Cambridge University Press, 1985, p 1.
3. Leiper RT. Report on the result of bilharziasis in Egypt 1915. J R Army Medical Corps 1915;25:1–55 (as referenced in Jordan P. Schistosomiasis – the St Lucia Project. Cambridge: Cambridge University Press, 1985).
4. Behbehani K. Candidate parasitic diseases. MMWR 1999;48(1):80–85.
5. WHO. Report of WHO informal consultation on schistososmaisis control. WHO/CDS/CPC/S10/99.2. Geneva: World Health Organization, 1999.
6. Warren KS. The relevance of schistosomiasis. N Engl J Med 1980;303:203–206.
7. http://www.who.int/ctd/schisto/disease.htm.
8. Oyediran AB. Renal disease due to schistosomiasis of the lower urinary tract. Kidney Int 1979;16:15–22.
9. Farley J. Bilharzia: A History of Imperial Tropical Medicine. Cambridge: Cambridge University Press, 1991, p 5.
10. Tomaszewsk JE. Cystitis: schistosomiasis. In: Hill GS (ed.) Uropathology, Vol. 1. New York: Churchill Livingstone, 1989, pp 440–443.
11. Arean VM. Schistosomiasis: a clinicopathologic evaluation. In: Sommers S (ed.) Pathology Annual, Vol. 1. New York: Appleton-Century-Crofts, 1966, p 68.
12. Pike EG. Engineering against Schistosomiasis/Bilharzia: Guidelines Towards Control of the Disease. London: Macmillan, 1987, pp 7–18.
13. von Lichtenberg F. Infectious disease: fungal, protozoal, and helminthic diseases and sarcoidosis. In: Cotran RS, Kumar V, Robbins S (eds.) Robbins' Pathologic Basis of Disease, 4th edn. Philadelphia: W.B. Saunders, 1989, p 424.
14. Conner DH, Gibson DW. Infectious and parasitic diseases. In: Rubin E, Farber J (eds.) Pathology. Philadelphia: J.B. Lippincott, 1988, p 441.
15. Smith JH, Christie DJ. The pathology of *Schistosoma haematobium* infection in humans. Hum Pathol 1986;17:333–345.
16. Smith JH, Kamel IA, Elwi A, von Lichtenberg F. A quantitative post mortem analysis of urinary schistosomiasis in Egypt. I. Pathology and pathogenesis. Am J Trop Med Hyg 1974;23:1054–1071.
17. Cheever AW, Kamel IA, Elwi AM, et al. *Schistosoma mansoni* and *S. haematobium* infections in Egypt. III. Extrahepatic pathology. Am J Trop Med Hyg 1978;27:55–57.
18. Christie JD, Crouse D, Pineda J, et al. Pattern of *Schistosoma haematobium* egg distribution in the human lower urinary tract. I. Non-cancerous lower urinary tracts. Am J Trop Med Hyg 1986;35:743–751.
19. Cheever AW, Young SW, Shehata A. Calcification of *Schistosoma haematobium* eggs: relation to radiographically demonstrable calcification to eggs in tissues and passages of eggs in urine. Trans R Soc Trop Med Hyg 1975;69:410–414.
20. Smith JH, Kelada AS, Khalil A. Schistosomal ulceration of the urinary balder. Am J Trop Med Hyg 1977;26:806–822.
21. Smith JH, Kelada AS, Farid Z. Schistosomal polyps of the urinary balder. Am J Trop Med Hyg 1977;26:85–88.
22. von Brunn A. Ueber drusenahnliche Bildungen in der Scheimhaut des Ureters und der Harnblase beim Menschen. Arch F Mikrosc Anat 1935;41:303.
23. Stoerk O, Zuckerkandl O. Ueber Cystitis glandularis and den Drusenkrebs der Harnvlase. Z Urol 1907;1:133.
24. Hill GS. Experimental production of pyeloureteritis cystica and glandularis. Invest Urol 1971;9:1–9.
25. Edwards PD, Hurm RA, Jaeschke WH. Conversion of cystitis glandularis to adenocarcinoma. J Urol 1972;108:568–570.
26. Lowry EC, Hamm FC, Bread DE. Extensive glandular proliferation of the urinary bladder resembling malignant neoplasm. J Urol 1944;52:133.
27. Bell TE, Wendel RG. Cystitis glandularis: benign or malignant? J Urol 1968;100:462–465.
28. Anthony PP. Malignant tumours of the kidney, bladder and urethra. In: Templeton AC (ed.) Tumours in a Tropical Country. Berlin: Springer-Verlag, 1973, pp 145–170.
29. Aly MS, Khaled HM. Chromosomal aberrations in early-stage bilharzial bladder cancer. Cancer Genet Cytogenet 2002;132(1):41–45.
30. Brawn PN. Interpretation of Bladder Biopsies. New York: Raven Press, 1984, p 39.
31. Dimmette RM, Sproat HF, Sayegh ES. The classification of carcinoma of the urinary bladder associated with schistosomiasis and metaplasia. J Urol 1956;75:680–686.
32. El-Bolkainy MN, Mokhtar NM, Ghoneim MA, Hussein MH. The impact of schistosomiasis on the pathology of bladder carcinoma. Cancer 1981;48:2643–2648.
33. Eissa S, Swelam M, Shaker Y, et al. Expression of p21WAF1/CIP1 in bladder cancer: relation to schistosomiasis. IUBMB-Life 1999;48(1):115–119.
34. Badawi AF. Nitrates, nitrite, and N-nitroso compounds in human bladder cancer associated with schistosomiasis. Int J Cancer 2000;86(4):598–600.
35. El-Rifai W, Kamel D, Larramendy ML, et al. DNA copy number changes in *Schistosoma*-associated and non-*Schistosoma*-associated bladder cancer. Am J Pathol 2000;156(3):871–878.
36. Khaled HM, Aly MS, Margrath IT. Loss of Y chromosome in bilharzial bladder cancer. Cancer Genet Cytogenet 2000;117(1):32–36.
37. Muscheck M, Abol-Enein H, Chew K, et al. Comparison of genetic changes in schistosome-related transitional and squamous bladder cancers using comparative genomic hybridization. Carcinogenesis 2000;21(9):1721–1726.
38. Fadl-Elmula I, Kytola S, Leithy ME, et al. Chromosomal aberrations in benign and malignant bilharzia-associated bladder lesions analyzed by comparative genomic hybridisation. BMC Cancer 2002;2:5.

39. Ghaleb AH, Pizzolo JG, Melamed MR. Aberrations of chromosomes 9 and 17 in bilharzial bladder cancer as detected by fluorescence in situ-hybridization. Am J Clin Pathol 1996;106(2):234–241.

40. Maker N. The bilharsial of ureter: some observations on the surgical pathology and surgical treatment. Br J Surg 1948;36:148.

41. Gelfand M, Weinberg R. Early inflammatory changes in the kidney in bilharziasis of the lower urinary tract. J Trop Med Hyg 1968;71:285–287.

42. Forsyth DM, MacDonald G. Urological complications of endemic schistosomiasis in schoolchildren. 2. Donge School, Zanzibar. Trans R Soc Trop Med Hyg 1966;60:568–578.

43. Bhagwandeen SB. The pathology of ureteric bilharziasis. S Afr Med J 1967;41:950–955.

44. Farid Z. Schistosomes with terminal-spined eggs: pathological and clinical aspects. In: Jordan P, Webbe G, Sturrock RF (eds) Human Schistosomiasis. Wallingford, Oxon: CAP International, 1993.

45. Christie JD, Crouse D, Smith JH, et al. Patterns of Schistosoma haematobium egg distribution in the human urinary lower tract in obstructive uropathy. Am J Trop Med Hyg 1986;35:752–758.

46. Elsebai I. Parasites in the etiology of cancer – bilharziasis and bladder cancer. CA Cancer J Clin 1977;27:100–106.

47. Wright ED, Chiphangwi J, Hutt MSR. Schistosomiasis of the female genital tract. A histopathological study of 176 cases from Malawi. Trans R Soc Trop Med Hyg 1982;76:822–829.

48. Marcial-Rojas RA, Fiol RE. Neurologic complications of schistosomiasis: review of the literature and report of two cases of transverse myelitis due to S. mansoni. Ann Intern Med 1963;59:215–230.

49. Scrimgeour EM, Gajdusek DC. Involvement of the CNS in S. mansoni and S. haematobium infection. Brain 1985;108:1023–1038.

50. Gelfand M. Schistosomal involvement of the brain and spinal cord. In: Schistosomiasis in South Central Africa: a clinico-pathological study. Cape Town: Post-Graduate Press, 1950, pp 194–202.

51. Alves W. The distribution of Schistosoma eggs in human tissues. Bull World Health Organ 1958;18:1092–1097.

52. Barlow CH, Meleney HE. A voluntary infection with Schistosoma haematobium. Am J Trop Med 1949;29:79–87.

53. Cowper SG. Clinical features and pathology of bilharziasis. In: A Symposium of African Bilharsiasis. London: H.K. Lewis, 1971, p 110–137.

54. Colley DG. Immunoregulatory Cells and Molecules indicating Helminthes Parasites. New York: Alan R. Liss, 1987, p 116.

55. Jansen-Rosseck R, Feldmeier H. Recent advances in diagnosis, treatment and prophylaxis of schistosomiasis and filariasis. Documentation of a training course sponsored by Department of Health and Social Affairs, The Senate of Berlin. Berlin: DSE/Westkreuz-Druckerei, 1988.

56. Tsang VCW, Wilkins PP. Immunodiagnosis of schistosomiasis: screen with FAST-ELISA and confirm with immunoblot. Clin Lab Med 1991;11:1029–1039.

57. Bergquist NR. Immunodiagnostic Approaches in Schistosomiasis. United Nations Industrial Development Organization (UNIDO). Chichester: Wiley, 1992.

58. Mott KE, Dixon H. Collaborative study on antigens for immunodiagnosis of schistosomiasis. Bull World Health Organ 1983;60:729–753.

59. Scrimgeour EM, Daar AS. Schistosomiasis: clinical relevance to surgeons in Australia and diagnostic update. Aust N Z J Surg 2000;70(3):157–161.

60. Samuel M, Misra D, Larcher V, Price E. Schistosoma haematobium in children in Britain. BJU Int 2000;85(3):316–318.

61. Gryseels B. Schistosomiasis vaccines: a devil's advocate view. Parasitol Today 2000;16:46–48.

62. WHO. Report on the WHO Informal Consultation on monitoring of drug efficacy in the control of schistosomiasis and intestinal nematodes. Geneva 8–10 July 1998. WHO/CDS/CPC/SIP/99/Chapter 3: Available drugs and measures of their efficacy. Geneva: Word Health Organization, 1999, p 17.

63. WHO. WHO/CDS/CPC/SIP/99/Chapter 5: Resistance of schistosomiasis and intestinal nematodes to antihelminthic drugs. Geneva: World Health Organization, 1999, p 23.

64. Blanchard TJ, Milne LM, Pollok R, Cook GC. Early chemotherapy of imported neuroschistosomiasis [Letter]. Lancet 1993;41:959.

18

PATHOLOGY OF THE NEUROPATHIC BLADDER CAUSED BY SPINAL CORD INJURY

Subramanian Vaidyanathan, Paul Mansour, Bakul M. Soni and Gurpreet Singh

INTRODUCTION

Spinal cord injury (SCI) causes limb paralysis and visceral dysfunction which, at least in our current state of knowledge and technology, are permanent in the vast majority of cases. It is not only a personal catastrophe for the patient and the family, but also a considerable economic drain on society as a whole: de Vivo[1] calculated the total annual cost of SCI in the United States to be $7.736 billion (Table 18.1).

SCI causes profound disturbances in the anatomy and physiology of many organ systems, including the urinary tract. A review of readmission of tetraplegic patients to the Regional Spinal Injuries Centre, Southport, UK, between January 1994 and December 1995 showed that the commonest reason for readmission was the management of urinary tract disorders. This accounted for 96 readmission episodes (43%) in 70 patients; 18 patients (26%) needed more than one readmission.[2] Pathologists reporting biopsies from patients with SCI, whether in the setting of a spinal injuries unit or not, should therefore be familiar with the spectrum of changes in the structure and function of the urinary tract, and particularly of the urinary bladder, seen in these patients. Some of these changes are direct or indirect consequences of denervation of the bladder, but others may be complications of treatment, and some knowledge of the expanding repertoire of treatments available is therefore also necessary.

Table 18.1 Total direct costs of US spinal injury cases in 1995 (US$)

Cause of spinal cord injury	New cases each year	First year charges per case	Recurring annual charges per case	Average lifetime charges per case	Annual aggregate direct costs (million)
RTAs	3590	233,947	33,439	969,659	3480
Assault	2950	217,868	17,275	613,345	1810
Falls	2030	185,019	26,238	630,453	1280
Sports	730	295,643	27,488	950,973	694
Other	700	208,762	23,510	673,749	472
Total	10,000	1,141,239	127,950	3,838,179	7736

RTA, road traffic accident. Figures are calculated by using (1) the average age at time of injury for each case, (2) a 2% real discount rate and (3) the most recent survival data from the National Spinal Cord Injury Statistical Center. All charges for emergency medical services, hospitalizations, attendant care, equipment, supplies, medications, environmental modifications, physician and outpatient services, nursing homes, household assistance, vocational rehabilitation, and miscellaneous items have been included. (From DeVivo MJ. Causes and costs of spinal cord injury in the US. Spinal Cord 1997; 35:809–813.)

PATHOGENESIS OF CHANGES IN THE URINARY BLADDER FOLLOWING SPINAL CORD INJURY

The major changes in the bladder following SCI comprise inflammation, fibrosis, bladder stone formation and the development of urothelial hyperplasia, metaplasia, dysplasia and neoplasia. These changes are caused by a combination of factors including recurrent urinary tract infection, the side effects of medical or nursing interventions, and possibly denervation per se.

Recurrent urinary tract infection

People with neuropathic bladder due to SCI often suffer from recurrent cystitis. Several physical or mechanical factors contribute to their increased susceptibility to urinary tract infection, including stasis of residual urine and the presence of indwelling catheters. In addition, it is feasible that denervation itself leads to changes at the molecular level which predispose to bacterial infection of the bladder.

Molecular pathology

The luminal surface of the normal bladder is lined by a layer of terminally differentiated, superficial umbrella cells that deposit on their apical surfaces a quasi-crystalline array of hexagonal complexes made up of four integral membrane glycoproteins known as uroplakins. In vitro binding assays have shown that uropathogenic *Escherichia coli* expressing type 1 pili can specifically bind to two of the uroplakins, UPIa and UPIb. Bacterial colonization of the normally innervated urinary bladder causes, as an innate host defense mechanism, the exfoliation and excretion of infected, damaged superficial cells, thereby exposing underlying, less differentiated urothelial cells. This exfoliation occurs through a rapid apoptosis-like mechanism involving activation of caspase (cysteine-containing aspartate-specific proteases) and fragmentation of host DNA (as revealed by terminal deoxytransferase-mediated deoxyuridine triphosphate nick end labeling (TUNEL) assays using infected mouse bladder).

The speed with which DNA fragmentation occurs after bacterial inoculation suggests that urothelial cells may be sensitized to undergo rapid programmed cell death (apoptosis). The process of apoptosis may be altered in the urothelium of SCI patients, thus increasing their susceptibility to recurrent cystitis; one mechanism by which this might occur involves changes in urothelial expression of parathyroid hormone-related protein (PTHrP). PTHrP acts mainly as a regulator of cellular differentiation, and in the urothelium is normally expressed only in the differentiating bladder. In bladder biopsies from SCI patients, however, using antibodies to different fragments of the PTHrP molecule, we have demonstrated the expression of PTHrP 43–52 in the urothelium in 9 out of 14 biopsies and of PTHrP 127–138 in 4 out of 14 biopsies, respectively.[3] If, as has been postulated (see below), denervation itself causes proliferation of the urothelium, then the expression of PTHrP in this immature 're-differentiating' epithelium would render it less susceptible to apoptosis.

Clinical effects

In our clinical practice, the commonest medical problem in SCI patients is urinary tract-related disease; three or four episodes of cystitis a year are not uncommon in some patients, accounting for much of the long-term personal, social and economic cost of SCI, for example:

- Patients are unwell and unable to socialize for 3 or 4 weeks a year.
- Antibiotics, sometimes expensive, are needed.
- Additional nursing care or hospitalization may be required.
- Earnings may be lost.
- Each episode of pyelonephritis causes progressive renal damage.

Transient bladder spasms occur during acute episodes, causing (depending on the catheterization regime used) either leakage of urine between intermittent catheterizations or the bypassing of an indwelling catheter. This leakage of urine can, where the person lies on urine-soaked sheets, contribute to the development of pressure sores. Cystitis can also cause autonomic dysreflexia, a serious complication necessitating hospitalization. Furthermore, repeated episodes of urinary tract infection may have a devastating consequence on the fertility of a young male patient; epididymitis can cause obstruction to the seminiferous tubules, while orchitis impairs spermatogenesis and rarely may require orchidectomy in those in whom it progresses to a testicular abscess.[4]

Although each clinical episode of cystitis usually lasts for only 5–10 days and inflicts no clinically discernible permanent bladder damage, there may be cumulative cellular changes at the molecular level which affect urothelial proliferation, maturation and apoptosis and thereby increase the risk of malignancy. The urothelium acts as a barrier, preventing leakage of urine into the bladder wall with consequent tissue damage (caused particularly by urea and potassium in high concentrations) and re-absorption of toxic excretion products. The properties of the urothelium responsible for this barrier function are the stratification and maintenance of polarity of the transitional epithelium, in which context the apical membrane and the junctions between superficial cells are particularly important.[5]

Infection can lead to loss of the barrier function of the urothelium, either by a direct effect of bacteria on the urothelial cells or as a secondary effect of inflammation. The consequent movement of toxic urine constituents into the underlying connective tissue and muscle layers may exacerbate the clinical effect of cystitis and may have a cumulative detrimental effect, predisposing the vesical urothelium to neoplastic transformation. An epidemiologic study was carried out on 2982 cases of bladder carcinoma (in the non-neuropathic bladder) and 5782 population controls from ten areas of the United States. The data from this study showed that a history of three or more episodes of urinary tract infection significantly elevated the risk of bladder cancer (relative risk = 2.0) and, in particular, the risk of squamous carcinoma (relative risk = 4.8). Chronic or recurrent infection in the neuropathic bladder carries a similarly increased risk, and prevention of cystitis is therefore one of the main aims of SCI patient management.[6]

Iatrogenic changes

Effects of bladder irrigation

A proportion of SCI patients with indwelling catheters use antiseptic solutions to irrigate the bladder in an attempt to minimize the chances of cystitis, the most commonly used antiseptics being chlorhexidine, kanamycin-colistin and povidone-iodine. These solutions are irritants and their use can cause erosive cystitis. This is particularly common with kanamycin-colistin and povidone-iodine solutions, but we have also observed erosive cystitis and severe hematuria in patients using chlorhexidine. A similar picture is seen in rats, in whom instillation of chlorhexidine digluconate causes changes in the bladder mucosa, ranging from regenerative epithelial atypia and degeneration to focal or widespread erosive cystitis and hemorrhage.[7,8] The clinical information accompanying bladder biopsies from SCI patients should therefore include any history of antiseptic bladder irrigation. Erosive cystitis may also occur in cases of severe bacterial cystitis.

Oxybutynin relaxes the detrusor muscle, and intra-vesical oxybutynin instillation is therefore recommended for control of bladder spasms (detrusor hyperreflexia) in SCI patients.[9] Recent studies have shown that oxybutynin also inhibits the proliferation of smooth muscle in the bladder wall induced by serum and mechanical stretch, possibly by downregulation of growth-promoting genes such as *c-jun*.[10] This observation raises the possibility that oxybutynin may also be useful for preventing permanent muscle hypertrophy in the neuropathic bladder. There is some experimental evidence of an inflammatory or allergic reaction to topical oxybutynin, with a mild mucosal infiltrate of eosinophils seen in five out of nine rabbits receiving intravesical instillation of crushed oxybutynin tablets, but it remains to be seen whether this constitutes a significant clinical problem in humans.[11]

Long-term catheter drainage

The ideal plan of management for bladder drainage in SCI patients would minimize the risk of urinary tract complications (including renal damage and urothelial neoplasia) without compromising quality of life (including comfort, convenience and independence). In practice, however, this is a difficult balancing act to achieve. Many SCI patients prefer long-term indwelling catheter drainage as it helps them maintain independence and does not require restriction of fluid intake. However, this regime causes more side effects than intermittent catheterization, which itself is less convenient for the patient. These side effects range from non-specific inflammation, mucosal hemorrhage and polypoid cystitis (see below), through urothelial hyperplasia and squamous metaplasia, to dysplasia and malignancy (particularly squamous carcinoma).[12]

The inflammation seen with indwelling catheters is consistently more severe than that associated with intermittent catheterization, probably due both to the chronic irritation produced by the indwelling catheter and to the increased incidence of cystitis in this group of patients (Figs 18.1, 18.2). The not uncommon end result is a small, painful, contracted, fibrotic bladder, as exemplified by the description by Janzen and colleagues

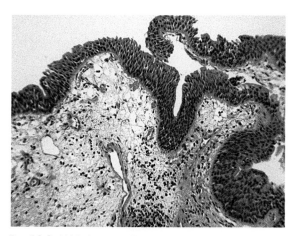

Fig. 18.2 Mild chronic inflammation in a spinal cord injury patient using intermittent catheterization.

of a cystectomy specimen from a 51-year-old woman who had used indwelling catheter drainage for 6 years.[13] Macroscopically, the mucosa was irregular, thickened and gray–white in colour, and the bladder wall was 3.5 cm thick and non-elastic. Histologically, the transitional epithelium showed multifocal squamous metaplasia. There was a dense, transmural, chronic inflammatory infiltrate, and severe fibrosis of the lamina propria and muscularis propria with areas of hyalinization. The fibrosis was causing dissociation of the smooth muscle cells of the muscularis, which also showed a pattern of hyperplasia resembling that of a leiomyoma. Immunohistochemical staining for S-100 antigen revealed marked hypertrophy and hyperplasia of the nerve fibers within both the lamina propria and muscularis.

The physical presence of an indwelling catheter can cause polypoid or papillary cystitis, by a combination of mechanical irritation and pressure effect.[14] Although entirely benign, polypoid or papillary cystitis can be confused both cystoscopically and histologically with carcinoma, and biopsy is usually indicated to exclude malignancy. It mainly affects the posterior wall or dome, and can be diffuse; it may involve the ureteric orifices with consequent hydronephrosis.[15] It is a reversible condition; in one study, removal of the catheter led to resolution of the polypoid cystitis in virtually all patients (13 out of 15) within 28 weeks.[16] Scanning electron microscopy of the polypoid areas shows the presence of pleomorphic microvilli on the surface layer of transitional cells, apparently specific to this condition.[17]

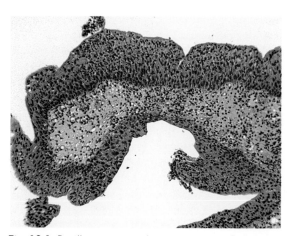

Fig. 18.1 Papillary cystitis with intense acute inflammation in a spinal cord injury patient with an indwelling catheter. Neutrophil polymorphs are present in both stroma and epithelium.

Denervation-induced changes

SCI patients are at high risk of developing both cystitis and bladder cancer; impaired regulation of urothelial proliferation may be a common predisposing factor for both. As in many other tissues, the increased urothelial turnover caused by chronic inflammation or mechanical irritation provides an environment in which the various steps along the path to malignancy are more likely to occur. In addition, however, denervation of the bladder in itself may, independently of the effects of inflammation, cause changes in the structure and function of the vesical urothelium which tend to increase its susceptibility to infection and neoplastic change.

Normal bladder innervation produces a trophic effect upon the urothelium. The biochemical basis of this trophic effect is not fully understood, but is likely to involve a complex interplay of molecules including growth factors and their receptors, cell adhesion molecules, secretory immunoglobulin (IgA), nitric oxide synthase and cytokines. We have shown, for example, abnormal immunohistochemical localization of epidermal growth factor receptor (EGFR-p) in the vesical urothelium of more than 70% of the SCI patients studied, with cytoplasmic staining rather than the linear cell membrane pattern considered necessary for effective receptor function. Normal EGFR-p staining was only seen in those patients with neither an indwelling urethral catheter nor bladder calculi, these patients also showing only minimal histologic evidence of cystitis.[18] These findings have some clinical relevance, supporting a regime of intermittent catheterization rather than long-term indwelling catheter drainage of the neuropathic bladder.

It is also known that the nervous system exerts a significant influence on lymphocyte distribution and function in certain mucosal tissues.[19] In a pilot study, we compared the intensity of secretory immunoglobulin A (sIgA) immunostaining in the urothelium of neuropathic bladders with normal controls. We observed a significant decrease in sIgA staining in about 50% of the neuropathic bladders, suggesting that the neural–immune interaction may affect the distribution, density or output of IgA-secreting cells in the bladder mucosa.[20]

We hypothesized that denervation, and consequent loss of this trophic effect, may initiate a cascade of events which disturb the normal regulation of urothelial proliferation, differentiation, maturation and apoptosis, contributing to an increased risk of infection and neoplasia.[6] This denervation-induced effect may be exacerbated by other factors commonly present in the neuropathic bladder such as recurrent cystitis, increased residual urine, bladder stones and long-term indwelling catheter drainage. Konety and colleagues[21] showed increased urinary levels of the nuclear matrix protein BLCA-4 in 96% of patients with bladder cancer and 19% of SCI patients compared with normal controls. Such raised BLCA-4 levels in SCI patients may be related to cystitis, chronic catheter-associated changes, denervation-induced urothelial proliferation, or to a combination of these factors.

Alipov and associates[22] have suggested that parathyroid hormone-related protein (PTHrP) acts as a cytokine for cell proliferation and tumor progression. Using an antibody to part of the PTHrP molecule, we showed the presence of PTHrP (1–34) in the majority of cases of neuropathic bladder (both in 'normal' and hyperplastic transitional epithelium and in metaplastic squamous epithelium), while it was absent from the urothelium of normal bladders.[23] Overexpression of PTHrP may be involved in the malignant transformation and progression of gastric carcinoma,[22] and it may play a similar role in the urothelium of the neuropathic bladder.

HISTOLOGIC CHANGES IN THE BLADDER MUCOSA OF SPINAL CORD INJURY PATIENTS

None of the histologic changes seen in the neuropathic bladder is specific to this condition, but certain patterns are characteristic.

Inflammation

Some degree of acute and chronic mucosal inflammation is very common, the inflammatory infiltrate including a combination of neutrophils, lymphocytes and plasma cells, and occasionally eosinophils and mast cells. Lymphoid aggregates may be present, and a diagnosis of follicular cystitis is appropriate when true follicles (including germinal centers) are seen (Fig. 18.3); these follicles are often numerous, giving a nodular appearance which can be confused with malignancy on cystoscopy. Severe inflammation may be associated with focal erosion or frank ulceration; erosive cystitis can be caused by certain irrigation fluids as well as by severe bacterial infection.

Other features of the inflammatory response may also be present, including stromal edema and conges-

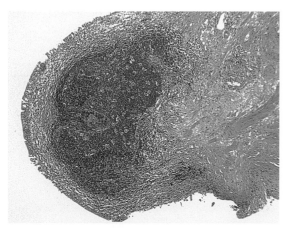

Fig. 18.3 Follicular cystitis: a large lymphoid follicle, including a germinal center, occupies much of the lamina propria, causing a nodular elevation of the mucosa evident on cystoscopy. Tingible body macrophages are visible even at this magnification.

tion. Edema can be marked focally in relation to local pressure or irritation from an indwelling catheter, causing the formation of cystoscopically apparent excrescences. This is termed polypoid cystitis if the protuberances are short and broad, and papillary cystitis if they are long and slender. Both may be confused with carcinoma macroscopically, but the potential for confusion on histologic examination is greater in papillary cystitis, especially during resolution when inflammation is less prominent (Fig. 18.4). The covering urothelium, and that of the adjacent mucosa, is usually normal but is occasionally metaplastic.[24] Fibrosis is usually a consequence of chronic inflammation, and

can be particularly marked in those patients using long-term indwelling (as opposed to intermittent) catheterization; fibrosis of the submucosa and muscularis can result in a small, contracted and inelastic bladder.

Janzen and associates[25] reviewed bladder biopsies in 61 SCI patients treated at the Swiss Paraplegic Centre in Nottwil. Chronic inflammation was present in 46 patients (75.4%) and subacute inflammation in 10 (16.4%). Fibrosis was seen in 34.4% of cases. Biopsies were normal in only five cases (8.2%).

Metaplasia

The transitional epithelium of the neuropathic bladder can undergo metaplasia to the same range of epithelial types seen in the normally innervated bladder, including squamous, columnar, intestinal and prostatic epithelium. Of these, the most important is squamous metaplasia, and in particular keratinizing squamous metaplasia, which is considered to be a premalignant condition and the background against which the majority of cases of squamous carcinoma arise (Fig. 18.5).

The presence of non-keratinizing squamous metaplasia, resembling vaginal-type glycogenated epithelium, is considered a variant of normal in the trigone of the postpubertal female. However, non-keratinizing squamous metaplasia can also occur elsewhere in the bladder as a response to chronic, low-grade inflammation, in which context it can also be seen in the male (Figs 18.6, 18.7). Non-keratinizing squamous metaplasia does not have the same implications as keratinizing metaplasia, and is not considered a premalignant condition.

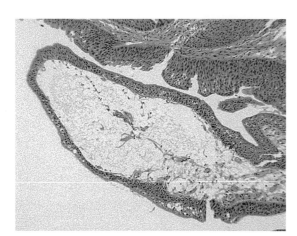

Fig. 18.4 Papillary cystitis: note the edematous fibrovascular core and normal overlying epithelium; inflammation in this case is minimal.

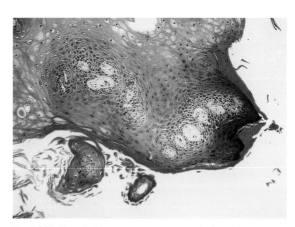

Fig. 18.5 Keratinizing squamous metaplasia with a papillomatous architecture. No atypia is present in this case.

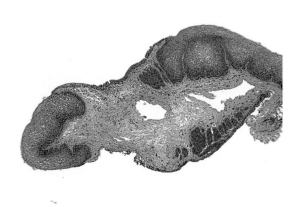

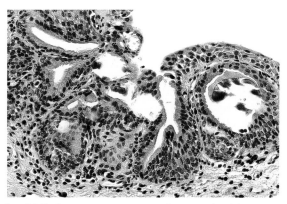

Fig. 18.8 Concretion in an area of cystitis glandularis: note the typical shattered or fractured appearance of the basophilic calcified nodule.

Fig. 18.6 Widespread non-keratinizing squamous metaplasia of 'vaginal' type in a male patient. Note the sharp transition from metaplastic to native epithelium.

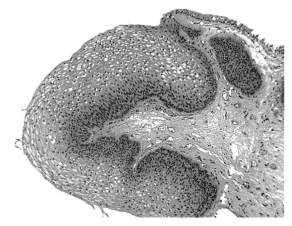

Fig. 18.7 A further example of a focus of non-keratinizing squamous metaplasia of 'vaginal' type also occurring in a male patient. Note the sharp transition from metaplastic to native epithelium (upper right).

Delnay and associates[26] observed either keratinizing squamous metaplasia or cystitis glandularis in 48 out of 208 SCI patients (23%) with chronic indwelling urinary catheters. While uncomplicated cystitis glandularis is probably not a premalignant condition, the presence of intestinal metaplasia does seem to predispose to subsequent adenocarcinoma, particularly if the metaplasia is widespread.

Concretions and calculi

Calcified concretions, usually with a typical shattered or fractured appearance in non-decalcified sections, are often seen on the surface or in the submucosa of bladder biopsies from patients with bladder calculi (Fig. 18.8). Mitsui and associates noted the formation of bladder stones in 65% of SCI patients with suprapubic cystostomy and 30% of those practicing intermittent catheterization, over a follow-up period of about 10 years.[27]

Dysplasia and malignancy

Patients with neuropathic bladder are at increased risk of developing bladder cancer. This increased risk is largely associated with recurrent infection, bladder calculi and the use of indwelling catheters; routine follow-up of patients with these risk factors should therefore include regular flexible cystoscopy and biopsy.

Between 1988 and 1992, West and colleagues identified 130 cases of bladder cancer in a total of 33,565 SCI patients; of these cancers, 23 were transitional cell carcinomas, 14 were squamous carcinomas, 4 were adenocarcinomas and 1 was mixed.[28] Squamous carcinomas were more common in the patients with indwelling catheters, while transitional carcinomas occurred more frequently in those using intermittent catheterization. Interestingly, malignancies developed earlier in those patients using intermittent catheterization (typically 8 years after cord injury) than in those with indwelling catheters (18 years after injury). It seems that those patients with the capacity and/or the opportunity to store urine in the bladder develop bladder cancer sooner. This might be because, in these patients, non-carcinogenic substances in the urine are converted to carcinogens when stored in the bladder, or because carcinogens in the urine are in contact with the urothelium for longer, or both. These putative carcinogens seem preferentially to cause transitional cell carcinoma, while the chronic irritation caused by indwelling catheters seems more likely to cause squamous carcinoma.

Squamous carcinoma usually develops against a background of keratinizing squamous metaplasia. Cytokeratin 14 (CK14), normally expressed in the basal cells of squamous epithelium, is a reliable and sensitive marker of the emergence of a squamous phenotype in the urothelium; in fact, Harnden and Southgate demonstrated its presence in areas of urothelium with no morphologic evidence of squamous differentiation.[29]

Dysplasia of the urothelium is the presumed precursor of transitional cell carcinoma; 19% of cases of isolated urothelial dysplasia (falling short of carcinoma in situ) followed up at the Mayo Clinic for up to 8 years showed histologic progression.[30] In common with other organs, the distinction between low-grade urothelial dysplasia and inflammatory or regenerative epithelial changes is subjective and sometimes difficult when assessment is limited to routine sections stained with hematoxylin and eosin. However, the morphologic stratification of the transitional epithelium, itself a reflection of increasing functional differentiation, is mirrored by a characteristic pattern of antigen expression at each level. Harnden and associates have shown that immunohistochemical staining for cytokeratin 20 (CK20) may provide an objective method for distinguishing reactive changes from true dysplasia.[31] In their study, normal transitional epithelium showed CK20 staining confined almost exclusively to the superficial cell layer, while dysplastic urothelium showed full-thickness expression in 89% of cases, with no false-positive results. Early detection of urothelial dysplasia by this method may not only prompt changes to management regimes (such as method of catheterization) but also allow follow-up schedules to be more precisely tailored to the individual needs of each patient.

Telomerase is an enzyme that contributes to the malignant phenotype in most malignant tumors by conferring immortality upon tumor cells; it is not usually detectable in normal somatic tissues. Its expression may be an early event in bladder carcinogenesis, preceding morphologic changes related to malignant transformation. In addition to its role as a prognostic marker of bladder tumor relapse or progression, therefore, telomerase activity may also be useful as an indicator of malignant potential in preneoplastic lesions such as intestinal metaplasia and dysplasia.[32]

Other than the predominance of squamous carcinoma, there are no special features of malignant tumors in the neuropathic bladder. As in the normally innervated bladder, transitional cell carcinomas can often show varying degrees of squamous differentiation, and squamous carcinoma should only be diagnosed where the carcinoma is overwhelmingly squamous in nature, as evidenced by either keratinization or by intercellular bridge formation. Squamous cell carcinoma (and, very rarely, mucinous adenocarcinoma) may occur in the suprapubic cystostomy tract,[33,34] and this possibility should be borne in mind in those patients who present with bloody drainage and/or masses arising from the suprapubic cystostomy site.

THE ROLE OF THE PATHOLOGIST IN THE GLOBAL MANAGEMENT OF SPINAL CORD INJURY PATIENTS

As in any other clinical setting, the main role of the pathologist is to provide relevant and timely information with which the clinical team can assess prognosis and base decisions about patient management. This role can be most effectively fulfilled by a pathologist who is a full member of the clinical team, and who participates where possible in the team's regular multidisciplinary meetings. Table 18.2 summarizes the most frequent practical issues faced by the pathologist; all have a direct

Table 18.2 The role of the pathologist in the management of neuropathic bladder in spinal cord injury patients

- Alert clinician to possible side effects of treatment:
  — polypoid cystitis, squamous metaplasia or widespread cystitis glandularis in patients with long-term indwelling catheters
  — erosive cystitis in patients using antiseptic bladder irrigation fluids
- Alert clinician to premalignant changes in a neuropathic bladder
  — keratinizing squamous metaplasia or intestinal metaplasia
  — urothelial dysplasia (immunohistochemistry may be helpful)
  — possible alterations in regulation of urothelial proliferation and/or apoptosis as revealed by immunohistochemistry and molecular pathology
- Accurate diagnosis and typing of malignancy

and immediate influence on patient management. In such a rapidly developing field as spinal injury medicine, the pathologist may also play an important role in evaluating new treatments, whether as part of a formal research program or not.

CONCLUSION

- Changes in the neuropathic bladder are caused by a combination of recurrent infection, iatrogenic factors such as the presence of indwelling catheters, and denervation per se.
- The main complications of neuropathic bladder in SCI patients are inflammation, bladder stone formation and neoplasia.
- Inflammation is more severe in neuropathic bladders drained by indwelling catheters than in those drained by intermittent catheterization.
- Recurrent cystitis and chronic inflammation in the neuropathic bladder can lead to fibrosis, small bladder capacity, hydronephrosis due to obstruction at the ureteric orifices and eventually to neoplasia.
- SCI patients with indwelling catheters and/or bladder stones have an increased risk of developing bladder cancer. Keratinizing squamous metaplasia is an important premalignant condition predisposing to the development of squamous carcinoma.
- Immunohistochemistry of bladder biopsy is a useful diagnostic aid in detecting early squamous metaplasia (CK14) and urothelial dysplasia (CK20).

REFERENCES

1. DeVivo MJ. Causes and costs of spinal cord injury in the United States. Spinal Cord 1997;35:809–813.
2. Vaidyanathan S, Soni BM, Gopalan L, et al. A review of the readmissions of patients with tetraplegia to the Regional Spinal Injuries Centre, Southport, United Kingdom, between January 1994 and December 1995. Spinal Cord 1998;36:838–846.
3. Vaidyanathan S, McCreavy DT, McDicken IW, et al. Immunohistochemical study of parathyroid hormone-related protein in vesical transitional epithelium of patients with spinal cord injury. Spinal Cord 1999;37:760–764.
4. Vaidyanathan S, Mansour P, Parsons KF, et al. Xanthogranulomatous funiculitis and epididymo-orchitis in a tetraplegic patient. Spinal Cord 2000;38:769–772.
5. Lewis SA. Everything you wanted to know about the bladder epithelium but were afraid to ask. Am J Physiol Renal Physiol 2000;278:F867–874.
6. Vaidyanathan S, McDicken I, Soni BM, Sett P, Krishnan KR. Possible role of denervation-induced changes in the urothelium in the pathophysiology of cystitis in patients with spinal cord injury: a hypothesis: Spinal Cord 1997;35:708–709.
7. Harper WES, Matz LR. The effect of chlorhexidine irrigation of the bladder in the rat. Br J Urol 1975;47:539–543.
8. Harper WES, Matz LR. Further studies on effects of irrigation solutions on rat bladders. Br J Urol 1976;48:463–467.
9. Vaidyanathan S, Soni BM, Brown E, et al. Effect of intermittent urethral catheterization and oxybutynin bladder instillation on urinary continence status and quality of life in a selected group of spinal cord injury patients with neuropathic bladder dysfunction. Spinal Cord 1998;36:409–414.
10. Park JM, Bauer SB, Freeman MR, Peters CA. Oxybutynin chloride inhibits proliferation and suppresses gene expression in bladder smooth muscle cells. J Urol 1999;162(3 Pt 2):1110–1114.
11. Landau EH, Fung LC, Thorner PS, et al. Histologic studies of intravesical oxybutynin in the rabbit. J Urol 1995;153:2022–2024.
12. Goble NM, Clarke T, Hammonds JC. Histological changes in the urinary bladder secondary to urethral catheterisation. Br J Urol 1989;63:354–357.
13. Janzen J, Vuong PN, Gonties D. Histopathological findings in a cystectomy specimen after six years of catheterisation. Spinal Cord 1997;35:860–861.
14. Norlen LJ, Ekelund P, Hedelin H, Johansson SL. Effects of indwelling catheters on the urethral mucosa (polypoid urethritis). Scand J Urol Nephrol 1988;22:81–86.
15. Valero Puerta JA, Medina Perez M, Valpuesta Fernandez I, et al. Bilateral hydronephrosis with papillary polypoid cystitis. Arch Esp Urol 1999;52:396–398.
16. Anderstrom C, Ekelund P, Hansson HA, Johansson SL. Scanning electron microscopy of polypoid cystitis – a reversible lesion of the human bladder. J Urol 1984;131:242–244.
17. Ekelund P, Anderstrom C, Johansson SL, Larsson P. The reversibility of catheter-associated polypoid cystitis. J Urol 1983;130:456–459.
18. Van Velzen D, Krishnan KR, Parsons KF, et al. Epidermal growth factor receptor in the vesical urothelium of paraplegic and tetraplegic patients: an immuno-histochemical study. Spinal Cord 1996;34:578–586.
19. Gonzalez-Ariki S, Husband AJ. The role of sympathetic innervation of the gut in regulating mucosal immune responses. Brain Behav Immun 1998;12:53–63.
20. Vaidyanathan S, McDicken IW, Soni BM, et al. Secretory immunoglobulin A in the vesical urothelium of patients with neuropathic bladder – an immunohistochemical study. Spinal Cord 2000;38:378–381.
21. Konety BR, Nguyen TS, Brenes G, et al. Clinical usefulness of the novel marker BLCA-4 for the detection of bladder cancer. J Urol 2000;164(3 Pt 1):634–639.

22. Alipov GK, Ito M, Nakashima M, et al. Expression of parathyroid hormone-related peptide (PTHrP) in gastric tumours. J Pathol 1997;182:174–179.

23. Vaidyanathan S, McDicken IW, Mansour P, et al. Parathyroid hormone-related protein (1–34) and urothelial redifferentiation in the neuropathic urinary bladder. Spinal Cord 2000;38:546–551.

24. Young RH. Papillary and polypoid cystitis: a report of eight cases. Am J Surg Pathol 1988;12:542–546.

25. Janzen J, Vuong PN, Bersch U, Michel D, Zaech GA. Bladder tissue biopsies in spinal cord injured patients: histopathologic aspects of 61 cases. Neurourol Urodyn 1998;17:525–530.

26. Delnay KM, Stonehill WH, Goldman H, Jukkola AF, Dmochowski RR. Bladder histological changes associated with chronic indwelling urinary catheter. J Urol 1999;161:1106–1108.

27. Mitsui T, Minami K, Furuno T, Morita H, Koyanagi T. Is suprapubic cystostomy an optimal urinary management in high quadriplegics? A comparative study of suprapubic cystostomy and clean intermittent catheterization. Eur Urol 2000;38:434–438.

28. West DA, Cummings JM, Longo WE, et al. Role of chronic catheterisation in the development of bladder cancer in patients with spinal cord injury. Urology 1999;53:292–297.

29. Harnden P, Southgate J. Cytokeratin 14 as a marker of squamous differentiation in transitional cell carcinomas. J Clin Pathol 1997;50:1032–1033.

30. Cheng L, Cheville JC, Neumann RM, Bostwick DG. Natural history of urothelial dysplasia of the bladder. Am J Surg Pathol 1999;23:443–447.

31. Harnden P, Eardley I, Joyce AD, Southgate J. Cytokeratin 20 as an objective marker of urothelial dysplasia. Br J Urol 1996;78:870–875.

32. Lancelin F, Anidjar M, Villette JM, et al. Telomerase activity as a potential marker in preneoplastic bladder lesions. BJU Int 2000;85:526–531.

33. Schaafsma RJ, Delaere KP, Theunissen PH. Squamous cell carcinoma of suprapubic cystostomy tract without bladder involvement. Spinal Cord 1999;37:373–374.

34. King DH, Barber DB, Farley NJ, Harris JM, Able AC. Mucinous adenocarcinoma arising from a suprapubic cystostomy site without bladder involvement. J Spinal Cord Med 1997;20:244–246.

19

UROTHELIAL PATHOLOGY FOLLOWING RECONSTRUCTIVE BLADDER SURGERY

Arnulf Stenzl and Hermann Rogatsch

CURRENT PRACTICE IN BLADDER SUBSTITUTION

More than a hundred years have passed since pioneer surgeons reported their first experiences with intestinal urinary diversion and reservoirs. Since then, numerous techniques and technical modifications have been introduced using various segments of the gastrointestinal tract. Apparently, however, urologists were not able completely to eradicate problems related to the use of bowel for urine storage. Complications continue to be reported from the donor site with regard to reduced bowel length, altered bowel motility and nutritional deficiencies[1-4] as well as from the gastrointestinal reservoirs in contact with urine.[5,6] An increasingly long-term follow-up is apparently responsible for reports about neoplastic changes in intestinal urinary reservoirs,[7-9] although the overall rate in any form of continent or non-continent diversion is not comparable to those seen with ureterosigmoidostomies.[10]

Reported long-term data of a single center looking at their 25-year experience in the management of more than 1300 patients with invasive bladder cancer by radical cystectomy regarding tumor progression and survival were superior to those where a multimodality organ-sparing treatment for advanced bladder neoplasms was attempted.[11,12] Even in patients older than 70 years[13] or in those with previous or planned adjuvant chemo- and/or radiation therapy,[14] an aggressive, curative, radical surgical approach with an orthotopic or continent cutaneous form of diversion is a viable treatment option leading to a 65% 5-year survival rate and a 92% continence rate in the elderly patient group.

An increasing number of radical cystectomies in recent years led to a growing desire for appliance-free urinary diversions to improve quality of life and body image. The results show that 96% and 79% of patients with orthotopic neobladders resume their daily living activities and occupational status, respectively, and that 85% are totally continent day and night while the remainder seem to manage a partial incontinence well with pads.[15,16] Continence as reported by these authors was by far better for the neobladder group than for the cutaneous continent diversions (85% versus 61%). Patients with continent cutaneous diversions when compared to wet stomas seem to respond almost equally positively, showing signs of enhanced vitality.[17] Recent studies assessing quality of life using validated questionnaires further demonstrated patients' preference for an orthotopic reservoir over a heterotopic diversion.[16,18]

ORTHOTOPIC NEOBLADDER

Orthotopic neobladders are the most natural way to reconstruct the urinary bladder. An increasing number of reports dealing with median-term experiences with ureterointestinal urethrostomy give us more information on how to select and follow patients, and how to reduce peri- and postoperative morbidity.[19]

As noted above, there is in some series a higher continence rate seen with orthotopic neobladders than with cutaneous continent diversions.[16] Continence rates of neobladders have increased in recent years and range (for both male and female patients followed for more than 6 months) between 80 and 90%. In some patients, however, diurnal or nocturnal incontinence will persist despite extensive conservative management. Turner et al., when looking at the factors influencing continence, found that autonomic nerve preservation – apart from enhancing potency – significantly improved postoperative continence.[20] Whether this is due to the meticulous dissection of the prostatic apex or whether the preserved autonomic nerves increase the tonus of the smooth musculature is unclear, but the results favor nerve preservation for patients where this can be safely done from an oncologic standpoint. Another factor influencing postoperative continence may be better patient selection using more refined imaging techniques such as transurethral ultrasound.[21]

Different visualization parameters on three-dimensional (3D) computerized tomography using various parameters and software techniques enable the illustration of the outline and position of neobladders and adjacent organs over time.[22] At 12 months postoperatively, 3D studies usually showed a spheroid,

bladder-like configuration of the urinary reservoir that was more or less centered in the pelvis in two-thirds of patients with an orthotopic neobladder. With 3D animation effects, an endoscopic fly-through effect not only of the pouch but also of the efferent ileal limb and ureters was possible.[23] Video sequences with these animation effects were created and became useful to demonstrate the technique of ureteroileal urethrostomy to students, nurses and patients.

Anatomy of the urethra in neobladder patients

With regard to the 'ends' to which the new pouch is anastomosed, the features of the anatomies of the male and female urethras and urethral sphincters must be taken into account in optimizing outcome. The male urethral sphincter is not a simple ring structure but is more or less 'omega-shaped'.[24] For surgery this means that adoption of a more cranial approach rather than dissecting at the prostatic apex can help to preserve some of the rhabdosphincter. When performing radical cystectomy it may be possible to preserve some of the intrinsic sphincter by careful dissection at the prostatic apex.

In the female patient, care should be taken when performing a cystectomy regarding neurovascular structures of the urethra. Previous studies have shown that the autonomic nerves supplying the smooth musculature of the urethra course from the hypogastric nerve plexus located dorsolaterally to the rectum distally close to the distal ureters, the lateral vaginal walls and the bladder neck.[25] Care should therefore be taken to preserve the lateral vaginal walls and carefully to 'peel out' the bladder neck and proximal urethra down to the level of its dissection.[26] Transverse vaginal reconstruction may be beneficial not only in young women who wish to remain sexually active but also in older women as the insertion of electrical devices for sphincter training is easier.[27]

Female orthotopic neobladders

During the last decade, neobladders in male patients have proven to enhance quality of life, whereas concepts regarding orthotopic urinary diversion in women with pelvic tumors have started to change only recently. This would not have been possible without meticulous anatomic and pathologic studies of the female urethra. The anatomic studies of Colleselli et al.[25] on the female urethral sphincter with regard to its morphology as well as the surrounding neural and pelvic floor structures have been the basis for several clinical reports.[28–31] It was demonstrated that the rhabdosphincter of the female urethra is preserved even if the bladder neck and a short segment of proximal urethra are removed during cystectomy. The majority of autonomous plexus fibers to the urethra should be preserved by careful dissection of the bladder neck and cranial urethra. This is an anatomic confirmation of the clinical experience of recent years that urinary continence of any bladder substitution in females can be maintained despite complete removal of the bladder neck because no prominent sphincteric structure is present in the female bladder neck.

Clinical series comprising female patients with orthotopic neobladders (in the majority due to bladder neoplasms) revealed results comparable to those obtained in male neobladder series. A complete daytime and night-time continence of 88% and 79–82%, respectively, was reported in the two largest series,[30,31] with a total of 64 patients followed for up to 70 months (median 30 months in one series). In this combined series, 6 of 64 patients (10%) required some form of intermittent catheterization – in the majority once in the morning or evening – to empty their neobladder completely.

A continent orthotopic ileal neobladder has also been reported in a female renal transplant patient[32] and has been performed as an undiversion in a female patient who had undergone prior cystectomy and cutaneous urinary diversion.[33] Old doctrines claiming that orthotopic neobladders are indicated only in male patients[34] therefore had to be reconsidered. Consequently, when counseling female patients for cystectomy, an orthotopic neobladder must be offered as an option of bladder reconstruction.

REMNANT URETHRA IN THE MALE

Several authors either suggested[35] or strongly recommended[36,37] urethrectomy in conjunction with radical cystectomy for bladder cancer. However, in recent years orthotopic reconstruction of the lower urinary tract has gained popularity with both patients and doctors,[38] which precludes a simultaneous prophylactic urethrectomy at the time of cystectomy.

Incidence of secondary urethral tumor

The reported incidence of secondary urethral tumors in patients with bladder cancer is diverging. This is in part due to the fact that this problem has been examined under various aspects. Gowing,[39] for example, autopsied patients who died with bladder cancer and found in 6 of 33 autopsies (18%) carcinoma in situ (CIS). On the other hand, most of the other authors looked at urethral tumor recurrences after radical cystoprostatectomy. They found urethral recurrences in around 10% of the patients and usually suggested a generous decision to perform primary prophylactic urethrectomy.[40]

Ashworth's series on 1307 patients with bladder tumors[41] was, for many years, the only report available where concomitant urethral tumors were related to the total number of cases treated for bladder cancer at the same institution. Out of 914 male patients with papillomatous lesions or solid tumor, 50 (5.4%) had urethral tumors which were preferentially treated by fulguration.

The most recent and largest retrospective study dealing with secondary urethral tumor occurrences in bladder tumors also deals with the incidence of urethral tumors in the overall population of patients treated for bladder cancer.[42] The majority of these patients (96.8%) were treated conservatively, i.e. without major surgery or radiation, thus allowing assessment of the incidence of urethral tumors of patients with primary and recurrent bladder tumors of all stages. A 6.1% overall incidence of urethral tumors found in this study was similar to several other studies dealing with this subject[41,43–47] (Table 19.1). A significant difference was evident between those patients where a solitary transitional cell carcinoma (TCC) occurred in the bladder for the first time (2.6%) and those with recurrent multifocal cancer (10.1%, Table 19.2). This may be a factor in the decision-making process, as to whether an orthotopic neobladder is prudent or whether a synchronous urethrectomy should be performed.

In the same study, only 17 of 87 patients with bladder cancer and concomitant urethral cancer treated endoscopically had recurrences in the urethra. Transurethral resection and/or fulguration may therefore be seen as a possible method of treatment for superficial papillary TCC in the urethra.

Radical surgery and orthotopic neobladder

Those patients which, according to their clinical staging, would nowadays be good candidates for radical surgery with the option of an orthotopic neobladder were also identified in the study by Erckert et al.[42] Patients with a clinically staged T2–3 N0, M0 TCC had a lower rate (4.2%) of urethral tumor occurrence than

Table 19.1 Review of the literature with documented cases of bladder cancer with urethral tumor involvement

Reference	Study period	No. of bladder tumor events	No. of urethral tumor events (%)	No. of bladder neck tumors	CIS in the bladder
Ashworth[41]	1946–54	1307	54 (4.1)	?	?
Levinson et al.[63]	1969–76	324	12 (3.7)	65	22
Hardeman & Soloway[50]	1975–87	102	14 (13.7)	37	20
Schellhammer & Whitmore[37]	1961–73	461	32 (7.2)	?	5
Beahrs et al.[43]	1965–74	349	28 (8)	?	?
Stöckle et al.[35]	1967–87	251	23 (9.2)	?	21
Tongaonkar et al.[28]	1981–90	177	15 (8.5)	35	?
Cordonnier & Spjut[44]	1953–60	174	7 (4)	?	2
Raz et al.[45]	1955–76	174	10 (5.4)	3	?
Zabbo & Montie[46]	1960–79	119	7 (5.9)	?	27
Hickey et al.[61]	1976–85	75	7 (10)	?	16
Faysal[47]	1963–77	59	8 (13.5)	1	6
Gowing[39]	?	33	6 (18)	?	6
Erckert et al.[42]	1969–94	2052	126 (6.1)	104	116
Total		5657	349 (6.2)		

?, no data given.

CIS, carcinoma in situ.

Table 19.2 Frequency of urethral tumors among primary versus recurrent and solitary versus multifocal bladder tumors*

Characteristic of tumor	No. of urethral tumors	Percentage
Primary unilocular	10	2.6
Recurrent unilocular	22	4.1
Primary multifocal	27	5.8
Recurrent multifocal	67	10.1

* 910 men with bladder cancer observed at a single institution over a period of 25 years.
Adapted from Erckert et al.[42]

the average 6.1% of the whole study group. If all node-positive patients (N0–2) were included in this group, the urethral tumor rate was still 4.3%. A tendency towards solitary primary tumors, a more aggressive initial therapy, and a decreased life expectancy resulting in shorter follow-up times may account for the lower urethral tumor rate in this group.[48,49]

CIS/papillary tumors after orthotopic neobladder

Another aspect is the occurrence of CIS or papillary tumors in the remaining urethra after an orthotopic neobladder. Contrary to other authors,[50–52] Erckert et al.[42] did not see an increased risk of urethral tumors in patients with CIS of the bladder. This may in part be due to the fact that dysplasia or CIS of the urethra may have been missed in conservatively treated patients. One might argue, however, that clinically important dysplasia or CIS left untreated, or treated conservatively and followed up long-term, would eventually result in overt and clinically important urethral cancer.

Urethral recurrence in heterotopic versus orthotopic urinary diversions

In most of the older studies, urethral recurrence is defined as tumor in the remnant, blind-ending urethra.[53] Apart from a longer follow-up there might have been other contributing factors responsible for a considerably higher incidence of secondary urethral tumors than that observed with the functioning remnant urethra

Table 19.3 Review of the literature regarding incidence of urethral tumor recurrence and time interval after cystoprostatectomy for bladder cancer

Reference	No. of patients	No. of urethral tumor recurrences (%)	Interval to recurrence
Steven & Poulsen[104]	166	2 (1.2)	n.g.
Slaton et al.[105]	210	4 (1.9)	median 15 months
Lebret et al.[106]	106*	0 (0)	N/A
Robert et al.[107]	185	8 (4.3)	6–36 months
Freeman et al.[40]	436:	34 (7.7):	
	174 (Neo)	5 (2.9)	median 2.3 years
	262 (HUD)	29 (11.1)	median 1.6 years
Freeman et al.[53] †	2062	208 (10.1)	mostly in the first 5 years

* Cystoprostatectomies with negative urethral margins on frozen sections; † review of 18 studies. HUD, heterotopic urinary diversion; Neo, Kock ileal neobladder; N/A, not applicable; n.g., no data given.

connected to a neobladder (Table 19.3). It may be speculated that scarring, chronic inflammation with certain *Escherichia coli* strains, absence of cancer-preventing properties of the urine, and a lack of careful follow-up may play a role. The only larger study comparing urethral recurrence in orthotopic and heterotopic diversions did reveal a significant advantage for orthotopic neobladders independent from the length of follow-up in each group.[40]

The outcome of patients with TCC in the prostatic urethra and/or parenchyma (Fig. 19.1) was assessed in two large studies. Freeman et al.[40] looked at 436 patients undergoing cystectomy and either a heterotopic or orthotopic urinary diversion. They demonstrated the highest probability of urethral recurrence in patients with invasive prostatic TCC followed by superficial TCC. Despite prostatic TCC, however, urethral recurrence was 5% in orthotopic neobladder patients versus 24% in patients with a blind-ending urethra after heterotopic urinary diversion. Iselin et al. looked at urethral recurrence in 70 men with prostatic TCC undergoing radical cystectomy for bladder cancer with a mean follow-up of 35 months.[54] The overall urethral recurrence rate was 3%. None of the patients with prostatic TCC in the cystectomy specimen died secondary to a urethral recurrence. The results presented are in line with other data in the literature,[55] suggesting that orthotopic neobladder reconstruction is not contraindicated in bladder cancer patients with prostatic involvement provided the margins of resection are negative.

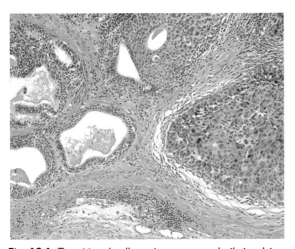

Fig. 19.1 Transitional cell carcinoma secondarily involving the prostate. There is expansion of the prostatic ducts by tumor cells (right). Note the preservation of the prostatic secretory cell layer (top).

REMNANT URETHRA IN THE FEMALE

Few data exist about urethral involvement in women with bladder cancer. The older literature concentrated on urethral tumor involvement of male patients with bladder cancer, and female cases are only rarely discussed. In a large cystoscopy study, Ashworth[41] found urethral tumor involvement in 1.4% of female patients compared to 4.1% of male patients presenting with bladder cancer. In a more recent report, retrospectively working up 22 female cystectomy specimens obtained over a period of 15 years, a much higher incidence of superficial or invasive urethral tumors was found and a strong argument for routine urethrectomy in all female patients with bladder cancer was made.[56] However, no details about the total number of women with bladder cancer treated during this period, the tumor sites in bladder and urethra in patients subject to study, or the number and type(s) of treatment prior to cystectomy were given in this study.

Numbers in many studies dealing with concomitant urethral tumors or urethral recurrence in patients with bladder cancer have been small and any conclusions or at least a trend for female patients has not been possible.[36,39,44,50,51,57] There has been focused interest, however, in data concerning the risk of secondary urethral tumors in female bladder cancer patients undergoing surgery.[58–60] If an adequate segment of the caudal urethra could be spared at cystectomy with a minimal risk of tumor recurrence, it might be used for continent orthotopic reconstruction of the lower urinary tract similar to that performed in male patients. Until recently no data existed in the literature about risk factors for urethral involvement in female bladder cancer patients.

Ashworth[41] found urethral tumors in 1.4% of 293 female patients presenting with bladder cancer in contrast to 4.1% of 1307 male patients. Until then this had been the only study that used a large, more or less unselected, female bladder cancer population for the study of urethral bladder tumor involvement. In a more recent study,[61] urethral tumor involvement was confirmed as being 2% in female patients with biopsy-proven bladder cancer of all grades and stages. The mean follow-up was 5.5 years.

Incidence of secondary urethral tumor

One of the reasons for the apparent lower incidence of secondary urethral tumors in females in comparison to males[35,42] may be the fact that transitional cell mucosa covers a much smaller urethral segment in females, whereas the rest is normal or metaplastic squamous cell mucosa. The area at risk in the female urethra is therefore small, and probably even diminishes with increasing age, because the demarcation line between squamous and transitional cell mucosa moves cephalad in the menopause.[62] In the sixth and seventh decades, when most of the bladder tumors occur, metaplastic squamous cell mucosa may cover the whole urethra, bladder neck and at times even a portion of the trigone.

Involvement of the bladder neck

The fact that tumor involvement of the bladder neck and prostatic urethra is a possible predictor for synchronous or recurrent urethral tumors in male patients has been shown by several authors.[35,50,63] Most recent reports also describe a close coincidence between tumor involvement of the bladder neck and urethra in females.[58–60] In these studies there was no urethral bladder cancer involvement without concurrent tumor involvement at the bladder neck, resulting in a statistically highly significance (Table 19.4). There was also a significant correlation between the primary tumor location in the trigone and concomitant urethral tumors, but only if the bladder neck was involved as well. In an unselected study of 356 female patients with different stages of bladder tumor followed for up to 33 years,[60] the incidence of urethral tumor involvement was 2% for the whole study group, 3.1% for a subgroup of invasive (T2–4) TCC, and 1% for localized (T2–3b, N0, M0) invasive cancer amenable to radical cystectomy. None of the patients with recurrent bladder tumors, whether progressing or not, had overt urethral

Table 19.4 Correlation of the location of primary bladder tumors with urethral tumor involvement in 356 patients (442 tumour locations in the bladder and 7 in the urethra due to solitary and multilocular tumors)

Location	No. of patients at specific location	Secondary urethral tumors	Percentage	p-value
Vault	35	1	2.8	0.77
Right bladder wall	89	1	1.1	0.51
Left bladder wall	96	1	1.0	0.39
Posterior bladder wall	121	1	0.8	0.18
Trigone	65	4	6.5	0.035
Bladder neck	36	7	19.4	0.000

Adapted from Stenzl et al.[60]

Table 19.5 Characteristics of seven patients with primary bladder cancer and urethral tumor involvement

Patient	Age (years)	Histo.	Stage	N/M	Grade	Solit.	Prim.	Locat.	Rx	F/U
1	73	Adeno	T3b	–/–	3	yes	yes	BN	Rad.	8
2	68	TCC	Ta	–/–	2	no	yes	V, BN	TUR	24
3	63	TCC	T4	+/–	3	no	yes	L, BN	Rad. + Chem.	30
4	87	Adeno	T4	no data	3	yes	yes	T, BN	Rad.	2
5	63	TCC	T2	+/+	3	no	yes	T, BN	Rad.	12
6	69	TCC	Ta	–/–	2	no	yes	P, R, T, BN	TUR	60
7	62	TCC	T3b	–/+	3	yes	yes	T, BN	Chem.	14

Adeno, adenocarcinoma; BN, bladder neck; Chem., chemotherapy; F/U, follow-up in months; L, left lateral wall; Locat., location within the bladder in addition to urethra; N/M, + positive or – negative lymph nodes/metastases; P, posterior wall; Prim., primary versus recurrent tumor(s) in the bladder; R, right lateral wall; Rad., radiation; Rx, treatment other than transurethral biopsy/resection of the tumor; Solit., solitary versus multiple tumor locations; T, trigone; TCC, transitional cell carcinoma; TUR, transurethral resection; V, vault.

Adapted from Stenzl et al.[60]

tumor at any of the recurrences over the years. There was no correlation between urethral cancer and any other prognostic factor: stage, multicentricity, number of tumors, presence of CIS or duration of the disease did not appear to play a predominant role (Table 19.5).

From these data one may conclude that female patients without tumor either at the bladder neck or at frozen section of the proximal urethra at the time of cystectomy can probably be spared a portion of the urethra to enable lower urinary reconstruction to the urethra without running a greater risk of developing recurrent urethral tumors than their selected male counterparts.

Reviewing the literature we found 32 cases of documented urethral tumor involvement, including CIS (Fig. 19.2), in female patients with bladder cancer (Table 19.6). The overall incidence according to this table would be 4% (32 out of 794 patients). With two exceptions, however, all authors used a highly selected group of only those patients undergoing cystectomy. The actual number of women seen and treated for all stages of bladder cancer at any of these institutions should have been higher than just an average of two cases per year. In order to obtain an overall urethral involvement rate for female bladder cancer patients it is therefore misleading to use percentages only out of the total number of cystectomized patients at a time when only a few patients had exenteration for highly advanced bladder tumors.

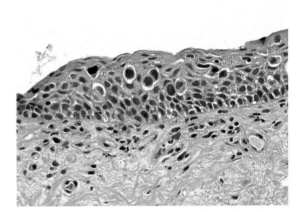

Fig. 19.2 Pagetoid intramucosal spread of urothelial carcinoma in the female urethra.

Radical surgery and orthotopic neobladder

Several biopsies of the bladder neck should be performed in those patients where a subtotal urethrectomy is considered.[64] Any woman with a finding of atypia or overt tumor at the bladder neck is at risk for developing recurrent urethral tumor after cystectomy and should therefore undergo simultaneous total urethrectomy. However, those patients in whom curative radical cystectomy is indicated and who are good candidates for an orthotopic reconstruction of the lower urinary tract

Table 19.6 Review of the literature with documented cases of urethral tumor involvement or carcinoma in situ in female patients with bladder cancer

Reference	Study period	No. of patients	BN tumors	Urethral tumors	CIS	Tumors + CIS
Riches & Cullen[57]	n.g.	19*	3	3	–	3
Ashworth[41]	n.g.	293	n.g.	4	–	4
Richie & Skinner[51]	1969–71	21*	n.g.	–	1	1
Coutts et al.[36]	1974–83	18*	n.g.	2	1	3
De Paepe et al.[56]	1974–88	22*	n.g.	5	3	8
Stein et al.[59]	1982–92	65*	16	7	–	7
Stenzl et al.[60]	1973–92	356	49	6	–	6
Total		794		27 (3.4%)	5	32 (4%)

* Heterogeneously selected bladder cancer study populations.
BN, bladder neck; CIS, carcinoma in situ; n.g., no data given.
Adapted from Stenzl et al.[60]

may be spared a segment of the urethra for that purpose provided that preoperative biopsies of the bladder neck and frozen section of the urethra at the time of surgery are free of atypia or tumor.

Based on these pathologic studies and anatomic data of the continence mechanism of the female urethra, clinical protocols offering an ureteroileal urethrostomy to carefully selected female patients undergoing radical cystectomy for localized bladder cancer was initiated at several centers.[28,29,65–68] Their preliminary data and subsequent reports have been promising and have led to an increase in the number of centers where orthotopic neobladders are performed.[34] However, the urethra – or a portion of it – should not be left in unless it is used for reconstructive purposes, because it can easily be removed en bloc with the bladder specimen and it is difficult to follow oncologically when left in as a blind-ending sac.

Risk factors for urethral tumor occurrence

In conclusion, the incidence of urethral tumors in primary or recurrent bladder cancer in long-term studies is approximately 6% for male and 2% for female patients. Risk factors for urethral tumor occurrence are tumors at the bladder neck and recurrent multifocal tumors. CIS of the bladder not involving the bladder neck, and muscle-invasive tumors with or without lymph node involvement, are not significantly correlated with urethral cancer. Those patients at risk for urethral tumors should be worked up more carefully

(multiple urethral biopsies and/or urethral brushings, frozen section of the membranous urethra) before an orthotopic urinary diversion to the urethra is considered. The majority of patients with urethral tumors in our study group had a single conservative treatment session, and did not suffer any recurrence thereafter. A conservative approach for superficial urethral tumor recurrences in patients with an orthotopic neobladder to the urethra may therefore be feasible.

UPPER URINARY TRACT AFTER INTESTINAL BLADDER SUBSTITUTION

Undoubtedly enormous progress has been achieved since Simon's first report in the middle of the 19th century about ureteral diversion into the rectum by creating a fistula with the help of a silk thread. Subsequently, several techniques have been developed to restore continuity between the upper urinary tract and the reconstructed lower urinary tract which have helped to reduce the long-term morbidity and complication rate of intestinal urinary diversion.[69]

The advent of continent pouches put the upper urinary tract at increased risk due to intermittent pressure peaks within the reservoir. Long-term results in ureterosigmoidostomy[70,71] and ileal and colonic conduits[72–74] showed that reflux to the pelvicaliceal system, at times combined with infected urine, led to renal deterioration. Reflux, in contrast to obstruction, tends to damage the renal parenchyma at the poles.[75]

Experimental studies demonstrated that reflux nephropathy develops with concave or flat papillae due to the right-angle opening of Bellini's ducts, whereas convex papillae seem to be more resistant to reflux due to the oblique aperture of the ducts into the calyces.[76] This may explain the irregular patterns of intrarenal changes seen in patients with urinary diversion and reflux with or without additional obstruction.

Various techniques imitating the natural ureterovesical valve system have been suggested. Whereas antireflux protection could be achieved on the one hand, on the other stricture and functional stenosis occurred in some patients leading again to renal deterioration.[77–81]

Antireflux mechanisms

Orthotopic neobladders usually carry a lower risk of high-pressure development in the reservoir at maximal filling because of the limits of the urethral sphincter system. This prompted some authors to suggest that only a low-pressure antireflux mechanism was necessary in sphincter-controlled orthotopic bladder substitution. On the other hand, a simple, easy to learn, and time- and gastrointestinal tract-sparing method of connecting the native ureters to the pouch was sought.[82,83] Direct antirefluxive implantation of the ureters into the intestinal pouch, however, necessitates preservation of a great part of the distal ureters. This may compromise vascularization to an extent that distal ischemia and ureterointestinal stricture ensues.

Several authors suggested a tubular ileal segment to bridge the distance between the level of ureteral dissection and intestinal reservoir.[84–87] Whether an isoperistaltic tubular segment of ileum of certain length is sufficient for antireflux protection in orthotopic neobladders or whether a more sophisticated valve system is necessary is still a matter of debate.

Incidence and risk factors

The incidence of upper urinary tract tumors secondary to primary bladder cancer lies around 2–4%.[88–90] There is a higher risk in patients with multiple recurrences of superficial Ta or T1 tumors.[91] The incidence of upper tract tumors following cystectomy and urinary diversion has been reported as 2.4–17.4%[88,92–100] (Table 19.7). In our own series we have seen an incidence of 3% (3 of 89 patients). Multifocality, CIS and other superficial tumors in the bladder were considered risk factors in some series whereas a report from the Memorial Sloan-Kettering Cancer Center[99] put those patients with locally advanced tumor stage at a higher risk. Most likely tumor invasion of the intramural ureter, CIS in the distal ureter and/or the frozen section of the dissected ureter are additional risk factors. The median time between cystectomy and diagnosis of upper tract tumor lies between 8 and 69 months in most series, but upper tract cancer recurrences more than 10 years after cystectomy have been observed. A tendency for a higher incidence can be seen in those series with longer follow-up. A longer observation period in larger numbers of patients with an orthotopic neobladder and longer survival rates in general after cystectomy may therefore reveal an increase in the incidence of upper tract tumors over the next decade.

Table 19.7 Review of the literature regarding upper tract recurrences after cystectomy for bladder cancer			
Reference	No. of patients	No. of upper tract recurrences (%)	Interval to recurrence (months)
Balaji et al.[99]	529	16 (3)	median 37.2
Slaton et al.[105]	382	9 (2.4)	median 25
Solsona et al.[97]	179*	7 (3.9)	mean 28.3
	46†	8 (17.4)	mean 18.3
Tsuji et al.[98]	61	4 (6.5)	mean 69
Kenworthy et al.[93]	430	11 (2.6)	median 40
Schwartz et al.[90]	638	20 (3.1)	mean 8
Hastie et al.[92]	180	10 (5.5)	mean 44
Malkowicz & Skinner[94]	220	5 (2.4)	22–54
Zincke et al.[88]	425	14 (3.3)	mean 40

* Following cystectomy due to invasive bladder cancer; † following cystectomy due to bladder Tis.

Diagnosis and management

Most of the upper tract tumors in patients with urinary diversion are diagnosed following symptoms such as flank pain, macrohematuria or a positive cytology. A routine radiologic assessment of the upper urinary tract may not be worthwhile due to its poor detection rate according to this series.[99] Open surgical removal of the involved upper urinary tract was the preferred method of treatment, but successful management of the tumors by endourologic and conservative treatment has been reported.[100,101]

Suspicion of an upper tract recurrence in neobladder patients not clearly visible on radiographic examination, or small superficial tumors amenable to endourologic treatment, are usually a dilemma for the treating physician. Access to the upper urinary tract for diagnostic and therapeutic purposes is generally not easy in neobladder patients due to the antireflux valve, difficulties in localizing the ureteral neo-orifice(s), or the type and angle of the ureteroileal anastomosis.

A variation of the technique of the original T-pouch has been suggested to overcome these problems.[102] The T-pouch already has a wide, visible orifice of the tapered afferent segment in the pouch, which makes its localization and catheterization much easier compared with other forms of neo-orifices in neobladders.[103] Instead of an end-to-side ureteroileal anastomosis, the end-to-end Wallace-type anastomosis with the same preparation and coverage of periureteral adventitial tissue as described above was applied.[104,105] This facilitates retrograde catheterization and insertion of ureteroscopes should a diagnostic workup and/or treatment of upper tract tumors, strictures, etc. become necessary.[106] It may also enable the management of complicated upper tract urolithiasis without percutaneous nephrostomy.

REFERENCES

1. N'Dow J, Leung HY, Marshall C, Neal DE. Bowel dysfunction after bladder reconstruction. J Urol 1998;159(5):1470–1474, discussion 1474–1475.

2. Wood GA, Heathcote PS, Nicol DL. Bowel motility after enterocystoplasty. Br J Urol 1998;81:565–568.

3. Kalloo NB, Jeffs RD, Gearhart JP. Long-term nutritional consequences of bowel segment use for lower urinary tract reconstruction in pediatric patients. Urology 1997;50(6):967–971.

4. Racioppi M, D'Addessi A, Fanasca A, et al. Vitamin B12 and folic acid plasma levels after ileocecal and ileal neobladder reconstruction. Urology 1997;50(6):888–892.

5. Mansson W, Bakke A, Bergman B, et al. Perforation of continent urinary reservoirs – Scandinavian experience. Scand J Urol Nephrol 1997;32:70–72.

6. Palmer LS, Palmer JS, Firlit BM, Firlit CF. Recurrent urolithiasis after augmentation gastrocystoplasty. J Urol 1998;159:1331–1332.

7. Albertini JJ, Sujka SK, Helal MA, Seigne JD, Lockhart JL. Adenocarcinoma in a continent colonic urinary reservoir. Urology 1998;51(3):499–500.

8. Ahlstrand C, Herder A. Primary adenocarcinoma of distal ileum used as outlet from a right colonic urinary reservoir. Scand J Urol Nephrol 1998;32:70–72.

9. Malone MJ, Izes JK, Hurley LJ. Carcinogenesis. The fate of intestinal segments used in urinary reconstruction. Urol Clin North Am 1997;24(4):723–728.

10. Gittes RF. Carcinogenesis in ureterosigmoidostomy. Urol Clin North Am 1986;13:201.

11. Skinner DG, Stein JP, Lieskovsky G, et al. 25-year experience in the management of invasive bladder cancer by radical cystectomy. Eur Urol 1998;33(Suppl. 4):25–26.

12. Shipley U, Kaufman DS, Heney NM, Althausen AF, Zietman AL. An update of selective bladder preservation by combined modality therapy for invasive bladder cancer. Eur Urol 1998;33(Suppl. 4):32–34.

13. Figueroa A, Stein JP, Dickinson M, et al. Radical cystectomy for elderly patients with bladder carcinoma. Cancer 1998;83:141–147.

14. Ward AM, Olencki T, Peerboom D, Klein EA. Should continent diversion be performed in patients with locally advanced bladder cancer? Urology 1998;51(2):232–236.

15. Lee KT, Li MK, Cheng WS, Foo KT. The impact of a modified ileal neobladder on the lifestyle and voiding patterns in Asian patients. Br J Urol 1998;81:705–708.

16. Weijerman PC, Schurmans JR, Hop WC, Schroder FH, Bosch JL. Morbidity and quality of life in patients with orthotopic and heterotopic continent urinary diversion. Urology 1998;51(1):51–56.

17. Gerharz EW, Weingartner K, Dopatka T, et al. Quality of life after cystectomy and urinary diversion: results of a retrospective interdisciplinary study. J Urol 1997;158(3 Pt 1):778–785.

18. Hobisch A, Tosun K, Kienzel J, et al. Morbidity and quality of life after cystectomy and orthotopic neobladder versus ileum conduit: long term follow-up. Eur Urol 1999;35(Suppl. 2):62.

19. Studer UE, Zingg EJ. Ileal orthotopic bladder substitutes. What we have learned from 12 years' experience with 200 patients. Urol Clin North Am 1997;24(4):781–793.

20. Turner WH, Danuser H, Moehrle K, Studer UE. The effect of nerve sparing cystectomy technique on postoperative continence after orthotopic bladder substitution. J Urol 1997;158(6):2118–2122.

21. Strasser H, Frauscher F, Helweg G, et al. Transurethral ultrasound: evaluation of anatomy and function of the rhabdosphincter of the male urethra. J Urol 1998;159(1):100–104, discussion 104–105.

22. Frank R, Stenzl A, Frede T, et al. Three-dimensional computed tomography of the reconstructed lower urinary tract: technique and findings. Eur Radiol 1998;8(4):657–663.

23. Stenzl A, Frank R, Eder R, et al. 3-Dimensional computerized tomography and virtual reality endoscopy of the reconstructed lower urinary tract. J Urol 1998;159(3):741–746.

24. Strasser H, Ninkovic M, Hess M, Bartsch G, Stenzl A. Anatomical and functional studies of the male and female urethral sphincter. World J Urol 2000;18:324–329.

25. Colleselli K, Stenzl A, Eder R, et al. The female urethral sphincter: a morphological and topographical study. J Urol 1998;160(1):49–54.

26. Stenzl A, Colleselli K, Poisel S, et al. Rationale and technique of nerve sparing radical cystectomy before an orthotopic neobladder procedure in women. J Urol 1995;154(6):2044–2049.

27. Stenzl A, Colleselli K, Bartsch G. Update of urethra-sparing approaches in cystectomy in women. World J Urol 1997;15(1):134–138.

28. Tongaonkar H, Dala A, Kulkarni J, Kamat M. Urethral recurrences following radical cystectomy for transitional cell carcinoma of the bladder. Br J Urol 1993;72:910–914.

29. Stein J, Stenzl A, Esrig D, et al. Lower urinary tract reconstruction following cystectomy in women using the Kock ileal reservoir with bilateral ureteroileal urethrostomy: initial clinical experience. J Urol 1994;152:1404–1408.

30. Stein JP, Grossfeld GD, Freeman JA, et al. Orthotopic lower urinary tract reconstruction in women using the Kock ileal neobladder: updated experience in 34 patients [see comments]. J Urol 1997;158(2):400–405.

31. Stenzl A, Colleselli K, Poisel S, Feichtinger H, Bartsch G. Anterior exenteration with subsequent ureteroileal urethrostomy in females. Anatomy, risk of urethral recurrence, surgical technique, and results. Eur Urol 1998;33(Suppl. 4):18–20.

32. Perabo FG, Schultze-Seemann W. Continent orthotopic ileal neobladder after kidney transplant in a female patient with multifocal transitional cell carcinoma. J Urol 1998;159(5):1635–1636.

33. Stein JP, Ginsberg DA, Grossfield GD, et al. Orthotopic reconstruction in a women following cystectomy and cutaneous urinary diversion – the 1st reported case. Eur Urol 1997;32:499–502.

34. Stenzl A. Editorial comment: Orthotopic reconstruction in a women following cystectomy and cutaneous urinary diversion – the 1st reported case. Eur Urol 1997;32:502.

35. Stöckle M, Gökcebay E, Riedmiller H, Hohenfellner R. Urethral tumor recurrences after radical cystoprostatectomy: the case for primary cystoprostatourethrectomy? J Urol 1990;143:41–43.

36. Coutts A, Grigor K, Fowler J. Urethral dysplasia and bladder cancer in cystectomy specimens. Br J Urol 1985;57:535–541.

37. Schellhammer P, Whitmore W. Urethral meatal carcinoma following cystourethrectomy for bladder carcinoma. J Urol 1976;115:61–64.

38. Skinner DG, Boyd SD, Lieskovsky G, Bennett C, Hopwood B. Lower urinary tract reconstruction following cystectomy: experience and results in 126 patients using the Kock ileal reservoir with bilateral ureteroileal urethrostomy. J Urol 1991;146(3):756–760.

39. Gowing N. Urethral carcinoma associated with cancer of the bladder. Br J Urol 1960;32:428–438.

40. Freeman JA, Tarter TA, Esrig D, et al. Urethral recurrence in patients with orthotopic ileal neobladders. J Urol 1996;156(5):1615–1619.

41. Ashworth A. Papillomatosis of the urethra. Br J Urol 1956;28:3–11.

42. Erckert M, Stenzl A, Falk M, Bartsch G. Incidence of urethral tumor involvement in 910 men with bladder cancer. World J Urol 1996;14(1):3–8.

43. Beahrs J, Fleming T, Zincke H. Risk of local urethral recurrence after radical cystectomy for bladder carcinoma. J Urol 1984;131:264–266.

44. Cordonnier J, Spjut H. Urethral occurrence of bladder carcinoma following cystectomy. J Urol 1962;87(3):398–403.

45. Raz S, McLorie G, Johnson S, Skinner D. Management of the urethra in patients undergoing radical cystectomy for bladder carcinoma. J Urol 1978;120:298–300.

46. Zabbo A, Montie J. Management of the urethra in men undergoing radical cystectomy for bladder cancer. J Urol 1984;131:267–268.

47. Faysal M. Urethrectomy in men with transitional cell carcinoma of the bladder. Urology 1980;16(1):23–26.

48. Skinner D, Lieskovsky G. Contemporary cystectomy with pelvic node dissection compared to preoperative radiation therapy plus cystectomy in management of invasive bladder cancer. J Urol 1984;131:1069–1072.

49. Stöckle M, Alken P, Engelmann U, et al. Radical cystectomy – often too late? Eur Urol 1987;13(6):361–367.

50. Hardeman S, Soloway M. Urethral recurrence following radical cystectomy. J Urol 1990;144:666–669.

51. Richie J, Skinner D. Carcinoma in situ of the urethra associated with bladder carcinoma: the role of urethrectomy. J Urol 1978;119:80–81.

52. Mahadevia P, Koss L, Tar I. Prostatic involvement in bladder cancer. Cancer 1986;58:2096–2102.

53. Freeman JA, Esrig D, Stein JP, Skinner DG. Management of the patient with bladder cancer. Urethral recurrence. Urol Clin North Am 1994;21(4):645–651.

54. Iselin CE, Robertston CN, Webster GD, Vieweg J, Paulson DF. Does prostate transitional cell carcinoma preclude orthotopic bladder reconstruction after radical cystoprostatectomy for bladder cancer. J Urol 1997;158:2123–2126.

55. Stenzl A. Editorial comment: Does prostate transitional cell carcinoma preclude orthotopic bladder reconstruction after radical cystoprostatectomy for bladder cancer? J Urol 1997;158:2126.

56. De Paepe M, André R, Mahadevia P. Urethral involvement in female patients with bladder cancer. A study of 22 cystectomy specimens. Cancer 1990;65:1237–1242.

57. Riches E, Cullen T. Carcinoma of the urethra. J Urol 1951;23:209.

58. Coloby P, Kakizoe T, Tobisu K, Sakamoto M. Urethral involvement in female bladder cancer patients: mapping of 47 consecutive cysto-urethrectomy specimens. J Urol 1994;152:1438–1442.

59. Stein J, Cote R, Freeman J, et al. Lower urinary tract reconstruction in women following cystectomy for pelvic malignancy: a pathologic review of female cystectomy specimens. J Urol 1994;151:304A, abstract 308.

60. Stenzl A, Draxl H, Posch B, et al. The risk of urethral tumors in female bladder cancer: can the urethra be used for orthotopic reconstruction of the lower urinary tract? J Urol 1995;153(3):950–955.

61. Hickey D, Soloway M, Murphy W. Selective urethrectomy following cystoprostatectomy for bladder cancer. J Urol 1986;136:828–830.

62. Packham D. The epithelial lining of the female trigone and urethra. Br J Urol 1971;43:201.

63. Levinson A, Johnson D, Wishnow K. Indications for urethrectomy in an era of continent urinary diversion. J Urol 1990;144:73–75.

64. Stenzl A, Colleselli K, Poisel S, Feichtinger H, Bartsch G. The use of neobladders in women undergoing cystectomy for transitional-cell cancer. World J Urol 1996;14(1):15–21.

65. Hautmann R, Paiss T, de Petriconi R. The ileal neobladder in women: 9 years of experience with 18 patients. J Urol 1996;155:76–81.

66. Cancrini A, de Carli P, Fattahi H, et al. Orthotopic ileal neobladder in female patients after radical cystectomy: 2-year experience. J Urol 1994;153(part 2):956–958.

67. Jarolim L, Babjuk M, Hanus T, Jansky M, Skrivanova V. Female urethra-sparing cystectomy and orthotopic bladder replacement. Eur Urol 1997;31(1):173–177.

68. Tobisu K-I, Coloby P, Fujimoto H, Miutani T, Kakizoe T. An ileal neobladder for a female patient after radical cystectomy to ensure voiding from the urethra: a case report. Jpn J Clin Oncol 1992;22:359–363.

69. Lotheissen G. Ueber Uretertransplantationen. Wiener Klin Wochenschrift 1899;12(36):883–889.

70. Clarke B, Leadbetter W. Ureterosigmoidostomy: collective review of results in 2,897 reported cases. J Urol 1955;73:999–1008.

71. Goodwin WE, Scardino PT. Ureterosigmoidostomy. J Urol 1977;118(1 Pt 2):169–174.

72. Richie JP, Skinner DG. Urinary diversion: the physiological rationale for non-refluxing colonic conduits. Br J Urol 1975;47(3):269–275.

73. Sullivan JW, Grabstald H, Whitmore WF Jr. Complications of ureteroileal conduit with radical cystectomy: review of 336 cases. J Urol 1980;124(6):797–801.

74. Hendren WH, Radopoulos D. Complications of ileal loop and colon conduit urinary diversion. Urol Clin North Am 1983;10(3):451–471.

75. Djurhuus J, Frokiaer J, Christensen L. Renal function considerations in bladder substitution. In: Webster G, Goldwasser B (eds) Urinary Diversion: Scientific Foundations and Clinical Practice. Oxford: ISIS Medical Media, 1995, pp 77–90.

76. Ransley PG. Intrarenal reflux: anatomical, dynamic and radiological studies – part I. Urol Res 1977;5(2):61–69.

77. Roth S, van Ahlen H, Semjonow A, Oberpenning F, Hertle L. Does the success of ureterointestinal implantation in orthotopic bladder substitution depend more on surgeon level of experience or choice of technique? J Urol 1997;157(1):56–60.

78. Shaaban A, Gaballah M, el-Diasty T, Ghoneim M. Urethral controlled bladder substitution: a comparison between the intussuscepted nipple valve and the technique of Le Duc as antireflux procedures. J Urol 1992;148:1156–1161.

79. Studer U. Ileal bladder substitute: antireflux nipple or afferent tubular segment? Eur Urol 1991;20(4):315–326.

80. Flohr P, Hefty R, Paiss T, Hautmann R. The ileal neobladder – updated experience with 306 patients. World J Urol 1996;14(1):22–26.

81. Stein JP, Freeman JA, Esrig D, et al. Complications of the afferent antireflux valve mechanism in the Kock ileal reservoir [see comments]. J Urol 1996;155(5):1579–1584.

82. Le Duc A, Camey M, Teillac P. An original antireflux ureteroileal implantation technique: long-term follow-up. J Urol 1987;137:1156–1158.

83. Sarosdy MF, Rochester M, Feng YP. A new technique for continent urinary diversion. J Urol 1987;137(5):1020–1023.

84. Kock N, Nilson A, Nilsson L. Urinary diversion via a continent ileal reservoir: clinical results in 12 patients. J Urol 1982;128:469–475.

85. Skinner D, Lieskovsky G, Boyd S. Technique for creation of a continent internal ileal reservoir (Kock pouch) for urinary diversion. Urol Clin North Am 1984;11:741.

86. Studer U, Ackermann D, Casanova G, Zingg E. Three years experience with an ileal low pressure bladder substitute. Br J Urol 1989;63:43–52.

87. Stein JP, Lieskovsky G, Ginsberg DA, Bochner BH, Skinner DG. The T pouch: an orthotopic ileal neobladder incorporating a serosal lined ileal antireflux technique. J Urol 1998;159(6):1836–1842.

88. Zincke H, Garbeff PJ, Beahrs JR. Upper urinary tract transitional cell cancer after radical cystectomy for bladder cancer. J Urol 1984;131(1):50–52.

89. Shinka T, Uekado Y, Aoshi H, Hirano A, Ohkawa T. Occurrence of uroepithelial tumors of the upper urinary tract after the initial diagnosis of bladder cancer. J Urol 1988;140(4):745–748.

90. Schwartz CB, Bekirov H, Melman A. Urothelial tumors of upper tract following treatment of primary bladder transitional cell carcinoma. Urology 1992;40(6):509–511.

91. Ferriere JM, Pariente JL, Mettetal PJ, et al. [Tumors of the upper urinary tract in patients following bladder tumors: multicentric locations or seeding? Apropos of 14 cases]. Prog Urol 1994;4(4):563–568.

92. Hastie KJ, Hamdy FC, Collins MC, Williams JL. Upper tract tumours following cystectomy for bladder cancer. Is routine intravenous urography worthwhile? Br J Urol 1991;67(1):29–31.

93. Kenworthy P, Tanguay S, Dinney CP. The risk of upper tract recurrence following cystectomy in patients with transitional cell carcinoma involving the distal ureter [see comments]. J Urol 1996;155(2):501–503.

94. Malkowicz SB, Skinner DG. Development of upper tract carcinoma after cystectomy for bladder carcinoma. Urology 1990;36(1):20–22.

95. Lindell O. Ileal conduit urinary diversion: a review of 148 patients. Ann Chir Gynaecol 1986;75(4):229–235.

96. Silver DA, Stroumbakis N, Russo P, Fair WR, Herr HW. Ureteral carcinoma in situ at radical cystectomy: does the margin matter? J Urol 1997;158(3 Pt 1):768–771.

97. Solsona E, Iborra I, Ricos JV, et al. Upper urinary tract involvement in patients with bladder carcinoma in situ (Tis): its impact on management. Urology 1997;49(3):347–352.

98. Tsuji Y, Nakamura H, Ariyoshi A. Upper urinary tract involvement after cystectomy and ileal conduit diversion for primary bladder carcinoma. Eur Urol 1996;29(2):216–220.

99. Balaji KC, McGuire M, Grotas J, Grimaldi G, Russo P. Upper tract recurrences following radical cystectomy: an analysis of prognostic factors, recurrence pattern and stage at presentation. J Urol 1999;162(5):1603–1606.

100. Batista JE, Palou J, Iglesias J, et al. Significance of ureteral carcinoma in situ in specimens of cystectomy. Eur Urol 1994;25(4):313–315.

101. Kramolowsky EV, Clayman RV. Advances in endosurgery. Treatment of ureteral–enteric anastomotic strictures. Urol Clin North Am 1988;15(3):413–418.

102. Neururer R, Stenzl A, Hobisch A, Bartsch G. Experience with the T-pouch in patients undergoing cystectomy and ureteroileal urethrostomy. J Urol 1999;161:348A.

103. Steven K, Poulsen AL. The orthotopic Kock ileal neobladder: functional results, urodynamic features, complications and survival in 166 men. J Urol 2000;164(2):288–295.

104. Slaton JW, Swanson DA, Grossman HB, Dinney CP. A stage specific approach to tumor surveillance after radical cystectomy for transitional cell carcinoma of the bladder. J Urol 1999;162(3 Pt 1):710–714.

105. Lebret T, Herve JM, Barre P, et al. Urethral recurrence of transitional cell carcinoma of the bladder. Predictive value of preoperative latero-montanal biopsies and urethral frozen sections during prostatocystectomy. Eur Urol 1998;33(2):170–174.

106. Ravery V, de la Taille A, Hoffmann P, et al. Balloon catheter dilatation in the treatment of ureteral and ureteroenteric stricture. J Endourol 1998;12(4):335–340.

20

PHENOTYPIC AND GENOTYPIC ANALYSIS OF NEOPLASTIC LESIONS OF THE URINARY BLADDER

Joe Philip, Jennifer Temple, Pradip Javle, Youqiang Ke, Christine Gosden, Andrew Dodson and Christopher S. Foster

INTRODUCTION

Bladder cancer accounts for at least 6.5% of all cancers reported annually throughout the world and is the most common malignancy of the urinary tract.[1] In the general population in both the UK and the USA, approximately 15 cases are reported per 10,000 persons and those between the ages of 50 and 70 are most at risk.[2] Males are three times more likely to be affected than females,[3] making bladder cancer the fourth most common malignancy in men and the eighth most common malignancy in women in the UK and the USA.[4] Two distinct morphologic types of bladder cancer are recognized: squamous cell carcinoma and transitional cell carcinoma (TCC).

Squamous cell carcinoma

Squamous cell carcinoma is most common in the Middle and Far East. In the UK only 2% of bladder cancers are of this type,[5] although the incidence in the USA is somewhat higher. In these countries, squamous carcinoma is caused by infection of the urinary tract by the parasite *Schistosoma haematobium* as a consequence of drinking or bathing in infected water.[4]

Transitional cell carcinoma

TCCs (urothelial carcinoma) can be divided into *papillary lesions*, which are less likely to invade rapidly or deeply into the bladder wall but have a high tendency to recur, and the less common *flat lesions* which directly invade the bladder wall and are related to poor prognosis.[6] Following initiation of these different morphologic types of urothelial neoplasm by changes within distinct spectra of genes, the genotypic and phenotypic factors which promote invasion and metastasis of individual bladder cancers are likely to be similar. Although genetically encoded, many of the factors that control the behavioral phenotype of an individual cancer are likely to be epigenetic.

Bladder TCCs become clinically apparent as either superficial papillary tumors or flat invasive lesions. The majority of papillary lesions initially run a superficial course, recurring frequently and necessitating multiple resections. Presently, these are classified into three morphologic grades (International Union Against Cancer (UICC) criteria) according to their architectural pattern, nuclear pleomorphism and mitotic figures. In contrast, morphologically flat lesions can be reactive, dysplastic or neoplastic. Reactive lesions may contain inflammatory changes in the lamina propria beneath a hyperplastic or metaplastic urothelium. A comprehensive assessment of the status of the current World Health Organization (WHO) classification of urothelial neoplasms is presented in Chapter 9. Cytologic abnormalities occur in dysplasia and include cellular and nuclear pleomorphism restricted to the basal and intermediate layers. Urothelial carcinoma in situ (CIS) is frequently multifocal and is characterized by a flat proliferation of disordered urothelial cells with marked atypia. Flat malignant lesions tend to be invasive and aggressive with a poor clinical outcome (Fig. 20.1).

Invasive TCC can arise de novo,[7] occur following progression of a flat lesion[8] or develop from the progression of a superficial papillary tumor.[9,10] Nevertheless, identification of the invasive potential of particular papillary or flat lesions remains a dilemma, particularly in the pre-invasive stage. Morphologic similarities between superficially invasive papillary tumors that are recurrence-prone, and invasive tumors with deep bladder wall penetration, presently confound diagnostic and prognostic prediction.

Identification of genes associated with bladder cancer

Many studies have been conducted to identify genes associated with bladder cancer development.[11] Several molecular studies[12,13] of transitional cell bladder tumors have revealed characteristic chromosomal abnormalities. Spruck et al.[12] proposed two distinct molecular pathways for bladder cancer development with acquisition of particular chromosomal defects responsible for invasive capability. The genes considered permissive for malignant transformation comprised several oncogenes and tumor suppressor genes. Initially quiescent, proto-oncogenes may be activated by critical genetic events which can include mutation, altered expression due to hypermethylation or novel insertion of viral DNA. Such events could occur in isolation or following inactivation of a tumor suppressor gene, thus causing a disturbance in the cell cycle leading to malignant transformation.[11] However, it is beyond the scope of this chapter to present a detailed appraisal of the different genetic mechanisms affecting gene function.

Two major chromosomes involved in bladder cancer, of both squamous and papillary types, are chromosomes 9 and 17.[14,15] Loss of heterozygosity (LOH) on chromosome 9 characterizes 60–65% of TCCs and is considered by some to be the earliest event in the genesis of transitional cell bladder cancer.[13,15] Functional assays of transitional assays have demonstrated lack of protein expression of cells containing mutations of the p16 gene[16] or on the short arm (region p21) of chromosome 9.[17] A high frequency of allelic loss on chromosome 9p21 appears to be frequently involved in bladder cancer progression.[18] Damage to chromosome 17 is suggested to be a late event. LOH of chromosome 17 short arm was noted in 40% of bladder tumors, mainly of high grade and high stage.[19] Tumors found to penetrate into muscle and beyond the bladder wall contained losses on chromosomes 3, 4, 5, 6, 8, 11, 13 and 18. Halachmi et al.[20] compared the probable (suggested) genetic events with pathologic stage and

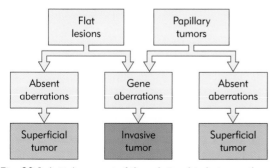

Fig. 20.1 Initial concept of the relationship between the origins of superficial and invasive tumors.

Normal urothelium

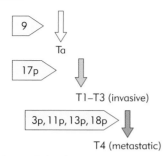

Fig. 20.2 Proposed association between progression of genetic events and evolution of the aggressive phenotype of bladder neoplasms.

proposed a unified genetic pathway of bladder cancer progression (Fig. 20.2).

ALTERATIONS IN GENE EXPRESSION AND ACTIVITY

Investigations to try to elucidate the early changes in bladder cancer and to understand the fundamental processes underlying the transition from initial genetic changes to invasion and metastasis have been complex. Initial thoughts on the genetic pathways involved in bladder cancer were based largely on chromosomal (cytogenetic) mechanisms such as deletion or duplication of entire chromosome arms, or even whole chromosomes. The key events detected by this process showed the importance of the loss of the short arm of chromosome 9 (9p) and the subsequent loss of the short arm of chromosome 17 (17p). It is now known that the tumor suppressor gene p16 is located on chromosome 9p and p53 (another key tumor suppressor) is on chromosome 17p. Gains or amplification of chromosomal regions were associated with oncogene amplification such as that of the *ras* genes.

According to current understanding, mutations of tumor suppressor genes (e.g. p16, p53, pRb and PTEN) diminish control of proliferation and are permissive for accelerated growth. Thus, the dynamic equilibrium between cell proliferation and apoptosis becomes disturbed following deregulation of the cell cycle, allowing events favoring tumorigenesis to dominate. The rate of cell proliferation is an important factor contributing to initiation of a malignancy. Expression of Ki-67 protein is a widely accepted measure of this activity.[21] Apoptosis

(programmed cell death) and regulation of cell division are recognized to be controlled by a number of proteins including Bcl-2, Bcl-X (L and S forms), Bax, Bad and Noxa, amongst others. In their non-mutated forms, tumor suppressor genes such as p53 and pRb inhibit cell proliferation and repress factors that might otherwise stimulate tumor development. Thereafter, malignancy is exploited by changes in cell–cell and cell–matrix adhesions of isoforms of CD44, and is undetected by the reduced frequency of major histocompatibility complex (MHC) antigens.

The genes currently considered to be some of the most important in the etiopathogenesis of bladder cancers, particularly those of transitional cell type, will be assessed in the remainder of this chapter. Wherever possible, their practical diagnostic utility, and limitations, are discussed and illustrated. While still highly fragmented, a picture is now emerging of these genes, their complexity and their interactions, that promotes and modulates individual malignant urothelial phenotypes, although the events initiating involvement of these genes remain stubbornly obscure.

More recent knowledge of gene structure and function, gene mapping and gene sequencing, culminating in the Human Genome Project, has given much greater insights into the genetic changes that underlie tumor progression. It is now known that, although chromosome loss is still one of the major components contributing to loss of function of tumor suppressor genes, there are other mechanisms that can contribute to loss (or gain) of function of genes that play critical roles in oncogenesis. It is now recognized that gene deletion or amplification may involve small microscopic deletions that are difficult to detect at the gross chromosomal level unless specific gene probes are used (examples of this are the tumor suppressor genes and HER2/*neu*). Genes may be inactivated or changed by mutation. Even single base changes can affect gene function, through mechanisms such as producing a stop codon (thus initiating premature termination of the messenger RNA produced) or by affecting splice sites and thus splice variants. Genes can also be silenced by methylation, or their function altered by translocation so they are adjacent to other genes and control systems that may result in their under- or overproduction (this latter process is particularly important in the amplification of oncogenes). It is for these reasons that more detailed information about some of the major genes involved in bladder cancer progression aids understanding of the most fundamental processes at each stage of progression. From this, pathways of the processes underlying

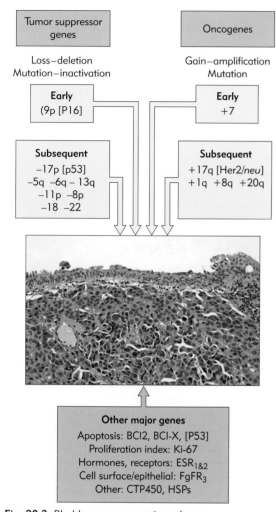

Fig. 20.3 Bladder cancer genetic pathways.

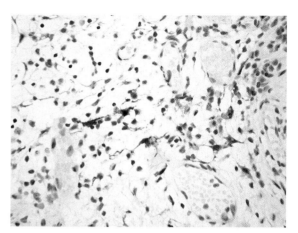

Fig. 20.4 Suburothelial mucosal connective tissue containing an extensive plexus of p16-positive neurons. The overlying urothelium did not express this gene product.

the major transitions in bladder cancer pathology have evolved from those of basic mechanisms utilizing chromosomal changes alone, to those involving this rapidly expanding molecular genetic knowledge, shown in Figure 20.3.

Tumor suppressor genes

Gene: CDKN2A (protein: p16)

Gene CDKN2A, also known as p16, MTS1, TP16, CDKN2 or INK4a, maps on chromosome 9, at 9p21. The products of these genes localize in the nucleus where they have cyclin-dependent protein kinase inhibitor, tumor suppressor activities and are involved in cell-cycle arrest, cell-cycle checkpoint, negative regulation of cell proliferation, regulation of CDK activity and oncogenetic functions.

The gene generates several transcript variants which differ in their first exons and utilize alternate poly-adenylation sites. The gene sequence produces, by alternative splicing, 12 different transcripts, together encoding 11 different protein isoforms. There are seven likely alternative promoters and three non-overlapping alternative last exons. Four alternatively spliced variants encoding distinct proteins have been reported, three of which encode structurally related isoforms known to function as inhibitors of CDK4 kinase. The remaining transcript includes an alternate first exon located upstream of the remainder of the gene and contains an alternate open reading frame (ARF) that specifies a protein which is structurally unrelated to the products of the other variants. This ARF product functions to stabilize p53 protein and is able to interact with protein MDM1 responsible for p53 degradation. Although there are significant structural and functional differences, the CDK inhibitor isoforms and the ARF product encoded by this gene are commonly involved in cell-cycle control at G1 through regulation of the activities of CDK4 and p53. This gene is frequently mutated or deleted in a wide variety of tumors, including bladder cancer, and is recognized to be an important tumor suppressor gene (Fig. 20.4).

Gene: WAF1/CIP1 (protein: p21)

The gene encoding protein CDKN1A is known as p21, CIP1, WAF1 or CDKN1 and maps on chromosome 6, at 6p21. The products localize in the nucleus and have potent cyclin-dependent protein kinase inhibitor, cell-cycle regulator activities involved in cell-cycle arrest.

The gene is expressed at a very high level and produces, by alternative splicing, 13 different transcripts, together encoding 12 different protein isoforms. The encoded protein binds to, and inhibits, the activity of cyclin–CDK2 or –CDK4 complexes, thus functioning as a regulator of cell-cycle progression at G1. Expression of this gene is tightly controlled by tumor suppressor protein p53, through which this protein mediates the p53-dependent cell-cycle G1 phase arrest in response to a variety of stress stimuli. The WAF1/C1P1 gene contains at least two p53-responsive sites in its promoter region, responsible for transcription of p21 when bound to p53, thus suggesting protein p21 to be a potent downstream mediator of the antiproliferative function of wild-type p53.[22] Conversely, a p53-independent pathway has been associated with p21 induction observed in various normal tissues during development or differentiation, in the absence of p53 activation as well as in tumor cells with mutated p53.[23–25]

Controversy persists concerning the prognostic utility of p21 expression in bladder cancer. Maintenance of p21 has been suggested to reduce the deleterious effects of altered p53 in TCCs.[26] Conversely, an associated p53 mutation appears to enhance chemosensitivity.[27] An inverse correlation has been suggested between p21/WAF1 immunoreactivity and tumor stage, tumor grade, p53 accumulation and Ki-67 expression in muscle-invasive tumors.[28,29] However, the value of immunohistochemically derived data is now questionable (Fig. 20.5). This study caveat applies not only to the WAF1/C1P1 gene, but also to the products of other genes with multiple-spliced products. Nevertheless,

Qureshi et al. showed distinct prognostic groups with p21-positive, p53-positive tumors associated with the best survival advantage and p21-negative, p53-negative tumors the worst.[30] Zlotta et al. reported increased p21 expression with the grade and stage of superficial tumors, attributing a lower recurrence-free survival and a positive correlation with p53 but not with Ki-67.[31] Studies of p21 immunoexpression by Waldman et al. reported better chemo- and radiosensitivity in p21-negative bladder cell lines, raising the possibility of an anti-apoptotic function.[32]

Gene: TP53 (protein: p53)

Gene TP53, also known as p53 or TRP53, maps on chromosome 17, at 17p13.1. The gene product, tumor protein Tp53, is a nuclear protein that plays an essential role in regulating the cell cycle, specifically during transition from G0 to G1. In normal cells, it is found in very low levels but in a variety of transformed cell lines it is expressed in high amounts, and is believed to contribute to neoplastic transformation and to malignancy. Tp53 is a DNA-binding protein containing DNA-binding and transcription activation domains. It is postulated that p53 activates expression of downstream genes that inhibit growth and/or invasion, thus functioning as a tumor suppressor. Alterations of the TP53 gene occur not only as somatic mutations in human malignancies, but also as germline mutations in some cancer-prone families.

Protein p53 regulates progression through the cell cycle in G1 and G2 in response to DNA damage and to apoptosis which occurs following a range of DNA-damaging agents.[33] In non-transformed cells, p53 causes arrest after G1, allowing time for cell repair or apoptosis. The gene is inactivated in up to 50% of all cancers,[34] and is the most frequently modified gene in bladder cancer. It is possibly the most important gene involved in the progression of this disease.[1] Although many different mutations are recognized to occur within the genome, mutated p53 usually differs by a single point mutation from the wild type, resulting in an amino acid substitution. All such mutations occur in areas of the gene conserved by evolution. One particular region ('hotspot') comprises four codons in which more than 30% of mutations are known to occur. Inactivation of this gene inhibits activity of the normal protein, resulting in a proliferative advantage to affected cells,[35] causing them to become unstable. The retarded degradation and nuclear accumulation conferred upon abnormal p53 proteins is a reflection of elevated stability and self-aggregation of the mutated mole-

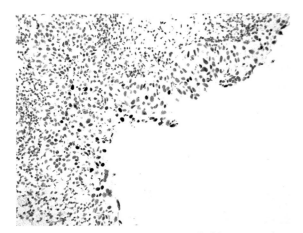

Fig. 20.5 Heterogeneous expression of p21 gene product by a flat urothelial lesion that is p53 mutation-positive and also PTEN downregulated (see Fig. 20.11).

cules.[36] Thus, mutant p53 products are more likely to be detected using immunohistochemical analysis.

The TP53 gene has been studied in TCC with mutations correlating with tumor grade and stage,[37,38] recurrence,[39] progression[12] and survival.[40] Dahse et al. found TP53 abnormalities to be more frequent in high-grade, muscle-invasive lesions (Fig. 20.6) and hypothesized that low-grade bladder TCCs (Fig. 20.7) proceed through another genomic pathway associated with the inactivation of CDK inhibitors p15, p16 and p21.[41] Sarkis et al. showed a significant decrease in the survival rate of patients with muscle-invasive cancer and altered p53 function.[42] Bladder tumors with TP53 alterations

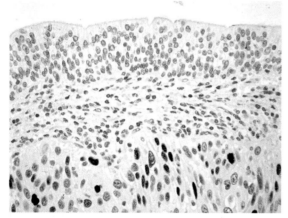

Fig. 20.6 p53 expression by invasive transitional cell carcinoma penetrating deep within the submucosa beneath apparently normal overlying urothelium that is p53 negative. These appearances demonstrate the value of taking random biopsies in the comprehensive assessment of a bladder neoplasm.

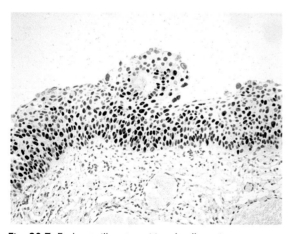

Fig. 20.7 Early papillary transitional cell carcinoma containing a p53 mutation, but no RB1 mutation (see Fig. 20.9).

exhibited more aggressive phenotypes and gene mutation rates, correlated with higher grading and/or staging together with muscle invasiveness.[43]

Gene: RB1 (retinoblastoma protein: pRb)

The RB1 gene maps on chromosome 13, at 13q14.2, where it consists of 27 exons.[44] It encodes a retinoblastoma-associated protein that has tumor suppressor activity. The gene sequence produces, by alternative splicing, 11 different transcripts, together encoding 10 different protein isoforms. Retinoblastoma-like and retinoblastoma-associated proteins have regulatory functions in the cell cycle. The proteins form a complex with adenovirus E1A and SV40 large T antigen, and may bind and modulate the activities of certain cellular proteins with which E1A and T antigen compete for pocket binding. These proteins may also act as tumor suppressors and are potent inhibitors of E2F-mediated transactivation.

Retinoblastoma protein regulates cell-cycle progression according to its own state of phosphorylation which reaches its peak at the beginning of S phase and is lowest after mitosis. Retinoblastoma protein pRb is a target for the enzymatic activity of cyclin–CDK complexes.[45,46] Phosphorylation of pRb occurs as cells progress from G1 through late G1, early S phase and G2. The active underphosphorylated form of pRb exerts a negative regulatory effect on gene expression in G0 to middle G1 through complex formation with DNA-binding proteins.[47] Stimulation of quiescent cells with mitogens induces phosphorylation of pRb, whereas differentiation of the same cells induces hypophosphorylation. It is the hypophosphorylated form that suppresses cell proliferation.[48] Mutations to the retinoblastoma gene can occur through a number of different mechanisms, all causing inactivation of pRb. Large-scale deletions account for 30% of mutations, the remaining 70% being caused by splicing errors, point mutations and small deletions in the promoter region.

Mutagenic deactivation of RB1 produces a spectrum of altered expression patterns, from undetectable pRb levels (Fig. 20.8) to heterogeneous cytoplasmic localization of truncated pRb products that have lost their nuclear localization signal.[49,50] Thus, in any bladder carcinoma, the precise levels of pRb are not static but are in constant flux (Fig. 20.9). Furthermore, pRb is subject to splice variation, making single-agent detection highly unreliable. Cordon-Cardo et al. found significant associations between undetectable pRb and tumor stage, tumor grade, disease progression and reduced survival.[51] Altered RB1 expression, identified

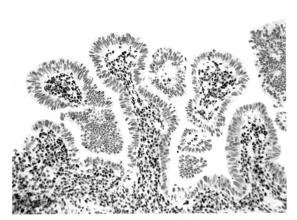

Fig. 20.8 Early papillary transitional cell carcinoma containing an RB1 mutation in which the urothelial cells appear morphologically unremarkable.

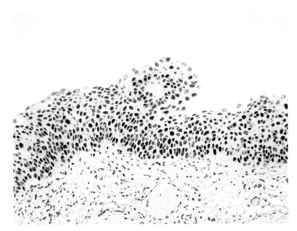

Fig. 20.9 An early papillary transitional cell carcinoma that is RB1 positive (non-mutated with respect to the epitope identified by this antibody) but is p53 positive (see Fig. 20.7).

immunohistochemically, was associated with a high rate of recurrence and poor outcome in T1 tumors.[52] Mutated expression of the retinoblastoma gene found in association with muscle-invasive tumors suggests a functional importance during acquisition of an invasive capability.[53]

There is a significant association between p53 nuclear overexpression and undetectable pRb,[51] including a synergistic carcinogenic effect between mutated pRb and p53 such that patients with both alterations manifest an advanced tumor grade, marked progression and decreased survival. TP53 appears to target p21/WAF1, which encodes a CDK inhibitor,[22] pRb being a substrate for cyclin–CDK complexes.[45,46]

Gene: *PTEN*

The gene PTEN, also known as BZS, MHAM, TEP1, MMAC1 or PTEN1, maps on chromosome 10, at 10q23.3. The gene sequence produces, by alternative splicing, nine different transcripts, together encoding nine different protein isoforms. It encodes a phosphatase tensin homolog family member. The products localize in cytoplasm, have tumor suppressor, protein tyrosine phosphatase activities and are involved in regulation of CDK activity, development, cell proliferations and protein amino acid dephosphorylation.

PTEN is a major tumor suppressor gene, frequently mutated or deleted in a wide range of tumors. It encodes a dual-specific phosphatase which, when non-mutated and active, can restrain the capacity of tumor cells to invade through a basement membrane matrix (Fig. 20.10). PTEN overexpression leads to changes in cell adhesion and in spreading, and inhibits cell migration.[54] Studies have found involvement of PTEN protein in the regulation of cell migration and invasion with its loss being significant in late stages of tumor progression.[54,55] The response of PTEN in bladder neoplasia is complex and its role remains to be elucidated in individual cancers. Immunohistochemical studies confirm the protein to be modulated in an individual and idiosyncratic manner. In non-neoplastic transitional epithelium, PTEN is strongly expressed by many basal cells. However, in some neoplasms, early PTEN expression becomes diminished (Fig. 20.11), only to recur at high intensity as the tumor becomes invasive. Unfortunately, immunohistochemistry is insufficiently sensitive to discriminate whether there is a

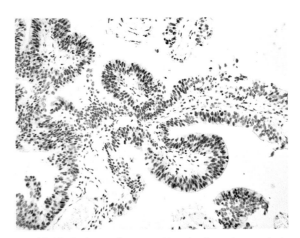

Fig. 20.10 Early papillary transitional cell carcinoma that is strongly PTEN positive, but which contains foci of downregulation, identified as the unstained epithelial nuclei.

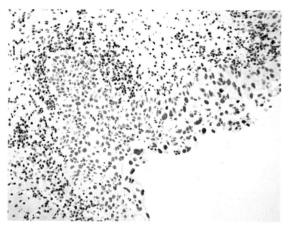

Fig. 20.11 Early flat neoplastic lesion that is PTEN negative but p21 positive (see Fig. 20.5).

quantitative or qualitative change in expression of the products of this gene.

Oncogenes

Oncogenic sequences encode proteins that have normal function and are described as 'proto-oncogenes'. However, when the gene is mutated ('oncogene'), the abnormal protein product becomes a strong independent oncogenic stimulus that operates outwith normal cellular regulatory mechanisms.

Ras genes

The *ras* gene maps on the X chromosome where it encodes *ras*-related protein Rab-6B. It is expressed at low level in normal cells and produces, by alternative splicing, two different transcripts, together encoding two different protein isoforms. There are two probable alternative promoters. The transcripts appear to differ by truncation of the N-terminus, because an internal intron is not always spliced out.

The *ras* branch of the *ras* superfamily consists of small GTPases most closely related to *ras* and include the r-ras, Rap, Ral, Rheb, Rin and Rit proteins. Although the understanding of *ras* signaling and biology is now considerable, recent observations suggest that the function of these proteins is more complex than previously believed, i.e.:

- the different ras proteins may not be functionally identical
- ras protein function involves interactive cross-talk with their close relatives.

The mammalian *ras* gene family consists of the Harvey and Kirsten *ras* genes (c-Hras1 and c-Kras2), an inactive pseudogene of each (c-Hras2 and c-Kras1) and the N-*ras* gene. The proteins differ significantly only in their C-terminal 40 amino acids. These ras genes have GTP/GDP binding and GTPase activity, and their normal function may be as G-like regulatory proteins involved in the normal control of cell growth. Point mutations in the three members of the RAS proto-oncogene family (H-*ras*, K-*ras*, N-*ras*) are common in human cancers[56] and are suspected in the development and progression of many human bladder cancers. A high incidence of both H-*ras* and K-*ras* mutations at codon 12 has been reported in histochemically confirmed bladder cancers.[56,57] In these tumors, Przybojewska et al. found frequent N-*ras* gene mutation at codon 61 associated with H-*ras* mutations.[56] Fontana et al. demonstrated a significant relationship between enhanced c-ras oncogene expression and early recurrence in superficial bladder cancer.[58]

Gene: H-RAS1

The Harvey *ras* gene (H-RAS), also known as HRAS1 or RAS111, maps on chromosome 11, at 11p15.5. The gene encodes transforming protein products that have GTP-binding properties, GTPase activities and are involved in small GTPase-mediated signal transduction. The gene is expressed at very high level and its sequence produces, by alternative splicing, nine different transcripts, together encoding five different protein isoforms.

Gene: K-RAS2

The Kirsten *ras* gene (K-RAS2), also known as RASK2, KI-RAS, C-K-RAS, K-RAS2A or K-RAS2B, maps on chromosome 12, at 12p12.1. It encodes transforming GTPase protein products that have GTPase activity and are involved in small GTPase-mediated signal transduction. The gene sequence produces, by alternative splicing, three different transcripts, together encoding three different protein isoforms. Single amino acid substitutions are responsible for activating mutations. Alternative splicing leads to variants encoding two isoforms that differ in the C-terminal region.

Gene: N-RAS

The N-RAS gene, also known as N-*ras* or NRAS1, maps on chromosome 1, at 1p13.2. It encodes transforming protein products predicted to have small GTP-binding ability and GTPase activities, and to be involved in small GTPase-mediated signal transduction. Mutations that change amino acid residues 12, 13 or 61 activate the potential of N-*ras* to transform cells in tissue culture and are implicated in a variety of human tumors.

Gene: c-ERBB-2

The ERBB2 gene, also known as NEU, NGL, HER2 or TKR1, maps on chromosome 17, at 17q21.1.[59,60] The protein product is a transmembrane glycoprotein within the receptor protein-tyrosine kinase family.[61] Specifically, the protein exhibits Neu/ErbB-2 receptor activity in addition to protein kinase, transmembrane receptor protein tyrosine kinase, epidermal growth factor receptor and ATP-binding activities. The protein

products of the gene localize in membrane and are involved in protein amino acid phosphorylation and transmembrane receptor protein tyrosine kinase signaling pathways. The gene sequence produces, by alternative splicing, 19 different transcripts, together encoding 19 different protein isoforms.

C-erbB-2 (also known as HER2/*neu*) is a proto-oncogene implicated in a number of tumors.[62] Some of these proto-oncogenes are related to growth factors or to growth factor receptors (e.g. c-sis, c-fms, c-erbB-1 and c-erbB-2).[63–65] Overexpression and amplification in bladder cancer (Fig. 20.12) correlate with tumor grade, recurrence and disease progression.[66,67] Several

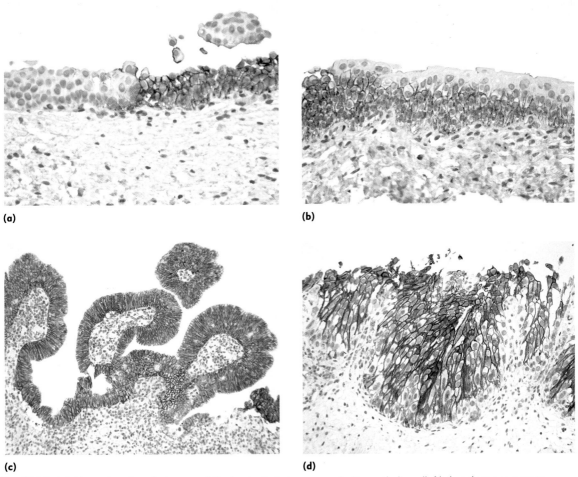

(a)

(b)

(c)

(d)

Fig. 20.12 **(a)** Abrupt interface between mildly dysplastic but non-neoplastic urothelium (left) that does not express HER2/*neu*. In contrast is the morphologically dysplastic and phenotypically neoplastic epithelium (right) expressing HER2/*neu* that is spreading along the mucosa. **(b)** Morphologically dysplastic and phenotypically neoplastic (HER2/*neu* positive) urothelial cells (left) invading along the mucosa beneath overlying non-neoplastic urothelium. **(c)** Papillary lesion composed of morphologically dysplastic urothelium strongly expressing HER2/*neu*. **(d)** Transitional cell carcinoma (grade 2) containing a few residual, basal and non-neoplastic epithelial cells (unstained) that is pushing downwards towards, but is not yet invading, the submucosa.

reports indicate a significant relationship between c-erbB-2, p53 and increased cell proliferation,[68,69] with these oncoproteins rarely expressed in superficial tumors.[69–72] C-erbB-2 overexpression appears to precede disease progression, suggesting prognostic value.[67]

Tumor-modulating genes

Gene: MK167 (protein: Ki-67)

Ki-67 is the protein product of gene MK167, also known as KIA, that maps on chromosome 10, at 10q25. It is expressed at very high levels in all cells. The gene sequence produces, by alternative splicing, three types of transcript predicted to encode three distinct proteins. Protein Ki-67, detected by immunohistochemically murine monoclonal antibody MCB1, is a good indicator of proliferation in a variety of tumors, including bladder.[73,74] This proliferation-associated nuclear antigen is expressed in all cells in G1, S and G2M phases but not by cells in G0, thus allowing assessment of the entire proliferating cell pool.[75] Ki-67 expression studies have shown a strong overall correlation with tumor stage and grade.[76] High-grade TCCs (Fig. 20.13) tend to have a higher Ki-67 index than low-grade tumors (Fig. 20.14), although this is not a universal or invariable relationship. Studies have also shown a correlation with tumor aggressiveness, both recurrence and progression to invasive disease,[77] and metastasis. Ki-67 index can help distinguish grade 2 tumors with a favorable outcome from clinically unfavorable tumors of identical morphology.[78] A Ki-67 labeling index over 20% predicts that morphologically well-differentiated tumors (Fig. 20.15) of pathologic stage pTa/pT1 will recur within a year of diagnosis.[79]

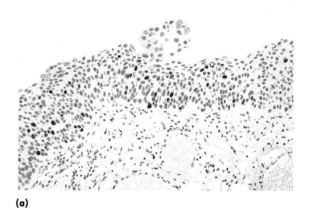

(a)

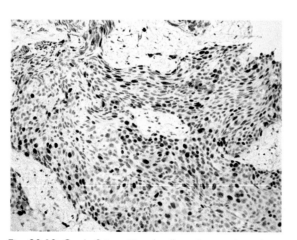

(b)

Fig. 20.14 (a) Early papillary transitional cell carcinoma in which an elevated rate of cell division is confirmed by Ki-67 expression. This lesion is known to be strongly p53 positive (see Fig. 20.7) but RB1 negative (see Fig. 20.9). In addition, the lesion is Bcl-2 negative but strongly HER2/*neu* positive. These parameters together indicated a likely aggressive course for this lesion, confirmed by its subsequent behavior, despite its apparent indolent appearance at the outset. **(b)** Highly elevated Ki-67 expression in an apparently indolent papillary lesion expressing PTEN (see Fig. 20.10) despite the elevated level of cell division, absence of p53 or RB1 mutation, together with continued strong expression of PTEN indicated a likely benign course for this lesion, which continues to behave in an indolent manner.

Fig. 20.13 Grade 3 transitional cell carcinoma strongly expressing nuclear Ki-67 protein. The tumor is invading deep to the mucosa but not involving detrusor (pT1).

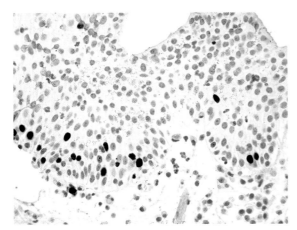

Fig. 20.15 Mildly hyperplastic, but not significantly dysplastic, urothelial lesion in which there is focal elevation of Ki-67 expression. Although cell division is not restricted to the basal layer of epithelium, there is no proliferation into the mid or upper zones, in contrast to those lesions illustrated in Figure 20.14.

Gene: CYP2B6 encoding cytochrome P450

Gene CYP2B6, also known as CPB6, IIB1, P450 or CYPIIB6, maps on chromosome 19, at 19q13.2. The gene encodes a member (P-450 2B-BX) of the cytochrome P450 superfamily of enzymes, and is moderately expressed. There are two probable alternative promoters, although these have yet to be confirmed by functional studies. The transcripts appear to differ by truncation of the N-terminus, or by the presence or absence of a cassette exon. By alternative splicing the gene sequence produces two types of transcript, predicted to encode two distinct protein isoforms. It contains nine confirmed introns, four of which are alternative. The products are involved in electron transport.

Cytochrome P450 proteins are mono-oxygenases which catalyze many reactions involved in drug metabolism, in the synthesis of cholesterol, steroids and other lipids, and hence are indirectly involved in maintaining cellular homeostasis. This protein localizes to the endoplasmic reticulum and its expression is induced by phenobarbital. The enzyme is known to metabolize some xenobiotics, such as the anticancer drugs cyclophosphamide and ifosfamide. Transcript variants for this gene have been described. However, it has not been confirmed whether these transcripts are produced by this gene or by a closely related pseudogene, CYP2B7. Both the gene and the pseudogene are located in the middle of a CYP2A pseudogene found on chromosome 19q within a large cluster of cytochrome P450 genes

from the CYP2A, CYP2B and CYP2F subfamilies. The cytochrome P450 motif is found in two isoforms from this gene; 62 other genes in the database also contain this motif. The cytochrome P450 enzymes usually act as terminal oxidases in multicomponent electron transfer chains. The significance of this observation is self-evident with respect to the production of monoclonal antibodies to specific proteins and to possible overlapping functions of apparently dissimilar proteins.

Gene: FGFR3 encoding fibroblast growth factor receptor 3

Gene FGFR3, also known as ACH, CEK2, JTK4 or HSFGFR3EX, maps on chromosome 4, at 4p16.3. It encodes a growth factor receptor with ATP-binding and protein kinase activities. It is involved in protein amino acid phosphorylation. The gene is expressed at high level and produces, by alternative splicing, seven different transcripts, together encoding seven different protein isoforms. There are two probable alternative promoters and two non-overlapping alternative last exons. The transcripts appear to differ by truncation of the N-terminus, truncation of the C-terminus, presence or absence of four cassette exons, or common exons with different boundaries, because an internal intron is not always spliced out.

The protein encoded by this gene is a member of the fibroblast growth factor receptor family, where amino acid sequence is highly conserved between family members and throughout evolution. FGFR family members differ from one another in their ligand affinities and tissue distribution. A full-length representative protein comprises an extracellular region containing three immunoglobulin-like domains, a single hydrophobic membrane-spanning segment and a cytoplasmic tyrosine kinase domain. The extracellular portion of the protein interacts with fibroblast growth factors, initiating a cascade of downstream signals, ultimately influencing mitogenesis and differentiation. This particular family member binds acidic and basic fibroblast growth hormone.

Gene: ESR1 encoding estrogen receptor 1 (ER alpha)

Gene ESR1, also known as ER, ESR, Era, ESRA or NR3A1, maps on chromosome 6, at 6q25.1. It encodes an estrogen receptor localized in nucleus with DNA binding, transcription factor, steroid hormone receptor and steroid-binding activities. The products are involved in the regulation of transcription. Estrogen receptor (ESR) is a ligand-activated transcription factor composed of several domains that are important for hormone binding, DNA binding and activation of transcription. It is expressed at high level in many cells and produces, by alternative splicing, 11 different transcripts, together encoding 11 different protein isoforms. There are five probable alternative promoters and five non-overlapping alternative last exons. The transcripts appear to differ by truncation of the N-terminus, truncation of the C-terminus, presence or absence of five cassette exons, or common exons with different boundaries.

The ligand-binding domain of this nuclear hormone receptor motif is found in seven isoforms from this gene; at least 47 other genes are known to contain this motif. The steroid hormones and their receptors are involved in the regulation of eukaryotic gene expression and affect cellular proliferation and differentiation in target tissues. In the absence of ligand, steroid hormone receptors are thought to be weakly associated with nuclear components. Hormone binding greatly increases receptor affinity. The hormone–receptor complex appears to recognize discrete DNA sequences upstream of transcriptional start sites. The estrogen receptor motif is found in five isoforms from this gene. No other gene in the database contains this motif.

Gene: ESR2 encoding estrogen receptor 2 (ER beta)

Gene ESR2, also known as Erb, ESRB, NR3A2, ER-BETA or ESR-BETA, maps on chromosome 14, at 14q. It encodes estrogen receptor beta that is well expressed in many different cell types. The gene produces, by alternative splicing, nine types of transcript, predicted to encode seven distinct protein isoforms. It contains 28 confirmed introns, 27 of which are alternative. There are six probable alternative promoters and four non-overlapping alternative last exons. The transcripts appear to differ by truncation of the N-terminus, truncation of the C-terminus, or by the presence or absence of eight cassette exons.

The products have a wide range of properties including steroid binding, transcription coactivator, transcription factor, receptor antagonist, and estrogen receptor activities. The gene products are involved in regulation of transcription, DNA-dependent signal transduction, cell–cell signaling, negative regulation of cell growth, and estrogen receptor signaling pathway; they localize in the nucleus. Estrogen receptor beta (ESR2) is a member of the superfamily of nuclear receptors that transduce extracellular signals into transcriptional responses. The gene is antisense to gene SYNE2.

The possibility that its mRNAs may be present and stable only in the absence of matching mRNAs from the gene on the other strand and vice versa is a distinct possibility.

Gene: EGF-R encoding epidermal growth factor receptor

The EGF-R gene, also known as ERBB or ERBB1, maps on chromosome 7, at 7p12, and encodes an epidermal growth factor receptor with protein kinase, transmembrane receptor protein tyrosine kinase and ATP-binding activities. The receptor is involved in protein amino acid phosphorylation, transmembrane receptor protein tyrosine kinase signaling and localizes in membrane. The gene is expressed at very high level and produces, by alternative splicing, 10 different transcripts, together encoding 10 different protein isoforms. EGF-R is a 170 kD protein product of a proto-oncogene with three domains that are extracellular, transmembrane and intracellular. Activation of EGF-R by ligands such as epidermal growth factor, transforming growth factor alpha, betacellulin and amphiregulin results in stimulation of the ras/raf, phosphatidylinositol-3-kinase and protein kinase C pathways, culminating in increased nuclear transcription and cellular proliferation[80] as well as increased angiogenesis and reduced apoptosis.

EGF-R immunoexpression, normally confined to the basal cell layer of urinary bladder epithelium,[81,82] is reported to be overexpressed in the entire urothelium involved in bladder TCC.[70,72,83–85] Overexpression of EGF-R correlates with a shorter interval to recurrence, higher recurrence rate and an increased rate of progression in patients with superficial bladder cancer but not in patients with muscle-invasive disease.[86] Its expression suggests that the phenotype of an individual bladder cancer is not static but evolves with the stage of disease progression. Stein et al.[86] suggested that increased expression of EGF-R in histologically normal urothelium or the presence of high EGF-R levels in normal urothelium distant to a tumor site[82] are early events in bladder tumorigenesis.

HOMEOSTATIS MODULATORS

Gene: heat shock proteins

There are two known genes encoding homeostatic regulatory proteins in this family:

- The gene HSPB1, also known as HSP27, HSP28 or HSP25, maps on chromosome 7, at 7q11.23. The protein products have heat shock protein (HSP) activity and are involved in regulation of translational initiation and localize in the cytoplasm. The gene is expressed at a very high level and produces, by alternative splicing, 16 different transcripts, together encoding 13 different protein isoforms. There are two probable alternative promoters.

- The gene HSPB2, also known as MKBP, HSP27, HSP72, HS.78846, FLJ25219 or MGC14839, maps on chromosome 11, at 11q22–q23. The products localize within the cytosol, have enzyme activator, protein binding, HSP activities and are involved in response to cellular 'stress'. The gene is expressed at high level and produces, by alternative splicing, six different transcripts, together encoding six different protein isoforms. Its regulation may use antisense and co-regulation, with neighboring genes organized in an operon-like structure.

HSP modulation is an essential cellular defense mechanism found in both prokaryotic and eukaryotic organisms as a response to a variety of stress insults. HSP-27, -60, -70 and -90, present in all living cells, play key cytoprotective roles as molecular chaperones of other proteins. They participate in developing cellular resistance and intracellular protein stabilization.[87,88] By inhibiting apoptosome formation, HSP-70 inhibits the receptor or mitochondrial pathways hampering the caspase cascade that leads to apoptosis.[89] HSP-70 interacts with p53 protein, stabilizing the mutant form, thus permitting cell proliferation that is thereafter unregulated by this pathway.[90]

HSPs act as antigen presenters and play an important role in antibody assembly. Overexpression of HSPs has been associated with poor prognosis but may increase immunogenicity in some tumors, potentiating immune response and improved overall survival.[91] In superficial bladder cancers with a propensity to recur,[92] studies have shown that HSP overexpression may be an important prognosticator of bacillus Calmette–Guérin (BCG) response. The universal expression of HSP-27 in normal urothelium makes this a powerful immunohistochemical reagent with which to detect early invasive disease (Fig. 20.16). However, some TCCs express HSP-27 only at very low level, although immunoreactivity may be dependent upon the expression of individual splice variants and the reactivity of particular monoclonal antibodies with these variants. Nevertheless, relative absence of this protein from these tumors appears to be a strong (but hitherto unconfirmed) indicator of their potential aggressiveness (Fig. 20.17).

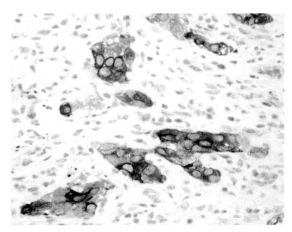

Fig. 20.16 Small clusters of invasive transitional cell carcinoma within the submucosa identified by strong HSP-27 expression. This is an invaluable marker in discriminating pTa from pT1 disease.

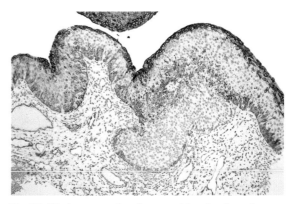

Fig. 20.17 An aggressive, flat, transitional cell carcinoma invading within the urothelium. The tumor does not express HSP-27, and is also negative for bcl-2 (see Fig. 20.20). The residual HSP-27-positive cells within the basal layers and the surface epithelium are residual non-neoplastic cells from pre-existing non-neoplastic epithelium.

Gene: CD44 (CD44 adhesion molecule)

Gene CD44, also known as IN, MC56, MDU2, MDU3, MIC3, Pgp1 or CD44R, maps on chromosome 11, at 11p13, and contains at least 20 exons.[6,109,110] It encodes cell surface glycoprotein CD44 that has collagen binding, hyaluronic acid binding and cell adhesion receptor activities. The gene is expressed at very high level and its sequence produces, by alternative splicing, 21 different transcripts, together encoding 21 different protein isoforms.

The term 'CD44' refers to a family of widely distributed cell surface (cluster differentiation) glycoproteins with an array of functions and many isoforms. The inappropriate and overabundant expression of this gene is of potential value in tumor diagnosis and in prognostic evaluation,[111,112] as well as in further understanding of adhesion aspects of tumor biology. A correlation has been identified in the altered quantity and distribution of CD44 variant isoforms (CD44v) and in the progression of a number of different tumors.[113] CD44v6 isoform expression is reduced in poorly differentiated, invasive TCC cell lines when compared to moderately or well-differentiated non-invasive tumors.[114–116] In bladder cancer it has been reported that overexpression of the CD44 locus is seen early in malignancy; this progressively diminishes as the tumor invades deeper into the bladder wall and is linked to loss of function of cell–cell cohesion, detachment of the basement membrane and infiltration of the surrounding muscle. The pattern of CD44 expression confirms that the environment surrounding a tumor cell affects its regulation.[6]

Correlation between CD44 expression and prognosis has been reported, with strong expression related to high survival probability in muscle-invasive tumors.[114] Toma et al. found that focal loss of immunostaining against CD44v3 and -v6 was a significant factor in identifying patients with superficial TCC at high risk of recurrence.[116] Sugino et al. found that detection of CD44 overexpression was of importance not only in detecting early bladder cancer but also in evaluating borderline lesions.[6]

Apoptotic modulators

Gene: bcl-2

The chromosomal localization and sequence of the bcl-2 gene has not yet been mapped. However, the principal product of the bcl-2 gene is a $\cong 25$–26 kD integral membrane protein, mainly located in the outer mitochondrial membrane and to a lesser extent in the endoplasmic reticulum and nuclear envelope. It is known that presence of the bcl-2 protein promotes cell survival, even when the rate of cell proliferation is not high, thus providing a growth advantage that may eventually lead to neoplastic transformation.[93] This may be of particular importance in the normal bladder where the proliferation index of normal urothelium is extremely low. Krajewski et al. suspected that bcl-2 influences the activity of Ca^{2+}-dependent enzymes involved in apoptosis by regulating the activity of Ca^{2+}

pumps or channels in the endoplasmic reticulum, and in mitochondrial and nuclear membranes.[94]

Nakopoulou et al.[95] observed an increased bcl-2 expression in low-grade TCCs and in superficial rather than invasive TCCs. Conversely, high-grade, aggressive and advanced tumors tend to show non-basal bcl-2 overexpression.[96–99] This finding suggested a deregulation of mechanisms controlling bcl-2 expression. The prognostic significance of bcl-2 expression is controversial, with Atug et al.[97] and Kirsh et al.[99] concluding an unfavorable outcome, refuted by Li et al.[96] and Lipponen et al.[97] The common expression of bcl-2 in normal (Fig. 20.18) and dysplastic urothelium but its loss from low-grade TCC (Fig. 20.19) suggests that bcl-2 expression may be an early event in TCC tumorigenesis.[101] Also, a reciprocal relationship between bcl-2 and p53 has been reported, with the presence of p53 implying greater probability of invasion.[102–105] These earlier findings are at some variance with respect to current findings from this laboratory (Fig. 20.20).

Apoptosis (programmed cell death) plays an important role in physiologic processes such as embryogenesis, organ development and cell proliferation. It is also an important function in pathologic processes including autoimmune disease and cancer development.[3] Bcl-2 belongs to a family containing both pro- and anti-apoptotic genes.[106] Bcl-2 inhibits apoptosis induced by a number of stimuli such as radiation, chemotherapeutic agents and growth factor deprivation. It is unusual in that its function assists neoplastic growth by prolonging cell survival through inhibition of apoptosis rather than accelerating cell proliferation,

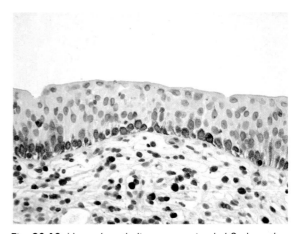

Fig. 20.18 Normal urothelium expressing bcl-2 along the basal layer. Loss of bcl-2 expression is an early phenomenon of urothelial neoplasia, but should be assessed together with other parameters of neoplasia.

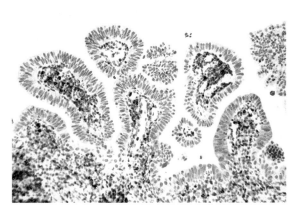

Fig. 20.19 Early bcl-2 negative papillary transitional cell carcinoma. This tumor contains an RB1 mutation (see Fig. 20.8). Without further identifiable mutation or expression–loss of PTEN or p21, this proliferative lesion is likely to behave in an indolent manner.

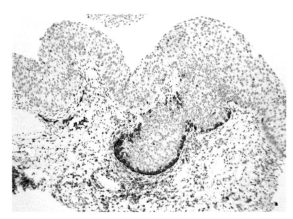

Fig. 20.20 An aggressive flat transitional cell carcinoma invading within the urothelial compartment. This tumor does not express HSP-27 (see Fig. 20.17). This illustration shows a basal layer of epithelial cells that continue to express bcl-2. These cells are of residual non-malignant mucosal epithelial origin and have not yet been replaced by the mucosally pagetoid-invasive tumor.

thus enhancing the metastatic potential of a tumor.[3] Bcl-X_L, from the same family, is also an anti-apoptotic gene which displays distinct patterns of expression to bcl-2 in TCCs, suggesting that the proteins from these two genes regulate different cellular functions at specific stages of cell differentiation.[100]

Gene: Bcl-X

The BCK2L1 gene, also known as BCLX, BCL2L, Bcl-X, bcl-xL, bcl-xS or BCL-XXL/S, maps on chromosome 20,

at 20q11.21. The gene sequence produces, by alternative splicing, 21 different transcripts, together encoding nine different protein isoforms. There are four probable alternative promoters. The transcripts appear to differ by truncation of the N-terminus, the presence or absence of three cassette exons, or common exons with different boundaries. As a result of alternate splicing, the gene encodes two functionally different proteins. The longer Bcl-X_L is anti-apoptotic while the shorter Bcl-X_S facilitates apoptosis by interfering with the action of Bcl-2.[100,107,108]

The proteins encoded by this gene are located at the outer mitochondrial membrane, and have been shown to regulate outer mitochondrial membrane channel (VDAC) opening. VDAC regulates mitochondrial membrane potential, and thus controls the production of reactive oxygen species and release of cytochrome C by mitochondria, both of which are the potent inducers of cell apoptosis.

Two alternatively spliced transcript variants, which encode distinct isoforms, have been reported. These homologs of the bcl-2 gene family have been demonstrated to show a high degree of overexpression in TCC but only a moderate degree in normal urothelium.[94] Kirsh et al. found that immunohistochemical staining of bladder cancer cell lines reflected a comparatively higher expression of Bcl-X_L than Bcl-X_S.[100]

In this laboratory, evidence from immunohistochemical studies is at variance with some findings reported elsewhere. Previously, strong expression of bcl-2 in the basal cells of normal transitional epithelium (see Fig. 20.18) becomes attenuated as an early event in bladder neoplasia, even when the architecture is not overtly dysplastic. Surprisingly, expression of this protein occurs infrequently in established bladder cancers – whether in situ or invasive. This consistent lack of immunohistochemical staining may be due to a number of factors including the specificity of the particular antibody employed and possible splice variants of the proteins expressed in bladder neoplasia. Nevertheless, there is a distinct reciprocal correlation between diminished expression of bcl-2 and enhanced expression of HER2/*neu*, suggesting that the observed loss of identified splice variants of the protein is a real phenomenon.

Gene: major histocompatibility complex antigens

The MHC superfamily of molecules are heterodimeric cell surface receptors that function to present antigen peptide fragments to T cells responsible for cell-mediated immune responses. MHC molecules can be subdivided into two groups on the basis of their structure and function:

- Class I molecules present intracellular antigen peptide fragments (~10 amino acids) on the surface of the host cells to cytotoxic T cells.
- Class II molecules present exogenously derived antigenic peptides (~15 amino acids) to helper T cells.

MHC molecules comprise two chains:

- In Class I, the alpha chain is composed of three extracellular domains, a transmembrane region and a cytoplasmic tail. The beta chain (beta-2-microglobulin) is composed of a single extracellular domain.
- In Class II, both the alpha and the beta chains are composed of two extracellular domains, a transmembrane region and a cytoplasmic tail.

It is known that the immunoglobulin constant chain domains and a single extracellular domain in each type of MHC chain are related. These homologous domains are approximately 100 amino acids long and include a conserved intradomain disulfide bond. Members of the immunoglobulin superfamily are found in hundreds of proteins of different functions. The existence of such regions of structural homology predicate an identification system of adequately high sensitivity to distinguish these similar proteins. Antibodies are unlikely to provide sufficient discrimination. Such a system requires the precision of a molecular biological hybridization technique.

Gene: HLA-A (Class I)

The HLA-A gene, also known as HLA-A.1 or HLA-J, maps on chromosome 6, at 6p21.3. It encodes protein products that localize in membrane and are involved in immune response. The gene sequence produces, by alternative splicing, 34 different transcripts, together encoding 34 different protein isoforms. There are 10 probable alternative promoters and seven non-overlapping alternative last exons. The transcripts appear to differ by truncation of the N-terminus, truncation of the C-terminus, the presence or absence of 37 cassette exons, or common exons with different boundaries.

HLA-A belongs to the MHC Class I heavy chain paralogs. This Class I molecule is a heterodimer consisting of a heavy chain and a light chain (beta-2 microglobulin). The heavy chain is anchored in the membrane. Class I molecules play a central role in the

immune system by presenting peptides derived from the endoplasmic reticulum lumen. They are expressed in nearly all cells. The heavy chain is approximately 45 kDa and its gene contains eight exons. Exon 1 encodes the leader peptide, exons 2 and 3 encode the alpha-1 and alpha-2 domains (which both bind the peptide), exon 4 encodes the alpha-3 domain, exon 5 encodes the transmembrane region, and exons 6 and 7 encode the cytoplasmic tail. Polymorphisms within exons 2 and 3 are responsible for the peptide-binding specificity of each Class I molecule.

Gene: B2M (protein: beta-2 microglobulin)

Gene B2M, also known as RNF36 or Trif, maps on chromosome 15, at 15q21–q22.2. The gene is expressed at very high level in a wide range of epithelial and reticuloendothelial cells. The gene sequence produces, by alternative splicing, 40 different transcripts, together encoding 35 different protein isoforms, all of which are involved in the presentation of endogenous antigen. There are seven probable alternative promoters and five non-overlapping alternative last exons. The transcripts appear to differ by truncation of the N-terminus, truncation of the C-terminus, the presence or absence of 22 cassette exons, or common exons with different boundaries.

The MHC plays a vital role in the interaction between a number of cells including those of the immune system. Reduction of Class I antigens has been reported in a number of tumors. In bladder cancer, this reduction is associated with poor survival.[117] These antigens are the main target for natural killer (NK) cells which destroy cells displaying foreign genetic material after cell interactions such as those infected by viruses or which have undergone malignant transformation. In situations where expression of MHC Class II molecules becomes downregulated, or 'masked' by sialic acid, affected cells appear to remain immunologically undetected and therefore not susceptible to immune attack. Such situations are common to all malignancies.[118]

Gene: HLA-A (Class II)

Gene HLA-DOB.2.2, also known as HLA-DRB3, HLA-DR3B, HLA-DOB.2, HLA-DRB2 or TAP2.2, maps on chromosome 6, at 6p21.3. It encodes an HLA DR-beta-1 precursor. The products have Class II MHC antigen activity and are involved in immune response; they localize in membrane.

HLA-DRB3 belongs to the HLA Class II beta chain paralogs. This Class II molecule is a heterodimer consisting of an alpha (DRA) and a beta (DRB) chain, both anchored in the membrane. It plays a central role in the immune system by presenting peptides derived from extracellular proteins. Class II molecules are expressed in antigen-presenting cells. The beta chain is approximately 26–28 kD and its gene contains six exons. Exon 1 encodes the leader peptide, exons 2 and 3 encode the two extracellular domains, exon 4 encodes the transmembrane domain and exon 5 encodes the cytoplasmic tail. Within the DR molecule the beta chain contains all of the polymorphisms defining the peptide-binding specificities.

CONCLUSION

In urinary bladder epithelium, both papillary and flat neoplastic lesions contain two cell populations, one superficial and the other invasive, the latter portending an aggressive phenotype with poor prognosis. It is likely that these different cell subsets could (and should) be differentiated by gene expression and gene mutation analysis. This is the subject of greatest diagnostic and prognostic dilemma and also the area in which bladder cancer may prove to be a paradigm for many other epithelial neoplasms, thereby yielding insights into general mechanisms of cancer progression that currently elude study of more complex glandular malignancies.

At present, immunohistochemical reagents (antibodies, lectins, etc.) are widely used in analyzing malignancies. In this laboratory, staining of bladder tumor samples is routinely performed using a panel of monoclonal antibodies, including those to the protein products of many of the genes discussed in this chapter. There are numerous examples, particularly in the bladder, of the adjunctive value (both clinical and pathologic) of knowing detailed phenotypic features of each individual malignancy (see Chapters 21 and 23). These markers are not only valuable in discriminating normal from reactive and neoplastic, but also in identifying tumors that will progress rapidly from those that are relatively quiescent. For example, a high level of the proliferation marker Ki-67 is seen in metastasizing cells, as is the overexpression of HER2/*neu*. Decreased levels of pRb indicate that a mutation has occurred and that the related tumor suppressor gene has been inactivated. The reverse is seen in p53 since increased levels indicate the mutated form because it is more stable than the wild type, resists degradation and accumulates in the nucleus. Loss of expression of CD44, and decreased levels of Class I HLA antigens,

are both expected in samples where bladder cancer is present.

Knowledge of gene structure, particularly from the Human Genome Database, has revolutionized our understanding of genetic factors in many neoplasms including bladder tumors. This knowledge has particularly emphasized the limitations of all antibodies employed to phenotype solid tumors and the necessity to transfer to molecular biologically based analytical systems as quickly as possible, for example:

- Immunohistochemical systems are labor-intensive and cannot be readily automated. They generate data which are derived from different parts of a tumor and hence are not exactly identical.
- The antibodies currently employed are frequently poorly defined with respect to their precise epitopes. Such lack of precision is no longer acceptable. It is important to understand the biological function(s) of the individually spliced domains of many of the proteins involved in the different stages of neoplasia, invasion and metastasis.
- To continue to employ current immunohistochemical techniques, splice variants that differ between different tumors as well as between a tumor and its normal tissue counterpart require, for their detection, a separate antibody for each distinct spliced variant peptide sequence. Generation of antibodies with the necessary levels of specification and sensitivity represents an enormous task and may even be biologically impossible. However, it is the expression and assembly of each spectrum of splice variants that determines the individuality of each tumor.

Finally, during the evolution and progression of an individual cancer, involved genes are frequently both heterogeneous and in flux with respect to their expression. Throughout this chapter, it has been adequately demonstrated that many genes contain numerous sequences that are not only differentially spliced but may also be under the control of different promoters at different times. Some regions are replicated in many different proteins. Meaningful analysis of such complexity requires the use of techniques significantly different from those currently employed. Those novel techniques will not only provide the necessary specificity to distinguish neoplastic from normal (hence refining the pathologic diagnosis), but will also provide the basis for biologically appropriate therapeutic modulation of bladder cancers – and thereafter of other tissue malignancies.

REFERENCES

1. Yung-Chang Lin, Shi-Ming Tu. Medical oncology: a comprehensive review – bladder cancer. www.intouchlive.com/textbook/morev28.htm

2. Muller M. Telomerase: its clinical relevance in the diagnosis of bladder cancer. Oncogene 2002;21:650–655.

3. Miyake H, Hara I, Yamanaka K, et al. Overexpression of Bcl-2 enhances metastatic potential of human bladder cancer cells. Br J Cancer 1999;79:1651–1656.

4. www.urologychannel.com/bladdercancer/index.shtml.

5. www.cancerhelp.org.uk.

6. Sugino T, Gorham H, Yoshida K, et al. Progressive loss of CD44 gene expression in invasive bladder cancer. Am J Pathol 1996;149:873–882.

7. Schalken JA, Van Moorselaar RJA, Bringuier PP, et al. Critical review of the models of study of the biologic progression of bladder cancer. Semin Surg Oncol 1992;8:274–278.

8. Lamm DL. Carcinoma in situ. Urol Clin North Am 1992;19:499–508.

9. Heney NM, Ahmed S, Flanagan MJ, et al. Superficial bladder cancer: progression and recurrence. J Urol 1983;130:1083–1086.

10. Malmstrom P-U, Busch C, Norlen BJ. Recurrence, progression and survival in bladder cancer: a retrospective analysis of 232 patients with >5 year follow-up. Scand J Urol Nephrol 1987;21:185–195.

11. Ruppert JM, Tokino K, Sidransky D. Evidence for two bladder cancer suppresser loci on human chromosome 9. Cancer Res 1993;53:5093–5095.

12. Spruck CH, Ohneseit PF, Gonsales-Zulueta M, et al. Two molecular pathways to transitional cell carcinoma of the bladder. Cancer Res 1994;54:784–788.

13. Dalbagni G, Presti J, Reuter V, et al. Genetic alterations in bladder cancer. Lancet 1993;342:469–471.

14. Ghaleb AH, Pizzolo JG, Melamed MR. Aberrations of chromosomes 9 and 17 in bilharzial bladder cancer as detected by fluorescence in situ hybridization. Am J Clin Pathol 1996;106:234–241.

15. Miyao N, Tsai YC, Lerner SP, et al. Role of chromosome 9 in human bladder cancer. Cancer Res 1993;53:4066–4070.

16. Williamson MP, Elder PA, Shaw ME, et al. p16 (CDKN2) is a major deletion target at 9p21 in bladder cancer. Hum Mol Genet 1995;4:1569–1577.

17. Cairns P, Mao L, Merlo A, et al. Rates of p16 (MTS1) mutations in primary tumours with 9p loss. Science 1994;265:415–416.

18. Orlow I, Lacombe L, Hannon GJ, et al. Deletion of the p16 and p15 genes in human bladder tumours. J Natl Cancer Inst 1995;87:1524–1529.

19. Poddighe PJ, Bringuier PP, Vallinga M, et al. Loss of chromosome 9 in tissue sections of transitional cell carcinomas as detected by interphase cytogenetics. A comparison with RFLP analysis. J Pathol 1996;179:169–176.

20. Halachmi S, Madeb R, Kravtsov A, et al. Bladder cancer – genetic overview. Med Sci Monit 2001;7:164–168.

21. Tsuji K, Kojima K, Murakami Y, et al. Prognostic value of Ki-67 antigen and p53 protein in urinary bladder cancer: immunohistochemical analysis of radical cystectomy specimens. Br J Urol 1997;79:367–372.

22. El-Deiry WS, Tokino T, Velculescu V, et al. WAF1, a potential mediator of p53 tumour suppression. Cell 1993;75:817–825.

23. MacLeod KF, Sherry N, Hannon G, et al. p53-dependent and independent expression of p21 during cell growth, differentiation and DNA damage. Genes Dev 1995;9:935–944.

24. Parker SB, Eichele G, Zhang P, et al. P53-independent expression of p21 Cip1 in muscle and other terminally differentiating cells. Science 1995;267:1024–1027.

25. Johnson M, Dimitrov D, Vojta PJ, et al. Evidence for a p53-independent pathway for upregulation of SDI1/CIP1/WAF1/p21 RNA in human cells. Mol Carcinog 1994;11:59–64.

26. Stein JP, Ginsberg DA, Grossfeld GD, et al. Effect of p21 WAF1/CIP1 expression on tumour progression in bladder cancer. J Natl Cancer Inst 1998;90:1072–1079.

27. Cote R, Esrig D, Groshen S, et al. p53 and treatment of bladder cancer (letter to the Editor). Nature 1997;385:123–125.

28. Pfister C, Flaman JM, Dunet F, et al. p53 mutations in bladder tumours inactivate the transactivation of the p21 and Bax genes, and have a predictive value for the clinical outcome after bacillus Calmette–Guérin therapy. J Urol 1999;162:69–73.

29. Braithwaite KL, Mellon JK, Neal DE. WAF1 expression in transitional cell carcinoma (TCC) of the bladder: inverse relationship to p53 accumulation and association with good prognosis. Proc Am Assoc Cancer Res 1997:3534.

30. Qureshi KN, Griffiths TRL, Robinson MC, et al. Combined p21 WAF1/CIP1 and p53 overexpression predict improved survival in muscle-invasive bladder cancer treated by radical radiotherapy. Int J Radiat Oncol Biol Phys 2001;51:1234–1240.

31. Zlotta AR, Noel JC, Fayt I, et al. Correlation and prognostic significance of p53, p21 WAF1/CIP1 and Ki-67 expression in patients with superficial bladder tumours treated with bacillus Calmette–Guérin intravesical therapy. J Urol 1999;161:792–798.

32. Waldman T, Zhang Y, Dillehay L, et al. Cell-cycle arrest versus cell death in cancer therapy. Nat Med 1997;3:1034–1036.

33. www.oncodox.com/markers/p53.htm.

34. Cooper GM. The Cell: A Molecular Approach. Washington DC: ASM Press, 1997, p 625.

35. Horwich A. Oncoclogy: A Multidisciplinary Textbook. London: Chapman and Hall Medical, 1995.

36. Halevy O, Hall A, Oren M. Stabilisation of the p53 transformation related protein in mouse fibrosarcoma cell lines: effects of protein sequence and intracellular environment. Mol Cell Biol 1989;9:3385–3392.

37. Fujimoto K, Yamada Y, Okajima E, et al. Frequent

association of p53 gene mutation in invasive bladder cancer. Cancer Res 1992;52:1393–1398.

38. Sidransky D, Von Eschenbach A, Tsai YC, et al. Identification of p53 gene mutations in bladder cancers and urine samples. Science 1991;252:706–709.

39. Serth J, Kuczyk MA, Bokemeyer C, et al. p53 immunohistochemistry as an independent prognostic factor for superficial transitional cell carcinoma of the bladder. Br J Cancer 1995;71:201–205.

40. Esrig D, Elmajian D, Groshen S, et al. Accumulation of nuclear p53 and tumour progression in bladder cancer. N Engl J Med 1994;331:1259–1264.

41. Dahse R, Utting M, Werner W, et al. TP53 alterations as a potential diagnostic marker in superficial bladder carcinoma and in patients' serum, plasma and urine samples. Int J Urol 2002;20:107–115.

42. Sarkis AS, Dalbagni G, Cordon-Cardo C, et al. Nuclear overexpression of p53 protein in transitional cell bladder carcinoma: a marker for disease progression. J Natl Cancer Inst 1993;85:53–59.

43. Bernardini S, Adessi GL, Billerey C, et al. Immunohistochemical detection of p53 protein overexpression versus gene sequencing in urinary bladder carcinomas. J Urol 1999;162:1496–1501.

44. Miyamoto H, Shuin T, Torigoe S, et al. Retinoblastoma gene mutations in primary human bladder cancer. Br J Cancer 1995;71:831–835.

45. Decaprio JA, Ludlow JW, Lynch D, et al. The product of the retinoblastoma susceptibility gene has properties of a cell cycle regulatory element. Cell 1989;58:1085–1095.

46. Buchkovich K, Duffy LA, Harlow E. The retinoblastoma protein is phosphorylated during specific phases of the cell cycle. Cell 1989;58:1097–1105.

47. Mittnacht S, Weinberg RA. G1/S phosphorylation of the retinoblastoma protein is associated with an altered affinity for the nuclear compartment. Cell 1991;65:381–393.

48. www.web.indstate.edu/theme/mwking/tumor-suppressors.html.

49. Cordon-Cardo C, Wartinger D, Petrylak D, et al. Altered expression of the retinoblastoma gene product: prognostic indicator in bladder cancer. J Natl Cancer Inst 1992;84:1251–1256.

50. Logothetics CJ, Xu H-J, Ro JY, et al. Altered expression of the retinoblastoma protein and known prognostic variables in locally advanced bladder cancer. J Natl Cancer Inst 1992;84:1256–1261.

51. Cordon-Cardo C, Zhang ZF, Dalbagni G, et al. Cooperative effects of p53 and pRB alterations in primary superficial bladder tumours. Cancer Res 1997;57:1217–1221.

52. Benedict WF, Lerner SP, Zhou J, et al. Level of retinoblastoma protein in expression correlates with p16 (MTS-1/INK4A/CDKN2) status in bladder cancer. Oncogene 1999;18:1197–1203.

53. Xu HJ, Cairns P, Hu SX, et al. Loss of RB protein expression in primary bladder cancer correlates with loss of heterozygosity at the RB locus and tumour progression. Int J Cancer 1993;53:781–784.

54. Tamura M, Gu J, Matsumoto K, et al. Inhibition of cell migration, spreading and focal adhesions by tumour suppresser gene PTEN. Science 1998;280:1614–1617.

55. Gu J, Tamura M, Pankov R, et al. Shc and FAK differentially regulate cell motility and directionality modulated PTEN. J Cell Biol 1999;146:389–404.

56. Przybojewska B, Jagiello A, Jalmuzna P. H-RAS, K-RAS and N-RAS gene activation in human bladder cancers. Cancer Genet Cytogenet 2000;121:73–77.

57. Haliassos A, Liloglou M, Likourinas M, et al. H-ras oncogene mutations in the urine of patients with bladder tumours: description of a novel non-invasive method for the detection of neoplasia. Int J Oncol 1992;1:731–734.

58. Fontana D, Bellina M, Scoffone C, et al. Evaluation of c-ras oncogene product (p21) in superficial bladder cancer. Eur Urol 1996;29:470–476.

59. Coussens L, Yang-Feng TL, Liao YC, et al. Tyrosine kinase receptor with extensive homology to EGF receptor shares chromosomal location with neu oncogene. Science 1985;230:1132–1139.

60. Fukushige S, Matsubara KI, Yoshida M, et al. Localisation of a novel v-erbB-related gene, c-erbB-2 on human chromosome-17 and its amplification in a gastric cell line. Mol Cell Biol 1986;6:955–958.

61. Schechter AL, Stem DF, Vaidyanathan L, et al. The neu oncogene: an erbB related gene encoding a 185,000-Mr tumour antigen. Nature 1984;312:513–516.

62. Underwood M, Bartlett J, Reeves J, et al. C-erb-2 gene amplification: a molecular marker in recurrent bladder tumours? Cancer Res 1995;55:2422–2430.

63. Waterfield MD, Scrace GT, Whittle N, et al. Platelet-derived growth factor is structurally related to the putative transmembrane protein p28 sis of simian sarcoma virus. Nature 1983;304:35–39.

64. Sherr CJ, Rettenmier CN, Sacca R, et al. The c-fms proto-oncogene product is related to the mononuclear phagocyte growth factor, CSF-1. Cell 1985;41:665–676.

65. Downward J, Yarden Y, Mayes E, et al. Close similarity of epidermal growth factor receptor and v-erb-B oncogene protein sequences. Nature 1984;37:521–528.

66. Coombs LM, Knowles MA, Milroy E. Her2 (cerbB-2, neu, Mac 117) amplification and expression in transitional cell carcinoma. Urol Res 1989;17:345–348.

67. Coombs LM, Pigott DA, Sweeney E, et al. Amplification and over-expression of c-erbB-2 in transitional cell carcinoma of the urinary bladder. Br J Cancer 1991;63:601–608.

68. Kallionemi OP, Holli K, Visakorpi T, et al. Association of c-erbB-2 protein overexpression with high rate of cell proliferation, increased risk of visceral metastasis and poor long-term survival in breast cancer. Int J Cancer 1991;49:650–655.

69. Lipponen P. Expression of c-erbB-2 oncoprotein in transitional cell bladder cancer. Eur J Cancer 1993;29:749–753.

70. Neal DE, Sharples L, Smith K, et al. The epidermal growth factor receptor and the prognosis of bladder cancer. Cancer 1990;65:1619–1625.

71. Moriyama M, Akiyama T, Yamamoto T, et al. Expression of c-*erb*B-2 gene product in urinary bladder cancer. J Urol 1991;145:423–427.

72. Sauter G, Haley J, Chew K, et al. Epidermal growth factor receptor expression is associated with rapid tumour proliferation in bladder cancer. Int J Cancer 1994;57:508–514.

73. Bush C, Price P, Norton J, et al. Proliferation in human bladder carcinoma measured by Ki-67 antibody labelling: its potential clinical importance. Br J Cancer 1991;64:357–360.

74. Mulder AH, Van Hootegem JC, Sylvester R, et al. Prognostic factors in bladder carcinoma: histologic parameters and expression of a cell cycle-related nuclear antigen (Ki-67). J Pathol 1992;166:37–43.

75. Lee AKS, Wiley B, Loda M, et al. DNA ploidy, proliferation and *neu*-oncogene protein overexpression in breast carcinoma. Mod Pathol 1992;5:61–67.

76. Michieli P, Chedid M, Lin D, et al. Induction of WAF1/CIP1 by a p53-independent pathway. Cancer Res 1994;54:3391–3395.

77. Asakura T, Takano Y, Iki M, et al. Prognostic value of Ki-67 for recurrence and progression of superficial bladder cancer. J Urol 1997;158:385–388.

78. Wu TT, Chen J, Lee Y, et al. The role of bcl-2, p53 and Ki-67 index in predicting tumour recurrence for low grade superficial transitional cell bladder carcinoma. J Urol 2000;163:758–760.

79. Gontero P, Casetta G, Zitella A, et al. Evaluation of p53 protein overexpression, Ki67 proliferative activity and mitotic index as markers of tumour recurrence in superficial transitional cell carcinoma of the bladder. Eur Urol 2000;38:287–296.

80. Colquhoun AJ, Mellon JK. Epidermal growth factor receptor and bladder cancer. Postgrad Med J 2002;78:584–589.

81. Liebert M. Growth factors in bladder cancer. World J Urol 1995;13:349–355.

82. Messing EM. Clinical implications of the expression of epidermal growth factor receptors in human transitional cell carcinoma. Cancer Res 1990;50:2530–2537.

83. Berger MS, Greenfield C, Gullick WJ, et al. Evaluation of epidermal growth factor receptors in bladder tumours. Br J Cancer 1987;56:533–537.

84. Neal DE, Marsh C, Bennett MK, et al. Epidermal growth factor receptors in human bladder cancer: comparison of invasive and superficial tumours. Lancet 1985;1:366–368.

85. Messing EM, Hanson P, Ulrich P, et al. Epidermal growth factor – interactions with normal and malignant urothelium: in vivo and in situ studies. J Urol 1987;138:1329–1335.

86. Stein JP, Grossfeld GD, Ginsberg DA, et al. Prognostic markers in bladder cancer: a contemporary review of the literature. J Urol 1998;160:645–659.

87. De Maio A. The heat-shock response. New Horiz 1995;3:198–207.

88. Kaufmann SHE. Heat shock proteins and the immune response. Immunol Today 1990;11:129–136.

89. Saleh A, Srinivasula SM, Balkir L, et al. Negative regulation of the Apaf-1 apoptosome by Hsp70. Nat Cell Biol 2000;2:476–483.

90. Jolly C, Morimoto RI. Role of the heat shock response and molecular chaperones in oncogenesis and cell death. J Natl Cancer Inst 2000;92:1564–1572.

91. Welch WJ. Mammalian stress response: cell physiology, structure/function of stress proteins and implications for medicine and disease. Physiol Rev 1992;72:1063–1081.

92. Lebret T, Watson RW, Fitzpatrick JM. Heat shock proteins: their role in urological tumours. J Urol 2003;169:338–346.

93. Vaux D, Cory S, Adams J. *Bcl*-gene promotes haematopoietic cell survival and co-operates with c-*myc* to immortalize pre-B cells. Nature 1988;335:440–442.

94. Krajewski S, Tanaka S. Investigations of the subcellular distribution of the bcl-2 oncoprotein: residence in the nuclear envelope, endoplasmic reticulum, and outer mitochondrial membranes. Cancer Res 1993;53:4701–4714.

95. Nakopoulou L, Michalopoulou A, Giannopoulou I, et al. bcl-2 protein expression is associated with a prognostically favourable phenotype in breast cancer irrespective of p53 immunostaining. Histopathology 1999;34(4):310–319.

96. Li B, Kanamaru H, Noriki S, et al. Reciprocal expression of bcl-2 and p53 oncoproteins in urothelial dysplasia and carcinoma of the urinary bladder. Urol Res 1998;26:235–241.

96. Lipponen PK, Aaltomaa S, Eskelinen M. Expression of the apoptosis suppressing bcl-2 protein in transitional cell bladder tumours. Histopathology 1997;28:135–140.

97. Atug F, Turkeri L, Ozyurek M, et al. Bcl-2 and p53 overexpression as associated risk factors in transitional cell carcinoma of the bladder. Int Urol Nephrol 1998;30:455–461.

98. Liukkonen TJ, Lipponen PK, Helle M, et al. Immunoreactivity of bcl-2, p53 and EGFr is associated with tumour stage, grade and cell proliferation in superficial bladder cancer. Finn-bladder III Group. Urol Res 1997;25:1–7.

99. Kirsch EJ, Baunoch DA, Stadler WM. Expression of bcl-2 and bcl-x in bladder cancer. J Urol 1998;159:1348–1353.

100. Pezzella F, Turley H, Kuzu I, et al. Bcl-2 protein in non-small cell lung carcinoma. N Engl J Med 1993;329:690–694.

101. Chiou S-K, Rao L, White E. bcl-2 blocks p53 dependent apoptosis. Mol Cell Biol 1994;14:2256–2263.

102. Miyashita T, Harigai M, Hanada M, et al. Identification of a p53 dependent negative response element in the bcl-2 gene. Cancer Res 1994;54:3131–3135.

103. Haldar S, Negrini M, Monne M, et al. Down regulation of *bcl*-2 by p53 in breast cancer cell lines. Cancer Res 1994;54:2095–2097.

104. Marin MC, Hsu B, Meyn RE, et al. Evidence that p53 and bcl-2 are regulators of a common cell death pathway important for in vivo lymphomagenesis. Oncogene 1994;9:3107–3112.

105. www.oncodox.com/markers/bcl2.htm.

106. Cooper GM. Oncogenes, 2nd edn. Boston: Jones and Bartlett, 1995, pp 336–338.

107. Krajewski S, Krajewski M, Shabaik A, et al. Immunohistochemical analysis of in vivo patterns of Bcl-x expression. Cancer Res 1994;54:5501–5507.

108. Cohen MB, Griebling TL, Ahaghotu CA, et al. Cellular adhesion molecules in urologic malignancies. Am J Clin Pathol 1997;107:56–63.

109. Woodman AC, Goodison S, Drake M, et al. Non-invasive diagnosis of bladder cancer by enzyme linked immunosurbent assay detection of CD44 isoforms in exfoliated urothelia. Clin Cancer Res 2000;6:2381–2392.

110. Matsumura Y, Tarin D. Significance of CD44 gene products for cancer diagnosis and disease evaluation. Lancet 1992;340:1053–1058.

111. Tarin D, Bolodeoku J, Hatfill SJ, et al. The clinical significance of malfunction of the CD44 locus in malignancy. J Neurol Oncol 1995;26:209–219.

112. Sugiyama M, Woodman A. Sugino T, et al. Non-invasive detection of bladder cancer of abnormal CD44 proteins in exfoliated cancer cells in the urine. J Clin Pathol 1995;48:M142–M147.

113. Lipponen P, Aaltoma S, Kosma VM, et al. Expression of CD44 standard and variant – v6 proteins in transitional cell bladder tumours and their relation to prognosis during a long-term follow-up. J Pathol 1998;186:157–164.

114. Hong RL, Pu YS, Chu JS, et al. Correlation of expression of CD44 isoforms and E-cadherin with differentiation in human urothelial cell lines and transitional cell carcinoma. Cancer Lett 1995;89:81–87.

115. Ross JS, del Rosario AD, Bui HX, et al. Expression of the CD44 cell adhesion molecule in urinary bladder transitional cell carcinoma. Mod Pathol 1996;9:854–860.

116. Toma V, Hauri D, Schmid U, et al. Focal loss of CD44 variant protein expression is related to recurrence in superficial bladder carcinoma. Am J Pathol 1999;155:1427–1432.

117. Klein B, Levin I, Klein T. HLA Class I antigen expression in human solid tumors. Israel J Med Sci 1996;32:1238–1243.

118. Foster CS. Processing of N-linked oligosaccharide glycoproteins in human tumours. Br J Cancer 1990;62:57–63.

21

VALUE OF ANALYZING p53 STATUS, OR OTHER OBJECTIVE MARKERS, WHEN DETERMINING MANAGEMENT STRATEGIES

Jessica L. J. Vriesema, Johannus A. Witjes, Frans M. J. Debruyne and Jack A. Schalken

INTRODUCTION

Bladder cancer is the fourth most common malignancy in men and the seventh most common malignancy in women in the United States. More than 90% of bladder cancers are urothelial cell carcinomas (UCCs), although the incidence varies markedly in different countries. About two-thirds of UCCs will present upon initial diagnosis as superficial tumors (carcinoma in situ (CIS); Ta, T1); the remaining one-third is muscle-invasive (T2–T4) or disseminated (N+ and/or M+). The clinical course of primary superficial UCC of the bladder is characterized by the tendency to recur after transurethral resection (approximately 70%, most frequently in the first year after the operation). Unfortunately, about 3–4% of the superficial tumors progress to a muscle-invasive and/or disseminated process with a poor prognosis.[1,2]

In the past, prognostic factors in bladder cancer were predominantly clinically and histopathologically defined. With the recent progress in molecular biological technology, however, research is focusing on revealing the molecular mechanisms associated with bladder carcinogenesis. A better understanding of molecular pathways implicated in the development of tumors may lead to new diagnostic and prognostic applications. These can be used not only in the assessment of the biological behavior of tumors, but also for the response to treatment, i.e. in directing management strategies.

Molecular studies, in relation to the etiology of bladder cancer, have focused on proto-oncogenes and tumor suppressor genes, as well as metastasis-associated genes. After the early revelation of *ras* p21 activation in a bladder cancer cell line, further identification of relevant oncogenes in bladder cancer have been less successful, albeit that EGFR and HER2 are still candidate oncogenes. The most important implications came from studies identifying the tumor suppressor gene p53 as a candidate. It is the most common mutated gene in all human malignant tumors.[3] Research on p53 in bladder cancer is aimed at diagnosis, predicting treatment outcome after intravesical therapy, predicting the risk of tumor progression and determining the benefits of (adjuvant) chemo- and/or radiotherapy. Not only are oncogenes and tumor suppressor genes studied, but cell adhesion molecules (e.g. E-cadherin) and their adhesion and signaling pathways are also investigated. This will contribute to a better understanding of bladder cancer biology. Molecular markers, such as the p53 tumor suppressor gene, may lead to a better approach in the management of patients with bladder cancer in the 21st century. In this chapter a review is provided on the research and applicability of p53 and some other markers in bladder cancer.

p53: 'GUARDIAN OF THE GENOME'

Introduction

The p53 gene is located on the short arm of chromosome 17 (17p13.1) and encodes for a 53 kD nuclear phosphoprotein with specific DNA binding properties. Mutations in and loss of the p53 gene are the most common genetic defects in human malignant tumors.[3] The p53 protein is encoded by 11 exons, and more than 90% of the mutations are found in four conserved domains (exons 5–8) encoding the DNA binding domain.[4] The wild-type protein p53 acts as a cell cycle control protein at the level of G1 to S phase transition.[5] If cellular stresses such as DNA damage occur, p53 protein levels rise and block cells in the G1 phase. The DNA damage can subsequently be eliminated either by DNA repair or by initiation of programmed cell death (apoptosis).[6] This decreases the chance of propagating mutant cells and hence of cancer formation.

It should be stressed that p53 is more involved in regulating and controlling the cell cycle than in playing a direct role in the mechanism of cell cycle progression. Studies using knockout mice have demonstrated that functional p53 is not essential for mitotic or meiotic cell cycles, but the high incidence of tumor development in p53-null mice[7] strongly suggests that p53 provides an important checkpoint that prevents aberrant growth, division and neoplastic transformation. The p53 gene seems to function as a transcription factor capable of regulating the expression of a growing list of downstream genes, as showed in Table 21.1. Hence, p53 is involved in pathways of cell cycle control, angiogenesis, growth factor signaling, etc.[8]

Alterations of the p53 gene result in loss of function. Cells that lose the wild-type p53 function fail to show growth arrest if DNA damage occurs, which can lead to replication of incorrect DNA, resulting in genetic instability.[9,10] The mutated protein undergoes conformational changes, resulting in a prolonged half-life and subsequently in accumulation of the protein.[11] Because of the minute amounts and rapid turnover of wild-type p53, it has been suggested that overexpression of immunodetectable p53 is synonymous with mutation, because the immunohistochemical detection of mutated p53 is based upon the extended half-life of the protein.

Table 21.1 The interaction of p53 with other genes[8]

Gene	Function
Activated by p53	
Bax	Inducer of apoptosis
Gadd45	Growth arrest and DNA damage inducible gene
Fas/Apo 1	Inducer of apoptosis
GD-AIF	Angiogenesis inhibitory factor
IGF-BP3	Insulin growth factor-binding protein 3
MCK	Muscle creatine kinase
MDM2	Feedback inhibition regulator of p53
p21$^{waf1/cip1}$	Cell cycle inhibitor
Thrombospondin	Inhibitor of angiogenesis
Repressed by p53	
bcl-2	Inhibitor of apoptosis
c-fos	Cellular oncogene
c-myc	Cellular oncoprotein
FGF	Fibroblast growth factor
HSP70	70-kDa heat shock protein
IL-6	Interleukin 6
MDR1	Multidrug resistance glycoprotein 1
PCNA	Proliferating cell nuclear antigen

However, overexpression of wild-type p53 has been found. Several studies have shown a considerable discrepancy (20–30%) between molecular genetic alterations in the p53 gene and overexpression of the protein.[12–15] Loss of wild-type p53 function can be the result of complexing with viral oncoproteins, for example adenovirus 5 Elb protein[16] and E6 protein of human papilloma virus 16 and 18.[17] In addition, many cellular proteins are capable of binding and inactivating p53, for example the MDM2 protein (also known as the 'big brother of p53').[18]

Detection methods

Methods used to demonstrate the presence of p53 mutations can be divided into three groups:

- Indirect mutation analysis using immunohisto-chemistry (IHC)
- Direct mutation analysis of DNA using direct sequencing
- The use of a screening method (e.g. single-strand conformation polymorphism) followed by sequence confirmation.

Indirect mutation analysis

The large majority of bladder tumor studies have used immunohistochemical detection of p53 protein accumulation as an indirect marker for the presence of p53 mutations. Difficulties arise in comparing these studies. Standardization of the immunohistochemical techniques used, the assessment of positive staining, the definitions of end-points such as recurrence and progression, the statistical analysis used and careful recording of the treatments which patients receive are required to aid comparison between studies.

The International Study Initiative on Bladder Cancer (ISBC), coordinated by Schmitz-Dräger, is undertaking a multi-institutional retrospective study to analyze present data concerning p53 accumulation and prognosis of bladder cancer. They have already concluded after detailed analysis that differences between various studies, with regard to the prognostic impact of p53, can be partly explained by the differing study designs and heterogeneous study populations.[19] McShane et al.[20] studied the reproducibility of p53 IHC in bladder tumors. They also concluded that standardization of staining protocols and selection of a uniform threshold for binary interpretation of results might improve assay reproducibility between laboratories.

Direct mutation analysis

Direct sequencing is still considered to be the best mutation detection method, although direct DNA sequencing has not been frequently used in p53 mutation detection. The classical sequencing method is manually performed and time-consuming, and mutation detection is hampered when DNA mixtures of wild-type and mutant DNA containing less than 50% mutant DNA are analyzed. As stated above, more than 90% of the mutations are found in exons 5–8. In most studies only these exons are analyzed because of time and costs; possible mutations in the other exons may therefore be missed. However, significant progress has been made in the last few years in developing automated DNA sequencing methods. These methods perform with lower costs, increased speed and increased sensitivity.

Screening

The use of a screening method before sequencing, such as single-strand conformation polymorphism (SSCP), is less costly and time-consuming than direct sequencing. However, under optimal conditions only 80–90% of potential mutations are detected.[21] Hence, SSCP is less sensitive than direct sequencing.

p53 in the diagnosis of (superficial) bladder cancer

Most studies are based on the prognostic value of p53 in bladder cancer instead of on its diagnostic value. Sidransky and colleagues[22] were the first to report detection of p53 mutations in urine of patients with primary invasive bladder cancer. These findings were in agreement with other reports suggesting that loss of heterozygosity on chromosome 17p and mutations in the p53 gene are late events in the progression of bladder cancer, and hence not suitable as an early marker for superficial bladder cancer.[23]

Molecular and immunohistochemical techniques for p53 mutation detection have been used to diagnose bladder cancer in urine. Righi et al.[24] investigated the use of p53 IHC to increase the diagnostic accuracy of urinary cytology. The sensitivity and specificity of this method were 24% and 75%, respectively, thus demonstrating that p53 IHC did not improve the diagnosis of bladder cancer. Molecular techniques such as blunt-end SSCP[25] and loss of heterozygosity detection by polymerase chain reaction (PCR) and agarose gel electrophoresis[26] are also used, with better results. However, larger series of patients are needed to confirm the accuracy of these techniques in urine of patients with bladder cancer.

Bladder wash samples form another medium for detection methods. Vet et al.[27] concluded that the analysis of p53 mutations in at least two bladder washings gives insight into the p53 status of the synchronous tumors. Bladder washings enable the harvest of more and better-preserved material compared to voided urine, but the main disadvantage is the invasive character of this method.

The main limiting factor for this clinical implication of p53 mutation detection is the observation that p53 mutations appear to be a late event in bladder tumor progression. This appears to limit this assay to screening patients for recurrences rather than for primary tumors.

In bladder cancer, mutations of the p53 gene are common events, and this has been shown to be strongly associated with tumor grade and stage.[28–31]

p53 and other predictors for recurrence

From Table 21.2 it is clear that controversy exists about the role of p53 in the prediction of recurrence in superficial bladder cancer. Some studies say that p53 expression is associated with recurrence in superficial disease. Controversial studies such as the one from Nakopoulou et al.[32] and recent ones from the group of Gontero[33] or Wu et al.[34] did not find any predictive relationship between the p53 status of a tumor and recurrence-free survival of the patient. However, there are large differences between these studies (e.g. the used cut-off level for immunohistochemical detection of positive nuclei). In addition, the analysis methods for calculation of correlation differ widely – for example in the study performed by Tetu et al.,[35] positive p53 staining was a prognostic indicator for recurrence in univariate analysis, but not in multivariate analysis, even if other thresholds for the number of positive cells and staining intensity were used. Moreover, Iakim-Liossi et al.[36] only compared the number of patients that recurred in the p53 positive group and in the p53 negative group.

Markers of proliferation, for example Ki-67 and proliferating cell nuclear antigen (PCNA), have also served as useful tools to determine the rate of tumor replication. PCNA has been shown to correlate with recurrence and progression to muscle invasion in superficial tumors of the same stage and grade.[37] Asakura and co-workers[38] found that the Ki-67 labeling index was an independent predictive factor for recurrence of superficial bladder cancer in 104 patients using multivariate analysis. Nevertheless, proliferation factors like PCNA and Ki-67 are not always demonstrated as being independent predictors of tumor recurrence. Additional studies are therefore needed to increase understanding in their role.

Clinical and histopathologic factors (e.g. multiplicity, tumor extent and tumor grade) are still used as prognostic markers for recurrence of superficial bladder cancer in daily clinical practice.[1]

Table 21.2 Studies correlating p53 alterations with recurrence in patients with superficial bladder tumors

Authors	Journal	Method of analysis	Patient group	Correlation?
Nakopoulou et al.	Urology 1995; 46:334–340	IHC (>10%)	n = 45; Ta-T1	No
Tetu et al.	J Urol 1996; 155:1784–1788	IHC (>0%)	n = 265; Ta-T1	Yes
Underwood et al.	Br J Urol 1996; 77:659–666	IHC (o.s.s.)	n = 164; Ta-T1	No
Casetta et al.	Eur Urol 1997; 32:229–236	IHC (>0%)	n = 59; TaGI	Yes
Inagaki et al.	Int J Urol 1997; 4:172–177	IHC (o.s.s.)	n = 128; Ta-T1	No
Ye et al.	J Urol 1998; 160:2025–2028	PCR-SSCP sequencing	n = 43; Ta-T1	Yes
Pister et al.	Clin Cancer Res 1999; 5:4079–4084	IHC (>5%)	n = 244; Ta-T1	No
Toktas et al.	Int Urol Nephrol 1999; 31:327–334	IHC (>?%)	n = 52; T1	Yes
Wu et al.	J Urol 2000; 163:758–760	IHC (>20%)	n = 93; Ta-T1/G1-G2	No
Iakim-Liossi et al.	Cytopathology 2000; 11:96–103	IHC (>10%)	n = 80; Ta-T1	Yes
Gontero et al.	Eur Urol 2000; 38:287–296	IHC (>20%)	n = 192; Ta-T1	No

IHC, immunohistochemistry; PCR-SSCP, polymerase chain reaction–single-strand conformation polymorphism; o.s.s, own scoring system

OTHER MOLECULAR MARKERS

The retinoblastoma gene

Another tumor suppressor gene potentially involved in bladder cancer is the retinoblastoma (Rb) gene located on chromosome 13q14. It encodes a 110 kD nuclear protein that acts to silence specific S phase genes.[39] Hence, like the p53 protein, it plays a pivotal role in cell cycle control. The Rb protein functions downstream of p53 in the same regulatory pathway. p53 influences the activity of cyclin-dependent kinases that phosphorylate pRb, via p21 production.[40] High levels of p21 inhibit cyclinE-Cdk2, which in turn results in decreased pRb phosphorylation and a G1/S cell cycle arrest. Loss of Rb protein function occurs in approximately one-third of human bladder cell lines.[41] Rb gene alterations occur in 30–37% of primary bladder cancers and are associated with muscle-invasive disease.[42,43]

Gross structural deletions of the Rb gene as well as point mutations have been documented, but detailed mutation analysis of this gene has so far not been reported, presumably because of the practical constraints of analyzing such a large gene. Loss of heterozygosity at the Rb locus is strongly associated with absence of protein expression.[44] However, immunohistochemical analyses have been performed, mainly to study the prognostic value of loss of Rb protein expression in progression and in response to radiation therapy.

E-cadherin: a key molecule in cell adhesion and invasion

A protein that marks epithelial integrity is E-cadherin. It belongs to the cadherin superfamily, which comprises transmembrane glycoproteins involved in calcium-dependent cell–cell adhesion. The cadherins are crucial for establishing and maintaining intercellular connections.[45] They are divided into several subclasses, all of which share a common basic structure, including an extracellular domain, a transmembrane sequence and an intracellular domain. It is through this intracellular portion of the molecule that the cadherins associate with proteins of the cytoskeleton, via the catenins (α, β and γ, a group of cytoplasmic proteins).

E-cadherin is restricted to epithelial tissues[46,47] and is homogeneously expressed in the urothelium at cell–cell contacts.[48] The functional importance of E-cadherin in preserving epithelial tissue integrity was demonstrated by using so-called blocking antibodies against E-cadherin. This leads to dissociation of epithelial cell layers in cell culture and, more significantly, to an increased invasive potential of cells.[49]

Introducing E-cadherin antisense DNA into cells can also induce increased invasive behavior.[50] Conversely, introduction of E-cadherin cDNA into invasive cells can result in a more differentiated and less invasive phenotype.[51] These studies provide evidence that E-cadherin can act as an invasion suppressor.

PROGNOSTIC MARKERS FOR PROGRESSION

Long-term survival is greatly reduced once a tumor has invaded the muscle of the bladder wall, or disseminates. The ability to stratify those superficial tumors with invasive or metastatic capabilities, and those unlikely to become invasive or clinically threatening, would be of great clinical benefit. Superficial tumors that maintain a more malignant phenotype may be better treated with early aggressive therapy (e.g. radical cystectomy).

Currently used prognostic markers in superficial bladder cancer are predominantly clinical and histopathologic parameters, such as tumor grade and especially stage, presence of CIS, recurrence rate, multiplicity, size and localization.[1] Although these 'classical' clinical and histopathologic indicators are useful in separating high- and low-risk groups, they are not specific enough to define individual risk. For example, most patients with (presumed aggressive) multiple stage pT1 grade 3 tumors do not have progressive disease (approximately 75%).[52] Better prediction of progression of pT1 tumors can be done with microstaging.[53] Even then, pT1cG3 tumors have a risk for progression of about 55% (within 3 years). Besides, there is also a significant possibility of both over- and under-staging, depending on the quality of the resected material.[54] This substantiates the urgent need for accurate (molecular) progression markers.

p53 as a marker for progression

The relatively high frequency of p53 mutations in pT2–T4 tumors compared to pT1 tumors suggests their involvement in the progression of T1 tumors to invasive disease.[23] Vet et al.[55] performed p53 mutation analysis in consecutive bladder washings from 26 patients at high risk for progression. p53 mutations were found in 6 out of 13 patients (46%) with progressive superficial UCC of the bladder. The positive predictive value of p53 mutations for progression of high-risk superficial

UCC was 86%. The observed negative predictive value was 63%.

The large majority of bladder tumor studies have used immunohistochemical detection of p53 protein accumulation as an indirect marker for the presence of p53 mutations. Overexpression of p53 has been shown to be an independent prognostic marker for progression.[56,57] Two reports have shown that > 20% staining was an independent predictor in pT1 tumors[58] and primary CIS.[59] There are a number of studies, however, that have failed to demonstrate p53 positivity as an independent predictive value over stage and grade (e.g. references 60 and 61). Clearly, these discrepant results are causing great confusion. As stated previously, difficulties arise in comparing and interpreting these studies. There is, for example, a wide range of cut-off levels to define abnormal p53 expression (up to 22%[62]), making comparisons difficult.

p53 status also forms a prognostic factor in invasive bladder cancer. Lipponen et al.,[63] Esrig et al.[64] and Sarkis et al.[65,66] investigated p53 expression in patients with invasive bladder cancer. They all found a significantly decreased survival in patients with an increased immunohistochemical detection of p53 in their tumor, in comparison to patients with a normal p53 expression pattern. However, p53 overexpression did not always have an independent prognostic value in a multivariate survival analysis over clinical stage. Again there are contradicting results found in other studies.[67–69] Larger prospective studies are needed in order to assess the clinical prognostic value of p53 in superficial and invasive bladder tumors.

Rb as a marker for progression

Loss of pRb expression is correlated with high-grade and high-stage tumors.[70] A few immunohistochemical studies have shown that an altered expression of the Rb protein, indicated by loss of pRb nuclear staining, is associated with a more aggressive biological behavior.[42,43] Hence, loss of Rb protein expression may be a prognostic marker in patients with invasive bladder cancer.

Grossman et al.[71] studied the staining pattern of the p53 and the Rb protein in T1 bladder tumors. They found a significant increase in progression in patients with abnormal expression of either or both proteins, compared to patients with normal expression of both proteins. Other studies[72,73] have confirmed this and suggestions are made that the p53 and the Rb protein act in an independent yet synergistic manner in patients with bladder cancer.

E-cadherin as a marker for progression

The role of E-cadherin in malignant progression had already been suggested by the late 1980s. Various research groups have studied the expression of E-cadherin in a great number of different human carcinomas. They found that a reduced expression of E-cadherin correlated with a poor degree of differentiation in many of these different types of human tumor, suggesting an important role for E-cadherin in the maintenance of the differentiated phenotype of carcinomas.[74–76] The overwhelming number of reports related to the inverse correlation between E-cadherin expression and progression in carcinomas underlines the potential relevance of this cadherin in cancer progression.

Several studies have examined the role of E-cadherin in UCC of the bladder using immunohistochemistry. These studies have uniformly demonstrated a significant association between decreased E-cadherin expression (as determined by IHC) and tumor grade and stage.[77–79] In contrast, increased levels of soluble E-cadherin (sE-cadherin) can be detected in the serum of patients with bladder cancer; this correlates with advanced grade[80] and also with the number of superficial lesions.[81] Patients with elevated serum E-cadherin levels had an increased risk of having recurrent disease at follow-up cystoscopy.

By a process of proteolytic cleavage, non-random soluble fragments of E-cadherin are produced, the major fragment having a molecular weight of 80 kDa (sE-cadherin). In epithelial cells of healthy individuals E-cadherin is regenerated at the cell surface at a rate sufficient to measure sE-cadherin in serum and urine. However, in neoplasms, rapid cellular proliferation is likely to result in increased turnover and proteolytic degradation of E-cadherin, accounting for the observed rise in sE-cadherin levels.[80] Hence, there could be a role for sE-cadherin as a new diagnostic tool in the follow-up of patients with bladder cancer.

Evidence available to date indicates that E-cadherin behaves as a suppressor of tumor cell invasion. The greater motility of invasive cells can also be affected by significant changes in the cadherin–catenin complex, which disturbs the junctional complex; E-cadherin and the catenins may therefore have potential as a prognostic marker. Bringuier et al.[77] found that decreased E-cadherin expression was found to be a predictor of poor survival in a group of bladder tumors. This has been confirmed by other studies.[82–84]

For patients with superficial bladder cancer, few studies have been conducted. Our own group analyzed

23 patients with progression and 22 patients with superficial tumors without progression. Immunohisto-chemical staining of E-cadherin was performed. In the progressive group 4 tumors were normal, 11 were abnormal and 8 were not evaluable due to technical reasons. In the non-progressive group 20 tumors showed normal expression, 0 were abnormal and 2 were not evaluable. Tumor grade, tumor stage and presence of CIS were confirmed as prognostic markers ($p < 0.005$). In addition, abnormal E-cadherin expression was shown to be a predictor of progression ($p < 0.001$) (unpublished data).

MOLECULAR MARKERS IN THE TREATMENT OF BLADDER CANCER

p53 and BCG

Intravesical instillations of bacillus Calmette-Guérin (BCG) are widely used following transurethral resection in the treatment of aggressive superficial bladder tumors. Especially for CIS, BCG is a highly effective treatment. A review of 34 clinical trials involving 1354 patients showed an average complete-response rate of over 70%.[85] Unfortunately, there still remains a patient group which does not react to BCG and in which superficial bladder cancer recurs and/or progresses. Histologic grading criteria cannot select this patient group. Several investigators have evaluated the immunoreactivity of p53 before and after BCG therapy in an attempt to determine non-responders. It would also be helpful to identify criteria that can determine patients who are likely to show progression of superficial bladder cancer

after failure of BCG therapy so that they can be offered early aggressive treatment.

A review of the literature available to date (Table 21.3) suggests that immunoreactivity of p53 protein does not identify patients who may fail BCG therapy.[86,87] However, positive p53 immunohistochemistry in bladder specimens after the failure of BCG therapy is associated with a high rate of disease progression and death.[88,89] In only one study was the post-therapy p53 overexpression an independent marker of disease-specific survival in a multivariate analysis.[89] If this finding is confirmed in larger studies, patients with p53 overexpression after BCG therapy should be offered aggressive therapy.

Markers for chemosensitivity and radiosensitivity in invasive bladder cancer

The optimal treatment of muscle-invasive bladder cancer remains controversial, albeit that the usual approach in locally confined cancer is a radical cyst-ectomy. However, bladder-sparing procedures, such as combined radiochemotherapy (RCT) following (complete) transurethral resection or neoadjuvant chemo-therapy, are optional for a select patient group. As stated previously, the biological behavior of bladder cancer is unpredictable. The current clinical and histopathologic parameters are inadequate to select the tumors responding to chemo- and/or radiotherapy. Molecular markers may give a better insight into the true biolo-gical potential of a tumor, as well as its response to specific cytotoxic therapies. For this purpose, regulators of the cell cycle and the apoptotic pathway have been investigated.

Table 21.3 Studies correlating p53 alterations with BCG-therapy in patients with superficial bladder tumors

Authors	Journal	Method of analysis	Patient group	Correlation?
Lacombe et al.	J Clin Oncol 1996; 14:2646–2652	IHC	n = 98; Ta,T1,CIS	No
Caliskan et al.	Br J Urol 1997; 79:373–377	IHC	n = 30; Ta,T1	Yes
Ovesen et al.	J Urol 1997; 157:1655–1659	IHC	n = 60; CIS	No
Lee et al.	Int J Urol 1997; 4:552–556	IHC	n = 32; T1/GII-III	No
Lebret et al.	J Urol 1998; 159:788–791	IHC	n = 35; T1GIII	No
Pages et al.	J Urol 1998; 159:1079–1084	IHC	n = 43; T1	No
Pfister et al.	J Urol 1999; 162:69–73	Functional yeast assay	n = 26; T1G3,CIS	Yes

IHC, immunohistochemistry.

p53 in the treatment of invasive bladder cancer

It is thought that cells with increased p53 steady state protein levels are more resistant to chemotherapy, because they are resistant to programmed cell death.[6] However, some laboratory studies suggest that alterations in the p53 gene may result in increased sensitivity to DNA-damaging agents.[90] This was confirmed in a clinical study by Cote et al.[91] They evaluated p53 nuclear reactivity in tumors of 88 patients with invasive bladder cancer who were enrolled in a randomized trial of adjuvant chemotherapy versus observation. In patients with p53 negative (wild-type) tumors no benefit in tumor recurrence was found due to adjuvant chemotherapy. However, in patients with p53 altered tumors a 3-fold lower risk of tumor recurrence and a 2.6-fold increase in survival was found in the group with adjuvant chemotherapy compared to those in the observation group. Therefore, the only patients to benefit from adjuvant chemotherapy in this series were those with p53 altered tumors. In contrast, there are many clinical studies showing no positive correlation between p53 positive immunostaining of the primary tumor and response to chemotherapy for patients with non-metastatic[66,92] or metastatic disease.[93–95] Therefore, selection of patients with advanced bladder cancer for chemotherapy, based on p53 status, remains controversial.

There is a great need for molecular markers that can predict chemotherapy outcome, because drug resistance is a major problem. Of the patients receiving methotrexate, vinblastine, doxorubicin and cisplatin (M-VAC) chemotherapy, 30% do not respond.[96] Some laboratory studies show that p53 alterations are associated with drug resistance.[97,98] In a study by Miyake et al.[99] the effects of introducing wild-type p53 on chemosensitivity of bladder cancer cells were evaluated. Both in vitro and in vivo the introduction enhanced the sensitivity of the cells to cisplatin. This suggests that the combined regimen of adenoviral-mediated p53 gene transfer and cisplatin may become an efficient and powerful tool in the treatment of bladder cancer.

In the response of bladder cancers to external beam radiotherapy, study results show heterogeneity.[100,101] Apoptosis is an important mechanism of radiation-induced cell death.[102] Therefore, defects in the apoptotic pathway should tip the balance between apoptosis and G1 arrest with repair of DNA damage. Wild-type p53 is essential for both cell growth regulation and apoptosis. Although the in vitro studies are inconclusive,[103–105]

the results of clinical studies suggest that abnormal p53 expression has no value in predicting radiation response.[106–108] Downstream factors of p53, such as the cell cycle regulators p21[wafl/cip1] and pRb, may be more determinant of cell fate due to radiation damage.

Retinoblastoma in the treatment of invasive bladder cancer

In clinical studies a strong correlation was found between altered immunohistochemical detectable Rb expression (pRb) and radiation response.[109] The study by Jahnson et al.[110] does not corroborate this finding. However, in the study they performed, radiotherapy was given without cystectomy being done; the effects of radiotherapy were therefore based upon radiologic, rather than pathologic staging.

It seems that pRb functions to limit apoptosis by promoting cell cycle arrest and DNA damage repair. In an immunohistochemical study, Pollack et al. demonstrated that bcl-2 complements pRb in predicting radiation response in muscle-invasive bladder cancer.[109] The overexpression of bcl-2 and the normal expression of pRb appeared to oppose the apoptotic response to radiation via independent mechanisms. Abnormalities in the expression of proteins that regulate apoptosis may help to establish a molecular phenotype to characterize which patients should receive radiotherapy.

Bcl-2 in the treatment of invasive bladder cancer

Bcl-2 is an apoptosis inhibitor, while its antagonist, bax, promotes cell death. The bcl-2/bax ratio has been the subject of much interest. A high ratio was a good predictor of recurrence in low-grade tumors, independent of stage and grade.[111]

Bcl-2 expression is elevated after irradiation,[112] and the apoptotic response to irradiation is ablated by bcl-2.[113–115] The action in the latter is complex, and seems to involve p53-dependent and -independent mechanisms.

Although early reports suggested that bcl-2 expression in bladder cancer was associated with lower-stage and grade tumors,[116] and with a less aggressive cancer phenotype,[117] a consensus seems to be emerging that bcl-2 expression is a marker of disease that is more likely to progress, and of poor prognosis. Because of its biological activity, bcl-2 may also be associated with resistance to radiotherapy, although the limited data available are conflicting (Table 21.4).

Table 21.4 Studies correlating the expression of bcl-2 with radiation response for muscle-invasive bladder cancer

Authors	Journal	Treatment	Patient group	Correlation?
Pollack et al.	Clin Cancer Res 1997; 3:1823–1829	Radiotherapy + radical cystectomy	n = 109; T2–T4 n × M0	Yes
Cooke et al.	BJU Int 2000; 85:829–835	Radiotherapy	n = 26; T2–T4 n × M0	No
Rodel et al.	Int J Radiat Oncol Biol Phys 2000; 46:1213–1221	Radiotherapy	n = 70; T2–T4 n × M0	No

However, bcl-2 expression has been shown to be relevant for other treatment modalities such as chemotherapy.[118] Cooke et al.[119] found a survival advantage for patients with bcl-2-negative tumors who received neoadjuvant cisplatin after radiotherapy. In vitro, UCC cell lines expressing high levels of bcl-2 have been shown to be resistant to adriamycin-triggered apoptosis. The use of bcl-2 antisense oligonucleotides (short single-stranded DNA molecules which are complementary to an essential region in the mRNA of the target gene) reduced the bcl-2 protein level.[120] This may be a useful tool for overcoming drug resistance in future.

CONCLUSION

To date, not one molecular marker has been proven useful for daily urologic practice. Most research has been done on the tumor suppressor gene p53 and its protein, although new molecular markers are being investigated every day. The results of these studies lead to a better understanding of bladder cancer biology, which may provide new diagnostic or therapeutic possibilities.

Clearly, the literature is controversial, for example concerning the prognostic value of p53. Among other reasons, p53 immunohistochemistry alone cannot determine whether the p53 pathway is intact. This requires assessment of cell cycle control, including cell cycle associated molecules (e.g. p15, p16, p21 and p27), proteins implicated in apoptosis or MDM2 status. That is why, in future, the management of bladder cancer patients will probably be partly directed not by one molecular marker, but by a panel of markers.

Especially with the new technical developments in molecular research (e.g. DNA microchips), the introduction of clinically valuable molecular markers will soon become feasible. The determination of a cohort of markers will then be less time-consuming and more reliable than nowadays. However, before this becomes reality, the true clinical value of various molecular markers should be assessed. Large prospective studies are necessary, in which the emphasis should lie on standardized use of (immunohistochemical) methods, and uniformly determined treatment for patients should be included.

REFERENCES

1. Kiemeney LA, Witjes JA, Heijbroek RP, et al. Predictability of recurrent and progressive disease in individual patients with primary superficial bladder cancer. J Urol 1993;150:60–64.
2. Van der Poel HG, Hessels D, Van Leenders GJ, et al. Multifocal transitional cell cancer and p53 mutation analysis. J Urol 1998;160:124–125.
3. Hollstein M, Sidransky D, Volgelstein B, Harris CC. p53 mutations in human cancers. Science 1991;253:49–53.
4. Soussi T, Caron de Fromentel C, May P. Structural aspects of the p53 protein in relation to gene evolution. Oncogene 1990;5:945–952.
5. Kastan MB, Onyekwere O, Sidransky D, et al. Participation of p53 protein in the cellular response to DNA damage. Cancer Res 1991;51:6304–6311.
6. Lowe SW, Ruley HE, Jacks T, Housman DE. p53-dependent apoptosis modulates the cytotoxicity of anticancer agents. Cell 1993;74:957–967.
7. Donehower LA, Harvey M, Slagle BL, et al. Mice deficient for p53 are developmentally normal but susceptible to spontaneous tumors. Nature 1992;356:215–221.
8. Velculescu VE, El-Deiry WS. Biological and clinical importance of the p53 tumor suppressor gene. Clin Chem 1996;42:858–868.
9. Livingstone LR, White A, Sprouse J, et al. Altered cell cycle arrest and gene amplification potential accompany loss of wild-type p53. Cell 1992;70:923–935.
10. Yin Y, Tainsky MA, Bischoff FZ, et al. Wild-type p53 restores cell cycle control and inhibits gene amplification in cells with mutant p53 alleles. Cell 1992;70:937–948.

11. Finlay CA, Hinds PW, Tan TH, et al. Activating mutations for transformation by p53 produce a gene product that forms an hsc70–p53 complex with an altered half-life. Mol Cell Biol 1988;8:531–539.

12. Cesarman E, Inghirame G, Chadburn A, Knowles DM. High levels of p53 protein expression do not correlate with p53 gene mutations in anaplastic large cell lymphoma. Am J Pathol 1993;143:845–856.

13. Hall PA, Lane DP. p53 in tumor pathology: can we trust immunohistochemistry?---Revised! [editorial]. J Pathol 1994;172:1.

14. Matsushima AY, Cesarman E, Chadburn A, Knowles DM. Post-thymic T cell lymphomas frequently overexpress p53 protein but infrequently exhibit p53 gene mutations. Am J Pathol 1994;144:573–584.

15. Wynford TD. p53 in tumor pathology: can we trust immunocytochemistry? [editorial]. J Pathol 1992;166:329.

16. Sarnow P, Ho YS, Williams J, Levine AJ. Adenovirus E1b-58kd tumor antigen and SV40 large tumor antigen are physically associated with the same 54 kD cellular protein in transformed cells. Cell 1982;28:387–394.

17. Werness BA, Levine AJ, Howley PM. Association of human papillomavirus types 16 and 18 E6 proteins with p53. Science 1990;248:76–79.

18. Momand J, Zambetti GP. MDM-2: 'big brother' of p53. J Cell Biochem 1997;64:343–352.

19. Schmitz-Dräger BJ, Goebell P, Heidthausen M. The International Study Initiative on Bladder Cancer (ISBC). p53 immunohistochemistry as a prognostic marker for bladder cancer: results of the ISBC meta-analysis [abstract]. Eur Urol 1999;35 (Suppl. 2):666.

20. McShane LM, Aamodt R, Cordon-Cardo C, et al. Reproducibility of p53 immunohistochemistry in bladder tumors. National Cancer Institute, Bladder Tumor Marker Network. Clin Cancer Res 2000;6:1854–1864.

21. Sheffield VC, Beck JS, Kwitek AE, et al. The sensitivity of single-strand conformation polymorphism analysis for the detection of single base substitutions. Genomics 1993;16:325–332.

22. Sidransky D, Von Eschenbach A, Tsai YC, et al. Identification of p53 gene mutations in bladder cancers and urine samples. Science 1991;252:706–709.

23. Spruck CH, Ohneseit PF, Gonzalez-Zulueta M, et al. Two molecular pathways to transitional cell carcinoma of the bladder. Cancer Res 1994;54:784–788.

24. Righi E, Rossi G, Ferarri G, et al. Does p53 immunostaining improve diagnostic accuracy in urine cytology? Diagn Cytopathol 1997;17:436–439.

25. Sugano K, Tsutsumi M, Nakashima Y, et al. Diagnosis of bladder cancer by analysis of the allelic loss of the p53 gene in urine samples using blunt-end single-strand conformation polymorphism. Int J Cancer 1997;74:403–406.

26. Friedrich MG, Erbersdobler A, Schwaibold H, et al. Detection of loss of heterozygosity in the p53 tumor-suppressor gene with PCR in the urine of patients with bladder cancer. J Urol 2000;163:1039–1042.

27. Vet JA, Hessels D, Marras SA, et al. Comparative analysis of p53 mutations in bladder washings and histologic specimens. Am J Clin Pathol 1998;110:647–652.

28. Fujimoto K, Yamada Y, Okajima E, et al. Frequent association of p53 gene mutation in invasive bladder cancer. Cancer Res 1992;52:1393–1398.

29. Cordon-Cardo C, Sheinfeld J. Molecular and immunopathology studies of oncogenes and tumor-suppressor genes in bladder cancer. World J Urol 1997;15:112–119.

30. Vet JA, Bringuier PP, Poddighe PJ, et al. p53 mutations have no additional prognostic value over stage in bladder cancer. Br J Cancer 1994;70:496–500.

31. Sauter G, Deng G, Moch H. Physical deletion of the p53 gene in bladder cancer. Detection by fluorescence in situ hybridization. Am J Pathol 1994;144:756–766.

32. Nakopoulou L, Constantinides C, Papandropoulos J, et al. Evaluation of overexpression of p53 tumor suppressor protein in superficial and invasive transitional cell bladder cancer: comparison with DNA ploidy. Urology 1995;46:334–340.

33. Gontero P, Casetta G, Zitella A, et al. Evaluation of p53 protein overexpression, Ki67 proliferative activity and mitotic index as markers of tumour recurrence in superficial transitional cell carcinoma of the bladder. Eur Urol 2000;38:287–296.

34. Wu TT, Chen JH, Lee YH, et al. The role of bcl-2, p53, and ki-67 index in predicting tumor recurrence for low grade superficial transitional cell bladder carcinoma. J Urol 2000;163:758–760.

35. Tetu B, Fradet Y, Allard P, et al. Prevalence and clinical significance of HER/2neu, p53 and Rb expression in primary superficial bladder cancer. J Urol 1996;155:1784–1788.

36. Iakim-Liossi A, Pantazopoulos D, Karakitsos P, et al. DNA ploidy and p53 protein expression in superficial transitional cell carcinoma of the bladder. Cytopathology 2000;11:96–103.

37. Blasco-Olaetxea E, Belloso L, Garcia-Tamayo J. Superficial bladder cancer: study of the proliferative nuclear fraction as a prognostic factor. Eur J Cancer 1996;32A:444–446.

38. Asakura T, Takano Y, Iki M, et al. Prognostic value of Ki-67 for recurrence and progression of superficial bladder cancer. J Urol 1997;158:385–388.

39. Goodrich DW, Wang NP, Qian YW, et al. The retinoblastoma gene product regulates progression through the G1 phase of the cell cycle. Cell 1991;67:293–302.

40. el-Deiry WS, Kern SE, Pietenpol JA, et al. Definition of a consensus binding site for p53. Nat Genet 1992;1:45–49.

41. Horowitz JM, Park SH, Bogenmann E, et al. Frequent inactivation of the retinoblastoma anti-oncogene is restricted to a subset of human tumor cells. Proc Natl Acad Sci USA 1990;87:2775–2779.

42. Cordon-Cardo C, Wartinger D, Petrylak D, et al. Altered expression of the retinoblastoma gene product: prognostic indicator in bladder cancer [see comments]. J Natl Cancer Inst 1992;84:1251–1256.

43. Logothetis CJ, Xu HJ, Ro JY, et al. Altered expression of retinoblastoma protein and known prognostic variables in locally advanced bladder cancer [see comments]. J Natl Cancer Inst 1992;84:1256–1261.

44. Xu HJ, Cairns P, Hu SX, et al. Loss of Rb protein expression in primary bladder cancer correlates with loss of heterozygosity at the Rb locus and tumor progression. Int J Cancer 1993;53:781–784.

45. Takeichi M. Cadherin cell adhesion receptors as a morphogenetic regulator. Science 1991;251:1451–1455.

46. Behrens J, Birchmeier W, Goodman SL, Imhof BA. Dissociation of Madin–Darby canine kidney epithelial cells by the monoclonal antibody anti-Arc-1: mechanistic aspects and identification of the antigen as a component related to uromorulin. J Cell Biol 1985;101:1307–1315.

47. Shimoyama Y, Hirohashi S, Hirano S, et al. Cadherin cell-adhesion molecules in human epithelial tissues and carcinomas. Cancer Res 1989;49:2128–2133.

48. Witjes JA, Umbas R, Debruyne FMJ, Schalken JA. Expression of markers for transitional cell carcinoma in normal bladder mucosa of patients with bladder cancer. J Urol 1995;154:2185–2189.

49. Vleminckx K, Vakaet L Jr, Mareel M, et al. Genetic manipulation of E-cadherin expression by epithelial tumor cells reveals an invasion suppressor role. Cell 1991;66:107–119.

50. Birchmeier W, Behrens J. Cadherin expression in carcinomas: role in the formation of cell junctions and the prevention of invasiveness. Biochem Biophys Acta 1994;1198:11–26.

51. Frixen UH, Behrens J, Sachs M, et al. E-cadherin-mediated cell–cell adhesion prevents invasiveness of human carcinoma cells. J Cell Biol 1991;113:173–185.

52. Catalona WJ, Dresner SM, Haaff EO. Management of superficial bladder cancer. In: Skinner DG, Lieskovsky G (eds) Diagnosis and Management of Genitourinary Cancer. New York: Alan R. Liss, 1988, p 281.

53. Smits G, Schaafsma E, Kiemeney L, et al. Microstaging of pT1 transitional cell carcinoma of the bladder: identification of subgroups with distinct risks of progression. Urology 1998;52:1009–1013, discussion 1013–1014.

54. Freeman JA, Esrig DE, Stein JP, et al. Radical cystectomy for high risk patients with superficial bladder cancer in the era of orthotopic urinary reconstruction. Cancer 1995;76:833–839.

55. Vet JA, Witjes JA, Marras SE, et al. Predictive value of p53 mutations analyzed in bladder washings for progression of high-risk superficial bladder cancer. Clin Cancer Res 1996;2:1055–1061.

56. Cordon-Cardo C, Dalbagni G, Sarkis AS, Reuter VE. Genetic alterations associated with bladder cancer. Important Adv Oncol 1994;71–83.

57. Llopis J, Alcaraz A, Ribal MJ, et al. p53 expression predicts progression and poor survival in T1 bladder tumours. Eur Urol 2000;37:644–653.

58. Serth J, Kuczyk MA, Bokemeyer C, et al. p53 immunohistochemistry as an independent prognostic factor for superficial transitional cell carcinoma of the bladder. Br J Cancer 1995;71:201–205.

59. Sarkis AS, Dalbagni G, Cordon-Cardo C, et al. Association of p53 nuclear overexpression and tumor progression in carcinoma in situ of the bladder. J Urol 1994;152:388–392.

60. Thomas DJ, Robinson MC, Charlton R, et al. p53 expression, ploidy and progression in pT1 transitional cell carcinoma of the bladder. Br J Urol 1994;73:533–537.

61. Gardiner RA, Walsh MD, Allen V, et al. Immunohistological expression of p53 in primary pT1 transitional cell bladder cancer in relation to tumour progression. Br J Urol 1994;73:526–532.

62. Popov Z, Hoznek A, Colombel M, et al. The prognostic value of p53 nuclear overexpression and MIB-1 as a proliferative marker in transitional cell carcinoma of the bladder. Cancer 1997;80:1472–1481.

63. Lipponen PK. Over-expression of the p53 nuclear oncoprotein in transitional-cell bladder cancer and its prognostic value. Int J Cancer 1993;53:365–370.

64. Esrig D, Elmajian D, Groshen S, et al. Accumulation of nuclear p53 and tumor progression in bladder cancer. N Engl J Med 1994;331:1259–1264.

65. Sarkis AS, Dalbagni G, Cordon-Cardo C, et al. Nuclear overexpression of p53 protein in transitional cell bladder carcinoma:a marker for disease progression. J Natl Cancer Inst 1993;6:53–59.

66. Sarkis AS, Bajorin DF, Reuter VE, et al. Prognostic value of p53 nuclear overexpression in patients with invasive bladder cancer treated with neoadjuvant MVAC. J Clin Oncol 1995;13:1384–1390.

67. Glick SH, Howell LP, White RW. Relationship of p53 and bcl-2 to prognosis in muscle-invasive transitional cell carcinoma of the bladder. J Urol 1996;155:1754–1757.

68. Jahnson S, Karlsson MG. Predictive value of p53 and pRb immunostaining in locally advanced bladder cancer treated with cystectomy. J Urol 1998;160:1291–1296.

69. Plastiras D, Moutzouris G, Barbatis C, et al. Can p53 nuclear overexpression, Bcl-2 accumulation and PCNA status be of prognostic significance in high-risk superficial and invasive bladder tumours? Eur J Surg Oncol 1999;25:61–65.

70. Geradts J, Hu SX, Lincoln CE, et al. Aberrant RbB gene expression in routinely processed, archival tumor tissues determined by three different anti-RB antibodies. Int J Cancer 1994;58:161–167.

71. Grossman HB, Liebert M, Antelo M, et al. p53 and RB expression predict progression in T1 bladder cancer. Clin Cancer Res 1998;4:829–834.

72. Esrig D, Shi SR, Bochner B, et al. Prognostic importance of p53 and Rb alterations in transitional cell carcinoma of the bladder. J Urol 1995;153:abstract 536.

73. Lerner SP, Linn D, Charkraborty S, et al. Correlation of p53 and retinoblastoma protein expression with established pathologic prognostic features in radical cystoprostatectomy specimens. J Urol 1995;153:abstract 537.

74. Umbas R, Schalken JA, Aalders TW, et al. Expression of the cellular adhesion molecule E-cadherin is reduced or absent in high-grade prostate cancer. Cancer Res 1992;52:5104–5109.

75. Mayer B, Johnson JP, Leitl F, et al. E-cadherin expression in primary and metastatic gastric cancer: down-regulation correlates with cellular differentiation and glandular disintegration. Cancer Res 1993;53:1690–1695.

76. Oka H, Shiozaki H, Kobayashi K, et al. Expression of E-cadherin cell adhesion molecules in human breast cancer tissues and its relationship to metastasis. Cancer Res 1993;53:1696–1701.

77. Bringuier PP, Umbas RU, Schaafsma HE, et al. Decreased E-cadherin immunoreactivity correlates with poor survival in patients with bladder tumors. Cancer Res 1993;53:3241–3245.

78. Ross JS, del Rosario AD, Figge HL, et al. E-cadherin expression in papillary transitional cell carcinoma of the urinary bladder. Hum Path 1995;26:940–944.

79. Giroldi LA, Bringuier PP, Schalken JA. Defective E-cadherin function in urological cancers: clinical implications and molecular mechanisms. Invasion Metastasis 1994;14:71–81.

80. Durkan GC, Brotherick I, Mellon JK. The impact of transurethral resection of bladder tumour on serum levels of soluble E-cadherin. BJU Int 1999;83:424–428.

81. Griffiths TR, Brotherick I, Bishop RI, et al. Cell adhesion molecules in bladder cancer: soluble serum E-cadherin correlates with predictors of recurrence. Br J Cancer 1996;74:579–584.

82. Syrigos KN, Krausz T, Waxman J, et al. E-cadherin expression in bladder cancer using formalin-fixed, paraffin-embedded tissues: correlation with histopathological grade, tumour stage and survival. Int J Cancer 1995;64:367–370.

83. Lipponen, PK, Eskelinen MJ. Reduced expression of E-cadherin is related to invasive disease and frequent recurrence in bladder cancer. J Cancer Res Clin Oncol 1995;121:303–308.

84. Popov Z, Gil-Diez de Medina S, Lefrere-Belda MA, et al. Low E-cadherin expression in bladder cancer at the transcriptional and protein level provides prognostic information. Br J Cancer 2000;83:209–214.

85. Lamm DL. BCG immunotherapy for transitional-cell carcinoma in situ of the bladder. Oncology 1995;9:947–952, 955; discussion 955–965.

86. Lebret T, Becette V, Barbagelatta M, et al. Correlation between p53 over expression and response to bacillus Calmette-Guérin therapy in a high risk select population of patients with T1G3 bladder cancer. J Urol 1998;159:788–791.

87. Pages F, Flam TA, Vieillefond A, et al. p53 status does not predict initial clinical response to bacillus Calmette-Guérin intravesical therapy in T1 bladder tumors. J Urol 1998;159:1079–1084.

88. Lacombe L, Dalbagni G, Zhang ZF, et al. Overexpression of p53 protein in a high-risk population of patients with superficial bladder cancer before and after bacillus Calmette-Guérin therapy: correlation to clinical outcome. J Clin Oncol 1996;14:2646–2652.

89. Ovesen H, Horn T, Steven K. Long-term efficacy of intravesical bacillus Calmette-Guérin for carcinoma in situ: relationship of progression to histological response and p53 nuclear accumulation. J Urol 1997;157:1655–1659.

90. Waldman T, Lengauer C, Kinzler KW, Vogelstein B. Uncoupling of S phase and mitosis induced by anticancer agents in cells lacking p21 [see comments]. Nature 1996;381:713–716.

91. Cote RJ, Esrig D, Groshen S, et al. p53 and treatment of bladder cancer. Nature 1997;385:123–125.

92. Koga F, Kitahara S, Arai K, et al. Negative p53/positive p21 immunostaining is a predictor of favorable response to chemotherapy in patients with locally advanced bladder cancer. Jpn J Cancer Res 2000;91:416–423.

93. Sengelov L, Horn T, Steven K. p53 nuclear immunoreactivity as a predictor of response and outcome following chemotherapy for metastatic bladder cancer. J Cancer Res Clin Oncol 1997;123:565–570.

94. Kakehi Y, Ozdemir E, Habuchi T, et al. Absence of p53 overexpression and favorable response to cisplatin-based neoadjuvant chemotherapy in urothelial carcinomas. Jpn J Cancer Res 1998;89:214–220.

95. Siu LL, Banerjee D, Khurana RJ, et al. The prognostic role of p53, metallothionen, P-glycoprotein, and MIB-1 in muscle-invasive urothelial transitional cell carcinoma. Clin Cancer Res 1998;4:559–565.

96. Sternberg CN, Yagoda A, Scher HI, et al. M-VAC (methotrexate, vinblastine, doxorubicin and cisplatin) for advanced transitional cell carcinoma of the urothelium. J Urol 1988;139:461–469.

97. Yeager TR, Reznikoff CA. Methotrexate resistance in human uroepithelial cells with p53 alterations. J Urol 1998;159:581–585.

98. Miyake H, Hara I, Yamanaka K, et al. Synergistic enhancement of resistance to cisplatin in human bladder cancer cells by overexpression of mutant-type p53 and Bcl-2. J Urol 1999;162:2176–2181.

99. Miyake H, Hara I, Gohji K, et al. Enhancement of chemosensitivity in human bladder cancer cells by adenoviral-mediated p53 gene transfer. Anticancer Res 1998;18:3087–3092.

100. Pollack A, Zagars GK, Swanson DA. Muscle-invasive bladder cancer treated with external beam radiotherapy: prognostic factors. Int J Radiat Oncol Biol Phys 1994;30:267–277.

101. Pollack A, Zagars GK, Dinney CP, et al. Preoperative radiotherapy for muscle-invasive bladder carcinoma. Long-term follow-up and prognostic factors for 338 patients. Cancer 1994;74:2819–2827.

102. Stephens LC, Hunter NR, Ang KK, et al. Development of apoptosis in irradiated murine tumors as a function of time and dose. Radiat Res 1993;135:75–80.

103. Brachman DG, Beckett M, Graves D, et al. p53 mutation does not correlate with radiosensitivity in 24 head and neck cancer cell lines. Cancer Res 1993;53:3667–3669.

104. Baird DSF, Martin M, Rhun YL, et al. Concomitant p53 mutation and increased radiosensitivity in rat lung embryo epithelial cells during neoplastic development. Cancer Res 1994;54:3361–3364.

105. Ribeiro JC, Barnetson AR, Fisher RJ, et al. Relationship between radiation response and p53 status in human bladder cancer cells. Int J Radiat Biol 1997;71:11–20.

106. Ogura K, Habuchi T, Yamada H, et al. Immunohistochemical analysis of p53 and proliferating cell nuclear antigen (PCNA) in bladder cancer: positive immunostaining and radiosensitivity. Int J Urol 1995;2:302–308.

107. Wu CS, Pollack A, Czerniak B, et al. Prognostic value of p53 in muscle-invasive bladder cancer treated with preoperative radiotherapy. Urology 1996;47:305–310.

108. Pollack A, Czerniak B, Zagars GK, et al. Retinoblastoma protein expression and radiation response in muscle-invasive bladder cancer. Int J Radiat Oncol Biol Phys 1997;39:687–695.

109. Pollack A, Wu CS, Czerniak B, et al. Abnormal bcl-2 and pRb expression are independent correlates of radiation response in muscle-invasive bladder cancer. Clin Cancer Res 1997;3:1823–1829.

110. Jahnson S, Risberg B, Karlsson MG, et al. p53 and Rb immunostaining in locally advanced bladder cancer: relation to prognostic variables and predictive value for the local response to radical radiotherapy. Eur Urol 1995;28:135–142.

111. Gazzaniga P, Gradilone A, Vercillo R, et al. Bcl-2/bax mRNA expression ratio as prognostic factor in low-grade urinary bladder cancer. Int J Cancer 1996;69:100–104.

112. Harney JV, Seymour CB, Murphy DM, Mothersill C. Variation in the expression of p53, *c-myc*, and bcl-2 oncoproteins in individual patient cultures of normal urothelium exposed to cobalt 60 gamma-rays and N-nitrosodiethanolamine. Cancer Epidemiol Biomarkers Prev 1995;4:617–625.

113. Sentman CL, Shutter JR, Hockenbery D, et al. Bcl-2 inhibits multiple forms of apoptosis but not negative selection in thymocytes. Cell 1991;67:879–888.

114. Marin MC, Hsu B, Meyn RE, et al. Evidence that p53 and bcl-2 are regulators of a common cell death pathway important for in vivo lymphomagenesis. Oncogene 1994;9:3107–3112.

115. Mor F, Cohen IR. IL-2 rescues antigen-specific T cells from radiation or dexamethasone-induced apoptosis. Correlation with induction of Bcl-2. J Immunol 1996;156:515–522.

116. King ED, Matteson J, Jacobs SC, Kyprianou N. Incidence of apoptosis, cell proliferation and bcl-2 expression in transitional cell carcinoma of the bladder: association with tumor progression. J Urol 1996;155:316–320.

117. Shiina H, Igawa M, Urakami S, et al. Immunohistochemical analysis of bcl-2 expression in transitional cell carcinoma of the bladder. J Clin Pathol 1996;49:395–399.

118. Kong G, Shin KY, Oh YH, et al. Bcl-2 and p53 expressions in invasive bladder cancers. Acta Oncol 1998;37:715–720.

119. Cooke PW, James ND, Ganesan R, et al. Bcl-2 expression identifies patients with advanced bladder cancer treated by radiotherapy who benefit from neoadjuvant chemotherapy. BJU Int 2000;85:829–835.

120. Bilim V, Kasahara T, Noboru H, et al. Caspase involved synergistic cytotoxicity of bcl-2 antisense oligonucleotides and adriamycin on transitional cell cancer cells. Cancer Lett 2000;155:191–198.

22

DETECTING RECURRENT BLADDER CANCER: NEW METHODS AND BIOMARKERS

Jeffrey S. Ross and Michael B. Cohen

INTRODUCTION

The diagnosis of tumors of the urinary bladder and urinary tract accounts for 6% of new cancer cases in men and 3% of new cancer cases in women in the United States each year.[1,2] Two distinct clinical forms of the disease are recognized:

- a non-invasive or superficially invasive papillary tumor prone to recurrence, but featuring a favorable prognosis
- invasive flat tumors with deep bladder wall penetration and a poor prognosis.

Of the 54,000 new diagnoses of urinary bladder cancer in the United States each year, 75% are at an early stage at the time of presentation with no invasion of the smooth muscle wall of the bladder.[3,4] Of these superficial bladder tumors, 50–70% will recur and 10–20% will progress to muscle-invasive disease.[5] The relatively high new case rate coupled with the high recurrence rate results in an extremely high overall disease prevalence and a significant cost to the health care system for the continued surveillance, follow-up and management of these patients. Thus, there is considerable interest in the development of new ancillary techniques that could detect recurrent urothelial neoplasia with higher sensitivity and specificity, lengthen the time intervals between cystoscopic surveillance, and allow for curative surgical intervention prior to the development of life-threatening tumor invasion of the bladder wall.

CYTOLOGY AND THE DETECTION OF RECURRENT UROTHELIAL NEOPLASIA

Cytologic examination of urothelial cells from voided urine, urinary bladder washings and upper urinary tract brushings specimens, in combination with cystoscopic examination, has been the gold standard for the detection of recurrent urothelial neoplasia.[6,7] The sensitivity for detection of recurrent urothelial neoplasms (papillomas, urothelial neoplasms of low malignant potential, urothelial carcinomas and urothelial carcinoma in situ) has shown a wide variation in the published literature.[8,9] For higher grades of urothelial carcinoma, cytologic examination can achieve a high sensitivity and specificity[10] (Table 22.1). However, for lower-grade tumors, false-positive and false-negative rates can be higher than 10%.[10]

The detection of low-grade urothelial neoplasia, a continuing challenge for cytopathologists, can be improved when experts use vigorous cytomorphologic criteria to separate low-grade lesions from benign urothelial cells.[10,11] Yet, when used by non-experts in a general pathology practice setting, exfoliative cytology has been criticized for having a high false-negative rate in low-grade lesions.[12] In addition, the atypical cytomorphology of the urothelium associated with the use of intravesical chemotherapeutic agents can complicate the interpretation of urothelial cytologic specimens.[13] Moreover, despite a published range from 0 to 73% for the sensitivity for detection of low-grade urothelial neoplasia by cytologic methods, substantial increases can be achieved when key cytologic criteria for detection are identified and effectively applied.[13] The multifocal nature of urothelial neoplasia must also be considered, together with the impact of specimen type: a voided urine sample versus a bladder washings specimen has a major impact on the cytologic detection of significant lesions.[14]

In summary, despite the high sensitivity and specificity for detection of both low- and high-grade urothelial neoplasms achievable in laboratories directed by expert cytopathologists, the general consensus is that cytologic techniques are not capable of identifying all cases of recurrent disease. The development of ancillary techniques to complement the relatively inexpensive and convenient cytologic methods has relevance for both clinical patient outcome and financial outcome in an era of health care cost containment.

ANCILLARY METHODS FOR THE DETECTION OF RECURRENT UROTHELIAL NEOPLASIA

A variety of wet laboratory immunoassays, on-slide immunoassays, in situ hybridization procedures and post-nucleic acid extraction molecular techniques have been designed to complement cytology and improve the overall sensitivity and specificity for the detection of recurrent urothelial neoplasia[2,3,7,15–17] (Table 22.2). Although the current consensus is that no new individual marker can eliminate the need for follow-up cysto-

Table 22.1 Features of low-grade and high-grade urothelial carcinomas

Feature	Low-grade urothelial carcinoma	High-grade urothelial carcinoma
Tumor configuration	Papillary	Sessile
Histologic grade	Low	High
Pathologic stage	Low	High
Recurrence rate	High	Not applicable
Progression rate	Low	High
Mortality	Low	High
Cytologic detection:		
Sensitivity	Moderate	High
Specificity	Moderate	High

Table 22.2 Ancillary methods of detection of recurrent urothelial neoplasia

- Polymedco BTA™ (bladder tumor antigen) test
- NMP22™ (nuclear matrix protein) test
- Telomerase assays
- Microsatellite instability assays
- Tests for aneuploidy, aneusomy and morphometrics
- Miscellaneous markers:
  - cytokeratins
  - blood group antigens and glycoproteins
  - tumor-associated proteins
  - hyaluronidase
  - growth factors
  - cell adhesion molecules
  - fibrinogen degradation products (e.g. AuraTek FDP™)
  - cell proliferation markers and cell cycle regulatory genes and proteins

scopy, there is significant agreement that, with the use of the ancillary tests, the sensitivity and specificity of cytologic diagnosis can be increased and the intervals between surveillance cystoscopy for the management of urothelial neoplasia can be lengthened.[15]

The Polymedco bladder tumor antigen test

The Polymedco™ (bladder tumor antigen) test is a US Food and Drug Administration (FDA)-approved latex agglutination test designed to detect bladder cancer in voided urine samples. Two new improved versions – the BTA Stat™ test, performed as a point of care test at

the bedside, and the BTA Track™ test, which is mailed away to a reference laboratory – have recently been introduced.[3] Table 22.3 lists a series of studies of the BTA test for the detection of urothelial neoplasia and compares the results to other methods. The sensitivity for this technique has ranged from a low of 32% to a high of 74%, with a range in specificity from 40 to 92%.[15–27] Although most of the studies have indicated that the BTA test is superior in sensitivity compared to cytology,[18–21] one study found low sensitivity and specificity for high-grade urothelial carcinomas,[15] another reported high false-positive and false-negative rates,[24] and another concluded that the test was useful

Table 22.3 The Polymedco™ (bladder tumor antigen) test

Year	Author	Method	Sensitivity (%)	Specificity (%)	Comment
1995	Sarosdy et al.[18]	LA	40	96	
1996	D'Hallewin & Baert[19]	LA	65	–	60 patients; superior to bladder washings cytology at 32%
1997	Ianari et al.[20]	LA	54	91	104 patients; higher sensitivity than washings cytology at 23%; lower specificity than cytology
1997	Leyh & Mazeman[21]	LA	54	92	164 patients; superior to voided urine cytology at 28%; cytology was 97% specific
1997	Miyanaga et al.[22]	LA	58	–	132 patients; superior to voided urine cytology at 38%
1998	Wiener et al.[15]	LA	57	68	291 patients; better than voided urine cytology, but cannot replace cystoscopy due to low sensitivity and specificity for grade 3 TCC
1998	Van der Poel et al.[23]	LA	34	81	138 patients; washings cytology more specific, but less sensitive than BTA; karyometry (Quanticyt) more sensitive (69%) and specific (73%) than BTA
1998	Zimmerman et al.[24]	LA	65	40	71 patients; BTA too high false-positive (33%) and false-negative (62%) rates; no clinical value
1998	Abbate et al.[25]	LA	62	–	156 patients; higher sensitivity than NMP22
1998	Schamhart et al.[26]	LA	32	82	53 patients; BTA more sensitive with high-stage tumors; possible use to monitor aggressiveness, but cannot replace cystoscopy
1999	Ramakumar et al.[27]	LA	74	73	196 patients; intermediate sensitivity/ specificity for BTA, outperformed by telomerase assessment at 95% specificity

LA, latex agglutination; TCC, transitional cell carcinoma.

to monitor disease aggressiveness, but cannot replace cystoscopy for management of patients.[26]

In addition, the BTA test results have been compared to other ancillary methods and found to be less sensitive and specific than the Quanticyt™ karyometry assay[23] (see below) and significantly less specific than telomerase assays[27] (see below). One study, however, found the BTA test to have a higher sensitivity than the nuclear matrix protein NMP22™ test[25] (see below).

In general, studies of the Bard BTA test were performed on voided urine samples rather than bladder washings specimens, and the comparison of sensitivity and specificity used cytology reports from 'non-expert' cytopathologists. In summary, despite high false-positive results in the 4–34% range,[3] and variable accuracy for the detection of low-grade lesions,[11] the BTA test shows significant promise as an adjunct to the detection of early urothelial neoplasia in bladder wash and voided urine samples.[28] The impact of test improvements that are currently under clinical trial evaluation is not yet known.

Nuclear matrix protein (NMP22) test

Nuclear matrix protein 22 is a member of a family of nuclear matrix proteins involved in DNA configuration, structure and function regulating free replication and transcription of a variety of genes.[29] The NMP22™ detection method is an immunoassay currently performed in reference laboratory settings as a referred specimen. A summary of studies of the NMP22 assay or the early detection of urothelial neoplasia is shown in Table 22.4. The NMP22 test is a quantitative assay in which the setting of the cut-off point, ranging from 6 to 10 IU/ml in published series, is critical for optimizing the test performance. This test has been approved by the FDA as an adjunct to cystoscopy, but is not approved as a stand-alone test capable of replacing cystoscopy.

As seen in Table 22.4, published studies have reported a range in sensitivity from 38 to 81% and specificity from 60 to 86% for the detection of urothelial neoplasia by the NMP22 assay.[15,25,27,30–40] In general, the test has been listed as having a higher sensitivity than cytology and is useful for monitoring bladder cancer recurrence.[15,30–32] In one study the NMP22 assay had a higher sensitivity than the BTA test,[39] and in another the sensitivity was lower than the BTA test.[25] Of two studies combining NMP22 and telomerase assays, in one both were found to have a higher sensitivity than the BTA test and cytology,[39] whereas in the other telomerase assessment out-

performed the NMP22 test as well as the BTA test and conventional cytology.[27]

In a recent study of 107 patients, the positive predictive value for the NMP22 assay combined with conventional cytologic examination was 74% and the negative predictive value was 81%.[40] Recently, a novel nuclear matrix protein, BLCA-4, measured in urine samples by immunoassay, has shown significant improvements in sensitivity (96%) and specificity (100%) for the detection of bladder cancer.[38] The patients assessed, however, appeared to have advanced or invasive disease and the specific capabilities of this marker to identify well-differentiated lesions was not described.[40]

In summary, the NMP22 test – when compared with cytology performed on voided samples by non-expert cytopathologists – appears to provide additional information for the risk assessment of patients for recurrence for urinary bladder cancer. However, given the relatively high cost of the test and the necessity of mailing the specimen to a reference laboratory, it remains to be seen whether the marginal improvement in cytology can be justified by the inconvenience and cost of the procedure.

Telomerase assays

Telomerase is a ribonucleoprotein enzyme with reverse transcriptase activity that contains an RNA component, which provides a template for the synthesis of repeat telomeric sequences.[41] Tests for telomerase activity using the polymerase chain reaction (PCR)-based telomeric repeat amplification protocol (TRAP) assay (Fig. 22.1) have been positive in nearly all urothelial tumors.[41,42] Telomerase activity, when a semi-quantitative TRAP assay is used, has not correlated with the grade or stage of the disease.[41] The published range in sensitivity for the detection of urothelial carcinomas by telomerase measurement is from 70 to 93%, with a specificity ranging from 60 to 99%[27,41,43–47] (Table 22.5). Although the false-positive rate was high in one study,[45] the telomerase assay has generally outperformed cytology in several additional studies.[27,43,44,46,47] In a study of 196 patients, Ramakumar and co-workers[27] found that telomerase had the highest combined sensitivity and specificity of the ancillary procedures tested, and outperformed NMP22 and BTA assays, as well as conventional cytology.

In summary, although of significant potential, the routine use of telomerase assays in the management of patients with recurrent urothelial neoplasia is currently limited by the cost and cumbersome nature of the

Table 22.4 NMP22™ (nuclear matrix protein) test

Year	Author	Method	Sensitivity (%)	Specificity (%)	Comment
1996	Soloway et al.[30]	Immunoassay	70	86	90 patients; 100% sensitivity for invasive disease; helpful for monitoring recurrence
1997	Miyanaga et al.[31]	Immunoassay (10 IU/ml cut-off)	81	64	280 patients; NMP22 had significantly higher sensitivity than cytology
1998	Witjes et al.[32]	Immunoassay (10 IU/ml cut-off)	–	–	50 patients; negative predictive value 91%, positive predictive value 56%; outperformed karyometry
1998	Serretta et al.[33]	Immunoassay	71	61	179 patients; specificity too low for routine clinical use
1998	Abbate et al.[25]	Immunoassay	54	–	156 patients; lower sensitivity than BTA
1998	Stampfer et al.[34]	Immunoassay (6.4 IU/ml cut-off)	68	80	231 patients; more sensitive, operator-independent and less costly than cytology; useful for screening
1998	Wiener et al.[15]	Immunoassay	48	70	291 patients; better than voided urine cytology, but cannot replace cystoscopy due to low sensitivity and specificity for grade 3 TCC
1998	Landman et al.[39]	Immunoassay	81	77	47 patients; NMP22 and telomerase assays have higher sensitivity than BTA and cytology
1999	Ramakumar et al.[27]	Immunoassay	53	60	196 patients; telomerase assay outperformed cytology, BTA and NMP22 as well as hemoglobin/blood detection
1999	Hughes et al.[40]	Immunoassay	47	79	107 patients; positive predictive value for NMP22 plus cytology 74%; negative predictive value 81%
2000	Mian et al.[35]	Immunoassay	56	79	240 patients; UBC ELISA test outperformed NMP22
2000	Perez Garcia et al.[36]	Immunoassay	69	64	30 patients; low positive predictive value; cystoscopy cannot be avoided
2000	Menendez et al.[37]	Immunoassay	38	81	71 patients; cannot replace cytology with NMP22

TCC, transitional cell carcinoma; ELISA, enzyme-linked immunosorbent assay.

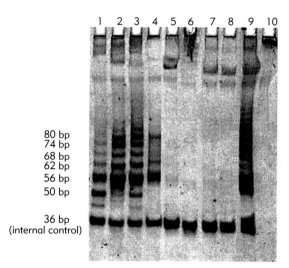

Fig. 22.1 Telomerase detection in cytologic specimens. Telomeric repeat amplification protocol (TRAP) method. Lanes 1, 2, 3 and 4 contain fluids with malignant cells and show a ladder of base pairs indicating the presence of telomerase activity. Lanes 5, 6, 7 and 8 are fluids that were negative for malignant cells and show no base-pair ladder. Lane 9 is the control cell line known to be positive for telomerase activity and lane 10 is the telomerase negative control fluid.

Table 22.5 Telomerase assays

Year	Author	Method	Sensitivity (%)	Specificity (%)	Comment
1998	Muller et al.[43]	TRAP	73	–	48 patients; TRAP test was not sensitive compared to other methods of telomerase detection
1997	Yoshida et al.[44]	TRAP	62	96	109 patients; relatively low sensitivity
1998	Lance et al.[45]	TRAP	81	60	66 patients; high false-positive rate for benign disease
1998	Ito et al.[46]	RT-PCR	80	–	59 patients; useful for detection of bladder cancer
1998	Lee et al.[47]	TRAP	93	–	15 patients with early-stage disease; telomerase-outperformed cytology in disease detection
1999	Ramakumar et al.[27]	TRAP	70	99	196 patients; telomerase had highest combination of sensitivity and specificity against NMP22, BTA and cytology
2000	Gelmini et al.[41]	TRAP (semi-quantitative)	82	–	33 patients; telomerase activity in tumor tissue correlated with levels in urine

RT-PCR, reverse transcriptase polymerase chain reaction; TRAP, telomeric repeat amplification protocol.

bioassay which requires intact tissue and use of the PCR-based TRAP procedure. The development of an on-slide method, utilizing either in situ hybridization or immunohistochemistry, appears necessary to create an easy (ideally automated) method that can be used on a routine basis for clinical material.

Microsatellite instability assays

Microsatellites are inherited short tandem repeat DNA sequences with low mutation rates unique to individuals.[48] Assays for abnormalities in microsatellites have generally included the detection of mutational copy errors and deletions of gene loci seen as loss of heterozygosity (LOH).[2] In addition, it has recently been recognized that low-grade papillary urothelial neoplasms are often associated with chromosomal instability and loss in parts of chromosome 9 in and near the p16[INK4A] (MTS1) tumor suppressor gene.[49] Abnormalities of chromosomes 3, 4, 8, 11, 13, 17 and 18 have also been associated with the development of urothelial malignancy. Microsatellite instability assays have been most frequently identified as LOH in the 9p region for low-stage tumors.[50] Additional mutations and genetic divergence appear to accumulate after the primary chromosome 9 alterations in most cases of low-grade, superficial urothelial neoplasia.[51]

Five studies of microsatellite instability (including LOH and mutational analyses) have demonstrated (Fig. 22.2) the apparent highest sensitivity (range 83–95%) and specificity (100%) for the early identification of recurrence of urothelial neoplasia in bladder washing and urinary cytology specimens[52-56] (Table 22.6). Microsatellite analysis has been successfully performed on stored frozen samples of urine specimens that lacked telomerase activity,[55] has achieved detection rates of twice the sensitivity of urine cytology,[53] and has been capable of detecting tumor recurrence months before cystoscopic examination became positive. In addition, the development of an automated low-cost method of microsatellite analysis appears feasible.[56] Recently, a study of microsatellite instability and LOH from Denmark found that a significant number of men with cystitis were also positive for the markers.[57]

A novel automated method for determining microsatellite status using a fluorescent PCR strategy has

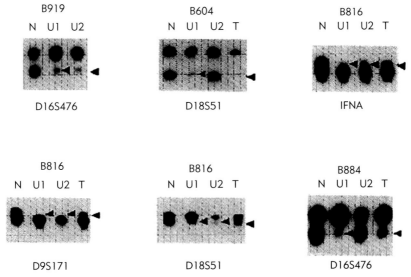

Fig. 22.2 Microsatellite instability assays in urine samples. The six blots shown were obtained from urinary sediments. In specimen B919, the arrows indicate a loss of heterozygosity (LOH) at the same locus in both the original sample and the sample at the time of recurrence. In cases B604 and B884, the initial urinary and tumor samples show similar LOHs (arrows), but the subsequent samples (U2) show restoration of both alleles and indicate that the patient was free of disease at follow-up. In specimen B816, continued LOHs are seen in the tumor, original and follow-up urine samples from three separate loci which were associated with confirmed disease recurrence at 6 months. N, normal; U1, urinary sediment prior to treatment; U2, urinary sediment obtained at 3–6 months after treatment started; T, the original first tumor tissue sample obtained at cystoscopy. (Adapted from Muller et al.[43])

Table 22.6 Assays for microsatellite instability

Year	Author	Method	Sensitivity (%)	Specificity (%)	Comment
1996	Mao et al.[52]	Loss of heterozygosity Mutational analysis	95	–	20 patients; near twice the sensitivity of urine cytology (50%)
1997	Steiner et al.[53]	Loss of heterozygosity Mutational analysis	90	100	21 patients; in two patients, MSI identified recurrence months before cystoscopy became positive
1997	Linn et al.[54]	Loss of heterozygosity Mutational analysis	87	–	15 patients; stored frozen urine samples; no telomerase activity in these specimens
1998	Mourah et al.[55]	Loss of heterozygosity Mutational analysis	83	100	59 patients; no false-positive cases; renal transplant patients had donor alleles identified
2000	Baron et al.[56]	Automated fluorescent PCR	78	84	25 patients; microsatellite analysis outperformed cytology

MSI, microsatellite instability; PCR, polymerase chain reaction.

been described, with a 78% sensitivity that was nearly twice that for conventional cytology.[58] Mismatch repair genes such as hMSH2 have also been studied in recurrent bladder cancer and have been shown to have an 81% sensitivity when measured by both immunohistochemistry and reverse transcriptase (RT)-PCR in urine samples.[59] Thus, assuming that assays can prevent loss of specificity due to inflammatory conditions, microsatellite analysis shows significant potential for clinical use to monitor early recurrence in urothelial neoplasia. If an inexpensive automated assay can be developed in the near future, this procedure may well become a part of the routine care of patients with urinary bladder and upper urinary tract tumors.

DNA aneuploidy and chromosomal aneusomy

In the early 1980s flow cytometry was introduced to detect abnormal total DNA content in urothelial cells obtained from urothelial cytology specimens.[60] Early hope that DNA aneuploidy would be a major adjunct to the cytologic detection of recurrent urothelial carcinoma ultimately gave way to the reality that the technique could improve on the sensitivity and specificity of cytology only to a marginal degree.[61,62]

Improvements in flow cytometric techniques, including dual-parameter immunoflow cytometry, have achieved an increased sensitivity for the detection of grade 1 transitional cell carcinomas (urothelial neoplasms of low malignant potential) to a level of 86%.[63] The introduction of DNA content measurements by digital static image analysis (Fig. 22.3) in the late 1980s also reported an increase in sensitivity and specificity for detection of recurrent urothelial malignancy.[64] Subsequently, it was reported that for patients with urothelial neoplasms, approximately one-third of cases with diploid urothelial cytology samples are ultimately associated with progression to muscle-invasive disease.[65] In addition, although the combination of conventional cytology with DNA ploidy measurements by image analysis has been capable of detecting up to 85% of cases of recurrent urothelial neoplasia, the combined modalities are not able to identify all of the patients with disease relapse.[66,67]

The Quanticyt karyometric analysis was developed in the Netherlands as an automated system for urothelial cell grading using Feulgen-stained cytospin preparations and a digital image analysis system.[68] This combined morphometric and DNA quantification system has been promoted as an adjunct that could reduce the need for surveillance cystoscopy.[68] A major application

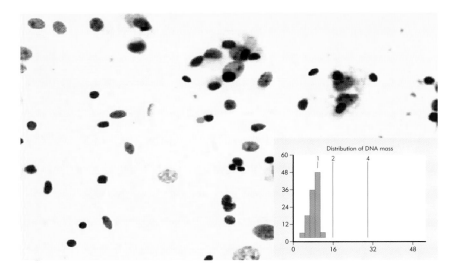

Fig. 22.3 DNA ploidy in urine cytology of chemotherapy-associated atypia. Although cytologic atypia of urothelial cells is present, the image analysis-based DNA ploidy histogram reveals a diploid pattern with DNA index of 1.02. Although diploid histograms are associated both with therapy atypia and low-grade urothelial carcinomas, aneuploidy is characteristic of high-grade tumors only.

of DNA ploidy analysis in urothelial cytology samples has been to differentiate recurrent urothelial malignancy (diploid or aneuploid) from cytologic atypia associated with intravesical instillation of chemotherapy and immunotherapy (uniformly diploid).

More recently the technique of fluorescence in situ hybridization (FISH) has been applied to urothelial cytology specimens to detect chromosomal aneusomy.[69] The success of this technique is dependent upon the number of chromosomal centromeric probes used to detect gains or losses[70] and will have relatively low sensitivity if insufficient numbers of probes are utilized.[70] In one study, routine ploidy analysis was combined with FISH-based assessment for chromosome 9 and resulted in an increase in sensitivity compared to that of either technique used alone.[71] Chromosome 9 has also been evaluated by single-strand conformational polymorphism analysis (SSCP), with LOH found to be a marker of recurrent urothelial cancer that was more sensitive than routine cytology.[72] However, urothelial carcinomas are a heterogeneous group of neoplasms and multiple probes must be used to detect recurrent disease. Thus, the FISH and SSCP methods are too complex, time-consuming and expensive for general use in most laboratories.[73]

Other markers utilized to detect recurrent urothelial neoplasia

Blood group antigens

The loss of cellular expression of the AB and O blood group antigens has long been recognized as a marker of urothelial neoplasia.[74] More recently, antibodies designed to detect Lewis X blood group expression in urothelial cytology have been evaluated as indicators of recurrent disease. However, blood group expression assays have not yet achieved significant levels of improvement in detection rates over conventional cytology to warrant their widespread clinical use.

Antigens associated with urothelial carcinomas

A variety of proteins, glycoprotein and other antigens have been studied for their ability to improve on the detection rates for recurrent urothelial neoplasia:[74,75]

- *Cytokeratin*: In one study, cytokeratin 20 staining achieved 91% sensitivity compared to 56% sensitivity for cytology alone,[76] and in another achieved an 87% sensitivity.[77] In a study of cytokeratin 19, using a quantitative assay, a sensitivity of 96% and specificity of 74% was achieved which more than doubled the 43% sensitivity for cytology alone.[78] When a receiver operating characteristics (ROC) curve was used, the cytokeratin 19 assay (also known as the CYFRA 21-1) achieved a 96% sensitivity and 67% specificity for bladder cancer detection in urine.[79] Another tissue polypeptide-specific antigen study based on urine cytokeratin levels reported 64% sensitivity and 84% specificity for the biomarker.[80]
- *Epithelial membrane antigen*: Studies of epithelial membrane antigen have yielded conflicting results in their ability to improve in the detection of urothelial neoplasia.[3]

- *AM43 and BB639*: AM43 and BB639 are two monoclonal antibodies utilized in a radioimmunoassay, which, although relatively sensitive, were associated with a 20% false-positive staining rate.[81]
- *486 P3/12*: The 486 P3/12 antigen has achieved a 89% sensitivity for detecting both high- and low-grade tumors and thus shows significant potential as an adjunct for detection of recurrent disease.[82]
- *M344 and 19A211*: The M344 and 19A211 antigens similarly show potential for use in the follow-up of patients due to their ability to detect low-grade lesions.[83]
- *Psorisian*: Psorisian is a squamous epithelial differentiation marker which has shown potential for the follow-up of patients with squamous cell carcinoma of the bladder.[84]
- *DD23*: The DD23 antigen is upregulated in approximately 80% of bladder neoplasms and may be of significant value for the early detection of recurrent bladder neoplasms.[85]
- *M344, LDQ10 and 19A211*: Recently, a panel of monoclonal antibodies (M344, LDQ10 and 19A211) comprising the ImmunoCyt™ test was found to be a highly sensitive detector of all grades of urothelial carcinomas which, when combined with cytologic examination, showed potential for reducing the need for cystoscopy in selected patients.[86]

Tumor-associated hyaluronic acid and hyaluronidase

Hyaluronidase and hyaluronic acid have been evaluated as predictors of urothelial neoplasia in urine samples. Although urinary hyaluronidase measurements have been associated with a sensitivity of 100% and specificity of 89% for the detection of high-grade bladder neoplasms,[87–89] the ability to detect low-grade lesions by hyaluronidase measurements has not, as yet, been proven. Recently, a study of 513 urine samples for hyaluronidase activity produced an 82% sensitivity and 90% specificity for bladder cancer detection, independent of tumor grade.[89]

Growth factors

A variety of growth factors have been measured in urine samples, both as adjuncts to the detection of urothelial neoplasia and as predictors of disease outcome:

- *Acidic fibroblast growth factor* (acidic FGF) is associated with proliferation, differentiation, angiogenesis and cell motility.[3] Urothelial cancers have

a significant increase in staining for acidic FGF compared to normal urothelium,[90] and urine samples from patients with bladder cancer contain significantly more acidic FGF than do samples from controls.[91,92] This marker appears more suited as a prognostic test than as a detector of low-grade lesions.

- *Basic fibroblast growth factor* (basic FGF) has also been evaluated as an adjunct to urothelial cancer detection.[92] Urinary basic FGF levels are higher in patients with bladder cancer than in control subjects and, in one study, this test was more sensitive than cytology for the detection of urothelial neoplasia.[93] Concerns about specificity and the ability to detect low-grade lesions have limited the adoption of basic FGF measurements into clinical practice.
- *Autocrine motility factor*: Urinary autocrine motility factor has been detected in 100% of patients with muscle-invasive urothelial carcinomas and in 80% of patients with superficial lesions.[94] Autocrine motility factor levels have also correlated with urothelial cancer stage and disease recurrence.[95] However, the 25% false-positive rate identified for control specimens[95] has created concern that the low specificity of this test would preclude its widespread clinical use.
- *Epidermal growth factor* (EGF) concentrations are lower in patients with urothelial neoplasia than in controls, possibly due to EGF binding to urothelial cells during carcinogenesis.[96] EGF measurements have not been used successfully for the early detection of recurrent urothelial carcinoma.
- *Transforming growth factor beta* (TGF-β) has also been studied in patients with urothelial neoplasia. TGF-β expression is higher in urothelial neoplasia than in normal urothelium and may be a significant marker of bladder cancer progression.[97] The use of TGF-β measurements for the detection of recurrent bladder cancer in urine samples has not yet been reported.

Cell adhesion molecules

- *E-cadherin/catenin*: The E-cadherin/catenin system has been extensively studied in patients with bladder cancer. Loss of expression of E-cadherin has been associated with high histologic grade, advanced pathologic stage, and adverse outcome in patients with urothelial neoplasia.[98,99] Elevated urinary E-cadherin measurements have been associated with the presence of papillary urothelial neoplasms (Fig. 22.4) which have featured upregulation of E-cadherin (which is subsequently downregulated in patients in whom the lower-grade papillary tumors

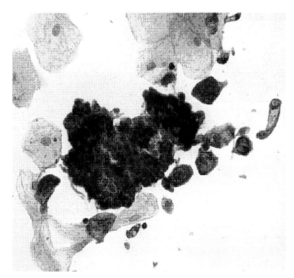

Fig. 22.4 E-cadherin cell adhesion molecule in urine cytology: overexpression in papillary low-grade urothelial neoplasms. Benign squamous cells surround the central darkly stained cluster of cells obtained from a patient with a papillary low-grade urothelial carcinoma. E-cadherin staining is increased in the cells from a low-grade papillary tumor, but progressively downregulated and completely lost in flat high-grade tumors with progressive invasion and subsequent metastasis (avidin-biotin immunoperoxidase × 400).

dedifferentiate), become flat lesions and invaded the bladder wall.[100] Widespread measurements of soluble E-cadherin by liquid immunoassay and cellular E-cadherin by immunocytochemistry have not been widely studied for the detection of recurrent urothelial neoplasia.

- *CD44*: The CD44 cell adhesion molecule has also been studied in bladder cancer. Similarly, loss of expression of the standard form of this molecule by immunohistochemistry has been associated with high-grade, high-stage disease.[101] However, attempts to use CD44 measurements in lysates of urine sediment were not successful in adding significant information for the detection of urothelial carcinoma.[102]
- *Integrins*: The study of integrins in urine samples has also shown a relationship between loss of cell adhesion expression and disease invasiveness.[103]

Fibrinogen degradation products

The shedding of fibrinogen degradation products (FDPs), reflecting focal disseminated intravascular coagulation associated with bladder neoplasia, has been

used as a method of detection of the disease.[3] The AuraTek FDP™ test uses an enzyme-linked immunosorbent assay (ELISA) method to detect FDPs in urine. The sensitivity and specificity of this method have been reported as 81% and 75%, respectively.[104] Similar to other markers, the ability of this method to detect well-differentiated early-stage tumors is not established. However, in a comparison of the AuraTek FDP test with the BTA test, urine hemoglobin detection and urothelial cytology, the AuraTek FDP test had the highest sensitivity for low-grade lesions.[104]

Fibrinolysis system

High levels of the urokinase type I plasmin activator (uPA), a protease associated with cancer invasion, have been detected in bladder tumor tissues.[2] Although elevated uPA levels have been associated with adverse outcome in bladder cancer independent of other prognostic factors,[105] the use of uPA measurements for the early detection of recurrent urothelial neoplasia has not been reported.

Glutathione S-transferase π

Glutathione S-transferase π-1 has been tested in urine as a marker for bladder cancer using an ELISA method. The sensitivity was relatively low and the potential of this marker to detect low-grade, early recurrent lesions is currently unproven.[106]

Cell-cycle regulators

- $p16^{INK4A}$: Genes and proteins regulating the transition from the G1 to the S phase of the cell cycle have frequently been implicated in both the development and the detection of urothelial neoplasia. LOH in the 9p21 region has confirmed that the $p16^{INK4A}$ tumor suppressor gene is associated with the development of papillary and low-grade urothelial neoplasms.[107] Large clinical trials evaluating the LOH at chromosome 9p to detect abnormalities of the p16 gene (point deletions), or loss of p16 protein production due to p16 promoter gene hypermethylation, are currently in progress. As discussed above, microsatellite instability assays are also focused in the 9p region and show substantial potential for the early detection of recurrent urothelial neoplasia. In addition, chromosomal abnormalities in the 9q region have also been associated with bladder cancer development and may generate a new series of molecular detection strategies.[108] Cell-cycle regulators are well established as prognostic factors for bladder cancer,[109] but their use as early detection markers is, to date, unproven.

- *p53*: The p53 tumor suppressor gene has been extensively studied as a cell cycle inhibitor at the G1 to S checkpoint, an apoptosis regulator, and a target for cancer therapy.[110] Mutations of the p53 gene (and resulting production of mutant p53 protein) have been associated with non-papillary, deeply invasive, high-stage disease.[110–112] However, attempts to use p53 immunostaining on urine cytology samples to enhance the detection of bladder cancer have shown a relatively low sensitivity and specificity.[113] Continued studies of p53 mutations for the management of bladder cancer appear likely to continue, but the use of this marker to aid the detection of low-grade disease appears unlikely to achieve clinical success.

- *pRb*: Mutations of the retinoblastoma tumor suppressor gene (pRb) have been studied in bladder cancer and identified in both superficial and invasive urothelial carcinomas.[114] The use of Rb protein detection or gene mutation analysis in urine samples to detect recurrent bladder cancer has not yet been reported.

- *Ki-67 and PCNA antigens*: Cell proliferation markers have been studied as prognostic factors in bladder cancer, including the Ki-67 and PCNA antigens.[115] The use of cell proliferation for the detection of recurrent urothelial neoplasia has not so far been performed on a wide scale. Ki-67 labeling can supplement the routine use of histologic grade and stage in predicting bladder cancer outcome, but has not been widely used to detect early disease recurrence.[116] Recently, when a 20% Ki-67 labeling index cut-off was used, Ki-67 immunostaining was a significant detector of recurrent early-stage disease.[116]

CONCLUSION

Recently, a series of ancillary tests have been introduced with claims that they can improve the sensitivity and specificity of routine urinary cytology, facilitate an earlier detection of relapse of urothelial carcinoma and reduce the number of cystectomies needed to monitor patients with this disease. Although the performance features of the ancillary tests have varied and the cytologic methods to which they have been compared have not been standardized, several of the procedures have received considerable support from urologists as assisting them in the management of their patients.

Over the next several years, the ancillary tests will continue to be measured prospectively against cytology alone in clinical trials designed to learn whether the additional costs of the new procedures can be overcome by the added benefits of a reduction in costly cystectomies and the earlier specific detection of disease relapses, leading to earlier therapy and reduced morbidity and mortality.

REFERENCES

1. Landis SH, Murray T, Bolden S, Wingo PA. Cancer statistics, 1999. CA Cancer J Clin 1999;49:8–31.
2. Foresman WH, Messing, EM. Bladder cancer: natural history, tumor markers, and early detection strategies. Semin Surg Oncol 1997;13:299–306.
3. Halachmi S, Linn JF, Amiel GE, Moskovitz B, Nativ O. Urine cytology, tumor markers and bladder cancer. Br J Urol 1998;82:647–654.
4. Lynch CF, Cohen MB. Urinary system. Cancer (Suppl.) 1995;75:316–319.
5. Koss LG. Diagnostic Cytology of the Urinary Tract. Philadelphia: JB Lippincott, 1995.
6. Rosenthal DL. Urologic cytology. In: Astarita RW (ed.) Practical Cytopathology. New York: Churchill Livingstone, 1990, pp 303–336.
7. Brown FM. Urine cytology. Is it still the gold standard for screening? Urol Clin North Am 2000;27:25–37.
8. Shenoy UA, Colby TV, Schumann GB. Reliability of urinary cytodiagnosis in urothelial neoplasms. Cancer 1985;56:2041–2045.
9. Raab SS, Lenel JC, Cohen MB. Low grade transitional cell carcinoma of the bladder. Cytologic diagnosis by key features as identified by logistic regression analysis. Cancer 1994;74:1621–1626.
10. Maier U, Simak R, Neuhold N. The clinical value of urinary cytology: 12 years of experience with 615 patients. J Clin Pathol 1995;48:314–317.
11. Hughes JH, Raab SS, Cohen MB. The cytologic diagnosis of low-grade transitional cell carcinoma. Am J Clin Pathol 2000;114 (Suppl.):S59–67.
12. Murphy WM. Current status of urinary cytology in the evaluation of bladder neoplasms. Hum Pathol 1990;21:886–896.
13. Raab, SS, Slagel DD, Jensen CS, et al. Transitional cell carcinoma: cytologic criteria to improve diagnostic accuracy. Mod Pathol 1996;9:225–232.
14. Tut VM, Hildreth AJ, Kumar M, Mellon JK. Does voided urine cytology have biological significance? Br J Urol 1998;82:655–659.
15. Wiener HG, Mian CH, Haitel A, et al. Can urine-bound diagnostic tests replace cystoscopy in the management of bladder cancer? J Urol 1998;159:1876–1880.
16. Buchardt M, Burchardt T, Shabsigh A, et al. Current concepts in biomarker technology for bladder cancers. Clin Chem 2000;46:595–605.

17. Han M, Schoenberg MP. The use of molecular diagnostics in bladder cancer. Urol Oncol 2000;5:87–92.

18. Sarosdy MF, deVere White RW, Soloway MS, et al. Results of a multicenter trial using the BTA test to monitor for and diagnose recurrent bladder cancer. J Urol 1995;154:379–383.

19. D'Hallewin MA, Baert L. Initial evaluation of the bladder tumor antigen test and superficial bladder cancer. J Urol 1996;155:475–476.

20. Ianari A, Sternberg CN, Rossetti A, et al. Results of Bard BTA test in monitoring patients with a history of transitional cell cancer of the bladder. Urology 1997;49:786–789.

21. Leyh H, Mazeman E. Bard BTA test compared with voided urine cytology in the diagnosis of recurrent bladder cancer. Eur Urol 1997;32:425–428.

22. Miyanaga N, Akaza H, Kameyama S, et al. Significance of the BTA test in bladder cancer: a multicenter trial. Int J Urol 1997;4:557–560.

23. Van der Poel HG, Van Balken MR, Schamhart DH, et al. Bladder wash cytology, quantitative cytology, and the qualitative BTA test in patients with superficial bladder cancer. Urology 1998;51:44–50.

24. Zimmerman RL, Bagley D, Hawthorne C, Bibbo M. Utility of the Bard BTA test in detecting upper urinary tract transitional cell carcinoma. Urology 1998;51:956–958.

25. Abbate I, D'Introno A, Cardo G, et al. Comparison of nuclear matrix protein 22 and bladder tumor antigen in urine of patients with bladder cancer. Anticancer Res 1998;18:3803–3805.

26. Schamhart DH, de Reijke TM, van der Poel HG, et al. The Bard BTA test: its mode of action, sensitivity and specificity, compared to cytology of voided urine, in the diagnosis of superficial bladder cancer. Eur Urol 1998;34:99–106.

27. Ramakumar S, Bhuiyan J, Besse JA, et al. Comparison of screening methods in the detection of bladder cancer. J Urol 1999;161:388–394.

28. Nasuti JF, Gomella LG, Ismail M, Bibbo M. Utility of the BTA Stat Test Kit for bladder cancer screening. Diagn Cytopathol 1999;21:27–29.

29. Hughes JH, Cohen MB. Nuclear matrix proteins and their potential applications to diagnostic pathology. Am J Clin Pathol 1999;111:267–274.

30. Soloway MS, Briggman V, Carpinito GA, et al. Use of new tumor marker, urinary NMP22, in the detection of occult or rapidly recurring transitional cell carcinoma of the urinary tract following surgical treatment. J Urol 1996;156:363–367.

31. Miyanaga N, Akaza H, Ishikawa S, et al. Clinical evaluation of nuclear matrix protein 22 (NMP22) in urine as a novel marker for urothelial cancer. Eur Urol 1997;31:163–168.

32. Witjes JA, van der Poel HG, van Balken MR, Debruyne FM, Schalken JA. Urinary NMP22 and karyometry in the diagnosis and follow-up of patients with superficial bladder cancer. Eur Urol 1998;33:387–391.

33. Serretta A, Lo Presti D, Vasile P, et al. Urinary NMP22 for the detection of recurrence after transurethral resection of transitional cell carcinoma of the bladder: experience on 137 patients. Urology 1998;52:793–796.

34. Stampfer DS, Carpinito GA, Rodriguez-Villanueva J, et al. Evaluation of NMP22 in the detection of transitional cell carcinoma of the bladder. J Urol 1998;159:394–398.

35. Mian C, Lodde M, Haitel A, et al. Comparison of the monoclonal UBC-ELISA test and the NMP22 ELISA test for the detection of urothelial cell carcinoma of the bladder. Urology 2000;55:223–226.

36. Perez Garcia FJ, Escaf Barmadah S, Fernandez Gomez JM, Rodriguez Martinez JJ, Martin Benito JL. Determination of NMP-22 as recurrence marker in bladder cancer. Preliminary study. Arch Esp Urol 2000;53:305–312.

37. Menendez V, Filella X, Molina R, et al. Usefulness of urinary nuclear matrix protein 22 (NMP22) as a marker for transitional cell carcinoma of the bladder. Anticancer Res 2000;20(2b):1169–1172.

38. Konety BR, Nguyen TS, Dhir R, et al. Detection of bladder cancer using a novel nuclear matrix protein, BLCA-4. Clin Cancer Res 2000;6:2618–2625.

39. Landman J, Chang Y, Kavaler E, Droller MJ, Liu BC. Sensitivity and specificity of NMP-22, telomerase, and BTA in the detection of human bladder cancer. Urology 1998;52:398–402.

40. Hughes JH, Katz RL, Rodriguez-Villanueva J, et al. Urinary matrix protein 22 (NMP 22): examination for the detection of recurrent transitional cell-carcinoma of the bladder. Diagn Cytopathol 1999;20:285–290.

41. Gelmini S, Crisci A, Salvadori B, et al. Comparison of telomerase activity in bladder carcinoma and exfoliated cells collected in urine and bladder washings, using a quantitative assay. Clin Cancer Res 2000;6:2771–2776.

42. Vasef MA, Ross JS, Cohen MB. Telomerase activity in human solid tumors: diagnostic utility and clinical applications. Am J Clin Pathol 1999;112 (1 Suppl 1):S68–75.

43. Muller M, Krause H, Heicappell R, et al. Comparison of human telomerase RNA and telomerase activity in urine for diagnosis of bladder cancer. Clin Cancer Res 1998;4:1949–1954.

44. Yoshida K, Sugino K, Tahara H. Telomerase activity in bladder carcinoma and its implication for noninvasive diagnosis by detection of exfoliated cancer cells in urine. Cancer 1997;79:362–366.

45. Lance, RS, Aldous WK, Blaser J, Thrasher JB. Telomerase activity in solid transitional cell carcinoma, bladder washings, and voided urine. Urol Oncol 1998;4:43–49.

46. Ito H, Kyo S, Kanaya T, et al. Detection of human telomerase reverse transcriptase messenger RNA in voided urine samples as a useful diagnostic tool for bladder cancer. Clin Cancer Res 1998;4:2801–2810.

47. Lee DH, Yang SC, Hong SJ, Chung BH, Kim IY. Telomerase: a potential marker of bladder transitional cell carcinoma in bladder washes. Clin Cancer Res 1998;4:535–538.

48. Brentnall TA. Microsatellite instability: shifting concepts in tumorigenesis. Am J Pathol 1995;147:561–563.

49. Orntoft TF, Wolf H. Molecular alterations in bladder cancer. Urol Res 1998;26:223–233.

50. Christensen M, Jensen MA, Wolf H, Orntoft TF. Pronounced microsatellite instability in transitional cell carcinomas from young patients with bladder cancer. Int J Cancer 1998;79:396–401.

51. Takahashi T, Habuchi T, Kakehi Y, et al. Clonal and chronological genetic analysis of multifocal cancers of the bladder and upper urinary tract. Cancer Res 1998;58:5835–5841.

52. Mao L, Schoenberg MP, Scicchitano M, et al. Molecular detection of primary bladder cancer by microsatellite analysis. Science 1996;271:659–662.

53. Steiner G, Schoenberg MP, Linn JF, Mao L, Sidransky D. Detection of bladder cancer recurrence by microsatellite analysis of urine. Nat Med 1997;3:621–624.

54. Linn JF, Lango M, Halachmi S, Schoenberg MP, Sidransky D. Microsatellite analysis and telomerase activity in archived tissue and urine samples of bladder cancer patients. Int J Cancer 1997;74:625–629.

55. Mourah S, Cussenot O, Vimont V, et al. Assessment of microsatellite instability in urine in the detection of transitional-cell carcinoma of the bladder. Int J Cancer 1998;79:629–633.

56. Baron A, Mastroeni FR, Moore PS, et al. Detection of bladder cancer by semi-automated microsatellite analysis of urine sediment. Adv Clin Pathol 2000;4:19–21.

57. Christensen M, Wolf H, Orntoft TF. Microsatellite alterations in urinary sediments from patients with cystitis and bladder cancer. Int J Cancer 2000;85:614–617.

58. Wang Y, Hung SC, Linn JF, et al. Microsatellite-based cancer detection using capillary array electrophoresis and energy-transfer fluorescent primers. Electrophoresis 1997;18:1742–1749.

59. Leach FS, Hsieh J-T, Molberg K, et al. Expression of human mismatch repair gene hMSH2. A potential marker for urothelial malignancy. Cancer 2000;88:2333–2341.

60. Klein FA, Herr HW, Sogani PC. Detection and follow-up of carcinoma of the urinary bladder by flow cytometry. Cancer 1982;50:389–395.

61. Cajulis RS, Haines GK, Frias-Hidvegi D, McVary K, Bacus JW. Cytology, flow cytometry, image analysis, and interphase cytogenetics by fluorescence in situ hybridization in the diagnosis of transitional cell carcinoma in bladder washes: a comparative study. Diagn Cytopathol 1995;13:214–224.

62. Badalament RA, Kimmel M, Gay H. The sensitivity of flow cytometry compared with conventional cytology in the detection of superficial bladder carcinoma. Cancer 1987;59:2078–2085.

63. Jankevicius F, Shibayama T, Decken K, et al. Dual-parameter immunoflow cytometry in diagnosis and follow-up of patients with bladder cancer. Eur Urol 1998;34:492–499.

64. De la Roza GL, Hopkovita A, Caraway NP, et al. DNA image analysis of urinary cytology: prediction of recurrent transitional cell carcinoma. Mod Pathol 1996;9:571–578.

65. Raitanen MP, Tammela TL, Kalloinen M, Isola J. p53 accumulation, deoxyribonucleic acid ploidy and progression of bladder cancer. J Urol 1997;157:1250–1253.

66. Mora LB, Nicosia SV, Pow-Sang JM, et al. Ancillary techniques in the follow up of transitional cell carcinoma: a comparison of cytology, histology and deoxyribonucleic acid image analysis cytometry in 91 patients. J Urol 1996;156:49–54.

67. Richman AM, Mayne ST, Jekel JF, Albertsen P. Image analysis combined with visual cytology in the early detection of recurrent bladder carcinoma. Cancer 1998;82:1738–1748.

68. Boon ME, Marres EM, van der Poel HG. Combining Quanticyt karyometric analysis with architectural confocal-aided cytology to prognosticate superficial bladder cancer. Diagn Cytopathol 1998;18:10–17.

69. Matsuyama H, Bergerheim US, Nilsson I, et al. Nonradom numeral aberrations of chromosomes 7, 9 and 10 in DNA diploid bladder cancer. Cancer Genet Cytogenet 1994;77:118–124.

70. Sauter G, Gasser TC, Moch H, et al. DNA aberrations in urinary bladder cancer detected by flow cytometry and FISH. Urol Res 1997;25 (Suppl. 1):S37–43.

71. Reeder JE, O'Connell MJ, Yang Z, et al. DNA cytometry and chromosome 9 aberrations by fluorescence in situ hybridization of irrigation specimens from bladder cancer patients. Urology 1998;51 (5A Suppl.):58–61.

72. Shigyo M, Sugano K, Fukayama N, et al. Allelic loss on chromosome 9 in bladder cancer tissues and urine samples detected by blunt-end single-strand DNA conformation polymorphism. Int J Cancer 1998;78:425–429.

73. Yokogi H, Wabba Y, Moriyama GN, Igawa M, Ishibe T. Genomic heterogeneity in bladder cancer as detected by fluorescence in situ hybridization. Br J Urol 1996;78:699–703.

74. Liebert M, Seigne J. Characteristics of invasive bladder cancers: histological and molecular markers. Semin Urol Oncol 1996;14:62–72.

75. Aprikian AG, Sarkis AS, Reuter VE, Cordon-Cardo C, Sheinfeld J. Biological markers of prognosis in transitional cell carcinoma of the bladder: current concepts. Semin Urol 1993;11:137–144.

76. Rotem D, Cassel A, Lindenfeld N, et al. Urinary cytokeratin 20 as a marker for transitional cell carcinoma. Eur Urol 2000;37:601–604.

77. Buchumensky V, Klein A, Zemer R, et al. Cytokeratin 20: a new marker for early detection of bladder cell carcinoma? J Urol 1998;160:1971–1974.

78. Pariente JL, Brodenave L, Jacob F, et al. Analytical and prospective evaluation of urinary cytokeratin 19 fragment in bladder cancer. J Urol 2000;163:1116–1119.

79. Pariente JL, Bordenave L, Michael P, et al. Initial evaluation of CYFRA 21-1 diagnostic performances as a urinary marker in bladder transitional cell carcinoma. J Urol 1997;158:338–341.

80. Sanchez-Carbayo M, Urrutia M, Silva JM, et al. Urinary tissue polypeptide-specific antigen for the diagnosis of bladder cancer. Urology 2000;55:526–532.

81. Barton H, Liebert M, Sakakibra N, et al. Evaluation of new bladder tumor marker. Urol Clin North Am 1991;18:509–513.

82. Huland H, Arndt R, Huland E, Loening T, Steffens M. Monoclonal antibody 486p 3/12: a valuable bladder carcinoma marker for immunocytology. J Urol 1987;137:654–659.

83. Cordon-Cardo C, Wartinger D, Lemaned M, Fair WR, Fradet Y. Immunopathology analysis of human urinary bladder cancer. Am J Pathol 1992;140:375–385.

84. Celis JE, Rasmussen HH, Vorum H, et al. Bladder squamous cell carcinoma expresses psoriasin and externalizes it to the urine. J Urol 1996;155:2105–2112.

85. Wilding G, Knabbe C, Zugmaier G, Flanders K. Differential effect of TGF beta on human prostate cancer cells in vitro. Mol Cell Endocrinol 1989;62:79–87.

86. Mian C, Pycha A, Wiener H, et al. ImmunoCyt: a new tool for detecting transitional cell cancer of the urinary tract. J Urol 1999;161:1486–1489.

87. Lokeshwar VB, Obek C, Pham HT, et al. Urinary hyaluronic acid and hyaluronidase: markers for bladder cancer detection and evaluation of grade. J Urol 2000;163:348–356.

88. Lokeshwar VB, Obek C, Soloway MS, Block NL. Tumor-associated hyaluronic acid: a new sensitive and specific urine marker for bladder cancer. Cancer Res 1997;57:773–777.

89. Pham HT, Block NL, Lokeshwar VB. Tumor-derived hyaluronidase: a diagnostic urine marker for high-grade bladder cancer. Cancer Res 1997;57:778–783.

90. Chopin DK, Caruelle JP, Colombel M, et al. Increased immuno-detection of acidic fibroblast growth factor in bladder cancer detectable in urine. J Urol 1993;150:1126–1130.

91. Ravery V, Jouanneau J, Gil Diez S, et al. Immunohisto-chemical detection of acidic fibroblast growth factor in bladder transitional cell carcinoma. Urol Res 1992;20:211–214.

92. Chow NH, Change CJ, Yeh TM, et al. Implications of urinary basic fibroblast growth factor excretion in patients with urothelial carcinoma. Clin Sci 1996;90:127–133.

93. Nguyen M, Watanabe H, Budson AE, Richie JP, Folkman J. Elevated levels of angiogenic peptide basic fibroblast growth factor in urine of bladder cancer patients. J Natl Cancer Inst 1993;85:241–242.

94. Korman HJ, Peabody JO, Cerny JC, et al. Autocrine motility factor receptor as a possible urine marker for transitional cell carcinoma of the bladder. J Urol 1996;155:347–349.

95. Guirguis R, Schiffmann E, Liu B, et al. Detection of autocrine motility factor in urine as a marker of bladder cancer. J Natl Cancer Inst 1988;80:1203–1211.

96. Messing EM, Murphy-Brooks N. Recovery of epidermal growth factor in voided urine of patients with bladder cancer. Urology 1994;44:502–506.

97. Mayamoto H, Kubota Y, Shuin T, et al. Expression of transforming growth factor beta 1 in human bladder cancer. Cancer 1995;75:2565–2570.

98. Bringuier PP, Umbas R, Schaafsma HE, et al. Decreased E-cadherin immunoreactivity correlates with poor survival in patients with bladder tumors. Cancer Res 1993;53:3241–3245.

99. Ross JS, del Rosario AD, Figi HL, et al. E-cadherin expression in papillary transitional cell carcinoma of the urinary bladder. Hum Pathol 1995;26:940–944.

100. Ross JS, Cheung C, Sheehan C, et al. E-cadherin cell-adhesion molecule expression as a diagnostic adjunct in urothelial cytology. Diagn Cytopathol 1996;14:310–315.

101. Ross JS, del Rosario AD, Bui HX, et al. CD44 cell adhesion molecule expression in urinary bladder transitional cell carcinoma. Mod Pathol 1996;9:854–860.

102. Muller M, Heicappell R, Habermann F, et al. Expression of CD44v2 in transitional cell carcinoma of the urinary bladder and in urine. Urol Res 1997;25:187–192.

103. Liebert M, Washington R, Stein J, Wedemeyer G, Grossman H. Expression of the DLAb1 integrin family in bladder cancer. Am J Pathol 1994;144:1016–1022.

104. Johnston B, Morales A, Emerson L, Lundie M. Rapid detection of bladder cancer: a comparative study of point of care tests. J Urol 1997;158:2098–2101.

105. Hsui Y, Marutsuka K, Asada Y, Osada Y. Prognostic value of urokinase-type plasminogin activator in patients with superficial bladder cancer. Urology 1996;47:34–37.

106. Lafuente A, Rodriguez A, Gibanel R, et al. Limitations in the use of glutathione S-transferase P1 in urine as a marker for bladder cancer. Anticancer Res 1998;18:3771–3772.

107. Liggett WH, Sidransky D. Role of the p16 tumor suppressor gene in cancer. J Clin Oncol 1998;16:1197–1206.

108. Sidransky D, Frost P, Von Eschenbach A, et al. Clonal origin of bladder cancer. N Engl J Med 1992;326:737–740.

109. Cordon-Cardo C. Cell cycle regulators as prognostic factors for bladder cancer. Eur Urol 1998;33 (Suppl. 4):11–12.

110. Wiman KG. p53: emergency brake and target for cancer therapy. Exp Cell Res 1997;237:14–18.

111. Esrig D, Elmajian D, Groshen S, et al. Accumulation of nuclear p53 and tumor progression in bladder carcinoma. N Engl J Med 1994;331:1259–1264.

112. Hudson MA, Herr HW. Carcinoma in-situ of the bladder. J Urol 1995;153:564–572.

113. Righi E, Rossi G, Ferrari G, et al. Does p53 immunostaining improve diagnostic accuracy in urine cytology? Diagn Cytopathol 1997;17:436–439.

114. Benedict WF. Altered Rb expression as a prognostic clinical marker involved in human bladder tumorigenesis. J Cell Biochem (Suppl.) 1992;161:769–771.

115. Stein JP, Grossfeld GD, Ginsberg DA, et al. Prognostic markers in bladder cancer: a contemporary review of the literature. J Urol 1998;160:645–659.

116. Gontero P, Casetta G, Zitella A, et al. Evaluation of p53 protein overexpression, Ki67 proliferative activity and mitotic index as markers of tumour recurrence in superficial transitional cell carcinoma of the bladder. Eur Urol 2000;38:287–296.

23

ANALYSIS OF BLADDER CANCER USING MODERN MOLECULAR TECHNIQUES: APPLICATIONS OF HIGH THROUGHPUT DNA MICROARRAYS

Marta Sánchez-Carbayo and Carlos Cordon-Cardo

INTRODUCTION

The biological behavior of bladder cancer has been assessed by clinical and pathological parameters, including stage, tumor grade, tumor size, suspicion of vascular invasion, presence of concomitant carcinoma in situ, and multicentricity.[1] The power of these standard histopathologic markers in predicting the clinical outcome of individual tumors has certain limitations. It has been very difficult to identify within each stage clinically useful parameters that can predict risk of disease recurrence or progression. These categorical variables are too unspecific to render predictive information for individual patients, especially those with superficial disease. Due to these limitations, multiple groups have examined a variety of additional phenotypic characteristics and molecular markers, some of which appear to have potential clinical significance.[2,3] Alterations of molecular regulators of critical programs involved in cellular homeostasis, such as p53 inactivating mutations affecting both proliferation and apoptosis, are now being validated in large, well-characterized cohorts of patients.

Cancer is being defined as a genetic disease, a product of the accumulation of alterations in certain genes or their encoded products, regulating critical programs such as those of cell growth and death. Owing to the relatively high incidence of bladder neoplasms, and their anatomic accessibility, bladder cancer has become an excellent model for the study of molecular pathogenesis and tumor progression. Application of low-throughput methods, such as allelotyping and sequencing, has provided evidence for the potential clinical relevance of some deregulated genes.[2–6]

Early-stage conventional transitional cell carcinoma has been classified into two groups with distinct behavior and different molecular profiles: low-grade tumors (always papillary and usually superficial), and high-grade tumors (either papillary or non-papillary, and often invasive).[2] The inactivation of both RB and p53 pathways has been shown to be required for the transformation and immortalization of uroepithelial cells; their alterations are common and of predictive nature in clinical studies of bladder cancer.[3–6] In the post-genome era, and in view of the advent of high-throughput methods of molecular analysis, it is expected that specific tumor types will have distinct gene expression profiles. The elucidation of the molecular pathogenesis of tumors and the events involved in tumor progression are leading directly to the discovery and application of novel biological markers. The diagnosis and prognosis of certain neoplasms are in many cases enhanced by the use of markers, and the markers themselves may constitute a therapeutic target.

MOLECULAR ANALYSES USING cDNA MICROARRAYS IN CANCER

Understanding the biology underlying tumorigenesis is essential for improving our capacity to diagnose and treat bladder cancer. An increase in this understanding can come in large part from describing the mechanisms and pathways controlling both normal and bladder cancer physiology. A first and key step in describing these pathways is identifying the genes that control and participate in them as well as by defining their function. Analysis of patterns of gene expression and abundance is one of the primary ways of identifying the genes that control specific biological processes. Until recently, the ability to identify and analyze gene expression patterns has been technically limited to relatively few genes per study. This limitation has largely been removed, however, with the development of a number of methods that allow for a more comprehensive analysis of these patterns. Some of the most powerful methods include differential display,[7] serial analysis of gene expression (SAGE),[8] sequencing expressed sequence tags (ESTs), and massively parallel signature sequencing (MPSS),[9] as well as protein composition-based approaches such as combined two-dimensional gel and mass spectral analysis.[10]

Concurrent with the development of these techniques has been the tremendous increase in the DNA sequence information available for a range of organisms through genome sequencing efforts. The accomplishments of these efforts are well known: in addition to a large number of prokaryotic genomes, the genome sequences of *Saccharomyces cerevisiae*, *Caenorhabditis elegans* and *Drosophila melanogaster* have been determined; both public and private programs to sequence the mouse genome should soon be finished, and nearly complete versions of the human genome have been recently published.[11,12] An important component of the mouse and human sequencing efforts has been the determination, by cDNA sequencing, of both full and partial sequences for tens of thousands of human and mouse genes (see, for example, the Sanger Institute, www.sanger.ac.uk; The Institute for Genomic Research, www.tigr.org; the National Center for Biotechnology Information, www.ncbi.nlm.nih.gov). In addition to increasing the utility of the techniques described above, this expansion of gene and genome information has served as the basis for the development of one of the most powerful new techniques available to provide both static and dynamic views of gene expression patterns in cells and tissues – DNA microarrays.[13,14]

A DNA microarray is a very precise grid of single-stranded nucleic acid samples attached to a solid support. Typically, microarrays are made with either oligonucleotides or polymerase chain reaction (PCR)-generated fragments of cDNA clones, such that each position in the grid contains many copies of the same DNA sequence. The utility of DNA in this format arises from the ability of single-stranded nucleic acids to hybridize with high specificity to a second strand containing the complementary sequence, thus forming double-stranded nucleic acid molecules. Because of this, DNA microarrays can be used to 'interrogate' complex mixtures of thousands of nucleic acids for both the presence and abundance of molecules of known sequence. Hybridization-based assays and the microarray format combine to make extremely versatile technology. There is an increasingly large and broad range of applications to which microarrays have been applied, including genotyping polymorphisms and mutations,[15,16] determining the binding sites of DNA-binding proteins[17] and comparative genome hybridization (CGH).[18] The most widespread use of this technology has none the less been in the analysis of gene expression.

As genetic alterations and the resulting changes in gene expression are primary determinants controlling the transition from the normal to the neoplastic state, it is not surprising that expression profiling using DNA microarrays has found wide application in cancer research and will provide critical clues for the management of bladder cancer patients. In this chapter, we describe the principal DNA microarray platforms in use today, discuss some practical considerations for their use, emphasizing the use of clinical material, and present the main applications of how this technology is being applied to the study of cancer in general and the studies already described in bladder cancer in particular.

TYPES OF ARRAY

Depending on the combination of the size of the arrayed nucleic acid used to construct the array – 20–25mer oligonucleotides or PCR-amplified cDNAs (ranging in size from 150 to 1500 bp in length) – and the solid support on to which the nucleic acid is attached (glass or nylon), three different types of DNA microarray are in common use:

* arrays of oligonucleotides
* arrays of cDNAs spotted on to nylon filters
* arrays of cDNAs spotted on to glass

Oligonucleotide microarrays are widely used for both RNA expression and DNA variation analysis, whereas spotted cDNA microarrays are primarily used for RNA expression analysis (Table 23.1).

Whatever the choice of microarray platform, there are five essential steps in the use of this technology, as outlined in Figure 23.1: the fabrication of the microarray, the generation from sample RNA of the hybridi-

zation probe, the hybridization of the probe to the microarray, the acquisition of the hybridization results, and the analysis of the results. In the case of oligonucleotide microarrays, Affymetrix is one of the main producer of the microarrays and the instrumentation that nearly completely automates the hybridization and washing steps of the protocol, as well as fluorescent scanner/data analysis software system for result acquisition and analysis.[14] This instrument and software system has been designed to function as an integrated unit that uniquely and exclusively supports the use of the Affymetrix oligonucleotide microarrays. In contrast, both of the spotted cDNA microarray platforms can be implemented in a number of ways using a variety of instrument options.[19]

Nylon microarrays have long been available, and commercial glass microarrays are becoming increasingly common. For investigators wanting to make their own microarrays, a number of different spotting robots are available; likewise, a number of distinct fluorescent and radioactive scanners are available for data acquisition.[19] Alternatively, publicly available spotting robot and fluorescent scanner designs exist for those willing or wanting to make their own instruments.[20] Because of the variety of instrument and protocol options that exist for spotted cDNA arrays, care must be taken to optimize each step of the process.

Oligonucleotide microarrays

High-density oligonucleotide microarrays are fabricated in situ on glass, using a combination of photolithography and solid-phase DNA synthesis tech-

Table 23.1 Types of DNA microarray					
Parameter	Nylon macroarrays	Nylon enzymatic microarrays	Nylon radioactive microarrays	Glass microarrays	Oligonucleotide chips
Probes	PCR products	PCR products	PCR products	PCR products	20-mer oligos synthesized in situ
Support	Nylon membrane	Nylon membrane	Nylon membrane	Glass slide	Glass chip
Format	50–2000	9600 spots	200–2000 spots	50–30,000 spots	6000–64,000 oligonucleotides
Labeling	^{32}P or ^{33}P	Enzymatic	^{33}P	Fluorescence	Fluorescence
Image acquisition	Imaging plate device	Flatbed scanner or digital camera	Imaging plate device	Laser scanning	Confocal scanning
Application	Expression analysis	Expression analysis	Expression analysis	Expression analysis	Expression and variation analysis

PCR, polymerase chain reaction.

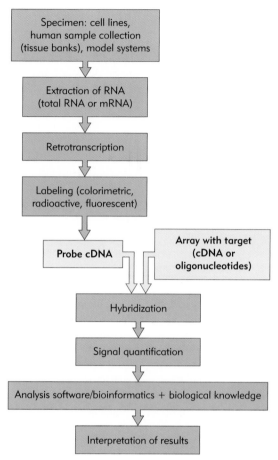

Fig. 23.1 Overall scheme of DNA microchips. The general procedure includes probe preparation, hybridization, and data acquisition and analysis steps. The complex mixture of nucleic acids (either cDNA or cRNA) derived from cellular RNA is referred to as 'probe' and the nucleic acid attached to the microarray surface as 'target'.

niques able to produce arrays of hundreds of thousands of precisely located oligonucleotides of distinct sequence in an area roughly 1 cm². [14] In this type of DNA microarray, each gene to be analyzed is represented by a set of 15–20 oligonucleotides that are perfectly complementary to the reference sequence. These oligonucleotides are chosen based on both gene sequence information and empirically derived design rules that improve the odds of selecting a sequence that will hybridize with high affinity and specificity. Choosing multiple oligonucleotides per gene improves the quantitation, specificity and reliability of the expression data. Specificity is further increased by distinguishing between true hybridization and non-specific hybridization by pairing each perfectly matched oligonucleotide target with a mismatch target oligonucleotide, identical

in sequence to the original, with the exception of a single base mismatch in the central position.

Hybridization samples are typically in vitro-transcribed cRNAs generated via a cDNA intermediate derived from either total or polyA-selected RNA. Biotin-conjugated nucleotides are incorporated into the in vitro transcription reaction, thus enabling the fluorescent labeling of hybridization products using fluorescence-conjugated streptavidin. The signal intensity at each different oligonucleotide target is determined using a laser confocal fluorescence scanner. The intensity of the hybridization signal at each target (corrected using the signal at the paired mismatch target) is related to the abundance of the corresponding RNA sequence in the original sample. In addition, the arrays contain an extensive set of internal controls that allow chip-to-chip comparison. In contrast to glass cDNA arrays, separate hybridization reactions are performed for each sample to be analyzed, raising the probability of introducing non-biological variability in expression comparisons between samples.

Although the first oligonucleotide microarrays were designed for re-sequencing applications (Fig. 23.2), their current primary application is for gene expression analysis. The target sequences for the human and mouse arrays were developed using GenBank database sequences, including those of the Unigene databases of EST sequences. The high array design and fabrication set-up costs make the design and use of custom targets unreasonably expensive for all but the most well-funded laboratories. For this reason, most users will be dependent upon the manufacturer for designing and releasing new arrays, which will most likely include only those that meet a large market demand. Current available expression profiling arrays have a maximum density in the range of $6 - 60 \times 10^3$ genes per array; this density is expected to increase due to continued improvements in the target design algorithms and fabrication technology.

cDNAs spotted on nylon filters

cDNAs spotted on nylon filters was the first commonly used microarray format applied to large-scale analysis of gene expression. [21] This technology grew from the many well-established methods for using nitrocellulose and nylon membrane-bound nucleic acids in the hybridization-based analysis of RNA and DNA. [22] The large amount of EST data being generated by the genome-sequencing programs served as the impetus both to miniaturize the format and to automate the

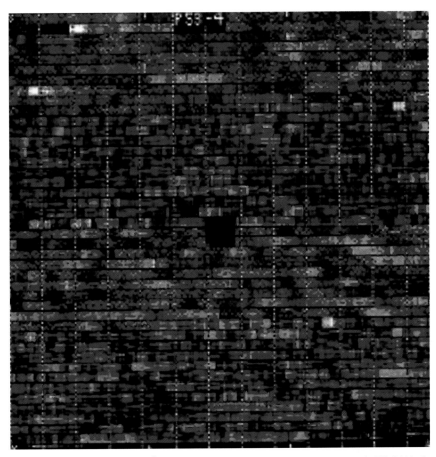

Fig. 23.2 Image of a p53 Affymetrix GeneChip®. Given a reference sequence for a region of p53 DNA, four probes are designed to interrogate every single position. The four differ only in that at the studied position there is a substitution of each of the four nucleotides, each of them containing the four bases. The probe complementary to the sample will obtain the highest fluorescence intensity. The presence of a unique sequence should hybridize only to the perfectly complementary probe rather than to the three probes containing a central mismatch. The variant array signals the presence of a sequence variation so that if two sequence species are present, the change in the fluorescence intensity will show the presence of a mutation at a certain position.

production of arrayed sets of EST clones. In spite of its relatively 'low-tech' nature, nylon filter microarrays continue to be an important and powerful expression profile platform. These microarrays continue to be used because of their accessibility and their flexibility in covering the demands of a broad range of research laboratories. High-density nylon membranes can include PCR products, and can contain hundreds to thousands of genes. Nylon microarrays can be bought or made in the user's laboratory;[23,24] they are comparatively inexpensive, and require relatively little investment in instrumentation such as appropriate spotting devices and robots. They provide reasonable sensitivity, not only when a radioactive label is incorporated in a cDNA probe generated from the RNA sample,[25] but also with

colorimetric detection.[26] Fluorescent detection methods cannot be used with nylon filter microarrays due to the intrinsic fluorescent emission of nylon, which results in unacceptably high levels of background signal. Depending on the labeling system, image acquisition can be performed with a flatbed scanner or a digital camera for enzymatic labeling, or image plate devices for radioactive specimens. As with oligonucleotide microarrays, it is not possible to carry out simultaneous hybridization of test and reference samples.

cDNAs spotted on glass

The introduction of a chemically treated glass microscope slide as the solid surface on to which the DNA

Fig. 23.3 cDNA microarray image after hybridization including approximately 8976 spots distributed into four quadrants. Red spots represents those genes which were highly expressed in the sample dyed with Cy5 whereas green spots represent those genes which were highly expressed in the sample dyed with Cy3. Yellow spots represent those genes similarly expressed in both samples dyed with Cy3 and Cy5. Gray or black faint spots are genes that did not hybridize with any of the samples.

target samples are printed brought many improvements to the spotted cDNA microarray format.[27] Using a rigid substrate as the printing surface led to the development of new printing technologies that allowed further miniaturization of the format. Densities of up to 30,000 DNA samples can be arrayed on a standard microscope slide with current spotting robots. The rigid, non-porous glass surface also enhances hybridization and washing steps, and improves post-hybridization image acquisition and processing. Finally, the negligible autofluorescence of glass makes possible the use of fluorescent detection methods. Fluorescent detection is responsible for one of the key advantages of the cDNA glass microarray format – the ability to do test sample–reference sample co-hybridizations. The test and reference probe samples are labeled with different fluorescent markers and then co-hybridized on a single microarray. Following high-stringency washes, the fluorescence intensities of each marker at each gene are determined using a laser scanner. The ratio of the fluorescence intensities at a given gene is a measure of the relative expression levels of that gene in the test and reference samples (Fig. 23.3).

PRACTICAL CONSIDERATIONS USING DNA MICROARRAYS

There are several issues to consider when choosing a DNA microarray platform, such as the selection of the most appropriate type of microarray for a particular study and sample preparation protocols. The importance of each of these issues depends heavily on the questions the investigator wishes to address and the resources available. For example, issues concerning slide and filter preparation will be irrelevant to users who opt for commercially available arrays, whereas RNA isolation may be the critical and limiting factor in studies involving human cancer tissue.

Selection of the type of array

Researchers can proceed either by buying commercial oligonucleotide, glass or nylon cDNA microarrays, or by making their own spotted cDNA microarrays. Issues of cost, set-up time, personnel available, flexibility and product range will influence this decision. The oligonucleotide and spotted cDNA formats each have unique advantages and disadvantages and thus offer investigators a distinct choice.

Oligonucleotide microarrays

Affymetrix is one of the major commercial provider of oligonucleotide microarrays (although a number of well-known companies are entering the field). The principal advantage of this platform is that it is an integrated system, providing array sets, optimized protocols, automated processing stations and data analysis software. The result is a 'plug-in and play' system requiring relatively little set-up and maintenance time. The main drawbacks of this approach are the relatively expensive price of the complete set of instruments necessary (hybridization system, scanner and software), the fact that expression chips are not reusable and, in most cases, that the user is restricted to arrays designed by the company (although the cost of custom arrays is decreasing).

Spotted cDNA microarrays

Microarrays consisting of cDNAs spotted on to treated microscope slides or nylon membranes are seen as a more flexible, less expensive alternative to the oligonucleotide arrays. These platforms allow the investigator extreme flexibility in the choice of PCR products to be arrayed, and can be implemented using any of a number of different spotting robots, scanners and analysis software. Because of this, cDNA microarrays are the most widely used platform in academic basic and clinical research laboratories. An important step in the production of spotted cDNA arrays is the choice of the cDNA clone library that will be used to generate the PCR fragment targets arrayed on to the slide or nylon membrane. Several companies sell individual IMAGE clones and have developed clone sets both as bacterial colonies in microtiter plates and as PCR products. The optimization of a protocol to generate the PCR fragment targets is essential in order to obtain reproducible and reliable results. Important considerations also include whether the clones used to produce the arrays are re-streaked and sequence-verified, whether DNA or lysed colonies are arrayed, and the number of known genes and ESTs include on the array.[27] Some ESTs correspond with known genes, but the majority represent partially sequenced novel genes.

Nylon microarrays

Nylon microarrays, with both colorimetric and radioactive labeling, offer a lower-cost alternative to glass microarrays. Certain configurations of spotting robots used in the fabrication of glass microarrays can also be used to prepare nylon microarrays, although care must be taken in choosing spotting pins that are compatible with nylon. A relatively expensive high-resolution imaging plate system is necessary for radioactive labeling, whereas cheaper and simpler devices, such as a flatbed scanner or a digital camera fitted on a low-power microscope, are sufficient for colorimetric detection.[26] In addition to cost, important advantages of nylon arrays are that they are reusable, and that the DNA to be spotted does not require elaborate purification.

Glass microarrays

The glass microarray is a well-established platform in the academic basic research environment and is starting to be used in clinical research projects. Various groups are designing and manufacturing their own arrays, representing sets of genes expressed in a specific organism, tissue or pathologic condition. Although they have been inaccessible to many academic scientists due to the high cost of the necessary equipment (robotic spotter and laser scanner) and the fact that they are non-reusable arrays, this situation is rapidly changing and a wide range of equipment is available commercially. As with nylon arrays, some companies are marketing ready-to-use glass microarrays containing thousands of targets derived from public or proprietary sequenced cDNA clones.

Sample preparation

A critical issue in microarray use that is sometimes overlooked is the control of the quantity and quality of the RNA from which the hybridization probe is prepared. This is particularly true when the RNA is isolated from clinical specimens and critical when studying bladder cancer specimens. Potential solutions to the quantitative limitation include:

- probe-labeling protocols that increase sensitivity through label signal amplification using dendrimers[28]
- probe amplification protocols that reduce the amount of RNA required through the use of highly efficient phage RNA polymerases or PCR amplification[29]
- post-hybridization amplication methods in which the target-probe duplexes are detected enzymatically.[30]

Currently, probe amplification is the most frequently used method to solve problems of starting material and to improve the detection of low-abundance gene transcripts. Although there are studies showing favorable data,[29,30] care must be taken when amplifying probe material, as this may introduce bias such that the hybridization probe does not accurately reflect the transcript representation of the original RNA sample.[31]

Problems of RNA quality can also be severe when working with archived samples, as many fixing and embedding protocols utilize aldehyde-based fixatives, which damage RNA integrity.[31,32] None the less, there have been studies that indicate RNA quality is not diminished, at least for certain tumors, following certain standard fixation protocols.[33] RNA quality is generally superior if tissue specimens are frozen at the time of surgery, although freezing often compromises sample histology. Finally, the tumor cells of interest are frequently limited in number and surrounded by normal cells. Laser capture microdissection appears to be a technique capable of isolating relatively pure sample cancer cells from clinical specimens.[33,34] The degree of the effect of laser beam on the quality of the RNA obtained is still controversial, although there are reports showing good results using PALM-type microdissectors.[33]

The establishment of suitable tissue banks is a logical adjunct to any in-depth RNA analysis of human tissue; repositories must address issues of appropriate collection and storage and must also ensure that samples are accompanied by appropriate patient information, including treatment, outcome, epidemiologic and family history data.[35]

EXPRESSION PROFILING AND THE STUDY OF CANCER

Microarray-based gene expression profiling has found a number of important applications in the study of carcinogenesis and cancer biology. Broadly speaking, these applications can be described as:

- gene and pathway discovery
- functional classification of genes
- tumor classification.

For the sake of simplicity, we have chosen to describe each of these applications separately. It should also be obvious that these applications are very closely related and that a particular experiment may involve more than one of these applications. The intention here is to describe the power and the range of uses of microarray-based expression profiling. Clearly, a larger number of laboratories than the ones mentioned here have contributed to both the development and use of this technology.

Gene and pathway discovery

The functional association of changes in gene expression with changes in cell state or phenotype is a well-established paradigm that has served as the basis for a multitude of studies in molecular biology. Based on this paradigm, functional assignments have been made for hundreds of genes. This use – associating a change in the expression of a gene with a change in physiologic state – is one the simplest ways in which gene expression profiling can be used to suggest or predict gene function. Clearly, because this is done on the scale of hundreds or thousands of genes at a time, the use of microarrays greatly accelerates the process compared to more traditional gene expression approaches. Another way in which expression profiling can be used in the functional classification of genes is often referred to as 'guilt by association'. This method is based on the observation that genes with related expression patterns – genes that presumably are co-regulated – are likely to be functionally related and involved in the control of the same biological processes or physiologic pathways.[36,37] When genes with similar expression profiles are grouped (a process referred to as clustering), novel genes (usually ESTs) are often grouped with genes of known function and a tentative function for the novel genes can be inferred by this grouping. Moreover, new functions can be ascribed to known genes when they are grouped with genes that have a distinct functional classification.[38] Similarly, previously unknown functions can be ascribed to pathways when expression changes in the genes that make up the pathway correlate with changes in the physiologic state of the cell.

Functional classification of genes

A traditional approach to assigning a functional role to a gene is to overexpress that gene and observe the effect(s) of its expression on known pathways or processes. This approach has been especially useful in identifying the downstream targets of transcription factors. The genes identified as either up- or down-regulated in these experiments are likely to play important roles in the functional pathways controlled by the gene under investigation. The microarray format offers a straightforward way to apply this approach on a large scale.

In these experiments, it is often critical to be able to tightly control expression of the gene under study. In the case of tumor suppressor genes, for example, death or poor cell growth resulting from their constitutive expression can render the generation and growth of such cell lines difficult or impossible. The use of a tightly controlled inducible expression system can circumvent this problem. Another potential problem, particularly in experiments in which cells are transiently transfected, can be in restricting the analysis to only those cells that actually express the gene of interest. This can be avoided using expression constructs in which the gene of interest is fused to a tag – (e.g. green fluorescent protein) that can be used to select and enrich for cells expressing the gene.

Tumor classification

One of the most exciting and potentially most powerful applications of expression profiling with DNA micro-arrays is the classification of human tumors. Two major goals and challenges for cancer treatment are the early and accurate diagnosis of tumor type and the establishment of prognosis, so that the appropriate and most effective treatment can be chosen at a time when treatment is still effective. The traditional histopathologic approach to tumor classification has used a mixture of morphologic, immunohistochemical and clinical criteria to classify malignancies. Despite significant progress, these methods very often fail to predict accurately the clinical course of many tumors as well as the response to and effectiveness of treatment. It was recognized early on that gene expression patterns determined using DNA microarrays could provide a means for classifying tumors into more biologically meaningful and clinically useful categories. In addition, expression profiling of well-curated tumor specimens has the potential to identify genes controlling tumorigenesis, including the various stages of tumor progression. And although the true clinical utility of expression profile-based tumor classification is controversial and still unproven, early results are encouraging.

When using spotted cDNA arrays, the choice of the common reference to which the experimental (i.e. tumor) samples will be compared is a very important issue for which a range of strategies have been adopted. A pooled common reference sample derived from multiple related cell types has been used when the expression profiles of multiple unrelated samples are compared.[39,40] For example, in a study in which the expression patterns of a group of diffuse large B cell lymphomas (DLBCL) were compared, a pool of mRNAs from nine different lymphoma cell lines was used as the reference.[40] A similar choice was made in a large study of breast tumors, in which the reference consisted of an mRNA pool from 11 different cultured cell lines derived from tissues likely to be present in the surgically dissected tumor samples.[39] The use of a common reference sample is not possible with oligonucleotide micro-arrays, as only a single sample can be tested per array. Instead, comparative scaling and normalization tools are used to allow comparisons to be made among samples. In one effective approach, the mean expression level of a gene across all samples is calculated, the change for each sample relative to this mean is determined, and the sizes of the changes across all the samples are then compared.[41]

It is common practice to include analyses of purified primary cells and cell lines to provide a framework within which to interpret the results obtained from tumor samples.[39,40] Comparisons between expression profiles of tumor and normal tissue can often provide insight into the biology of the malignancy as well as information concerning its cellular composition. For example, it is often possible to identify the contribution of the different cellular components of the sample – cancerous and non-cancerous – to the overall expression profile of a histologically complex tumor. Furthermore, knowledge of the expression patterns of untransformed cells from which the malignancy has potentially developed can greatly assist in assigning a cellular origin to tumor.[39,40] Experimental justification for this latter practice derives from the observation that the expression profiles of tumor cell lines often correlate with the profiles of their tissue of origin.[42]

The few large-scale studies published thus far indicate that gene expression patterns vary sufficiently to allow sample classification based upon expression profiles. In spite of this, assigning tumors to biologically and clinically meaningful subclasses is not necessarily a straightforward process – a significant challenge lies in choosing the best groups of genes with which to identify the biologically related tumor subclass. Certain groups (or 'clusters') of genes vary consistently in tumor samples, and these genes can frustrate attempts at subclassification.[39,40] For example, a group of genes known to be important in controlling cellular proliferation have similar expression profiles in different tumor types (the proliferation cluster), as do genes that are induced by interferons (the interferon-regulated cluster). Tumor classifications based upon these types of 'dominant' gene cluster are unlikely to identify useful tumor subclasses. Much care must be placed in the choice of genes used to subclassify tumors, and the choices must be thoroughly and rigorously verified and validated, both statistically and clinically. A general

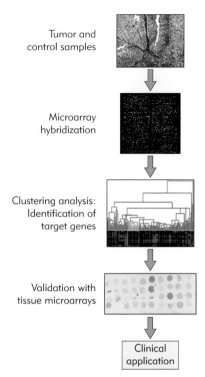

Tumor and
control samples

Microarray
hybridization

Clustering analysis:
Identification of
target genes

Validation with
tissue microarrays

Clinical
application

Fig. 23.4 The general procedure of a tumor expression profiling experiment includes: RNA isolation from tumor biopsy and control samples, preparation of the hybridization probe, hybridization with the DNA microarray, data acquisition and analysis, and verification of the results using, for example, tissue microarrays.

outline of the process of microarray expression profiling using tumor specimens, including the important step of result validation using tissue microarrays, is shown in Figure 23.4.

OLIGONUCLEOTIDE MICROARRAYS IN THE STUDY OF DNA VARIATION

The short length of oligonucleotide targets gives them the ability to discriminate between multiple probes that differ in sequence at a single base. Because of this, oligonucleotide microarray applications have been developed to identify simple polymorphisms and allelic variations in DNA.[16] The primary applications of these types of microarray have been in the genotyping of single nucleotide polymorphisms (SNPs) and in the identification of mutations in medically important genes. It is hoped that genetic analysis using SNPs will provide a means to identify the genes controlling the

development of many forms of human disease, including cancer,[43] through the analysis of either the SNPs responsible for coding sequence variations in genes (cSNP) or genetic analyses designed to scan the genome for SNP–disease associations.[43]

Oligonucleotide microarrays have also been used to analyze tumor samples for the presence of mutations in the TP53[44,45] and BRCA1[16] tumor suppressor genes. In these studies, the mutation status of the tumor samples was independently evaluated by conventional DNA sequencing. Although these two techniques were not in complete agreement, the speed and ease of the microarray analysis provided an argument for their use in this application on a larger scale. A principal drawback of the use of microarrays in mutation screening is the inherent inability of this technique to detect previously unidentified mutations – if the sequence is not represented on the array, it will not be detected.

APPLICATION OF DNA MICROARRAYS TO THE STUDY OF BLADDER CANCER

The main advantage of DNA arrays is that they allow the study of the multiple transcriptional events that take place when normal urothelium is transformed into tumor tissue in single experiments. Microarray technology is a reliable and powerful tool for profiling gene expression patterns in many biological systems related to cancer. Expression profiling using cell lines has been used to gain an insight into the molecular events associated with the disease. Here it is summarized as an example of how the technology can be applied to the discovery of gene function and pathway applied to bladder cancer. The tumor cell growth inhibition mediated by the soy isoflavone genistein was studied in the susceptible bladder tumor line TCCSUP, and expression profiling was analyzed at various periods of time, using cDNA chip containing 884 sequence-verified known human genes. The authors further describe the transient induction of egr-1, whose expression has been associated with proliferation and differentiation. The study detected many groups of genes with distinct expression profiles, most of them encoding for proteins that regulate the signal transduction or the cell cycle pathways. These genes warrant further investigation as regards their roles in the susceptibility of the tumor cell line to the antitumor drug.[46]

An example of the functional classification of genes applied to bladder cancer is the expression patterns of p53-mediated apoptosis-resistant tumor cell lines versus apoptosis-sensitive ones. The ECV-304 bladder carcinoma cell line was selected for resistance to p53 by repeated infections with a p53 recombinant adenovirus Ad5CMV-p53 and its expression pattern of 5730 genes using cDNA arrays was compared with p53-sensitive ECV-304 cells. A number of potential targets for p53 were identified that play roles in cell cycle regulation, DNA repair, redox control, cell adhesion, apoptosis and differentiation. Proline oxidase, a mitochondrial enzyme involved in the proline/pyrroline-5-carboxylate redox cycle, was upregulated by p53 in sensitive but not in resistant cells. Further experiments with pyrroline-5-carboxylate (P5C), a proline-derived metabolite generated by proline oxidase, inhibited the proliferation and survival of resistant and sensitive cells and induced apoptosis in both cell lines, showing the implication of proline oxidase and the proline/P5C pathway in p53-induced growth suppression and apoptosis.[47]

The classification of bladder cancer using expression profiling has not been reported by many studies to date using DNA microarrays. The most extensive one has monitored the expression patterns of superficial and invasive tumor suspensions prepared from bladder biopsies (36 normal, 29 tumor) and pools of cells made from normal urothelium and from pTa grade I and II and pT2 grade III and IV bladder tumors, using oligonucleotide arrays carrying probes for 6500 genes. Hierarchical clustering of gene expression levels not only identified the stage and/or grade of the samples studied but also identified several stage-characteristic, functionally related clusters, encoding proteins that were related to cell proliferation, oncogenes and growth factors, cell adhesion, immunology, transcription, proteinases and ribosomes. The study represents a first approach as to how gene expression patterns may provide a new biological insight, form a basis for the construction of molecular classifiers and be involved in developing new therapy for bladder cancer.[48]

Testing for mutations of the TP53 gene in bladder tumors is a valuable predictor for disease outcome. However, the time and cost of conventional sequencing limit its use as a common diagnostic tool in clinical daily practice. The analysis of P53 mutations has also been performed using variant oligonucleotide chips. The traditional manual dideoxy sequencing has been compared with the much faster microarray sequencing on a commercially available chip. DNA extracted from 140 human bladder tumors was subjected to a multiplex-PCR before loading on to the p53 chip. Each of the 1464 gene chip positions corresponded to an analyzed nucleotide in the p53 gene sequence. The authors report the presence of background signals not attributable to mutations and that the specificity of mutation calling can be increased using a mathematical correction considering each chip position as a separate entity with its own noise and threshold characteristics. The concordance with results obtained by traditional sequencing was 92%. Microarray-based sequencing is a novel option to assess TP53 mutations, representing a fast and inexpensive method compared with conventional sequencing.[44]

CONCLUSION

Genome sequencing programs have provided us with tremendous amounts of information about the genes and genomes of humans and model organisms. The challenge of those wanting to treat disease is to make efficient and maximal use of this information to understand the physiologic pathways and relationships that control the normal and diseased cell state and to translate that understanding into a clinical setting. The DNA microarray is one of the most powerful and flexible of the functional genomic technologies that have been developed to meet this challenge. In a short period of time, DNA microarrays have moved from being a technology restricted to a few well-funded or technically sophisticated laboratories to one that is more widely used and dispersed. This trend will continue as the quality and ease of use of the technology increase and the costs decrease.

Expression profiling using DNA microarrays is still in a relatively early stage of development and is changing and advancing at a rapid rate. The goal of having every human gene – including splice variants – on a single microarray should be realized in the next few years. The microarray protocols and technologies in use in 5 years' time will undoubtedly be quite different from those in use today (and we have only commented on those platforms currently in widespread use). Technical advances and improvements are being made at each step of the microarray experimental process. Lower cost and wider variety of commercial arrays options; improvements in the speed, reliability, and technologies of the spotting robots; improvements in probe labeling and hybridization techniques and protocols; changes in target design (e.g. longer oligonucleotides); improvements in data analysis and management – these and many more changes and improvements are imminent. The combined efforts of biologists and physicians, engineers, biostatisticians and bioinformaticians will ensure that the technology of DNA microarrays continues to evolve and mature.

The microarray is a convenient platform for assays involving biomolecules other than nucleic acids. Arrays of tissues, peptides, antibodies, proteins, and even cells have been developed,[35,49–52] demonstrating the format's strength and versatility for high-throughput screening. These should provide a means of rapidly validating, at the protein level, the genes identified by expression profiling using DNA microarrays.

The area of data analysis and management deserves special comment. Expression profiling experiments can produce data sets that are, at least by the standards of molecular biology, extremely large. A variety of numerical analysis approaches and algorithms have been used to cluster genes based upon their expression patterns. Various statistical approaches have likewise been used to perform the class predictions that identify expression patterns that correlate with phenotypic characteristics such as tumor type. Still, there exists a significant need and challenge to develop additional bioinformatic methods to extract all the information contained in these very rich, deep expression pattern data sets and to integrate it with other forms of biological information (e.g. the information contained in the published literature[53]). In addition, there is the hope that the raw data from (at least) published microarray experiments will be made available to the scientific community with unrestricted access in a uniform format. To this end, an international effort is underway to develop guidelines and consensus on data handling and annotation.[54]

Despite the relative youth of the technology, microarray use has already had a broad and significant impact on the study of cancer. As illustrated above, it has been possible to assign potential functional roles to novel genes in both the signaling pathways controlling, and the phenotypic changes associated with, cancer development. Microarray studies will continue to correlate changes in the expression of specific genes and groups of genes with cancer and cancer-related phenotypes. Following the biological validation of these expression–phenotype correlations, the result will be a more complete list of the genes controlling cancer development and progression. From this, a clearer view should emerge of the principles and pathways controlling cancer physiology.

The early studies indicate that expression profiling of a relatively small number of genes may provide a molecular means of identifying clinically important tumor subtypes not identified using standard methods and that these subtypes may identify specific subgroups

of patients that will benefit from distinct treatment regimes. What are needed are carefully controlled, large-scale expression profiling studies on large numbers of clinically well-described tumors before the true clinical utility of this technique can be accurately judged. It is clear that the results of these studies will add to our understanding of the mechanisms of carcinogenesis and may also improve our ability to diagnose and treat the disease. As interest in microarrays and their use in the study of cancer continue to increase, so does the likelihood that their use will have important clinical applications.

REFERENCES

1. Reuter VE, Melamed MR. The lower urinary tract. In: Sternberg SS (ed.) Diagnostic Surgical Pathology. New York: Raven Press, 1989, p 1355.
2. Dalbagni G, Presti J, Reuter V, Fair WR, Cordon-Cardo C. Genetic alterations in bladder cancer. Lancet 1993;342:469–471.
3. Orntoft TF, Wolf H. Molecular alterations in bladder cancer. Urol Res 1998;26:223–233.
4. Cordon-Cardo C, Cote RJ, Sauter G. Genetic and molecular markers of urothelial premalignancy and malignancy. Scand J Urol Nephrol Suppl 2000;205:82–93.
5. Mark ID, Jones PA. Presence and location of TP53 mutation determines pattern of CDKN2A/ARF pathway inactivation in bladder cancer. Cancer Res 1998;58:5348–5353.
6. Knowles MA. The genetics of transitional cell carcinoma: progress and potential clinical application. BJU Int 1999;84:412–427.
7. Liang P, Pardee AB. Differential display of eukaryotic messenger RNA by means of the polymerase chain reaction. Science 1992;257:967–971.
8. Velculescu VE, Zhang L, Vogelstein B, Kinzler KW. Serial analysis of gene expression. Science 1995;270:484–487.
9. Brenner S, Johnson M, Bridgham J, et al. Gene expression analysis by massively parallel signature sequencing (MPSS) on microbead arrays. Nat Biotechnol 2000;18(6):630–634.
10. Pandey A, Mann M. Proteomics to study genes and genomes. Nature 2000;405:837–846.
11. Interntional Human Genome Sequencing Consortium. Initial sequencing and analysis of the human genome. Nature 2001;409:860–921.
12. Venter JC, Adams MD, Myers EW, et al. The sequence of the human genome. Science 2001;291:1304–1351.
13. Duggan DJ, Bittner M, Chen Y, Meltzer P, Trent JM. Expression profiling using cDNA microarrays. Nat Genet 1999;21(1 Suppl.):10–14.
14. Lipshutz RJ, Fodor SP, Gingeras TR, Lockhart DJ. High density synthetic oligonucleotide arrays. Nat Genet 1999;21(1 Suppl.):20–24.
15. Fan JB, Chen X, Halushka MK, et al. Parallel genotyping

of human SNPs using generic high-density oligo-nucleotide tag arrays. Genome Res 2000;10(6):853–860.

16. Hacia JG. Resequencing and mutational analysis using oligonucleotide microarrays. Nat Genet 1999;21(1 Suppl.):42–47.

17. Iyer VR, Horak CE, Scafe CS, et al. Genomic binding sites of the yeast cell-cycle transcription factors SBF and MBF. Nature 2001;409:533–538.

18. Pinkel D, Segraves R, Sudar D, et al. High resolution analysis of DNA copy number variation using comparative genomic hybridization to microarrays. Nat Genet 1998;20:207–211.

19. Bowtell DD. Options available – from start to finish – for obtaining expression data by microarray. Nat Genet 1999;21(1 Suppl.):25–32.

20. Microarray Core Facility, Stanford School of Medicine: www.microarray.org

21. Lennon GG, Lehrach H. Hybridization analyses of arrayed cDNA libraries. Trends Genet 1991;7:314–317.

22. Southern E, Mir K, Shchepinov M. Molecular interactions on microarrays. Nat Genet 1999;21(1 Suppl.):5–9.

23. Nguyen C, Rocha D, Granjeaud S, et al. Differential gene expression in the murine thymus assayed by quantitative hybridization of arrayed cDNA clones. Genomics 1995;29:207–216.

24. Granjeaud S, Bertucci F, Jordan BR. Expression profiling: DNA arrays in many guises. Bioessays 1999;21:781–790.

25. Granjeaud S, Nguyen C, Rocha D, Luton R, Jordan BR. From hybridization image to numerical values: a practical, high throughput quantification system for high density filter hybridizations. Genet Anal 1996;12:151–162.

26. Chen JJ, Wu R, Yang PC, et al. Profiling expression patterns and isolating differentially expressed genes by cDNA microarray system with colorimetry detection. Genomics 1998;51:313–324.

27. Cheung VG, Morley M, Aguilar F, et al. Making and reading microarrays. Nat Genet 1999;21(1 Suppl.):15–19.

28. Stears RL, Getts RC, Gullans SR. A novel, sensitive detection system for high-density microarrays using dendrimer technology. Physiol Genomics 2000;3:93–99.

29. Eberwine J. Amplification of mRNA populations using RNA generated from immobilized oligo(dT)-T7 primed cDNA. Biotechniques 1996;20:584–591.

30. Zhao N, Hashida H, Takahashi N, Misumi Y, Sakaki Y. High-density cDNA filter analysis: a novel approach for large-scale, quantitative analysis of gene expression. Gene 1995;156:207–213.

31. Wang E, Miller LD, Ohnmacht GA, Liu ET, Marincola FM. High-fidelity mRNA amplification for gene profiling. Nat Biotechnol 2000;18:457–459.

32. Klimecki WT, Futscher BW, Dalton WS. Effects of ethanol and paraformaldehyde on RNA yield and quality. Biotechniques 1994;16:1021–1023.

33. Specht K, Richter T, Muller U, et al. Quantitative gene expression analysis in microdissected archival formalin-fixed and paraffin-embedded tumor tissue. Am J Pathol 2001;158:419–429.

34. Cerroni L, Minkus G, Putz B, Hofler H, Kerl H. Laser beam microdissection in the diagnosis of cutaneous B-cell lymphoma. Br J Dermatol 1997;136:743–746.

35. Kononen J, Bubendorf L, Kallioniemi A, et al. Tissue microarrays for high-throughput molecular profiling of tumor specimens. Nat Med 1998;4:844–847.

36. Eisen MB, Spellman PT, Brown PO, Botstein D. Cluster analysis and display of genome-wide expression patterns. Proc Natl Acad Sci USA 1998;95:14863–14868.

37. Alon U, Barkai N, Notterman DA, et al. Broad patterns of gene expression revealed by clustering analysis of tumor and normal colon tissues probed by oligonucleotide arrays. Proc Natl Acad Sci USA 1999;96:6745–6750.

38. Iyer VR, Eisen MB, Ross DT, et al. The transcriptional program in the response of human fibroblasts to serum. Science 1999;283:83–87.

39. Perou CM, Sorlie T, Eisen MB, et al. Molecular portraits of human breast tumours. Nature 2000;406:747–452.

40. Alizadeh AA, Eisen MB, Davis RE, et al. Distinct types of diffuse large B-cell lymphoma identified by gene expression profiling. Nature 2000;403:503–511.

41. Welsh JB, Zarrinkar PP, Sapinoso LM, et al. Analysis of gene expression profiles in normal and neoplastic ovarian tissue samples identifies candidate molecular markers of epithelial ovarian cancer. Proc Natl Acad Sci USA 2001;98:1176–1181.

42. Ross DT, Scherf U, Eisen MB, et al. Systematic variation in gene expression patterns in human cancer cell lines. Nat Genet 2000;24:227–235.

43. Risch NJ. Searching for genetic determinants in the new millennium. Nature 2000;405:847–856.

44. Wikman FP, Lu ML, Thykjaer T, et al. Evaluation of the performance of a p53 sequencing microarray chip using 140 previously sequenced bladder tumor samples. Clin Chem 2000;46:1555–1561.

45. Ahrendt SA, Halachmi S, Chow JT, et al. Rapid p53 sequence analysis in primary lung cancer using an oligonucleotide probe array. Proc Natl Acad Sci USA 1999;96:7382–7387.

46. Chen CC, Shieh B, Jin YT, et al. Microarray profiling of gene expression patterns in bladder tumor cells treated with genistein. J Biomed Sci 2001;8:214–222.

47. Maxwell SA, Davis GE. Differential gene expression in p53-mediated apoptosis-resistant vs. apoptosis-sensitive tumor cell lines. Proc Natl Acad Sci USA 2000;97:13009–13014.

48. Thykjaer T, Workman C, Kruhoffer M, et al. Identification of gene expression patterns in superficial and invasive human bladder cancer. Cancer Res 2001;61:2492–2499.

49. Reineke U, Volkmer-Engert R, Schneider-Mergener J. Applications of peptide arrays prepared by the SPOT-technology. Curr Opin Biotechnol 2001;12:59–64.

50. Haab BB, Dunham MJ, Brown PO. Protein microarrays for highly parallel detection and quantitation of specific proteins and antibodies in complex solutions. Genome Biol 2001;2(2):RESEARCH0004.

51. MacBeath G, Schreiber SL. Printing proteins as microarrays for high-throughput function determination. Science 2000;289:1760–1763.

52. Ziauddin J, Sabatini DM. Microarrays of cells expressing defined cDNAs. Nature 2001;411:107–110.

53. Jenssen TK, Laegreid A, Komorowski J, Hovig E. A literature network of human genes for high-throughput analysis of gene expression. Nat Genet 2001;28:21–28.

54. Microarray Gene Expression Data Society: www.mged.org.

Index